Pathology
Practicals and Quick Review

Second Edition

Pathology
Practicals and Quick Review

Second Edition

Ganga S Pilli MBBS, MD, PhD
Professor
Department of Pathology
Jawaharlal Nehru Medical College
KLE Academy of Higher Education and Research
Belagavi, Karnataka

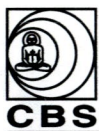

CBS
CBS Publishers & Distributors Pvt Ltd

New Delhi • Bengaluru • Chennai • Kochi • Kolkata • Mumbai
Bhopal • Bhubaneswar • Hyderabad • Jharkhand • Nagpur • Patna • Pune • Uttarakhand • Dhaka (Bangladesh)

Disclaimer
Science and technology are constantly changing fields. New research and experience broaden the scope of information and knowledge. The author has tried her best in giving information available to her while preparing the material for this book. Although all efforts have been made to ensure optimum accuracy of the material, yet it is quite possible some errors might have been left uncorrected. The publisher, the printer and the author will not be held responsible for any inadvertent errors or inaccuracies.

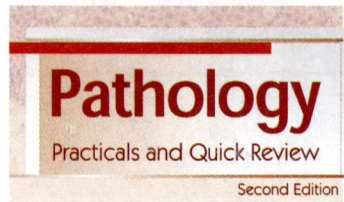

ISBN: 978-81-94125-40-2

Copyright © Author and Publisher

Second Edition: 2020

First Edition: 2015

All rights reserved. No part of this book may be reproduced or transmitted in any form or by any means, electronic or mechanical, including photocopying, recording, or any information storage and retrieval system without permission, in writing, from the author and the publisher.

Published by Satish Kumar Jain and produced by Varun Jain for
CBS Publishers & Distributors Pvt Ltd
4819/XI Prahlad Street, 24 Ansari Road, Daryaganj, New Delhi 110 002, India.
Ph: 23289259, 23266861, 23266867   Fax: 011-23243014   Website: www.cbspd.com
e-mail: delhi@cbspd.com; cbspubs@airtelmail.in.
Corporate Office: 204 FIE, Industrial Area, Patparganj, Delhi 110 092
Ph: 4934 4934   Fax: 4934 4935   e-mail: publishing@cbspd.com; publicity@cbspd.com

Branches

- **Bengaluru:** Seema House 2975, 17th Cross, K.R. Road, Banasankari 2nd Stage, Bengaluru 560 070, Karnataka
  Ph: +91-80-26771678/79   Fax: +91-80-26771680   e-mail: bangalore@cbspd.com
- **Chennai:** 7, Subbaraya Street, Shenoy Nagar, Chennai 600 030, Tamil Nadu
  Ph: +91-44-26680620, 26681266   Fax: +91-44-42032115   e-mail: chennai@cbspd.com
- **Kochi:** 42/1325, 1326, Power House Road, Opp KSEB Power House, Ernakulam 682 018, Kochi, Kerala
  Ph: +91-484-4059061-65   Fax: +91-484-4059065   e-mail: kochi@cbspd.com
- **Kolkata:** 6/B, Ground Floor, Rameswar Shaw Road, Kolkata-700 014, West Bengal
  Ph: +91-33-22891126, 22891127, 22891128   e-mail: kolkata@cbspd.com
- **Mumbai:** 83-C, Dr E Moses Road, Worli, Mumbai-400018, Maharashtra
  Ph: +91-22-24902340/41   Fax: +91-22-24902342   e-mail: mumbai@cbspd.com

Representatives

- Bhopal   0-8319310552   • Bhubaneswar   0-9911037372   • Hyderabad   0-9885175004
- Jharkhand   0-9811541605   • Nagpur   0-9421945513   • Patna   0-9334159340
- Pune   0-9623451994   • Uttarakhand   0-9716462459   • Dhaka (Bangladesh) 01912-003485

Printed at: Goyal Offset Printers, GT Karnal Road, Industrial Area, Delhi India

to

*my parents and family members
for their
constant encouragement
and
to my dear students*

Foreword

For any physician to give the appropriate care for his patients an appropriate diagnosis is to be made and for this, the investigations form an important component in the whole process. The investigations may be from pathology, microbiology or biochemistry departments.

Now for doing these investigations, one has to be up-to-date in procedures and interpretations. The diagnostic workups are usually done by the individual departments by the skilled people like postgraduates, undergraduates and medical laboratory students. These students have to learn the various laboratory procedures in great detail. This is usually done by referring to the various books on these topics. All these groups of students will be greatly in need of a comprehensive manual which would encompass all the procedures of investigations in a nutshell so that they can be referred on day-to-day basis.

The second edition of the earlier book with new title *Pathology: Practicals and Quick Review* by Dr Ganga S Pilli is one such attempt in which she has tried to cover all the topics and procedures which are required to be learnt by the students and also related important theory related aspects to understand the subject. She has worked hard for the preparation of this book. She has a rich experience in the field of pathology for having worked as lecturer, assistant professor, associate professor and professor of pathology for a period of almost 34 years in a reputed department of our college. She was heading the department during the years 2012 to 2014. She has made an excellent attempt to give the procedural details of all the investigations which will be of a real benefit to the students of medical/dental sciences, medical laboratory technology and AYUSH courses. This book deals with the practical aspects of the procedures and also necessary theory material which will enrich the knowledge and will improve the skills of the students. I am sure this book will be accepted by all the students and teaching fraternity of pathology. I congratulate Dr Ganga S Pilli for the bold venture and hope she will continue to bring out more books for the benefits of the students and wish her all the success in her future endeavors.

VD Patil
Registrar
KLE Academy of
Higher Education and Research
and
Former Principal
JN Medical College
Belagavi

Preface to the Second Edition

Pathology is a medical speciality concerned with the study of diseases which leads to the structural and functional changes in the human body. Today pathologists work mostly in the laboratory and examine the specimens including the surgically removed tissues, blood and other body fluids and hence, practical pathology plays a very important role in the field of medicine. Now it has grown to a great extent. There are many voluminous books dealing extensively with various aspects of practical pathology written by foreign and Indian authors. But most of them do not fully meet the academic requirements of the Indian students. It was felt that there is a need for a simple and comprehensive book for undergraduate and postgraduate students covering the syllabi prescribed by various health universities in India.

The first edition of this book was evolved while teaching practical pathology to the undergraduate and postgraduate students over a period of 30 years. This is the second edition. This has seen enormous changes with not only practical aspects but also with addition of theory related aspects in a particular exercise. The book has been written in an easy language and in a simple and lucid style with the help of illustrations for the benefit of wise as well as ordinary students studying pathology in various fields of medicine (medical, dental, laboratory technology and AYUSH courses).

The salient features of the book are

1. The book is divided into five parts, namely, Haematology, Clinical Pathology, General Pathology and Systemic Pathology, Histopathology Techniques and Cytology Techniques.
2. In each part different exercises are covered.
3. The book emphasizes on practical skills.
4. The book is also useful for the students in preparation of examination to answer long answers, short essays and short answers and to face viva voce as quick review in pathology.
5. After five main parts, at the end has similes in pathology, know your scientists and pearls to remember covering various topics which will help the students in preparation of competitive examination in medicine.
6. The book is re-designed with illustrations of gross and microscopic pictures with original as well as schematic diagrams.

The book has seen its second edition due to CBS Publishers & Distributors who have made the book to reach the students studying pathology nationwide and also coming out with a textbook.

The legacy of authoring a book is to follow the footprints of my father (Prof SS Nanjannavar) who is a retired Professor from Karnatak University, Dharwad and a noted author of many books in the field of geography. He is the main source of inspiration for me to continue this noble task of writing a book in order to serve the cause of student community in particular and medical education in general. It is hoped that this book would be of great help and guidance to the students and serve as a ready reference book.

I will be failing in my duty if I do not express my sincere gratitude to Shri Prabhakar Kore, Chancellor and Dr Vivek Saoji, Vice-Chancellor of KLE University, Belgaum for providing me all the facilities. I extend my grateful thanks to Dr VD Patil, Registrar, KAHER (deemed to be university), Belgaum, for writing Foreword to this book and constantly encouraging for this difficult task of authoring books. I sincerely thank my Principal, Dr Niranjana Mahantshetti, and my colleagues at the department.

I offer my special thanks to Dr (Mrs) AV Dhaded, former Professor (Pathology), JN Medical College, Belagavi and to Dr Bhagyashree Hungund, Professor (Pathology), JN Medical College, Belgaum, for giving valuable suggestions. I thank Prof Uday V Kokatnur, in spite of his busy schedule, stood next to me for drawing nice diagrams. I also thank Mahantesh Nanjannavar for editing the pictures. I am thankful to my postgraduate students for their timely help. I am grateful to my husband, Dr Sharanabasava C Pilli, for his constant encouragement and support. Similarly, I appreciate the patience and co-operation of my children Vijay and Veena and daughter-in-law and son-in-law during the preparation of this book.

Constructive suggestions from the teachers and students of pathology are most welcome for the improvement of this book in the subsequent editions.

Ganga S Pilli

Preface to the First Edition

Pathology is a medical speciality concerned with the study of diseases which leads to the structural and functional changes in the human body. Today pathologists work mostly in the laboratory and examine the specimens including the surgically removed tissues, blood and other body fluids, and hence practical pathology plays an important role in the field of medicine. Now it has grown to a great extent. There are many voluminous books dealing extensively with various aspects of practical pathology written by foreign and Indian authors. But most of them do not fully meet the academic requirements of the Indian students. It was felt that there is a need for a simple and comprehensive book for undergraduate and postgraduate students covering the syllabi prescribed by various health universities in India.

The concept of this book was evolved while teaching practical pathology to the undergraduate and postgraduate students over a period of 23 years. There have been enormous changes with not only practical aspects but also with the addition of theory-related aspects in some exercises. The book has been written in an easy language and in a simple and lucid style with the help of illustrations for the benefit of wise as well as ordinary students studying pathology in various fields of medical sciences (medical, dental, laboratory technology and AYUSH courses).

The salient features of the book are
1. The book is divided into six parts, namely, haematology, clinical pathology and basics of cytology, general pathology and systemic pathology, histopathology techniques, cytology techniques, and miscellaneous topics.
2. In each part different exercises are covered.
3. The book emphasises practical skills.
4. The book is also useful for the students in preparation of examination to answer long questions, short assays, short questions and to face *viva voce* as quick review in pathology.
5. The book is redesigned with illustrations of gross and microscopic pictures with original as well as schematic diagrams.

The book will surely reach all the students studying pathology nationwide and I am sure it will encourage me to take up many more such assignments in future.

The legacy of authoring a book is to follow the footprints of my father, Prof SS Nanjannavar, who is a retired professor from Karnataka University, Dharwad, and a noted author of many books in the field of geography. He is the main source of inspiration for me to continue this noble work of writing a book to serve the cause of student community in particular and medical education in general. It is hoped that this book would be of great help and guidance to the students and serve as a ready reference book.

I will be failing in my duty if I do not express my sincere gratitude to Shri Prabhakar Kore, Chancellor, and Dr Kokate, Vice-Chancellor, KLE University, Belgaum, for providing me all the facilities. I extend my grateful thanks to Dr VD Patil, Registrar, KLE University, Belgaum, for writing the Foreword to this book. I sincerely thank Dr AS Godhi, Principal of the college, and my colleagues at the department.

I am thankful to the following for helping me in the preparation of some of the topics.
- Dr Prasad Shenoy and Dr Ramesh Chavan: Automation in haematology
- Dr Resma Davangere: Acute glomerulonephritis, rapidly progressive glomerulonephritis, chronic pyelonephritis, and reflux nephropathy
- Dr Bhagyashree Hungund: Carcinoma oral cavity, gastric ulcer/peptic ulcer, and carcinoma stomach and cervix
- Dr Sunita Patil: Renal cell carcinoma and Wilms' tumour
- Dr Ashwini: Hodgkin's lymphoma

I offer my special thanks to Dr (Mrs) AV Dhaded, *ex*-Professor of Pathology, JN Medical College, Belgaum, and Dr Bhagyashree Hungund, Associate Professor, Pathology, JN Medical College, Belgaum, for going through the manuscript and giving valuable suggestions. I thank Prof Uday V Kokatnur, in spite of his busy schedule, stood next to me for drawing nice diagrams. I also thank Mahantesh Nanjannavar for editing the pictures. I am thankful to my postgraduate students for their timely help. I am grateful to my husband, Dr Sharanabasava C. Pilli, for his constant encouragement and support. Similarly, I appreciate the patience and cooperation of my children, Vijay and Veena, during the period of writing this book.

Constructive suggestions from the teachers and students of pathology are most welcome for the improvement of this book in the subsequent editions.

Ganga S Pilli

Acknowledgements

I acknowledge the help rendered by the following in preparation of the manuscript:
Automation in Haematology: Dr Prasad Shenoy, Consultant Pathologist, Goa and Dr Ramesh Chavan, presently Professor and Head, Department of Pathology, JN Medical College, KAHER, Belagavi.

I am also thankful to CBS Publishers & Distributors. I would like to put on record the sincere efforts of Mr YN Arjuna (Senior Vice President Publishing, Editorial and Publicity), and his team comprising of Ms Ritu Chawla (GM Production), Mr Parmod Kumar, Mr Prasenjit Paul and Mr Manish Raj, for bringing out the book in the present form.

Ganga S Pilli

Contents

Foreword by VD Patil — vii
Preface to the Second Edition — ix
Preface to the First Edition — xi
Abbreviations — xix

Section I. HAEMATOLOGY

Exercise 1. Haemopoiesis — 3
Exercise 2. Blood Collection — 8
Exercise 3. Anticoagulants — 10
Exercise 4. Peripheral Smear (Blood Film) Preparation and Staining — 12
Exercise 5. Haemoglobin (Hb) Estimation — 14
Exercise 6. Cell Counts — 17
Exercise 7. Red Cell Indices — 21
Exercise 8. Absolute Eosinophil Count — 22
Exercise 9. Differential Leukocyte Count — 23
Exercise 10. Packed Cell Volume (Haematocrit) — 26
Exercise 11. Erythrocyte Sedimentation Rate (ESR) — 28
Exercise 12. Blood Groups Related Exercises — 31
Exercise 13. Normal Blood Picture — 36
Exercise 14. Nutritional Anaemias — 37
Exercise 15. Haemolytic Anaemias and Tests Related to Haemolytic Anaemias — 44
Exercise 16. Leukaemias — 56
Exercise 17. Multiple Myeloma/Plasma Cell Dyscrasias — 64
Exercise 18. Bleeding Disorders — 66
Exercise 19. Tests Related to Bleeding Disorders — 67
Exercise 20. LE Cell Phenomenon — 70
Exercise 21. Romanowsky Stains, Buffer, Instruments and Cleaning of the Glassware — 72
Exercise 22. Automation in Haematology — 74

Section II. CLINICAL PATHOLOGY AND BASICS OF CYTOLOGY...

Exercise 23. Urine Examination — 81
Exercise 24. Pregnancy Test — 98
Exercise 25. Semen Analysis — 99

Exercise 26.	Glucose Tolerance Test (GTT)	101
Exercise 27.	Fractional Test Meal (FTM)	102
Exercise 28.	Renal Function Tests	103
Exercise 29.	Liver Function Tests	105
Exercise 30.	Thyroid Function Tests	107
Exercise 31.	Instruments	109
Exercise 32.	Malaria and Filariasis	115
Exercise 33.	Basics of Cytology	119
Exercise 34.	Haematology, Clinical Pathology and Cytology Charts/Case Studies	120

Section III. GENERAL PATHOLOGY AND SYSTEMIC PATHOLOGY

Exercise 35.	Fixation and Processing for Paraffin Section and Frozen Section	129
Exercise 36.	Cell Injury	133
Exercise 37.	Fatty Change (Liver, Heart) and Amyloidosis	139
Exercise 38.	Inflammation (Acute and Chronic) and Granulation Tissue	144
Exercise 39.	Chronic Venous Congestion, Thrombosis, Infarction, Myocardial Infarction (MI) and Lung Infarction Oedema and Shock	161
Exercise 40.	Neoplasia	176
Exercise 41.	Some Common Tumours	183
Exercise 42.	Atherosclerosis and Vascular Pathology in Hypertension	187
Exercise 43.	Heart Lesions	191
Exercise 44.	Lesions of Respiratory Tract	202
Exercise 45.	Salivary Gland Tumours	219
Exercise 46.	Lesions of Gastrointestinal Tract	222
Exercise 47.	Common Lesions of Liver	234
Exercise 48.	Neoplasms of Breast	244
Exercise 49.	Kidney Lesions	251
Exercise 50.	Neoplasms Arising from Stratified Squamous Epithelium	266
Exercise 51.	Tumours of Melanocytes	269
Exercise 52.	Endometrium and Uterus, Trophoblastic Diseases and Cervix the Normal Endometrium	273
Exercise 53.	Common Ovarian Tumours	283
Exercise 54.	Common Testicular Lesions	287
Exercise 55.	Lesions of Prostate	290
Exercise 56.	Common Bone Lesions	292
Exercise 57.	Lesions of Thyroid	296
Exercise 58.	Lesions of Lymph Node	299
Exercise 59.	Lesions of Brain	305

Section IV. HISTOPATHOLOGY TECHNIQUES

Exercise 60.	Accessing Procedures in Surgical Pathology	311
Exercise 61.	Fixatives	314
Exercise 62.	Processing	318
Exercise 63.	Haematoxylin and Eosin (H & E) Staining	320

Exercise 64.	Microtomes and Microtomy	322
Exercise 65.	Frozen Section	329
Exercise 66.	Decalcification	330
Exercise 67.	Special Stains	333
Exercise 68.	Theoretical Aspects of some of the Special Stains	336

Section V. CYTOLOGY TECHNIQUES

Exercise 69.	Cytological Fixatives	341
Exercise 70.	Lysing Fixatives	342
Exercise 71.	Criteria to Evaluate Screening Tests	343
Exercise 72.	Different Staining Techniques in Cytology	344
Exercise 73.	Cytopreparatory Techniques	347
Exercise 74.	Technique of Fine Needle Aspiration Cytology (FNAC)	349
Exercise 75.	Pleural, Pericardial and Peritoneal Fluids	352
Exercise 76.	Cerebrospinal Fluid (CSF)	356
Exercise 77.	Synovial Fluid	359
Exercise 78.	Sampling, Cytopreparatory Techniques and Cytology of Oral Cavity and Alimentary Tract (Oesophagus, Stomach and Duodenum)	362
Exercise 79.	Sampling, Cytopreparatory Techniques and Cytology of Respiratory Tract	364
Exercise 80.	Sampling, Cytopreparatory Techniques and Cytology of Urinary Tract	369
Exercise 81.	FNAC of Thyroid, Salivary Gland and Breast Lesions	371
Exercise 82.	Cytology of Female Genital System	375
Exercise 83.	Hormone Cytology	380
Exercise 84.	Barr Body	384

Similes in Pathology	385
Know your Scientists	391
Pearls to Remember	393
Normal Values	413
References	415
Index	417

Abbreviations

ACR	Urinary Albumin Creatinine Ratio
ADCC	Antibody-Dependent Cell-mediated Cytotoxicity
ADH	Anti-Diuretic Hormone
AD	Autosomal Dominant
ADP	Adenosine Diphosphate
AIHA	Auto-Immune Hemolytic Anaemia
AFP	Alpha Feto Proteins
ALIP	Abnormal Localisation of Immature Precursors
APLA/APS	Antiphospholipid Antibody
APTT	Activated Partial Thromboplastin Time
AR	Autosomal Recessive
BCC	Basal Cell Carcinoma
CCF	Congestive Cardiac Failure
CaCl2	Calcium Chloride
CIN	Carcinoma *In Situ*
CFTR	Cystic Fibrosis Transmembrane Conductance Regulator
CMV	Cytomegalo Virus
CNS	Central Nervous System
CRAB	Calcium (elevated), Renal failure, Anaemia, Bone Lesions
CT	Computerised Tomography
DCIS	Duct Carcinoma *In Situ*
DVT	Deep Vein Thrombosis
ECM	Extra Cellular Matrix
ER	Estrogen Receptors
FSGS	Focal Segmental Glomerulo Sclerosis
GCT	Giant Cell Tumour
GERD	Gastro Esophageal Reflux Disease
GGT	Gamma Glutamyl Transpeptidase
G6PD	Glucose 6 Phosphate Dehydrogenase
HA	Hemolytic Anaemia
HCC	Hepatocellular Carcinoma
HCG	Human Chorionic Gonadotropin
HCl	Hydrochloric Acid
HD	Hodgkin Disease
HDN	Hemolytic Disease of Newborn
HELLP	Hemolysis, Elevated Liver enzymes, Low Platelet count
HLA	Human Leukocyte Antigen
HNPCC	Hereditary Non-Polyposis Colorectal Cancer
HPV	Human Papillomavirus
HS	Hereditary Spherocytosis

HSIL	High Grade Squamous Intraepithelial Lesion
IC	Integrated Circuit
IL	Interleukin
INF	Interferon
IHC	Immunohistochemistry
ITP	Idiopathic Thrombocytopenic Purpura
JSB	J Singh and Bhattacharji
KOH	Potassium hydroxide
LDH	Lactate Dehydrogenase
LDHD	Lymphocyte Depleted Hodgkin Disease
L&H	Lymphocytic and Histiocytic
LN	Lymph Node
LSIL	Low Grade Squamous Intraepithelial Lesion
MCD	Minimal Change Disease
MCHC	Mean Corpuscular Haemoglobin Concentration
MCV	Mean Corpuscular Volume
MDS	Myelo Dysplastic Syndrome
MGN	Mesangial Glomerulonephritis
MEN	Multiple Endocrine Neoplasia
MGG Stain	May-Grünwald Giemsa Stain
MM	Multiple Myeloma
MPGN	Membrano-proliferative Glomerulonephritis
NaOH	Sodium hydroxide
NADPH	Nicotinamide Adenine Dinucleotide Phosphate
NO	Nitric Oxide
NP	Niemann-Pick Disease
OD	Optical Density
OS	Osteosarcoma
PCV	Packed Cell Volume
PAS Stain	Periodic acid–Schiff Stain
Pf HRP$_2$	*P. falcifarum*-Histidine Rich Protein-2
PLAP	Placental Alkaline Phosphatase
POEMS	Polyneuropathy, Organomegaly, Endocrinopathy, Myeloma protein and Skin changes
PSGN	Post-Streptococcal Glomerulonephritis
PT	Prothrombin Time
QBC	Quantitative Buffy Coat
RBC	Red Blood cell
ROS	Reactive Oxygen Species
RPGN	Rapidly Progressive Glomerulonephritis
RS cells	Reed-Sternberg cells
SBC	Simple Bone Cyst
SIADH	Syndrome of Inappropriate secretion of ADH
TNF	Tumour Necrosis Factor
US	Ultrasound
V	Voltage
W	Watt
vWD disease	von Willebrand disease

Section 1

Haematology

Exercise 1. Haemopoiesis
Exercise 2. Blood Collection
Exercise 3. Anticoagulants
Exercise 4. Peripheral Smear (Blood Film) Preparation and Staining
Exercise 5. Haemoglobin (Hb) Estimation
Exercise 6. Cell Counts
Exercise 7. Red Cell Indices
Exercise 8. Absolute Eosinophil Count
Exercise 9. Differential Leukocyte Count
Exercise 10. Packed Cell Volume (Haematocrit)
Exercise 11. Erythrocyte Sedimentation Rate (ESR)
Exercise 12. Blood Groups Related Exercises
Exercise 13. Normal Blood Picture
Exercise 14. Nutritional Anaemias
Exercise 15. Haemolytic Anaemias and Tests Related to Haemolytic Anaemias
Exercise 16. Leukaemias
Exercise 17. Multiple Myeloma/Plasma Cell Dyscrasias
Exercise 18. Bleeding Disorders
Exercise 19. Tests Related to Bleeding Disorders
Exercise 20. LE Cell Phenomenon
Exercise 21. Romanowsky Stains, Buffer, Instruments and Cleaning of the Glassware
Exercise 22. Automation in Haematology

Exercise 1

Haemopoiesis

Formation of Blood Elements from Gestational Life to Adult Life

Cellular differentiation, proliferation and maturation of blood cells take place in the haematopoietic tissue, i.e. in the bone marrow (Fig. 1.1). Mature cells are released into the peripheral blood.

Development of haematopoiesis takes place at different places during gestational period and after birth and it is as follows:
1. Yolk sac—begins on 19th day of gestation and lasts up to 3 months.
2. Liver along with spleen, kidney, thymus, and lymph nodes—3rd month of gestation to 24 weeks.
3. Bone marrow—3rd trimester onwards and throughout life.

HAEMATOPOIETIC MARROW ARCHITECTURE

Nucleated cells of RBC series constitute 25–30% of marrow cells and are produced near the sinusoids. Erythroblastic island is composed of erythoblasts in varying states of maturation. Least mature cells are towards the centre of the island and more mature cells towards the periphery.

Granulocytes are produced in the nests, close to the trabeculae. At the metamyelocyte stage they begin moving towards the sinusoids.

Lymphocytes are produced in lymphoid tissues (nodules) which are randomly dispersed throughout marrow. Lymphoid stem cells may leave the bone marrow and travel to thymus where they mature into T-lymphocytes. Some lymphocytes remain in bone marrow where they mature into B-lymphocytes.

Megakaryocytes lie adjacent to the endothelium of sinusoidal walls and discharge platelets directly into lumen of sinuses. Cytoplasmic processes of megakaryocyte penetrate the sinus wall and pinch off to form platelets.

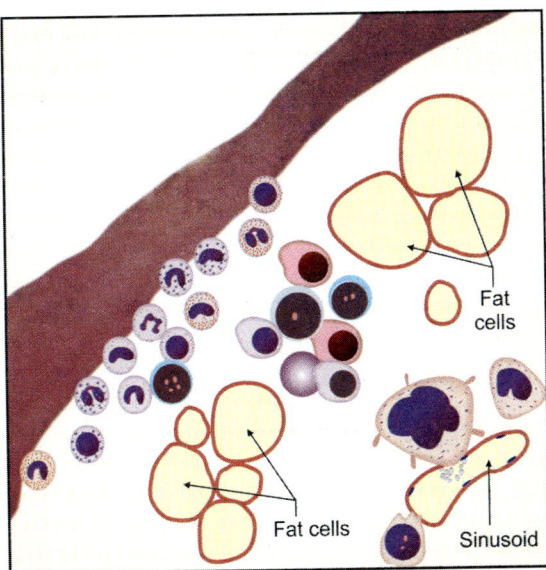

Fig. 1.1: Schematic diagram of topography of bone marrow cells of different series (paratrabecular area—myeloid series, near the sinusoids—megakaryocytic series, in between area—erythroid series)

ERYTHROID SERIES

It is an orderly process through which peripheral concentration of RBCs is maintained in a steady state.

Bone marrow maturation of normoblast occurs in orderly and well-defined sequence.

The process involves gradual decrease in cell size, together with condensation and eventual expulsion of nucleus.

As normoblasts mature, there is gradual increase in haemoglobin production. Normoblast generally spends 5–7 days in proliferating and maturing compartment of the marrow.

After maturation in the marrow the reticulocytes are released into the marrow sinuses and gain access to peripheral blood. It continues to mature in blood for 1 or 2 days.

Description of Erythroid Series Cells (Fig. 1.2)

Erythroblast (Normoblast/pronormoblast)

- 14–20 µ, round shaped, nucleus round
- Nucleus large occupies 4/5th of the cell and cytoplasm is 1/5th of the cell

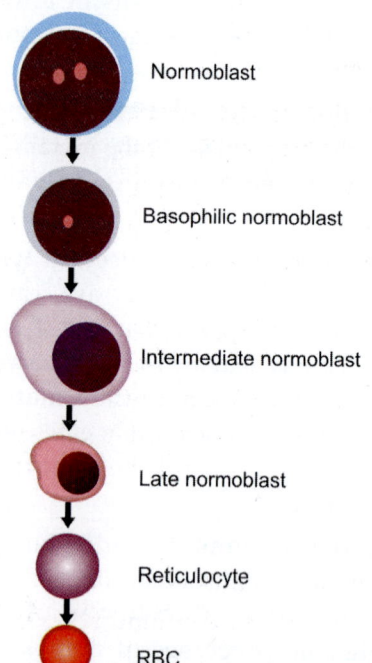

Fig. 1.2: Schematic diagram of eythroid series cells

- The cytoplasm is basophilic
- The nucleus has nucleoli
- Dividing cell.

Basophilic Erythroblast (Basophilic/Early normoblast)

- 12–15 µ
- Round-shaped
- Basophilic cytoplasm
- Nucleus-chromatin is dense
- Dividing cell.

Polychromatic Erythroblast (Intermediate normoblast)

- 12–14 µ
- Round-shaped
- Cytoplasm is polychromatic (purplish pink)
- Pink tint is because of haemoglobin
- Nucleus–chromatin clumped
- No division, cell develops by maturation.

Orthochromatic Erythroblast (Late normoblast)

- 12–14 µ
- Round-shaped
- Cytoplasm—more pinkish because of increased content of Hb
- Nucleus small and pyknotic with blue black colour
- The cell matures produce next cell.

Reticulocyte

- 8 µ
- Slightly larger than normal RBCs
- Biconcave discoid-shaped
- Cytoplasm–polychromatic, contains RNA material which can be stained with supravital stains
- Matures to RBC in 1–2 days.

Red Blood Cell

- 7.2 µ
- Biconcave, discoid-shaped
- Centre 1/3rd is pale, peripheral 2/3 coloured pinkish.

MYELOID SERIES (Fig. 1.3)

Myeloblast
- 15–20 μ, round-shaped
- Nucleus-round, occupies 4/5th of the cell and cytoplasm is 1/5th of the cell
- Nuclear chromatin less coarser than that of lymphoblast
- The cytoplasm is basophilic
- The nucleus has 4–5 nucleoli
- Dividing cell
- Sometimes Auer rod is found in the cytoplasm. It is purplish pink in colour.

Promyelocyte
- Nucleus-round
- Nuclear chromatin coarse
- Cytoplasm has primary granules which are dusty and purplish pink
- Nucleoli are few, 1–2 min number
- Other features are similar to myeloblast
- Dividing cell.

Myelocyte
- Nucleus is round
- Nuclear chromatin still coarser, no nucleoli
- Cytoplasm less basophilic and abundant
- Specific granules also appear in the cytoplasm. Depending upon these granules, the cells are called neutrophilic myelocyte, basophilic myelocyte and eosinophilic myelocyte.

Metamyelocyte
- Nucleus is kidney-shaped
- Cytoplasm is similar to earlier cell.

Band Form (Stab form)
- Nucleus more bent and attains U-shape. The degree of indentation is greater than 50% of the nuclear diameter
- Cytoplasm is similar to earlier cell
- These band forms mature to segmented forms.

Neutrophil (Polymorphonuclear leukocyte, segmented neutrophilic granulocyte)
- 12–14 μ
- Nucleus lobulated, has 2–5 lobes
- Cytoplasm has primary and secondary granules which are dusty and purplish pink coloured
- A sex chromatin (drumstick) may be present in some of the neutrophils attached to one of the lobes.

Eosinophil
- 14–16 μ
- Nucleus has two lobes (spectacular-shaped), cytoplasm has coarse granules which stain reddish or orange-coloured
- The granules do not overlap the nucleus.

Basophil
- 14–16 μ
- Nucleus has two lobes
- Cytoplasm has large round to oval deeply staining basophilic granules.

Note: Eosinophil and basophil are slightly larger than neutrophil.

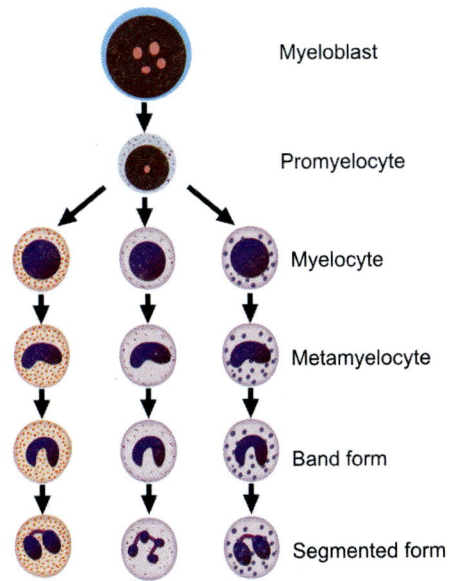

Fig. 1.3: Schematic diagram of myeloid series cells

LYMPHOID SERIES (Fig. 1.4)

Lymphoblast
- Nucleoli are 1–2
- Other features are similar to myeloblast.

Prolymphocyte
- Nucleoli are 0–1
- This cell divides and produces a large lymphocyte which matures to small lymphocyte.

Large Lymphocyte
- 12–16 µ
- Nucleus-round or indented
- Cytoplasm abundant, sky blue or pale blue coloured, a few azurophilic granules may be present.

Small Lymphocyte
- 6–10 µ
- Nucleus-round or indented
- Cytoplasm scanty and pale blue-coloured.

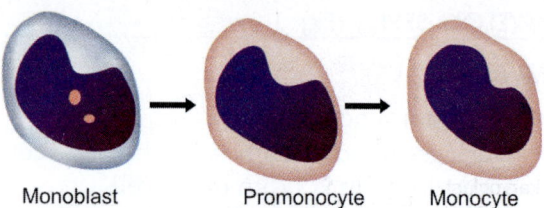

Fig. 1.5: Schematic diagram of monocyte series cells

MONOCYTE SERIES (Fig. 1.5)

Monoblast
- Nucleus-round or indented or convoluted
- Other features are similar to myeloblast.

Promonocyte
- Nucleus indented, can have clefts or convolutions
- Cytoplasm has azurophilic purplish pink granules
- Other features are similar to promyelocyte.

Monocyte
- 14–20 µ
- Nucleus lobulated, indented, kidney-shaped or has convolutions
- Nucleus has fine chromatin
- Cytoplasm grey blue, groundglass and abundant, fine azurophilic purplish pink
- Granules may be present sometimes cytoplasm has vacuoles.

MEGAKARYOCYTIC SERIES (Fig. 1.6)

Megakaryoblast
Nucleus and cytoplasmic features are similar to myeloblast.

Promegakaryocyte
- Nucleus is bigger than megakaryoblast
- Nucleus is lobulated because of endoreduplication of nucleus
- Cytoplasm basophilic, stains light blue and has azurophilic purplish pink granules.

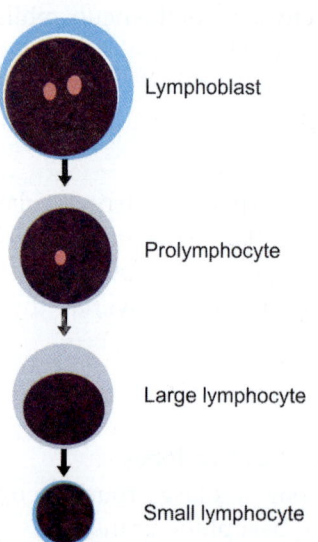

Fig. 1.4: Schematic diagram of lymphoid series cells

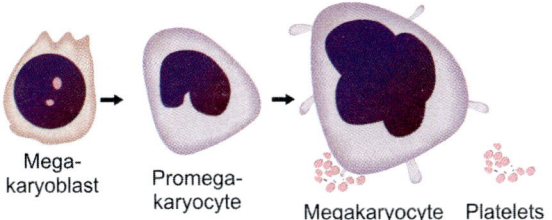

Fig. 1.6: Schematic diagram of megakaryocytic series cells

Megakaryocyte
- Largest cell in the bone marrow
- 30–90 μ
- Nucleus lobulated (4–16 lobes)
- Chromatin clumped
- Cytoplasm has azurophilic granules
- Platelets are formed by the protrusion of the pseudopodia of the megakaryocyte cytoplasm into the bone marrow sinusoids.

Platelets
- 1–4 μ
- Approximately 1/3 of an RBC size
- No nucleus
- Cytoplasm is light blue, has azurophilic purplish pink granules.

Exercise 2

Blood Collection

In investigating physiological functions and diseases related to blood, it is essential that the tests do not give misleading information. It is important to avoid faults in the specimen collection, storage and transport to the laboratory. Venous blood is preferred for most haematological investigations. Capillary blood is usually restricted to children; however for certain investigations, sample of blood needed is less and this blood can be used. Different sources, their techniques of obtaining and uses are as follows:

Sources
 i. Capillary or peripheral blood
 ii. Venous blood

i. Capillary or Peripheral Blood
When small quantity of blood is needed, this blood is preferred.

Sites
a. Ear lobe (free margin).
b. Tips of fingers—palmar surface, usually ring finger of left hand is used.
c. In infants great toe or heel—medial or lateral portions of plantar surface is chosen.
   Skin which is oedematous, congested, cold and cyanotic should not be used.

Equipment
1. Gauze pads.
2. 70% alcohol.
3. Lancet (disposable or reusable).

Procedure
- The site chosen for collecting blood is cleaned with 70% alcohol which acts as disinfectant and also removes the dirt and epithelial cells.
- Allow it to dry.
- Give a firm quick stab with a sterile lancet.
- Ideal depth is 1 to 3 mm.
- Allow the blood to collect at the puncture site. Do not squeeze, as with squeezing tissue juices will contaminate and dilute the blood.
- Blood collects in the form of a drop.
- Wipe away first drop, as it may be contaminated with tissue juices.
- Allow free flow of blood.
- Collect the blood for necessary investigations.
- To stop the flow of blood, apply light pressure with gauze pad after necessary amount of blood is collected.

Uses
Capillary blood is used for the following investigations:
1. Cell counts—total WBC count, RBC count, absolute eosinophil count.
2. Peripheral smear.
3. Hb% estimation.
4. Micro ESR.

Note: Before puncturing immerse the heel in warm water or apply hot water compression. Otherwise, values may be significantly higher than the venous blood.

ii. Venous Blood

This blood is used when many tests are to be done and when quantity of blood required is more.

Site: Median cubital vein

Equipment

Syringe: Syringes of 2 ml, 5 ml or 10 ml capacity depending on the quantity of blood needed are to be used. Disposable plastic syringes are used. The gauge of the needle chosen depends upon the amount of blood needed; usually 21 or 22 gauge needle can be used. The length of the needle used is shorter for superficial veins (Fig. 1.7). If deep veins are selected the needle should be longer. The needle tip should be sharp. If blunt, it may cause trauma and pain to the patient.

Procedure

- Assure the patient with a few good words.
- Make the patient to lie down or give him/her comfortable sitting position.
- Do not make the patient to stand or make him/her to sit on high stool, as there are chances of fainting.
- Arm, which is to be venipunctured should be firmly supported.
- Inspect and evaluate the veins.
- Apply the tourniquet above the vein (lower part of arm), which makes the vein more prominent. The pressure should not be maintained for longer time than necessary as it produces haemoconcentration.
  If tourniquet is not used, ask the patient to close the fist firmly for some time. Another person can be asked to apply pressure over the vein. These steps are meant to make the vein prominent.
- Clean the site with 70% alcohol.
- Fix the vein in position by supporting the patient's forearm. Instruct the patient to hold the pad. Request him/her to raise the outstretched arm for a few minutes.
- Hold the syringe between the thumb and last 3 fingers of right hand, resting the back of these fingers on the patient's arm.
- Rest the free index finger against the hub of the needle and this serves as a guide.
- Push the needle into the prominent vein with a single direct puncture of skin and vein.
- This is known as one step procedure which is less painful.
- Entrance into the vein is followed by appearance of blood into the hub.
- After the desired amount of blood is obtained, withdraw the syringe and the needle.
- Apply gentle pressure to the puncture with dry cotton or gauze.
- About 5 to10 ml of blood can be obtained for different investigations.
- The blood in the syringe is used for investigations directly or it can be maintained in fluid state by putting it in an anticoagulant.

Differences between Capillary Blood and Venous Blood

Venous blood and the capillary blood are not the same; even if the latter is freely flowing as it is more nearly arteriolar in origin. The packed cell volume (PCV), red blood cell count (RBC count) and haemoglobin (Hb) of capillary blood are slightly higher than those of venous blood. The total leukocyte count (TLC/TC), neutrophil count and monocyte count are higher especially among children.

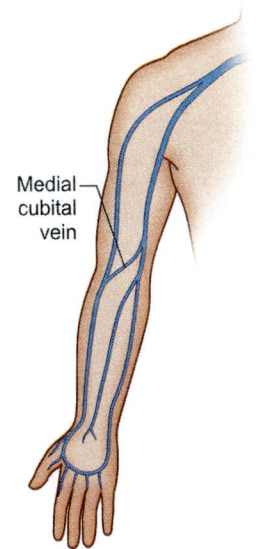

Fig. 1.7: Superficial veins of upper limb

Exercise 3

Anticoagulants

Different kinds of anticoagulants are available for various purposes. Following are the commonly used anticoagulants in the haematology laboratory. These anticoagulants can be prepared in the laboratory or recently plain and containing different anticoagulant vacutainers are available commercially (Fig. 1.8).

 i. Double oxalates—widely used
 ii. EDTA—widely used
 iii. Tri-sodium citrate—used in coagulation studies
 iv. Heparin

Action of Anticoagulants

Oxalates prevent clotting by precipitating calcium (Ca) ions in the plasma. Sodium citrate and EDTA convert Ca ions into unionized form. Heparin acts as antithrombin and prevents formation of thrombin.

i. Double Oxalates (Wintrobe's salt/mixture)

Ammonium oxalate   2.4 g
Potassium oxalate   1.6 g
Distilled water   100 ml

Three parts of ammonium oxalate and 2 parts of potassium oxalate are used to balance the swelling effect of ammonium oxalate and the shrinkage effect of potassium oxalate. About 0.2 ml of solution (8 mg of chemicals) is used to prevent clotting of 4 ml of blood. The bottles with the solution are heated in an incubator at 60 to 80°C for one hour.

Use
Used for Hb%, cell counts and ESR.

Disadvantages
1. WBC's morphology is not preserved well, so the double oxalate anticoagulants are not to be used for peripheral smear preparation.
2. As it is toxic, it is not used for blood transfusion.

ii. Ethylenediaminetetra-acetic (EDTA) Acid

It is also known as versene. Disodium and dipotassium salts are preferred by International Council for Standardization in Haematology (ICSH). Calcium is converted to unionised form and forms a soluble complex. It is a powerful anticoagulant.

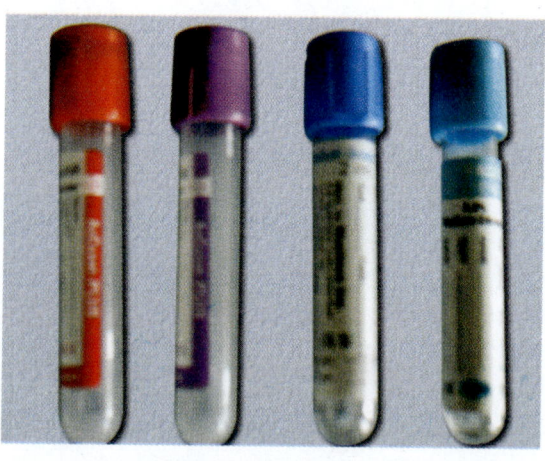

Fig. 1.8: Vacutainers

Dipotassium salt is easily soluble (1650 g/L) and hence preferred over to disodium salt (108 g/L) which is less soluble.

4 g/100 ml solution is prepared. About 0.1 ml (4 mg) of EDTA is put in vials and evaporated. 4 mg EDTA/2 ml of blood or 2 mg EDTA/ml of blood is used.

Uses
1. Gives good cellular morphology.
2. Clumping of platelets is prevented and hence, it is preferred for platelet counts.
3. Used for Hb% and cell counts.

Disadvantages
1. Platelets swell and disintegrate giving high platelet count.
2. RBCs and leukocytes show shrinkage and degeneration.
3. Excess EDTA gives decreased PCV and increased MCHC and Hb%.
4. Not suitable for coagulation studies.

iii. Tri-sodium Citrate

It binds calcium. One part of sodium-citrate to 9 part of blood is used for coagulation studies. About 0.4 ml of 3.8 g/dl of tri-sodium citrate is added to 1.6 ml of blood for ESR determination in Westergren's method.

Disadvantages
It is in liquid form. It dilutes the blood and hence it is not suitable for estimation of Hb% and cell counts.

iv. Heparin

Heparin neutralizes the thrombin, thus inhibits coagulation. About 15–20 IU heparin/ml of blood is used.

Uses
1. Best anticoagulant for osmotic fragility.
2. Size alteration of RBCs is nil, lysis is less.
3. Used for open-heart surgeries and emergency determination of blood sugar, urea and electrolytes.

Disadvantages
1. It is expensive.
2. Unsuitable for counts and smears, prevents coagulation for a limited period only.
3. Gives blue tint background, hence not suitable for peripheral smear.

Exercise 4

Peripheral Smear (Blood Film) Preparation and Staining

Peripheral smear (blood film) should be made on clean glass slides. Smears made on coverglasses are unsuitable for modern laboratory practice. Smear can be made by two slide manual method or by means of an automated slide spreader. Romanowsky stains are routinely employed for staining these peripheral smears and satisfactory results are obtained.

Two-Slide Method (Fig. 1.9)

- Take a slide and a spreader. The slide should be clean and free from dust, lint and grease. The spreader should be clean slide with sharp and even edges; sometimes the corners of the spreader are cut; by doing so we get a smear of lesser width than the width of a slide.
- A drop of fresh blood is taken either from the finger prick or sole in case of infants or from venous blood.
- The drop should be of moderate size.
- The drop is placed at a point three-fourth inch away from one end of the slide.
- Then the spreader is held between the thumb and the forefinger of right hand and then the drop of blood is touched with one end of it.
- Thus, the drop spreads along the edge of the spreader.
- Push the spreader forward immediately with an even and moderate spread, such that the drop spreads into a moderately thin smear.
- Air dry the smear either by waving the slide in air or by holding the slide near a fan or in front of a tube light.
- A good smear should be 3 cm in length. It should not cover the entire surface of the slide. It should have even and smooth appearance. Further it should be free from ridges, waves and windows (holes). The tail should not have any fringes (ragged ends).
- The smear has head, body and tail (Fig. 1.10). The beginning part which is slightly thicker is called head. The cells are overlapped here. The middle part is the body part; the cells are evenly spread in this region. The tapered part is called the tail. The smear is studied mainly in the body part.

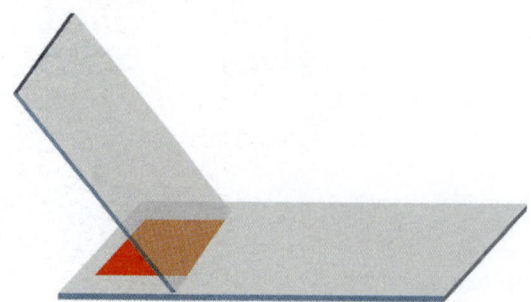

Fig. 1.9: Preparation of peripheral smear

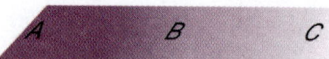

Fig. 1.10: Schematic diagram of different parts of peripheral smear. A. Head; B. Body; C. Tail

- The slide is labelled by marking with lead pencil on the head region.
- Once the smear is prepared, it has to be fixed.
- Fixing is done by keeping the slide in methyl alcohol for 1 to 2 minutes. Even 1 to 2 dips are sufficient. This prevents crenation and artifacts of the cells.
- If the staining is done immediately with Wright's stain, there is no need of fixation. But if delay is expected, then first it has to be fixed, and later stained.

Staining of Peripheral Smear (Fig. 1.11)

Commonly employed Romanowsky stains are: Wright's stain and Leishman's stain.

Procedure
- Place the slides on a stain rack.
- Put sufficient Wright's stain on the smear. If the stain is less, it evaporates and leaves some stain particles on the smear.
- Wait for 2 minutes. But the timing varies depending on the freshness of the stain. If the stain is old and prepared long back, it may need more time (2½ to 4 minutes).
- Add equal quantity of buffer.
- Blow gently (this step can be avoided).
- Wait for 7 minutes.
- Discard the stain and the buffer.
- The back of the slide is cleaned with gauze or wiped with a blotting paper.
- Excess water is drained off.
- Stained smear is then dried by leaving in a slanting position or by blotting gently with a filter paper.

Note: Instead of buffer, tap water also can be used; but the pH of the water should be around 6.4; a well-stained smear should look pink or purplish pink.

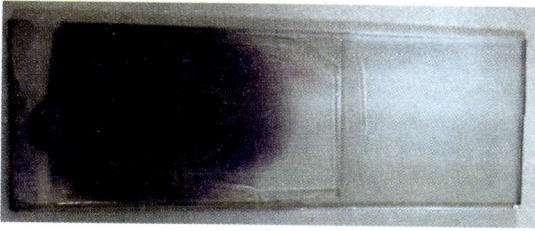

Fig. 1.11: Stained peripheral smear

Causes of Understaining
- More acidic pH of buffer or water
- If the staining period is shorter
- Too long wash
- Mounting the coverslip before the stained smear is dried.

In such smears the RBCs look red or orange. The nucleus and basophilic granules are not properly stained. The granules of the eosinophil are brilliant red. As the nucleus is not stained, the WBCs cannot be identified properly.

Causes of Overstaining
- More alkaline pH
- If the staining period is too long
- If washing time is too short or inadequate washing
- Thick films.

In such smears the RBCs are green or blue. The granules and nuclei are stained too dark even the granules of eosinophils stained blue grey.

Buffer Used

Refer to the topic on buffer.

Wright's Stain

Refer to Romanowsky stains.

Exercise

5

Haemoglobin (Hb) Estimation

The haemoglobin concentration can be estimated by various methods by measurement of colour, its power of combining with oxygen or carbon monoxide or by its iron content.

Acid Haematin Method (Sahli's method)

This is one of the colourimetric methods. Haemoglobin is converted into acid haematin by dilute HCl into brownish yellow coloured solution. This colour of the solution is matched with the colour comparator of Sahli's haemoglobinometer (Figs 1.12a and b).

Blood used: Direct or anticoagulated blood.

Procedure: N/10 HCl is taken up to '20' mark of the graduated tube. About 20 cc of blood is taken in the haemoglobin pipette. The tip of the pipette is wiped with blotting paper. The blood is added to the HCl in the dilution tube. Wait for 10 minutes, and then go on adding distilled water till the colour matches with the colour comparator of Sahli's haemoglobinometer.

Haemoglobin is expressed in g/dl.

Other Methods

1. In colourimetric methods:
   a. Alkali haematin method
   b. Cynmeth haemoglobin method
   c. Tallquist method.

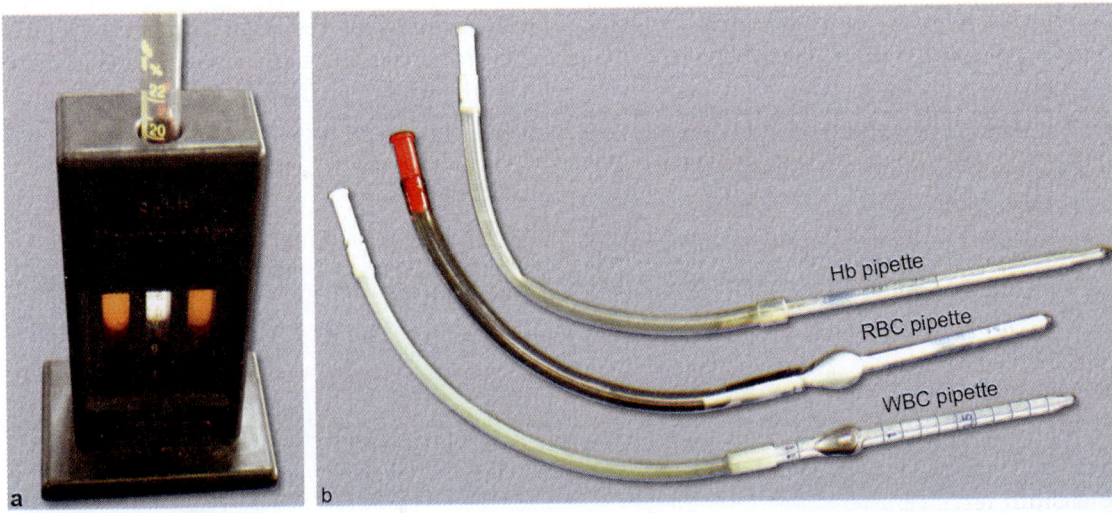

Figs 1.12a and b: (a) Haemoglobin estimation by Sahli's method; (b) Haemoglobin pipette with RBC and WBC pipettes

2. Specific gravity method.
3. Gasometric method.
4. Chemical method.

Normal Range

Men	13.5 to 15.5 g/dl
Women	12.5 to 13.5 g/dl
Newborn	16 to 18 g/dl
10 to 12 years of age	12 to 13 g/dl

Sources of Error in Sahli's Method

1. Non-haemoglobin substances like proteins and lipids in the plasma influence the colour of the blood that is diluted with acid.
2. About 2–12% of haemoglobin (sulphaemoglobin, methaemoglobin and carboxyhaemoglobin) is not converted into acid haematin.
3. Time has to be determined and every time the observation has to be made at the same interval.
4. Matching with glass standard may introduce some sources of error.
5. Variation from operator to operator in matching the colour is also possible.
6. The other possible errors are:
   - Errors of the sample
   - Errors of the equipment
   - Errors of pipette calibration
   - Unclean and wet pipette.

Cyanmethaemoglobin Method (Fig. 1.13)

Equipment
- Photoelectric colourimeter or photometer
- Drabkin's solution
- Haemoglobin pipette.

Composition of Drabkin's solution

Sodium bicarbonate (Sodium hydrogen carbonate)	1.0 g
Potassium cyanide	0.05 g
Potassium ferricyanide	0.20 g
Distilled water	1000.0 ml

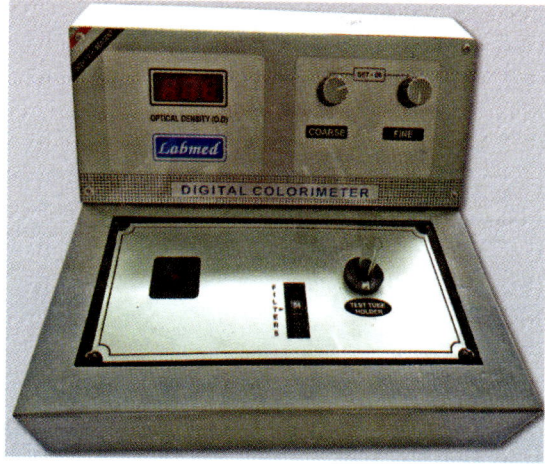

Fig. 1.13: Photocolourimeter for haemoglobin estimation by cyanmethaemoglobin method

Principle
Potassium ferricyanide converts haemoglobin iron from ferrous to ferric state and forms methaemoglobin. This combines with potassium cyanide to produce cyanmethaemoglobin which is stable.

Cyanmethaemoglobin (HiCN) standards are commercially available. The OD of this is measured at 540 nm (green filter) which corresponds to 15 g/dl of haemoglobin.

Procedure
Take 5 ml of Drabkin's solution, mix 20 cc (0.02 ml) of blood and wait for 5 min. Read the absorbance of test by setting blank to 100%.

$$\text{Hb g/dl} = (\text{OD test}/\text{OD STD}) \times 15$$

Draw a graph by plotting OD on Y-axis and concentration on Hb, i.e. 5 g, 10.0 g, 15.0 g on X-axis. A straight line, passing through the origin, agrees with Beer's law. This graph can be used as a standard graph for Hb determination.

Principle of Photocolourimeter

A 6V, 3W lamp fed from IC stabilized power supply forms source of light. The light passes through the filter, then onto test tube containing the sample solution. After this, light falls on the photocell which is sensitive.

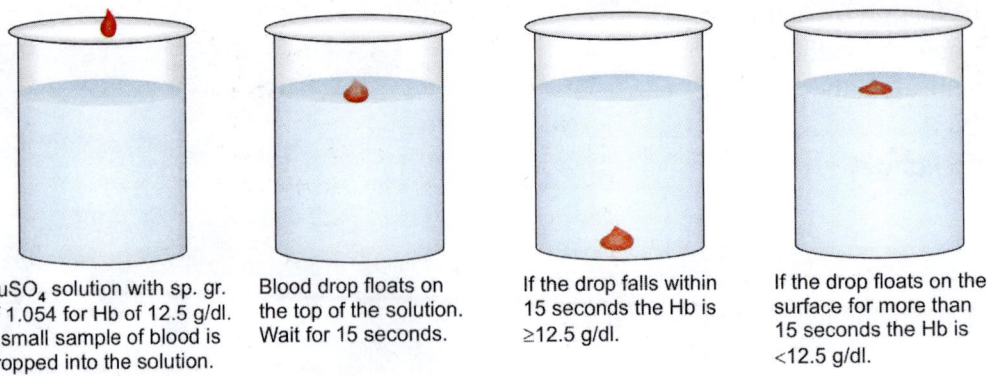

CuSO₄ solution with sp. gr. of 1.054 for Hb of 12.5 g/dl. A small sample of blood is dropped into the solution.

Blood drop floats on the top of the solution. Wait for 15 seconds.

If the drop falls within 15 seconds the Hb is ≥12.5 g/dl.

If the drop floats on the surface for more than 15 seconds the Hb is <12.5 g/dl.

Fig. 1.14: Haemoglobin estimation by specific gravity method

Then the readings are read as log DPM. The DPM displays optical density from 0.00 to 1.99.

The working of photometer is based on Beer's or Lambert's law.

Beer's law states that optical density is directly proportional to the concentration of solution.

Lambert's law states that OD of coloured solution is directly proportional to the path of light (diameter of cuvette).

Tallquist Method

This is a colourimetric method. A drop of blood is put on a filter paper. The resulting colour is compared with the Tallquist plate; but this is not a reliable method.

Haldane's Method

In this method, a known volume of blood is converted into carboxyhaemoglobin by allowing it to act with carbon monoxide gas. The cherry red colour of carboxyhaemoglobin thus formed is compared with a standard tube of the same size containing carboxyhaemoglobin.

Specific Gravity Method (Fig. 1.14)

This method is used in blood donation camps. A drop of anticoagulated blood is dropped into copper sulphate solution of known specific gravity. In a few seconds (15–20 seconds), the drop begins to rise or continues to fall (rises if specific gravity of blood is less and falls if specific gravity is more). The accuracy depends upon the number of copper sulphate solutions of different specific gravity used.

The specific gravity of blood ranges from 1.048 to 1.066; the average for men is 1.057, and for women is 1.053. The values are lower by 0.003 in the afternoon and after meals. But after exercise and during night, the same values are higher. In cases of anaemias the specific gravity is less than the normal range.

Gasometric Method
(By using von Slyke's apparatus)

By saturating the blood with oxygen first, then driving off the oxygen and collecting it separately, one can calculate the amount of haemoglobin. One gram of haemoglobin binds to 1.34 ml of oxygen.

Exercise

6

Cell Counts

NEUBAUER COUNTING CHAMBER
(Figs 1.15 and 1.16)

Various cell counts are being done using counting chamber. The visibility of the ruling in the chamber is important for the accuracy of the counts. The Neubauer or improved ruling is recommended.

- Neubauer counting chamber is made of a thick glass slide. It has H-shaped grooves. On either side of the horizontal gutter, there are two counting chambers.
- The total area of each chambers is 9 sq. mm (3 × 3 mm) and the depth is 0.1 mm. The area of the chamber is divided into 9 squares. The four corner squares are divided into 16 squares which are used for absolute eosinophil count and total leukocyte count. The central square is divided into 25 small squares. Each of these squares is again divided into 16 smaller squares.
- The central square is usually used for platelet count, whereas, five of the small squares (secondary squares) in the central square are used for RBC count.
- The coverslips used for Neubauer chamber should be smooth with even surface. The thickness is 0.3 to 0.5 mm. The sizes are 16 × 22 mm and 22 × 23 mm.

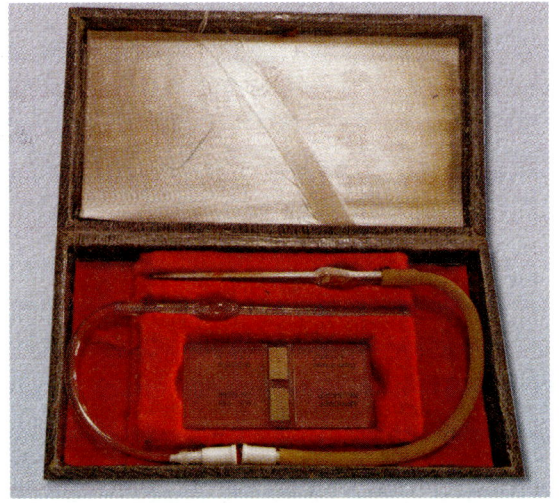

Fig. 1.15: Neubauer counting chamber with RBC and WBC pipettes in haemocytometer box

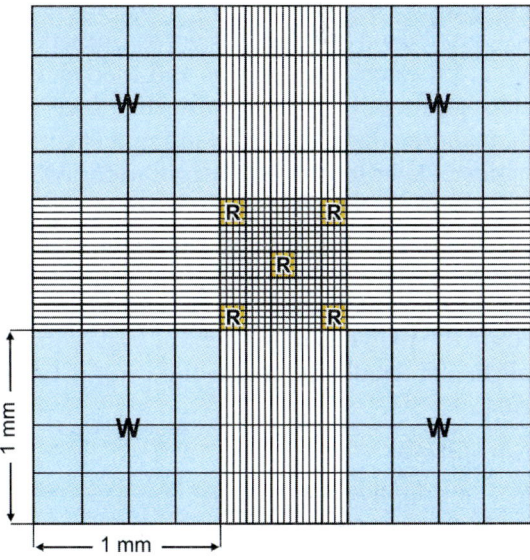

Fig. 1.16: Diagram of Neubauer counting chamber with markings W—WBC count, R—RBC count

Note:
- In improved Neubauer counting chamber, the 9 large squares are separated by solid black lines.
- Other counting chambers like Fuchus-Rosenthal and Speirs-Levy haemocytometers are with little modifications.

PLATELET COUNT

Reagents and Equipment

1. Counting chamber.
2. Anticoagulated blood (EDTA is the preferred anticoagulant).
3. RBC pipette.
4. Platelet diluting fluid (Rees-Ecker's fluid).

Composition of Rees-Ecker's Fluid

Brilliant cresyl blue	0.1 g
Sodium citrate	3.8 g
Neutral formaldehyde, 40%	0.2 ml
Distilled water to make	100 ml

Store in a refrigerator and filter before use.

Different diluent fluids like ammonium oxalate and formal-citrate red cell diluent fluids also can be used.

Procedure

Blood is drawn up to '1' mark of RBC pipette and diluting fluid up to '101' mark: these are properly mixed (Fig. 1.17). Wait for sometime, discard the first a few drops and then charge the chamber. It is preferable to place the chamber in a Petri dish containing wet cotton or filter paper to prevent evaporation. Allow some time for the cells to settle down.

The platelets appear as round to oval in structure. These should be differentiated from the debris, dust, etc. which are refractile. Count the platelets in the central large square (all the 25 small squares in the central large square).

Calculations

$$\frac{n \times \text{dilution factor}}{\text{Volume of chamber counted}}$$

$$= \frac{n \times 100}{0.1 \times 1 \times 1}$$

$$= n \times 1000 \text{ cells/cmm}$$

(n: Number of platelets counted)

Normal range: 1.5 to 4 lakh cells/cmm

RBC COUNT

Reagents and Instruments

1. RBC pipette.
2. Counting chamber.
3. RBC diluting fluid.

Composition of Hayem's Fluid

Mercuric chloride	2.5 g (to provide stability)
Sodium chloride	5.0 g (for isotonicity)
Sodium sulphate	25.0 g (to prevent rouleux)
Distilled water	1 litre (solvent)

Dissolve all the chemicals in distilled water and filter several times. Prepare a sufficient quantity to last only for 2–3 weeks, since deterioration may occur beyond this time, although Hayem's fluid remains fairly stable.

Procedure

Draw blood up to '0.5' mark of RBC pipette. Blood adhering to the tip is to be wiped off. Draw diluting fluid up to '101' mark. The pipette is shaken on the palms for about 30 seconds to facilitate mixing. Discard the first a few drops. Charge the chamber and wait for the cells to settle down. The chamber is visualised in low power and five of the 25 small squares of central large square are to be counted.

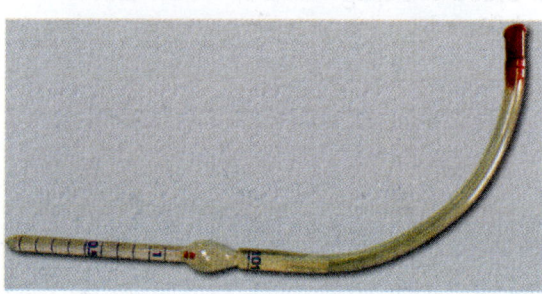

Fig. 1.17: RBC pipette

Calculation

$$\frac{n \times 200}{0.2 \times 0.2 \times 0.1 \times 5}$$
$= n \times 10{,}000 \text{ cells/cmm}$

(*n*: Number of RBCs counted)

Other diluting fluids

Gower's solution

Sodium sulphate	62.5 g
Glacial acetic acid	167 ml
Distilled water	to make 1 litre

Dacie's solution

3% tri-sodium citrate	99 ml
Conc. formalin	1 ml

TOTAL LEUKOCYTE COUNT

The total leukocyte count (TLC) is meant to determine the number of leukocytes per µl (cmm) of the blood.

Equipment

1. WBC pipette (Fig. 1.18)—It has a stem and a mixing chamber
   Markings on the pipette—0.5, 1 and 11
   The volume of the mixing chamber is 20 times of the blood drawn up to 0.5 mark.
2. WBC diluting fluid (Turk's fluid):

Glacial acetic acid	2 ml
1% aqueous solution of Gentian violet	1 ml
Distilled water to make	100 ml

   The solution is stable at room temperature. A pinch of thymol may be added as preservative.
3. Counting chamber.
4. Blood-anticoagulated or fresh blood could be used.

Procedure

Blood is drawn up to '0.5' mark of the WBC pipette. Wipe off the blood sticking at the tip. Draw diluting fluid up to '11' mark. Mix the contents well between the middle finger and thumb. Wait for 5 minutes. Discard the first few drops. Charge the chamber. Count the WBCs in the corner 4 squares of the chamber— '*n*' number of cells. Do not count the WBC touching the dividing lines to the right and below, but include the cells touching the dividing lines to the left and above.

Calculations

$n \times$ dilution factor/volume of squares counted, '*n*' being number of cells counted
$= n \times 20/0.4$
$= n \times 50 \text{ cells/cmm}$

WBC count is expressed as ... cells/cmm

Normal Values of Total Leukocyte Count

Adults	4000–11000 cells/cmm
At birth	10000–25000 cells/cmm
1–3 years	6000–18000 cells/cmm
4–7 years	6000–18000 cells/cmm
8–12 years	4500–13500 cells/cmm

Physiological Variations

- TLC is higher among females than among males. In females, TLC falls down after menopause.
- Oral contraceptive pills are reported to raise the TLC.
- *Diurnal variation:* Count is less in the morning and reaches maximum by afternoon.
- Physical exercise increases TLC up to 30,000 cells/cmm; the reason is that during

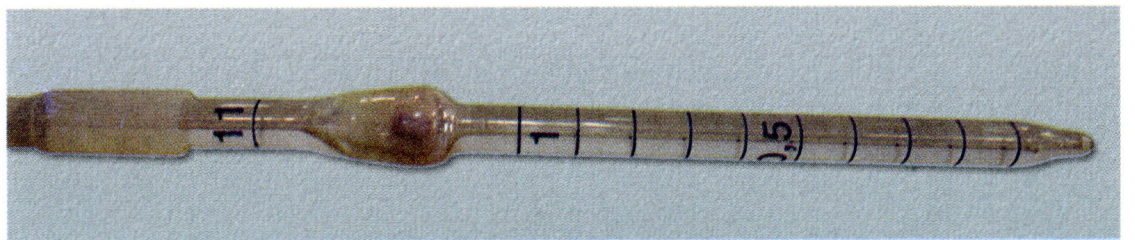

Fig. 1.18: WBC pipette

exercise splenic flow is reduced preventing sequestration of the cells. A large number of neutrophis, lymphocytes and monocytes enter the circulation during such exercise.
- Higher counts are observed with high temperature, severe pain, emotion, smoking, adrenaline administration and during pregnancy. Counts return to normal a week after delivery.
- At birth, the counts are high and gradually drop thereafter.

True Leukocyte Count/ Corrected Leukocyte Count

When the nucleated red cells are counted, they cannot be distinguished from leukocytes and if the number of nucleated red blood cells (NRBC) is higher in the stained smear, a correction is made according to the following formula:

True leukocyte count = $(TC \times 100)/(100 + NRBC)$

(NRBC: Number of nucleated red cells, counted in differential count per 100 leukocytes)

Exercise 7

Red Cell Indices

Mean Corpuscular Volume (MCV)

Indicates volume of red cells. It is expressed in femtolitres (fl).

$$MCV = \frac{Hematocrit \times 10}{RBC\ count\ in\ millions}$$

Normal range 80–98 fl: Normocytes
< 80 fl: Microcytes
> 100 fl: Macrocytes

Mean Corpuscular Haemoglobin (MCH)

MCH indicates amount of Hb per red cell. It is expressed in pg (picograms)

$$MCH = \frac{Hb\ (g/dl) \times 10}{RBC\ count\ in\ millions}$$

Normal range: 26–34 pg
Less than 26 pg: Decreased MCH
Seen in microcytic hypochromic anaemias
More than 34 pg: Increased MCH
Seen in macrocytic anaemia

Mean Corpuscular Haemoglobin Concentration (MCHC)

MCHC denotes average concentration of haemoglobin in the red cells.

$$MCHC = \frac{Hb\ (g/dl) \times 100}{Haematocrit\ (\%)}$$

MCHC is expressed in g/dl
Normal range: 31–37 g/dl
<31 g/dl—hypochromic
>37 g/dl—hyperchromic (spherocytes)

Red Cell Distribution Width (RDW)

Provides an assessment on variation in red cell volume.

In early iron deficiency anaemia RDW is increased with normal MCV.

In established case of iron deficiency anaemia RDW is increased with low MCV.

Vitamin B_{12} and folate deficiency anaemia RDW is increased.

In thalassaemia trait RDW is normal with low MCV. *Normal range:* 11.5–14.5%

Exercise 8

Absolute Eosinophil Count

Total eosinophil counts can be roughly calculated from the total and differential leukocyte counts, the staining properties make it possible to count them directly and more accurately in the counting chamber.

Reagents and Equipment

1. Eosinophil diluting fluid.
2. Neubauer counting chamber.
3. Anticoagulated blood.
4. WBC pipette.

Eosinophil Diluting Fluid (Dunger's fluid)

Eosin, aqueous 200 g/L	10 ml
Acetone	10 ml
Water	80 ml

Acid dye (eosin/phloxine) stains the granules, and water acts as a solvent; and also lysis the RBCs and other leukocytes. Eosinophils resist the lysis. Acetone prevents lytic action of water on eosinophil.

Procedure

Draw blood up to '1' mark of WBC pipette and eosinophil diluting fluid up to '11' mark (dilution factor 1:10) and wait for a few minutes. Discard the first few drops and charge the chamber. Allow some time for the cells to settle down and count the corner 4 large squares.

Calculation:

$$\frac{n \times 10}{0.1 \times 1 \times 4} = n \times 25 \text{ cells/cmm}$$

If the corner four large squares of both the chambers (totally 8 large squares) are counted, the accuracy of count is better and for calculation the formula $n \times 12.5$ cells/cmm is applied.

Normal range: 40–440 cells/cmm

Exercise 9

Differential Leukocyte Count

Differential leukocyte count (DLC) is the percent distribution of various WBCs in the peripheral blood so as to establish the relative frequency of different types of WBCs. But a limited number of cells are usually counted (100) in the peripheral smear and recorded in percentage. Counting of 200–500 leukocytes yields higher accuracy. This is carried out on Wright or Leishman stained smears.

In case of the smears prepared on glass slides, it is generally assumed that the distribution of leukocytes is random. The smears should not be too thin and the tail should be smooth. If the smear is too thin and rough edged spreader is used, the leukocytes accumulate at the edges and the tail. Even otherwise in a moderately thick smear, the polymorphs and the monocytes predominate at the margins and the tail. The lymphocytes would be in the middle region. This difference is mainly based on the stickiness, specific gravity and size of different WBCs. On unsatisfactory smears, DLC is not done. Various systems of performing DLC are adopted.

The film must be inspected from head to tail; 100 cells are counted in a longitudinal strip. If less than 100 cells are counted in one strip, then examine one or more additional strips. Each longitudinal strip represents the blood drawn from a small part of blood. If all the cells in such strips are counted, the DLC would approximate closely to the true DLC (Fig. 1.19a).

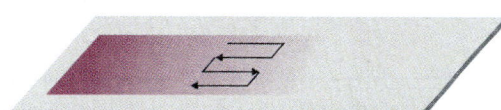

Fig. 1.19a: Method of inspection for doing DLC, peripheral smear

In the head part, sometimes it is difficult to identify the cells. The cells can be counted in a well spread area (body part of the smear) where the cells are clearly identifiable. The lateral edges are avoided.

Normal range

	Adults	Children
Neutrophils	60–70%	20–30%
Lymphocytes	20–40%	60–70%
Monocytes	02–08%	02–08%
Eosinophils	01–08%	01–08%
Basophils	00–01%	00–01%

Variations in Differential Count

Among children soon after birth for 3 days, polymorphs predominate and then they fall, whereas the lymphocytes predominate up to 5–7 years of age. However in tropical countries eosinophilia and monocytosis are common due to endemic parasites and protozoal diseases.

Causes for Variation in Leukocyte Counts

Neutrophilia (Fig. 1.19b)

The causes of neutrophilia
- Acute infections with cocci

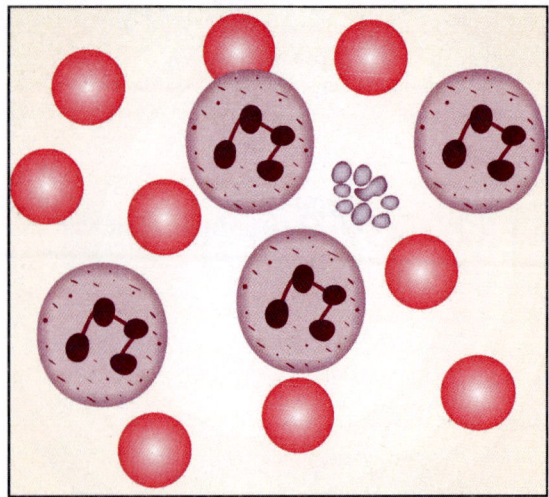

Fig. 1.19b: Neutrophilic leukocytosis

cell is a reactive lymphocyte with basophilic cytoplasm and it resembles plasma cell.

Chronic bacterial infections like tuberculosis, syphilis, typhoid and such other chronic infections.

Eosinophilia (Fig. 1.20)

The causes of eosinophilia
- Allergy to extrinsic agents such as vegetables, animal products, parasites, drugs and blood products
- Neoplasms-lymphoproliferative malignancies (Hodgkin's disease), carcinomas
- Certain vasculitis and collagen disorders—polyarteritis nodosa
- Dermatological conditions—pemphigus and dermatitis herpetiformis
- Löeffler's syndrome
- Familial
- Post-splenectomy
- Miscellaneous.

- Tissue injury—infarctions, burns, surgery and necrosis inducing processes
- Haemorrhage
- Neoplasms
- Stress states and hyperactivity conditions like convulsions, tachycardia, labour, severe colic, delirium-tremens
- Inflammatory disorders—collagen disorders, gout and rheumatic fever
- Metabolic disorders—diabetic ketoacidosis
- Corticosteroid administration
- Miscellaneous causes.

Monocytosis

When the absolute monocyte count exceeds the limit of 0.8×10^9 cells/L, then that condition is called monocytosis.

Lymphocytosis

Absolute lymphocyte count of about 4×10^9 cells/L is called lymphocytosis.

Relative lymphocytosis: Lymphocyte count is normal but when neutrophil count is reduced, there appears a relative increase in lymphocytes.

Causes of lymphocytosis
Viral—pertussis, mumps, measles, influenza and infectious mononucleosis. Atypical lymphocytosis is observed in EB virus infection, CMV infection and infective hepatitis. In atypical lymphocytosis, enlarged pleomorphic lymphocytes are observed. Turk

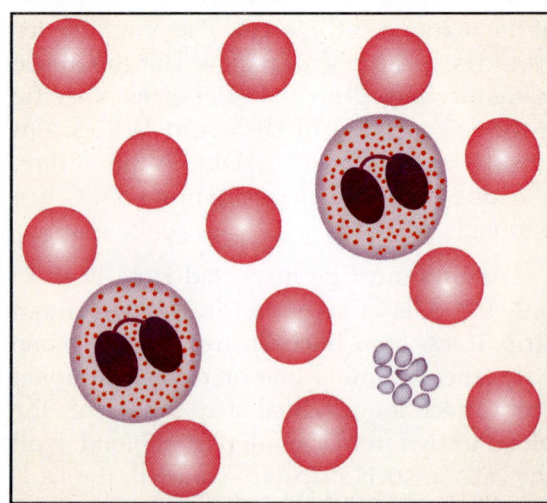

Fig. 1.20: Eosinophilia

Causes of monocytosis
- Infections like tuberculosis, malaria, bacterial endocarditis, typhoid, kala-azar, parasitic and protozoal diseases
- Ulcerative colitis
- Sarcoidosis
- Certain cases of acute myeloid leukemia
- Chronic myeloid leukemia
- Myelodysplastic syndrome.

Basophilia

Basophils are increased in chronic myeloid leukemia.

Lymphopenia

Absolute count below the limit of 1.5×10^9 cells/L is called lymphopenia.

Causes of lymphopenia
- Pancytopenia
- Advanced Hodgkin's disease
- Prodromal phase of viral infections due to depletion of helper T cells, e.g. AIDS
- Corticosteroid therapy.

Neutropenia

The causes of neutropenia
- Conditions that replace normal haemopoietic cells like acute leukemia, myelofibrosis, lymphoma, multiple myeloma, myelodysplastic syndrome
- Infections—typhoid, viral infections, sepsis
- Megaloblastic anaemia
- Aplastic anaemia
- Iron deficiency anaemia
- Drugs and radiation—marrow depression
- Chronic idiopathic neutropenia
- Hypersplenism
- Cytotoxic therapy
- Cyclic neutropenia.

Exercise 10

Packed Cell Volume (Haematocrit)

The volume of erythrocytes expressed as a percentage to the volume blood is called haematocrit (Fig. 1.21a).

Blood used: EDTA, double oxalate or heparinised blood.

Equipment
1. Wintrobe's haematocrit tube (110 mm long, internal bore—3 mm)
2. Pasteur's pipette
3. Centrifuging machine
4. Anticoagulated blood

Procedure

Mix the blood adequately and label the Wintrobe's tube (Fig. 1.21b). Fill the Wintrobe's haematocrit tube using Pasteur's pipette (Fig. 1.21c). As filling proceeds, the tip of the pipette is raised and filled up till 100 mark. Care is to be taken to see that there are no air bubbles present in the blood column. After the

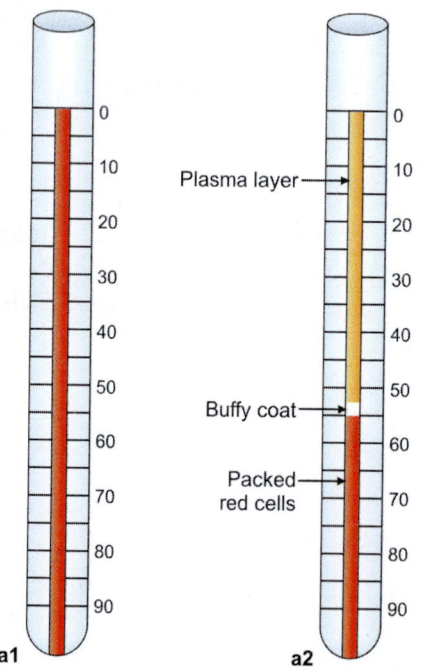

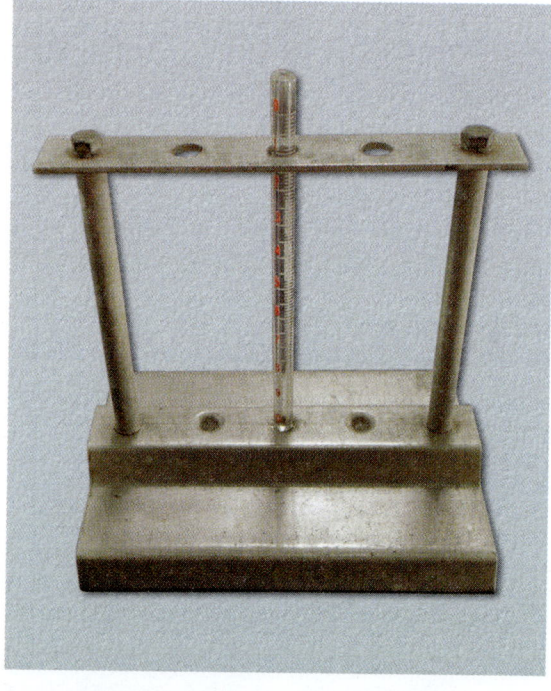

Fig. 1.21a: Schematic diagram of PCV (a1: Before centrifugation, a2: After centrifugation)

Fig. 1.21b Wintrobe's tube with stand

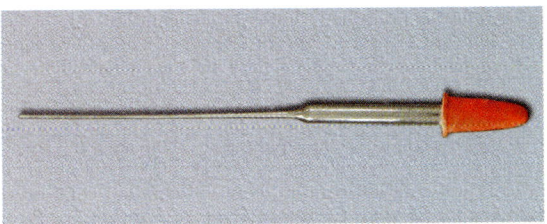

Fig. 1.21c: Pasteur's pipette for filling the Wintrobe's tube

blood is filled, it is preferred to cap the tube to avoid evaporation. Then the tube is placed in the centrifuging machine and centrifuged at 3000 RPM for 30 minutes. Reading is taken without disturbing the Wintrobe's tube. Read the red cell column and express in percentage or calculate by using the following formula.

Haematocrit percentage = 100 × L1/L2
L1 = Height of the red cell column in the tube
L2 = Height of whole blood (red cells + buffy coat + plasma layer)

While taking L1 reading, buffy coat layer is not included or read the red cell column and express in percentage.

Microhaematocrit Method

For this method a capillary haematocrit tube about 7.5 cm long with bore of 1 mm is used. Blood is filled by capillary action leaving 1.5 cm unfilled. The empty end is sealed by heating or filling soft wax/clay. It is centrifuged at 5000 to 12000 g/minute for 10 minutes for the former and 5 minutes for the latter. Special centrifuging machines are available for this method. The length of whole blood and length of RBC column are noted.

Normal values

Males	47 ± 7 (40–54%)
Females	42 ± 5 (37–47%)

PCV variations
- Decreased in anaemias and pregnancy.
- Increased in polycythemia, shock, dehydration, emphysema and congenital heart disease.

Errors in PCV could be due to
- Inadequate mixing of blood
- Improper reading of the levels of RBC column and plasma column
- Irregularity in the diameter of the bore of the tube
- Excess EDTA causes shrinkage of RBCs and PCV decreases
- PCV increases with tourniquet tied for longer duration while drawing blood.

PCV is simple screening test for anaemia. In conjunction with Hb% and RBC count, PCV helps in calculation of blood cell indices. Look for the RBC column, buffy coat and plasma layer in PCV carried out in Wintrobe's tube. Buffy coat is usually 0.5 to 1 mm; 0.1 mm denotes 1000 WBC cells/cmm.

Plasma layer

Reddish	Suggests haemolysis
Yellow	Suggests jaundice
Milky white	Suggests hypercholesterolemia
Cloudy	Indicates increased viscosity of plasma proteins as in multiple myeloma

Exercise 11

Erythrocyte Sedimentation Rate (ESR)

It is described as the rate of fall of column of the erythrocytes in a given period of time when blood is held in a vertical tube.

Westergren's Method (Fig. 1.22a)

Westergren's pipette with stand (Fig. 1.22b): Westergren's pipette is 30 cm long; its inside bore diameter is 2.5 mm; both ends are open; and markings are from 0 to 200 above downwards (graduated in the lower 20 cm). The pipette must be clean, dry and free from dust. It should be thoroughly washed with tap water, rinsed with acetone allowed to dry and it can be reused. Teat or mechanical devices for suction should be used. Mouth suction should be avoided. EDTA blood/citrated blood is used. As the length of the column is more, dilution is not much affected with the citrated blood.

Procedure

Pipette out the blood up to '0' mark. Allow it to stand in a vertical position in Westergren's

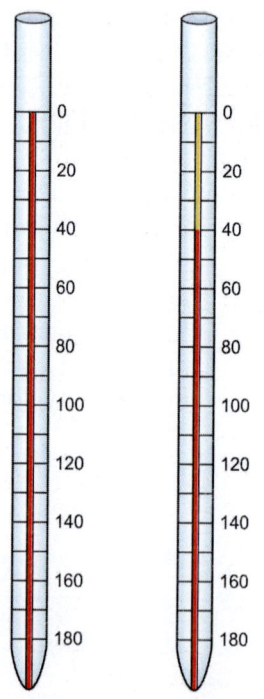

Fig. 1.22a: Schematic diagram of ESR by Westergren's method

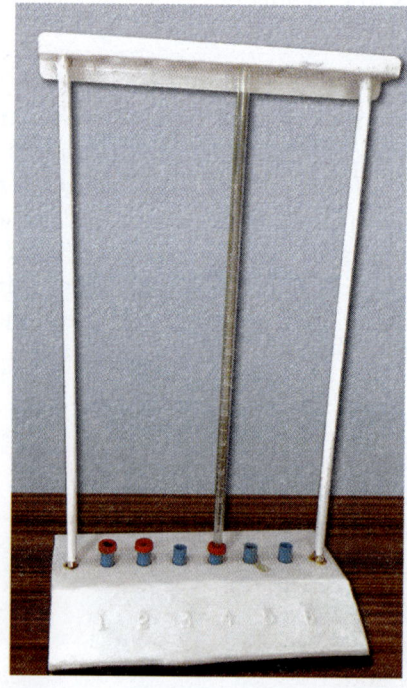

Fig. 1.22b: Westergren's pipette with stand

stand; read the upper level of the red cells exactly at the end of one hour. The reading is expressed as ... mm at the end of the first hour.

Normal range

Males	5 to 15 mm/1st hour
Females	5 to 20 mm/1st hour

Wintrobe's Method

- Blood used: EDTA blood
- Wintrobe's tube with stand and Pasteur's pipette.

Wintrobe's tube: Markings are 0 to 100 above downwards (for ESR) and below upwards (for PCV)

Procedure

Fill the blood up to '0' mark with Pasteur's pipette. Allow it to stand vertically for one hour in Wintrobe's stand. At the end of one hour note the upper level of red cells.

Normal values

Males	0–10 mm/1st hour
Females	0–20 mm/1st hour

Micro Method

A plastic disposable tube of 230 mm long with 1 mm bore diameter is used. About 0.2 ml blood is needed. This method is useful in paediatric patients; procedure and reading taken are similar to the other methods.

Landau Method
(Micro-sedimentation method)

Used in infants when blood is insufficient for the above methods. Capillary blood can be used.

Equipment

Landau pipette with stand—looks like RBC pipette with markings 0–50 mm.

5.0 g/dl sodium citrate is used as an anticoagulant.

Procedure

Draw sodium citrate up to the first mark on the stem and then blood up to the second mark. Wipe off excess blood on the tip of the pipette. Draw both the solutions in the bulb. Set the upper level of the mixture to '0' mark at the top. Detach the suction device, and then place the pipette in a vertical position on the stand. Note the reading at the end of the 1st hour.

Normal range

Male	0–5 mm/1st hour
Female	0–8 mm/1st hour

Stages in ESR

There are three stages in ESR.

- *Stage 1:* Stage of aggregation: During the first 10 minutes the red cells form rouleaux. The factors which influence rouleaux, greatly influence the ESR.
- *Stage 2:* Stage of sedimentation: In next 40 minutes the aggregated cells fall.
- *Stage 3:* Stage of packing occurs in last 10 minutes.

Factors Influencing ESR

1. Normally for ESR, room temperature of 18–25°C is preferred. With increase in temperature ESR also increases.
2. With the lapse of time and in stored blood, the ESR is reduced. Hence, it is preferable to do ESR within 4 hours of collection of blood.
3. Place the ESR pipette vertically; and free from vibrations and sunlight.
4. Length of tube: Sedimentation is better with long tubes.
5. Rouleaux formation is facilitated by globulins fibrinogen and acute phase proteins-haptoglobin, ceruloplasmin, α_1-antitrypsin, c-reactive protein, etc.
6. It is retarded by albumin.
7. Cholesterol to some degree increases ESR.
8. ESR is more in females than males because of the higher levels of fibrinogen.
9. ESR increases during pregnancy because of the increase in red cell aggregation.

10. ESR is influenced by stage of menstrual cycle and drugs like steroids and contraceptives.
11. With high blood cell counts, ESR is low and low blood cell counts increases the ESR by accelerating the rate of fall.
12. ESR is low in cases of polycythemia, hypofibrinogenemia, CCF, abnormalities of red cells such as poikilocytosis, spherocytosis and sickle cell anaemia. Microcytes resist rouleaux formation with the reduction in ESR.
13. ESR is low in infants.

Note

- Citrated blood (1 : 4 ratio) can be used for Westergren's method.
- Because of biohazard in cases of HIV, hepatitis B, etc. instead of open ended tubes, closed systems are highly recommended for ESR.

Exercise 12

Blood Groups Related Exercises

BLOOD GROUPS

There are several blood groups; they are ABO, MNSs, P, Rh, Lutheran, Kell, Lewis, Kidd, Duffy, Diego, Yt, Xg, Ii, Dombrock, etc. Amongst these, ABO and Rh systems are important.

ABO BLOOD GROUPS (Fig. 1.23)

The red cell surface has antigens. The antigenic characters of red cells are inherited. The antigen detection of blood groups is based upon haemagglutination reactions. This is a serological reaction of red cells with the corresponding antibody, as determined in the laboratory. There are naturally occurring ABO group antibodies of IgM type in the serum of the patients. The serum contains the antibody for that antigen missing on the cell surface.

Some information about ABO system is given below.

Blood group	General population	Antigens	Antibodies
AB	3%	A and B	Nil
A	42%	A	Anti-B
B	8%	B	Anti-A
O	47%	Nil	Anti-A, Anti-B

Note: Racial variations in the frequency of these groups are noticeable.

Purpose of ABO blood grouping
  i. Blood transfusion
  ii. Medicolegal purposes, i.e. in cases of disputed paternity.

Procedure

Red cell suspension with 0.9% NaCl is prepared. Take a slide with three concavities

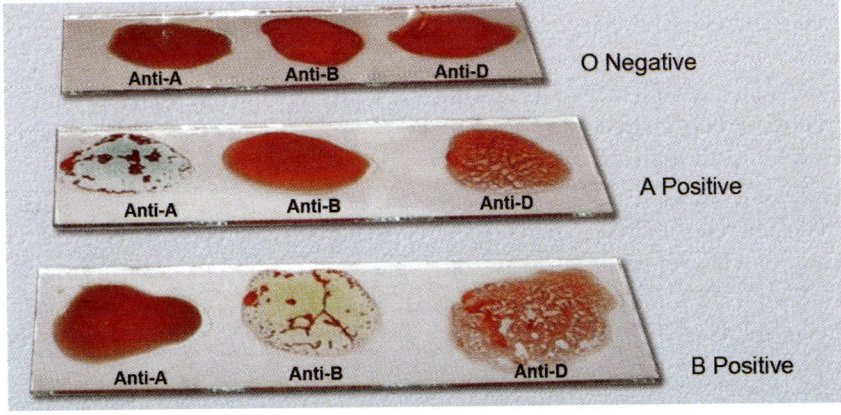

Fig. 1.23: Blood groups by slide method

or two concavities. Label the concavities as anti-A and anti-B. In a slide with three concavities, the central one is used for control.

One drop of anti-sera A (blue coloured) is put in the concavity labelled as anti-A and one drop of anti-sera B (yellow coloured) in concavity labelled as anti-B. Add one drop of blood diluted with normal saline to all the concavities. The central concavity containing only saline diluted blood acts as control. Take a glass rod; mix well, each time using different ends. Care is taken not to contaminate one another. Observe for agglutination after 5 to 10 minutes.

Agglutination	Blood group
Present in both anti-A, anti-B concavities	'AB'
Absent in both concavities	'O'
Present in only anti-A concavity	'A'
Present in only anti-B concavity	'B'

Note: When doubtful agglutination is present, the agglutination may be checked under microscope.

The antibodies in ABO system are naturally occurring complete antibodies and they can be easily detected by saline agglutination tests.

Blood Group Antigens

The antigenic determinants or epitopes are small portions of molecules recognised by antibodies.

ABO antigens are carbohydrate in nature. They are oligosaccharide chains anchored to glycoproteins or glycolipids of the RBC membrane.

They are highly immunogenic.

A and B antigens differ in only the terminal sugar.

There is terminal sugar N-acetyl galactosamine in A group.

And terminal sugar galactose in B group.

There is no A or B antigen in O blood group.

Antibodies

In ABO system there are natural antibodies.

They are present in the serum/plasma.

They are IgM type and have high molecular weight and hence cannot pass through the placenta.

These antibodies react well at 4°C, room temperature or at 37°C.

Sometimes IgG antibodies may be produced in O blood group patients which can cause hemolytic transfusion reactions and hemolytic disease of newborn.

UNIVERSAL DONORS AND RECIPIENTS

The earlier concept of 'O' blood group as universal donor and AB blood group as universal recipient does not hold good.

'O' blood group person have no antigens on the red cells but have anti-A and anti-B antibodies in the serum.

When given to recipient, these antibodies can destroy some of the recepient's red cells.

Hence, 'O' blood, better not to be given to A, B or AB persons. However, washed red cells can be given.

Earlier notion of AB person as a universal recipient, as they have A and B antigen on the red cells does not hold good. A or B blood groups will have antibodies against AB blood group antigens and can destroy some red cells of the AB recipient. Hence, A or B blood groups better not to be transfused to AB blood group patient. However, AB plasma can be given to A, B or O persons as it does not have any antibodies.

Hence, washed O red cell packs and AB plasma are universal donors.

ABO SUBGROUPS

Subgroups of A: A_1 and A_2

These two phenotypes are best differentiated using lectin that is extracted from the seeds of *Dolichos biflorus* which reacts only with A_1 cells.

A_1 accounts for 80% of blood group A.

A_2 accounts for 20% of blood group A.

Haematology

A_2 reacts weakly and misdiagnosed as 'O' blood group.

A_2 gene has two nucleotides different from A_1 gene which results in diminished enzymatic activity and subsequently weakened antigen expression.

If A_2 is misdiagnosed as 'O' blood group, there is no harm; however if A_2 is misdiagnosed as 'O' and if this blood is given to 'O' recipient, the anti-A and anti-B antibodies of the recipient might cause the early destruction of transfused blood.

A_2 and A_2B individuals can produce anti-A_1 antibodies.

Approximately 4% of A_2 individuals and up to 25% of the A_2B individuals can have Anti-A_1 antibodies in their serum.

The number of other subgroups of A has been described. This appears to result from inheritance of rare alleles of ABO locus and include A_{int}, A_3, A_x, A_m, A_{end}, A_{el}, A_{buntu} and A_{finn}. Except for A_{int} and A_3, many of these subgroups are weakly reactive or non-reactive with anti-A antibodies.

Subgroups of B

As described for A blood group, subgroups of B are also reported. Reactions of these red cells with anti-B are weak and variable.

BOMBAY BLOOD GROUP

This phenotype arises when two hh genes are inherited at the Hh locus. Such individuals are unable to convert type II paragloboside to H antigen. Hence, they are unable to make A or B antigens. These individuals produce anti-H, anti-A and anti-B as naturally occurring antibodies. On initial testing, Bombay blood group red cells appear to be of group 'O' but when this blood is transfused to 'O' blood group patients, these patients produce haemolytic reactions. This blood group occurs 1 in 13000 population all over.

LABORATORY TESTS DONE ON THE UNIT OF BLOOD DONATED

Following are the tests:
1. Haemoglobin estimation.
2. Blood grouping and cross matching.
3. Screening for unwanted antibodies.
4. Screening for transfusion transmissible infections: Indian Govt (Food and Drug Control Act) recommends following 5 tests to be mandatory. These are mentioned below.
   - HIV 1 and 2
   - Hepatitis B
   - Hepatitis C
   - Syphilis
   - Malaria.

Tests must be performed at each donation regardless of number of earlier donations.

TRANSFUSION REACTIONS

Transfusion reaction is defined as any unfavorable event that occurs during or after a transfusion of blood and its components.

The transfusion reactions can be classified as
Acute transfusion reactions—immunological
- Febrile non-hemolytic transfusion reactions (FNHTRs)
- Allergic reactions
- Anaphylactic and anaphylactoid reactions
- Acute hemolytic transfusion reactions (AHTRs)
- Transfusion related lung injury (TRALI).

Acute transfusion reactions—non-immunological
- Bacterial contamination
- Transfusion-associated
- Circulatory overload (TACO)
- Physical and chemical
- Hemolysis
- Metabolic derangements.

Delayed transfusion reactions—immunological
- Transfusion-associated graft-versus-host disease (TA-GVHD)
- Post-transfusion purpura.

Delayed transfusion reactions-non-immunological
- Iron overload
- Transfusion-transmitted diseases.

RH SYSTEM (RH TYPING)

The Rh system is so named because the original antibody was raised by injecting red cells of rhesus monkeys into rabbits and guinea pigs, also reacted with human cells. The Rh system is a gene complex which gives rise to various combinations of three alternative antigens C or c, D or d and E or e as originally suggested by Fisher. The Rh locus is on chromosome 1. Amongst these antigens, D antigen is the most immunogenic and it is convenient to classify the individual as Rh-D positive or Rh-D negative, depending on the presence of the Rh-D antigen. For Rh-D antigen detection, usually slide agglutination procedure is routinely done; whenever doubt arises tube technique is followed.

Slide Agglutination Method

One drop of anti-D and one drop of blood are mixed well, observe for agglutination after 2 minutes. This can be done along with ABO grouping as shown in Fig. 1.23.

Note: False negative result may be observed when room temperature is less and the test may need pre-warming of the slide.

Rh Confirmation by Tube Technique

This is done with controls; wash the cells with saline 3 times (5 drops of blood). Take 1 drop of cell suspension and 1 drop of anti-D; incubate at least for 30 minutes. Add anti-human globulin serum. Centrifuge for 1 minute and observe for agglutination.

WEAK D PHENOTYPE (DU PHENOTYPE)

Because of immunogenicity, the D antigen is the most clinically important antigen in the Rh blood group system. The donor and the recipient are tested for the presence or absence of the D antigen. The D positive recipients can receive D positive blood components and they can as well receive D negative blood components. On the other hand D negative recipients should be transfused with only D negative blood components. Although D typing on the vast majority of blood samples is straight forward, some variants of weak D typing may be encountered. These weak D typings are usually labelled as D negative on an immediate spin reading, but they are D positive when indirect antiglobulin test is conducted. This weak variant is described as Du phenotype (weak D). Reasons for this variant include a transposition effect, genetically transmissible Du and D categories.

When a C-producing Rh gene (without D) is in transposition, weakened expression of D antigen may be observed. These cells may fail to react with anti-D sera at immediate spin but they react strongly at antiglobulin phase of testing. This type of Du is also called high grade Du.

Some Du phenotypes arise from inheritance of specific Rh genes. This type Du is referred to as the low-grade Du. Among the blacks, a variant of R0 gene may produce lesser amounts of D antigen. Among the whites such diminished production is more frequently associated with variant R1 or variant R2 gene.

Among individuals with alloanti-D in the serum of D positive individuals, D Ag is proposed to be a mosaic, composed of genetically distinct pieces. A majority of D positive individuals have inherited Rh genes that produce all pieces of the mosaic; however some may inherit most of the pieces but not all the pieces of the antigen. Such individuals are at a risk during pregnancy and transfusion, to produce anti-D to the portion of D antigen, they lack on their red cells. These are grouped as D categories. Some of these are D positive on immediate spin, however others appear to be D-negative on immediate spin and demonstrate positive D with antiglobulin phase of testing. So most D category individuals are not apparent until they present with alloanti-D in their serum.

Hence, Du testing for donor cells is necessary to avoid immune response if transfused to D-negative recipient.

CROSS MATCHING

Purpose

This is done to ensure absence of incompatibility between the blood to be transfused and the blood of recipient.

Major cross matching is important, in which the serum of the recipient and the cells of the donor are mixed. The purpose of the major cross match is that the recipient's serum should not contain iso-antibodies to the donor's red cells. Minor cross matching is meant to detect iso-antibodies in the serum of the donor because they are capable of reacting with the recipient's red cells. This test is not mandatory.

Procedure of Major Cross Match

Prepare 2% red cell suspension of donor cells in saline. Add 2 drops of recipient's serum and 2 drops of red cell suspension, centrifuge at 1500 RPM for one minute and check for agglutination both macroscopically and microscopically. If positive the test detects IgM antibodies.

If there is no agglutination, then incubate in waterbath at 37°C for 15 minutes. Wash 3 times with saline. Thereafter follow the procedure of Coombs' test. Check for agglutination; if positive, it denotes IgG antibodies.

Procedure of Minor Cross Match

Similar procedure as above is followed using red cells of the recipient and the donor's serum.

COOMBS' TEST

Purpose: This test detects incomplete antibodies (IgG).

Requirements: Small glass test tubes (10 × 75 mm), pipettes, normal saline, centrifuging machine, Coombs' serum and the blood to be investigated into.

Coombs' serum (anti-human globulin serum): This is obtained by immunizing rabbits with human serum. Broad-spectrum antisera contains anti IgG and anti-complement components. Specific antisera against heavy chains of IgG, IgM and IgA can be prepared.

Direct Coombs' Test

Wash the test red cells 3–4 times with minimum of 3 ml of saline per wash and prepare 10–20% of red cell suspension in saline. About 2 drops of red cell suspension and 2 drops of Coombs' serum are mixed. Wait for 5 minutes. Centrifuge for 1 min/1500 RPM. Check for agglutination with naked eye or under microscope.

Test can be conducted with fourfold dilution of Coombs' serum (1:4, 1:16, 1:64, 1:256, 1:1024, and 1:4096).

Coombs' test with broad-spectrum antisera is non-specific. It would agglutinate a wide range of proteins, drugs and corresponding antidrug antibodies.

Indications

- Haemolytic disease of the newborn
- Auto-immune haemolytic anaemia
- Haemolytic transfusion reaction (incompatible blood transfusion).

Indirect Coombs' Test

Prepare red cell suspension of a known antigenicity ('O' cells). In a test tube place 2 drops of serum to be tested. To this add 2 drops of 10–20% red cells suspension ('O' blood group cells). Incubate for 30 minutes to 2 hours. If no agglutination, then wash for 3 times. Thereafter follow the steps of direct Coombs' test.

Indications

1. Detection of IgG antibodies to Rh factor (pregnant patients).
2. Detection of auto-antibodies in the serum of patients with auto-immune haemolytic anaemia.

Note: These tests should be conducted with controls.

Sources of errors

1. Red cells need to be washed adequately before adding anti-human globulin serum. Otherwise neutralization of anti-human globulin serum may occur.
2. Adequate incubation period is necessary.

Exercise

13

Normal Blood Picture

Reporting of Normal Blood Picture (Fig. 1.24)

RBCs: Normocytic and normochromic

WBCs: Normal in count and distribution.

Platelets: Adequate and seen in clumps

Note:
1. Normal blood picture does not show variation in size (anisocytosis) and shape (poikilocytosis) of the RBCs.
2. To comment on the RBC size, bring a small lymphocyte in the field and compare with its size. The RBC is called normocytic, if its size is almost same size as that of a small lymphocyte.
3. To label the RBC as normochromic, pallor should be central 1/3. This central pallor is due to biconcave shape of the RBC.
4. Usually one WBC per oil immersion (100 X magnification) is seen when WBC count is within normal limits.
5. Platelets are always seen in clumps in peripheral smear and one clump per oil immersion may be seen when platelet count is within normal limits.

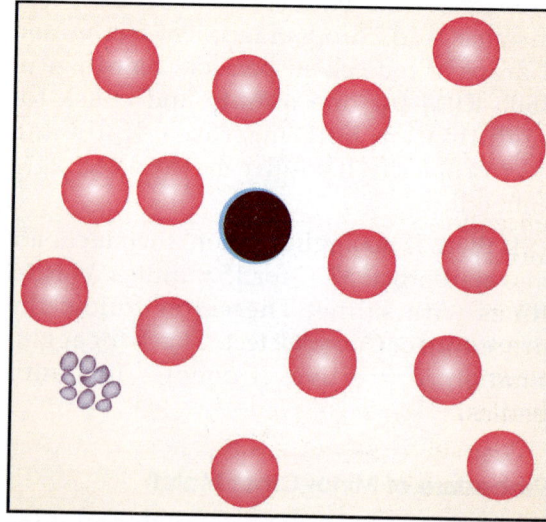

Fig. 1.24: Peripheral smear of normal blood picture (schematic)

Exercise 14

Nutritional Anaemias

IRON DEFICIENCY ANAEMIA

Iron deficiency anaemia occurs due to either reduced intake, decreased intestinal absorption, increased utilization or chronic blood loss. As a result, there is reduction in concentration of Hb in circulating blood below normal for that particular age and sex.

Causes

Major etiological factors for iron deficiency anaemia are:

Females in reproductive life
- Pregnancy—number and frequency
- Miscarriages
- Lactation
- Pathological blood loss
  - Deficient diet
  - Inadequate iron intake.

Adult males and postmenopausal females
- Pathological blood loss—causes are mentioned below.

Infants and children
- Deficient diet/inadequate iron intake (mentioned below)
- Diminished iron stores at birth.

Inadequate iron intake: This is the major cause of iron deficiency anaemia in infants and children. In adults it may occur due to:
- Poor economic status
- Iron content may be lower with vegetarian diet
- Dietary fads or dislikes.

Pathological blood loss
- Menorrhagia
- GI bleeding
  - Peptic ulcer
  - Carcinoma stomach
  - Carcinoma colon
  - Chronic aspirin ingestion/NSAID use
  - Oesophagitis
  - Oesophageal varices
  - Haemorrhoids
  - Hookworm infestation
  - Hiatus hernia
  - Angiodysplasia
  - Diverticulosis
  - Meckel's diverticula
  - Colitis or inflammatory bowel disease
- Bleeding disorder
- Pulmonary lesions with bleeding
- Haemoglobinuria—haemosiderinuria (chronic intravascular haemolysis)
- Haemodialysis
- Haematuria (chronic)
- Frequent blood donation each time 200–250 mg iron/unit-blood is lost.

The reasons for decreased absorption of iron are
- Gastric surgery
- Achlorhydria
- Sprue/coeliac disease
- Pica (non-nutritive substances like clay, chalk, sand, ice, etc.).

Clinical features: Clinical features most commonly occur with long-standing iron deficiency states.

Following are the clinical features
- Pallor, fatigue, weakness, dyspnoea
- Anxiety, irritability, angina, sleepiness, palpitations
- Changes in the tongue-like atrophy of papillae resulting in pale bald tongue
- Changes in the nails—longitudinal ridging, flattening and koilonychia (spoon-shaped nails) or nails that are weak or brittle
- Poor appetite
- Unusual obsessive food cravings, known as pica
- Plummer-Vinson syndrome (Paterson-Brown Kelly syndrome): Dysphagia due to formation of oesophageal webs, iron deficiency anaemia, glossitis, cheilitis and splenomegaly; most commonly seen in postmenopausal females
- Tayanc-Prasad syndrome (growth retardation, hypogonadism, hepatosplenomegaly, zinc and iron deficiency, geophagia).

Approach to a Patient with Iron Deficiency Anaemia

History

Females in reproductive period: Menorrhagia, pregnancies, number and frequency, miscarriages, iron deficient diet, GI blood loss, hematuria, epistaxis, haemoptysis, GI surgery, aspirin ingestion.

Males and postmenopausal females: Iron deficient diet, haematemesis, malaena or pre rectal bleeding (GI blood loss due to hemorrhoids, oesophageal varices, bleeding due to GI malignancies), haematuria, epistaxis, haemoptysis, GI surgery, aspirin ingestion.

Infants and children: Dietary history regarding supplementary feeding, prematurity, multiple births, iron deficiency in mother, GI disturbances, blood loss of any cause.

Physical and systemic examination: Examination any mass, rectal examination, pelvic examination in females, telangiectasias of face and mouth.

Relevant investigations commonly required

Examination of faeces for occult blood and hookworm.

Urine microscopy for haematuria

GI endoscopy or barium swallow study: Peptic ulcer, hiatus hernia, Ca stomach, oesophageal varices, Meckel's diverticulum.

Barium swallow studies in oesophageal varices in a cirrhotic patient show multiple serpiginous filling defects of lower one-third of the oesophagus.

Colonoscopy: Carcinoma colon, caecum, ulcerative colitis, diverticula, angiodysplasia

Sigmoidoscopy: Carcinoma rectum, ulcerative colitis.

Relevant investigations occasionally required

Chest X-ray and bronchoscopy (haemoptysis)

Cystoscopy (haematuria)

Liver function tests (cirrhosis).

Blood Picture, Bone Marrow and Biochemical Findings in Iron Deficiency Anaemia

1. *Complete blood count*
   - Low haemoglobin
   - Low haematocrit
   - Reduced RBC count.
2. *RBC indices*
   - Low MCV
   - Low MCH
   - Low or normal MCHC
   - Increased RDW.
3. *Peripheral smear* (Fig. 1.25)
   - RBCs: RBCs show anisocytosis and poikilocytosis.
   - Majority of the RBCs are microcytic hypochromic, ring/pessary type.
   - Pencil-shaped, target cells, tear drop cells polychromatic cells are present.
   - *WBCs:* Count and distribution normal.
   - *Platelets:* Count and morphology normal.

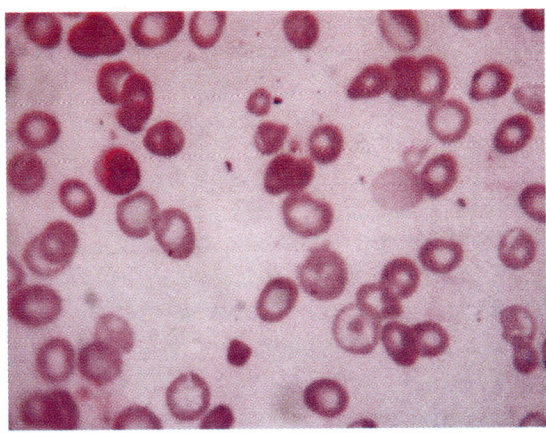

Fig. 1.25: Peripheral smear of microcytic RBCs in microcytic hypochromic anaemia

4. *Bone marrow examination:* Depleted iron stores (Perl's stain)
   - Erythroid hyperplasia
   - Micronormoblastic
   - Cytoplasm lags maturation
   - Granulopoiesis—normal
   - Megakaryopoiesis—normal.
5. *Iron studies*
   - Serum iron: ↓
   - Serum ferritin ↓ in general, values less than 10 µg/L are indicative of iron deficiency
   - TIBC: ↑, TIBC is 1/3 saturated under normal conditions
   - Plasma transferrin
   - *Transferrin saturation:* (Normal 6–33%), <5% definitely indicates iron deficiency
   - *Transferrin receptor:* Free erythrocyte protoporphyrin ↑.

Normal values

Serum iron: Male 27–138 µg/dl, female 33–102 µg/dl

Serum ferritin: Male 29–248 µg/L, female 10–150 µg/L

TIBC: Male 174–351 µg/dl, female 194–372 µg/dl

Plasma transferrin: Male 194–348 µg/dl, female 181–416 µg/dl

Free erythrocyte protoporphyrin: 17–27 µg/dl.

Differential diagnosis for microcytic anaemias (Fig. 1.26)
- Iron deficiency anaemia
- Thalassaemia, HbC, HbE, etc.
- Sideroblastic anaemia
- Lead poisoning
- Anaemia of chronic diseases (sometimes).

Grading of Iron Stores in Bone Marrow[1]

0	No iron granules seen
1+	Small granules in reticulum cells seen only with oil immersion
2+	Few small granules in reticulum cells seen only with low power
3+	Numerous small granules in all cells
4+	Large granules in small clumps
5+	Dense large clumps of granules
6+	Large deposits obscuring marrow picture.

MEGALOBLASTIC ANAEMIAS

Megaloblastic anaemias are macrocytic anaemias characterised by distinctive cytological and functional abnormalities in peripheral blood and bone marrow cells due to impaired DNA synthesis, resulting in erythroid precursors that are enlarged and show failure of nuclear maturation (megaloblasts).

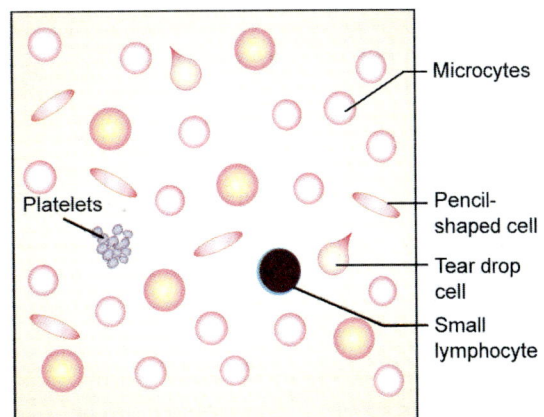

Fig. 1.26: Schematic diagram of microcytic hypochromic anaemia

Etiology: Megaloblastic anaemias result from conditions in which nucleic acid synthesis is abnormal as in:
- Vitamin B_{12} deficiency
- Folic acid deficiency.

Vitamin B_{12} is mainly obtained from foods of animal origin; kidney, heart and liver are richest sources. Lesser amounts are present in muscle meats, fish, eggs, cheese, and milk. Vegetarian diet has no B_{12}. The B_{12} is in the form of adenosylcobalamin and hydroxocobalmin and these are bound to proteins in the food. Folate is present in diet, largely attached to methyl group and is in inactive form. It is distributed in plant and animal tissues. The richest sources are liver, kidney, yeast and green leafy vegetables. Spinach and cabbage have good source of folates. Milk has low folate content (Table 1.1).

Absorption of vitamin B_{12}: When food passes through the stomach, vitamin B_{12} is released from the dietary proteins by the action of acid and proteolytic enzymes.

Vitamin B_{12} first combines with R protein released from the saliva. As this B_{12} and R complex proceeds to small intestine, the R protein is degraded by pancreatic enzymes and B_{12} is released. The B_{12} rapidly combines with the intrinsic factor (IF) secreted by parietal cells of fundus and body of stomach. B_{12} and IF complex as it passes in the ileum which is site of absorption. The B_{12} and IF complex binds to the receptors on the surface of the brush border cells and B_{12} is taken up. B_{12} in the circulation will be bound to transport protein called transcobalamine II. Transcobalamin I acts as storage protein. B_{12} is required for: Conversion of homocysteine to methionine.

Absorption of folate: Folate is absorbed from the duodenum and upper jejunum and to a lesser extent from lower jejunum and ileum. The polyglutamate are cleaved to monoglutamate and undergo further reduction and methylation and circulates in the blood as methyl tetrahydrofolate.

Folate is stored in the liver in polyglutamate form. It is required for
- Methylation of homocysteine to methionine
- Synthesis of thymidine monophosphate from deoxyuridilate monophosphate in DNA synthesis.

Role of Vitamin B_{12} and Folic Acid (Fig. 1.27)

Causes for megaloblastic anaemia due to B_{12} deficiency and folate deficiency are given in Tables 1.2 and 1.3.

Clinical Features

These patients present with general features of anaemia.

Following are the other features
- Glossitis
- Peripheral neuropathy and subacute combined degeneration of spinal cord in B_{12} deficiency anaemia
- Dementia
- Folate deficiency may also cause diarrhoea and glossitis.

Table 1.1: Information about vitamin B_{12} and folic acid

	B_{12}	Folic acid
Availability in diet	Vegetarian: Poor Non-vegetarian—meat: Rich	Vegetarian: Rich Non-vegetarian—meat: Moderate
Effect on cooking	10–30% loss	60–90% loss
Daily requirement in adults	2–4 µg	200 µg
Daily intake in adults	5–30 µg	100–500 µg
Absorption site	Ileum	Duodenum and jejunum
Body stores	2–5 mg	5–20 mg

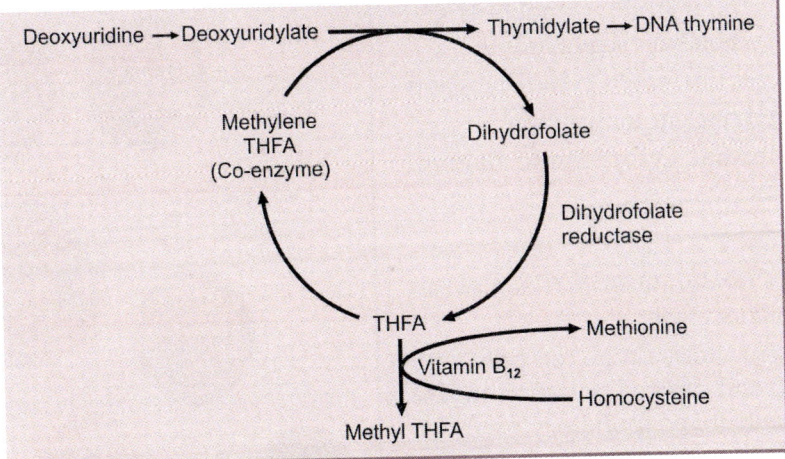

Fig. 1.27: Role of vitamin B_{12} and folate in DNA synthesis

Table 1.2: Causes of megaloblastic anaemia due to vitamin B_{12} deficiency

Mechanism	Disorder
Decreased intake	Nutritional deficiency
Impaired absorption	Gastric causes
	Pernicious anaemia
	Gastrectomy—total or partial
Intestinal causes	Lesions of small intestine
	Coeliac disease
	Tropical sprue
	Fish tapeworm infestation
	Bacterial overgrowth (blind loop syndrome)
	Surgical resection of Ileum

Table 1.3: Causes of megaloblastic anaemia due to folate deficiency

Mechanism	Disorder
Decreased intake	Nutritional deficiency
Impaired absorption	Lesions of small intestine
	Coeliac disease
	Tropical sprue
Increased demand	Pregnancy, puerperium, haemolytic anaemia, sideroblastic anaemia, MPDs, leukemias and lymphomas, carcinoma hyperthyroidism
Drugs	Anti-folate drugs (anti-epileptics), DHA reductase drugs (Methotrexate), alcohol

Pathology

Red cell changes

- Hb is moderately to markedly reduced, in the range of 5–10 g/dl, may go down as below as 2–3 g/dl
- PCV is reduced
- MCV >100 fl
- MCH is increased
- MCHC is normal
- Reticulocyte count is normal or slightly increased (2–3%).
- Erythropoiesis changes from normoblastic to megaloblastic.

Megaloblasts differ from normoblasts and show nuclear-cytoplasmic asynchrony.
- They are larger (increased cytoplasm) and
- Show delayed nuclear maturation
- But have normal cytoplasmic haemoglobinization.

Peripheral smear (Fig. 1.28)

RBCs: There is moderate to marked anisocytosis and poikilocytosis.

There is macrocytosis (large red cells with elevated MCV) and marked variation in size (anisocytosis) and shape (poikilocytosis)
- Oval forms (macro-ovalocytes) are prominent
- Evidence of dyserythropoiesis
  - Basophilic stippling
  - Cabot ring, Howell-Jolly bodies.

Megaloblastic anaemias are therefore macrocytic anaemias if morphologic classification is used.

Few nucleated RBCs with megaloblastic change may be seen.

Changes in white blood cells: Neutrophils show hypersegmented nuclei, with many cells showing more than 5 nuclear lobes.

Platelets: Normal or reduced.

Pancytopenia is seen in 10–20% cases of megaloblastic anaemias.

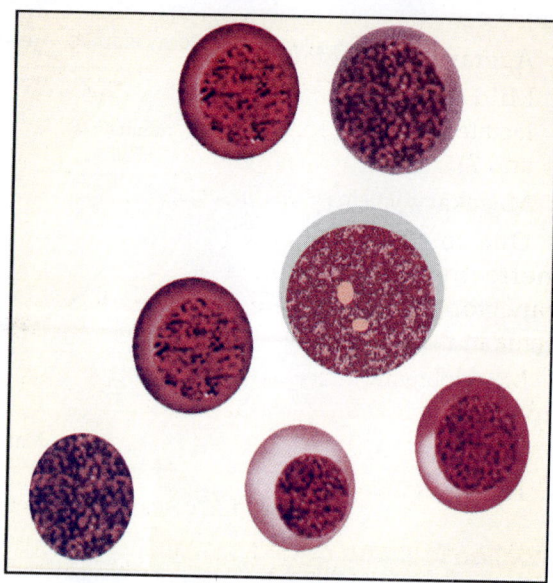

Fig. 1.29: Bone marrow in megaloblastic anaemia: Megaloblasts and other erythroid series cells with nuclei showing open chromatin

Bone Marrow Changes (Fig. 1.29)

Megaloblastic marrow
- These are large cells compared to normal nucleated erythroid precursors
- The nucleus has open-sieve like chromatin
- There is evidence of dyserythropoiesis
- Nuclear maturation lags behind the cytoplasmic maturation
- Late normoblasts have open chromatin
- Giant metamyelocytes are present
- Mitosis increased
- Marrow is hypercellular
- M:E ratio increased (1:1 or 2:1)
- Megakaryocytes may be reduced
- In pure megaloblastic anaemia iron stores may be increased.

Delayed maturation leads to accumulation of erythrocyte precursor cells. The bone marrow is hypercellular and contains large numbers of megaloblasts; as a result of intramedullary haemolysis or ineffective erythropoiesis, many megaloblasts undergo destruction in the bone marrow before maturation and this:

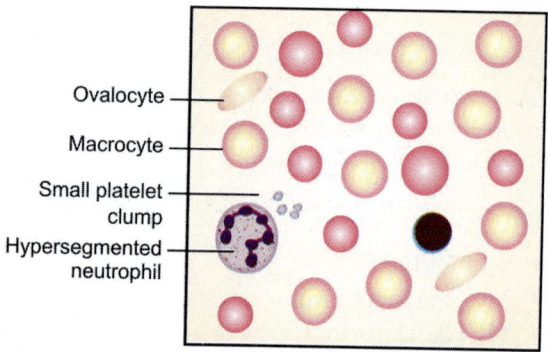

Fig. 1.28: Peripheral smear in megaloblastic anaemia to show macrocytes and hypersegmented neutrophil

Haematology

- Aggravates anaemia with
- Mild elevation of serum bilirubin and lactate dehydrogenase (LDH isoenzymes 1 and 2).

Megakaryocytic series are also affected.

Due to affection of all the series and ineffective erythropoiesis there may be pancytopenia, leukopenia or thrombocytopenia in these patients.

Megaloblastic anaemia should be suspected upon finding in the peripheral blood:
- Macrocytic anaemia with
- Hypersegmented neutrophils.

Biochemical and other Investigations

Serum B_{12} levels decreased in B_{12} deficiency anaemia.

Serum level and urinary excretion of methyl malonic acid are increased in B_{12} deficiency.

Homocysteine levels increased in both B_{12} and folic acid deficiency

Serum bilirubin increased in both B_{12} and folic acid deficiency.

Serum LDH is increased in both B_{12} and folic acid deficiency.

Serum ferritin levels are increased in both B_{12} and folic acid deficiency.

Normal values

Serum cobalamin levels—200–900 ng/L, <100 ng/L in megaloblastic anaemia due to vitamin B_{12} deficiency

Serum methyl malonic acid > 0.4 µmol/L

Serum folate levels up to 5.0 µg/L, < 3 µg/L in megaloblastic anaemia due to folate deficiency

Homocysteine levels—males 14–15 µmol/L, females—12–14 µmol/L

Red cell folate levels >160 µg/L.

Schilling Test in B_{12} Deficiency

1st step

Radioactive (RA) B_{12} (58 Co-B_{12}) is given orally.

Immediately 1,000 µg of non-RA B_{12} is given by IM to saturate B_{12} binding proteins.

Urine is collected for 24 hours

In normal health more than 10% of RA B_{12} is excreted in urine.

2nd step

If this is abnormal, the test is repeated with IF.

Interpretation: If the test turns normal with IF, the diagnosis of pernicious anaemia is made or IF deficiency may be because of gastrectomy.

If still abnormal it is because of Ileal pathology or blind loop syndrome.

Microbiological Assay

Two microorganisms *Euglena gracilis* and *Lactobacillus leichmani* are B_{12} dependent organisms and B_{12} in the serum is determined by comparing the growth of the organisms.

Deoxyuridine Suppression Test

Serum folate levels are decreased in folate deficiency anaemia.

Red cell folate levels—decreased

FIGLU an intermediate product in conversion of histidine to glutamate and is excreted in urine in folate deficiency.

Microbiological Assay

The folate activity can be assessed by methyl tetrahydrofolate; this compound is microbiologically active for *Lactobacillus casei* which is used for assay.

Diagnosis of Megaloblastic Anaemias

- Oval macrocytes in peripheral smear
- Hypersegmented neutrophils
- Megaloblastic hypercellular marrow
- Response to B_{12}/folate therapy.

Other Causes of Macrocytic Anaemia

- Alcoholism
- Hepatic causes
- Hypothyroidism
- Increased retic count—haemolysis
- Drugs.

Exercise 15

Haemolytic Anaemias and Tests Related to Haemolytic Anaemias

General Aspects

Haemolytic anaemia results from premature destruction of erythrocytes. The normal red cell lifespan is 120 days. In haemolytic anaemia the lifespan of RBCs is shortened by varying degrees and in many cases they survive only for a few days.

Patient may not always be anaemic because of bone marrow compensation.

Anaemia in haemolytic anaemia develops due to:
- Reduced lifespan
- Aplastic crises
- Haemolytic crises.

Clinical Features

- Pallor
- Intermittent jaundice
- Splenomegaly
- Gallstones—in chronic forms
- Crisis—aplastic, haemolytic
- Ankle ulcers.

Classification of Haemolytic Anaemia (HA)

HA due to intrinsic (intracorpuscular) abnormalities

Congenital
- Membrane abnormalities
  - Membrane skeleton proteins: Spherocytosis, elliptocytosis
  - Membrane lipids: Abetalipoproteinemia
- Disorders of haemoglobin synthesis
  - Deficient globin synthesis: Thalassaemia syndromes
  - Structurally abnormal globin synthesis (haemoglobinopathies): Sickle cell anaemia, unstable haemoglobins
  - Double heterozygous disorders: Sickle cell beta thalassaemia
- Enzyme deficiencies
  - Glycolytic enzymes: Pyruvate kinase, hexokinase, enzymes of hexose monophosphate shunt: Glucose-6-phosphate dehydrogenase, glutathione synthetase.

Acquired
Membrane defect: Paroxysmal nocturnal haemoglobinuria

HA due to extracorpuscular abnormalities

Acquired
- Immune mechanisms
  - Antibody mediated—warm antibodies/cold antibodies
  - Transfusion reactions: Incompatible blood transfusion
  - Erythroblastosis fetalis (Rh disease of the newborn)
  - Autoantibodies: Idiopathic (primary), drug-associated, systemic lupus erythematosus
- Non-immune mechanisms
- Mechanical trauma to red cells

Microangiopathic haemolytic anaemias: Thrombotic thrombocytopenic purpura, disseminated intravascular coagulation

- Miscellaneous causes
  - Infections: Malaria
  - Burns
  - Lead poisoning.

While investigating a case of haemolytic anaemia following questions needs to be answered
1. Is the anaemia of haemolytic nature?
2. If haemolytic anaemia is present, what is the site of destruction? Intravascular or extravascular?
3. What is the aetiology?

The haemolytic nature is determined by
1. Increased destruction of red cells with haemoglobin breakdown.
2. Bone marrow regeneration.

Site of destruction is determined by
In intravascular destruction, there is release of free haemoglobin due to destruction of RBCs in the circulation.

In extravascular haemolysis, there will be removal of senescent RBCs from reticuloendothelial cells (Fig. 1.30). Haemoglobin is released and catabolised within the macrophages. Indirect bilirubin may be increased but free haemoglobin is not detected in the plasma.

The aetiology is established by
- Clinical features
- Special investigations.

General Aspects

Age: Neonatal period H/O hyperbilirubinaemia
- Isoimmunisation
- Congenital haemolytic anaemia (HS, G6PD deficiency)
- Congenital infection.

3–6 months period H/O hyperbilirubinaemia
- Congenital disorder of haemoglobin synthesis
- Defects in haemoglobin structure.

Gender: X-linked disorders—G6PD deficiency, PK deficiency.

Race
Haemoglobin S and C—blacks
β-thalassaemias—whites
α-thalassaemias—black and yellow races.

Ethnicity
Thalassaemias—Mediterranean origin
G6PD deficiency—Jews, Greeks, Filipinos.

Infection
Infection induced HA (usually non-immune—malaria, babesiosis, *C. perfringens*).

Inheritance
Family history of anaemia, jaundice, gallstones, splenomegaly.

General Physical Examination

Skin: Jaundice, petechiae, purpura
Cavernous haemangioma, pregnancy (HELLP syndrome—haemolysis, elevated liver enzymes and low platelet count), microangiopathic HA.

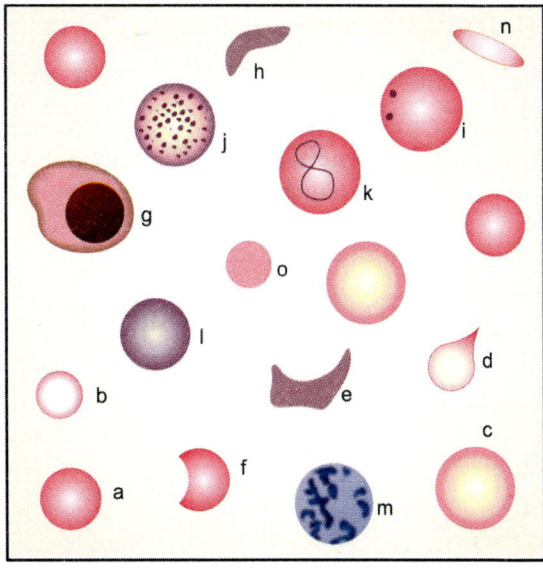

Fig. 1.30: Various red blood cells (poikilocytes): (a) Normal RBC, (b) microcyte, (c) macrocyte, (d) tear drop cell, (e) schistocyte, (f) bite cell, (g) nucleated RBC, (h) sickle cell, (i) Howell-Jolly body, (j) basophilic stipling, (k) Cabot ring, (l) polychromatophilic cell, (m) reticulocyte, (n) pencil-shaped cell, (o) spherocyte

Ulcers on lower limbs: S and C haemoglobinopathies, thalassaemias, sickle cell anaemia.

Facies and bones: Frontal bossing, prominence of molar and maxillary bones, thinning of cortical bone, spontaneous fractures, hand-foot syndrome.

Extra-medullary haematopoiesis
Eyes
Tortuosity of conjunctival and retinal vessels: HbS and HbC.

Microaneurysm of retinal vessels: S and C haemoglobinopathies.

Cataracts: G6PD deficiency, galactosaemia with HA in newborns.

Vitreous haemorrhage: S haemoglobinopathy.

Spleen and liver: Enlargement seen in most HAs.

Gallbladder: Stones (chronic hemolysis, congenital haemolytic anaemias).

LABORATORY EVIDENCE OF HAEMOLYSIS IN HAEMOLYTIC ANAEMIA

Thalassaemia

Thalassaemia was first recognised by Thomas B. Cooley. It is originally described in Italians, Greeks, and people of Mediterranean region. It also occurs in people of Middle East countries, South-East Asia and India.

It is a genetically determined disorder with autosomal dominant inheritance. There will be reduction in the rate of synthesis of normal haemoglobin polypeptide chains. Thus, there is less amount of adult haemoglobin (HbA) (Table 1.4).

Classification

Normally α and β chains are produced under separate genetic control and in normal state the synthesis is balanced.

There are two main groups of thalassaemia, one affecting synthesis of alpha chains is α thalassaemia and the other affecting beta chains is β thalassaemia.

Pathogenesis

In β thalassaemia there is less amount of HbA. There is production of gamma and delta chains, thus there is increased production of HbF and HbA2.

Due to lack of β chains the α chains accumulate, aggregate and interfere in erythroid cell maturation and function, resulting in premature destruction of RBCs.

In α thalassaemia the levels of HbA, HbF and HbA2 are reduced. The beta and gamma chains accumulate and form HbH (β4) and Hb Bart (γ4).

α thalassaemia and β thalassaemia are inherited co-dominantly and have homozygous and heterozygous states.

Clinical Features

Occurs in two forms: β thalassaemia major and β thalassaemia minor.

β thalassaemia major also called Cooley's anaemia is usually a severe illness characterized by total suppression of β chains. β thalassaemia minor or trait is mild form (Fig. 1.31).

If the severity falls in between the two, it is thalassaemia intermedia. These do not require transfusions or may require sporadically.

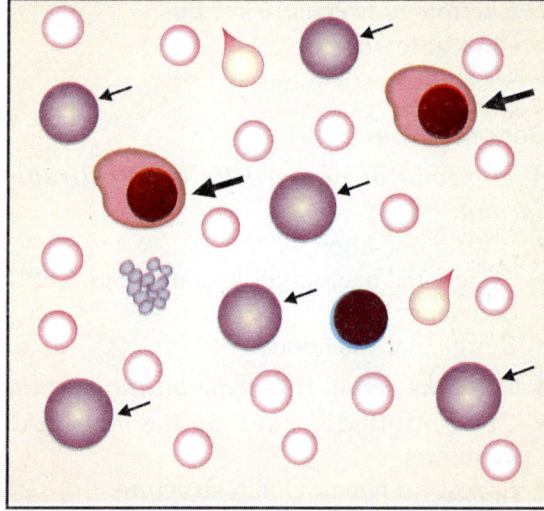

Fig. 1.31: Peripheral smear in thalassaemia major (thick arrow—nucleated RBCs, thin arrow—polychromatophilic cells)

Table 1.4: To show evidences for haemolysis

Evidence for increased red cell destruction
- Jaundice and hyperbilirubinaemia
- Reduced plasma haptoglobin (<250 mg/L) and haemopexin
- Increased plasma LDH (up to 800 IU/L) (N = 207 IU/L)
- Evidences of intravascular haemolysis
  - Haemoglobinaemia
  - Haemoglobinuria
  - Methaemoglobinaemia/methalbuminaemia
  - Increased urine and faecal urobilinogen
  - Decreased glycosylated haemoglobin
- Evidences of extravascular haemolysis
  - Positive Coombs' test
  - Splenomegaly

Evidence for compensatory erythroid hyperplasia

Peripheral smear
- Reduced haemoglobin
- Elevated reticulocyte count—marked polychromasia
- Nucleated RBCs

Bone marrow
- Erythroid hyperplasia
- Reduced M/E ratio

Radiological changes
- Deforming changes in the skull and long bones—frontal bossing

Evidences of red cell damage
- Spherocytosis—HS, immune HA
- Increased red cell fragility
- Fragmented RBCs
- Schistocytes—mechanical damage
- Heinz bodies, bite/blister cells
- Compensated erythroid hyperplasia
- *Compensated haemolytic state:* A state of haemolysis in which the resulting increased erythrocyte production is able to keep up with accelerated RBC destruction, thus preventing development of anaemia.
- Reticulocytosis
- Macrocytosis/polychromasia
- Nucleated RBCs in peripheral blood
- Leukocytosis
- Normoblastic erythroid hyperplasia—bone marrow

Reduced red cell lifespan
Measurement of red cell survival no longer routinely done—Cr 51 (N $T_{1/2}$ = 25–35 days)

Thalassaemia major manifests by first year of life. The anaemia is insidious. With regular blood transfusions the child can have normal growth and development.

Inadequately Transfused Child
- Retarded growth and development
- Anaemia—weakness, lethargy, fever, appetite

- Changes in the skeletal system with mongoloid facies with thinning of cortical bone and pathological fractures
- Osteoporosis
- Extramedullary haemopoiesis can form masses and can compress the spinal cord
- Brown pigmentation of skin
- Hepatosplenomegaly
- Infections (functional hyposplenism), pericarditis due to streptococcal infection
- Gallstones
- Bleeding tendencies
- Secondary leukopenia and thrombocytopenia
- Cardiac failure
- Recent years numerous reports of thrombotic complications—possibly procoagulant phospholipids are exposed on RBCs and platelets and haemostatic system is activated. Also endothelial injury and iron overload are possible pathological mechanisms.

The consequences of repeated transfusions like iron accumulation in liver, heart, pancreas, etc., haemochromatosis with organ dysfunction can develop and death is usually by 2–3 decades. Pancreatic haemosiderosis can lead to diabetes and cirrhosis develops with deposition of iron in liver. Cardiac haemosiderosis leads to arrhythmias, heart block and chronic congestive heart failure.

Bone Changes

- Hyperplastic marrow
- Frontal bossing, maxillary hypertrophy
- Hair-on-end appearance of skull on X-ray.

Lab Findings

Peripheral smear (Fig. 1.31)
- Microcytic hypochromic anaemia (Hb of 3–9 g/dl), anaemia is severe
- Anisopoikilocytosis
- Nucleated RBCs
- Polychromasia (reticulocytes increased)
- Schistocytes, dacrocytes, ovalocytes, target cells
- Basophilic stippling.

Other findings
- Decreased MCV, MCH, MCHC, PCV
- Decreased osmotic fragility
- Increased serum uric acid
- Normal free RBC protoporphyrin.

Bone Marrow

- Normoblastic erythroid hyperplasia
- Increased macrophages
- Inclusion bodies in normoblast—methyl violet
- Prussian blue stain—abundance of iron.

Lab Findings-Hb Electrophoresis

The following procedures can be done.
- Citrate agar electrophoresis at alkaline or acid pH
- Capillary electrophoresis
- Automated high performance liquid chromatography
- Isoelectric focussing
- Globin chain electrophoresis

This is done to establish which globin chain is affected.
1. α-migrate towards cathode
2. β-migrate towards anode.

Hereditary Spherocytosis (HS)

- Autosomal dominant
- Primary membrane skeletal disorder of vertical protein interaction
- Defective or absent spectrin molecule, protein 4.2, ankyrin and band-3 protein
- HS—most commonly deficient spectrin and ankyrin
- Membrane instability—membrane loss.

Laboratory Findings

- Moderate/mild/no anaemia
- Reticulocytosis (5–20%)
- Nucleated RBCs

- The peripheral blood smear shows characteristic micro-spherocytes, which appear small, dark, round with no central pallor and decreased diameter
- Polychromasia
- Normal/decreased MCV
- Increased MCHC—hyperhaemoglobin
- Hyperbilirubinaemia
- Negative antiglobulin test
- Increased osmotic fragility
- Mild cases with incubation, OF increased. Defibrinated blood to be used for this test. Blood incubated for 24 hours at 37°C. Normal RBCs also show increased fragility on incubation due to swelling. HS cells lose membranes more readily than normal RBCs when incubated. This test has increased sensitivity and is the most reliable diagnostic test for HS
- Autohaemolysis
- Cryohaemolysis.

RETICULOCYTE COUNT (Fig. 1.32)

This count is one of the important investigations in diagnostic haematology. It must be remembered that the reticulocytes are juvenile red cells (Fig. 1.32). They contain remains of ribosomes and ribonucleic acids which are present in large amounts in nucleated precursors. Ribosomes and RNA material react with certain dyes such as brilliant cresyl blue and new methylene blue to form a blue precipitate of granules or filaments. This reaction takes place in supravital stains. In Romanowsky stained smears the reticulocytes take up diffusely basophilic tint. Most immature reticulocytes have the largest amount of granules and filaments, whereas less immature cells have least granules and filaments.

The number of reticulocytes reflects the erythropoietic activity. After the cells have been released from the bone marrow, within one day they mature into RBCs. In some cases increased erythopoietin stimuli results in premature release of reticulocytes with longer time of maturation in circulation. In such cases reticulocyte maturation time and corrected reticulocyte count are to be deduced by using plasma iron turnover data.

Technique of Reticulocyte Count

1% brilliant cresyl blue

Brilliant cresyl blue	1.0 g
Sodium chloride	0.7 g
Sodium citrate	0.6 g
Distilled water	100 ml

New methylene blue can also be used instead of brilliant cresyl blue. New methylene blue stains reticulum filaments more deeply and more uniformly than the brilliant cresyl blue. New methylene blue is different from methylene blue; the latter is a poor reticulocyte stain.

Normal range

Adults and children	0.2 to 2.0%
Infants	2 to 6%

Note: Reticulocyte should be differentiated from
1. Pappenheimer bodies which are usually single and less commonly multiple.
2. HbH undergoes denaturation with brilliant cresyl blue or even with new methylene blue.

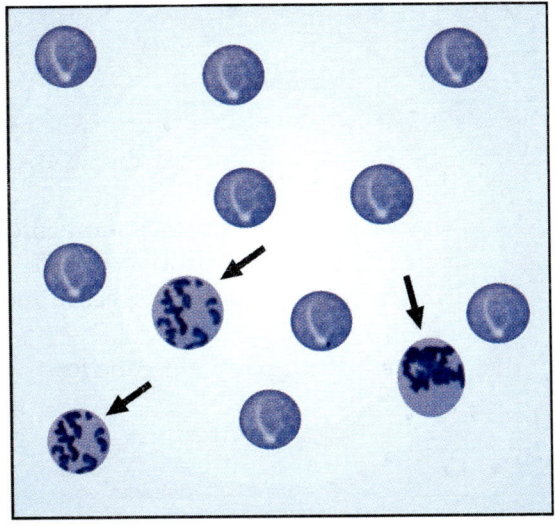

Fig 1.32: Reticulocytes (arrows)

3. Heinz bodies are stained lighter than reticulocytes with new methylene blue stain.

Reticulocytes also can be counted employing fluorescent microscopy. In that case, one volume of acridine orange to one volume of blood is mixed for 2 minutes, and then make smears and observe under fluorescent microscopy.

Procedure for demonstration of reticulocytes
2–3 drops of new methylene blue and equal drops of blood are added to 75 × 10 mm glass or plastic tube. After mixing well keep at 37°C in a incubator for 15–20 minutes. Mix well again before preparing smears; smears should be well spread and the cells should be well stained. Interpret under oil immersion.

Counting of Reticulocytes

Adjustable diaphragms, paper or cardboard diaphragms could be used for counting the reticulocytes. In paper or cardboard diaphragms circle/square is cut and inserted in the eyepiece. RBCs counted with this diaphragm should be roughly 50. Such 20 fields are observed, so that roughly 1000 RBCs are inspected. In all these 20 fields, the reticulocytes ('n' cells) are counted.

Calculation
In 1000 RBCs = 'n' reticulocytes
For 100 RBCs = 100 × n/1000

The result is expressed in percentage.

Example: In 20 fields (1000 RBCs) 20 reticulocytes are counted.

Hence reticulocytes count is: (100 × 20)/1000 = 2%.

Corrected Reticulocyte Count

Counting of circulating reticulocytes is the simplest and very reliable sign of accelerated erythrocyte production.

The percentage of reticulocytes can increase either because there are more reticulocytes in the circulation or because there are fewer mature cells. In anaemias, however some prefer to correct the reticulocyte count by multiplying the percentage of reticulocytes by patient's haematocrit and then dividing the result by normal haematocrit.

Corrected reticulocyte count = Reticulocyte percentage × Patient's haematocrit/0.45

However corrected counts are not the perfect indices of production, as the percentage of reticulocytes could be altered by premature release from the marrow (shift). A reticulocyte production index (RPI) has been proposed to correct this shift.

RPI = Corrected reticulocyte count/2 (maturation time correction)

SICKLING PHENOMENON (Fig. 1.33)

This test detects the presence of HbS; because of the decreased solubility of the abnormal haemoglobin at low oxygen tension.

Methods: The two methods followed are as under.
1. Mix equal volume of blood and freshly prepared 2% sodium metabisulphite (0.2 g in 10 ml distilled water) on a slide. Place a cover slip. Seal the coverslip edges with vaseline or paraffin wax. Inspect for the resulting sickling under low power.

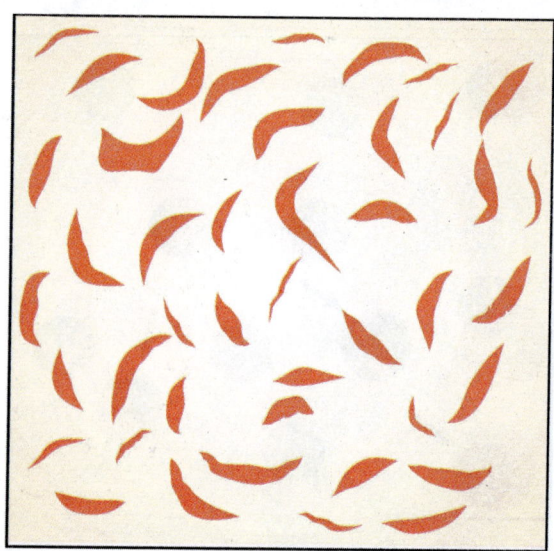

Fig 1.33: Schematic diagram of sickling

2. Two volumes of 0.114 M-sodium dithionite ($Na_2S_2O_4$) is mixed with three volumes of 0.114 M-disodium hydrogen phosphate (Na_2HPO_4) to give a final pH of 6.8. Sodium dithionite solution freshly prepared should be added to disodium hydrogen phosphate just before use. About 50 μl of the reagent is mixed with 10 μl of blood, then seal the sides of the coverslip and observed for sickling.

Sickling is visible immediately in HbS disease and within about 60 minutes in HbS trait. If this test is positive, then haemoglobin electrophoresis should be undertaken.

FOETAL HAEMOGLOBIN

1. Alkali Haematin Method

i. Take 10 drops of patient's blood and also the control blood in separate test tubes.
ii. Saline wash (2–3 changes) both of them.
iii. Add one and a half times (15 drops) of distilled water to the above, this is haemolysate.
iv. Add 1 ml of chloroform, mix well and centrifuge.
v. Take 3.2 ml of N/12 NaOH in a big test tube and 6.8 ml of precipitant reagent, i.e. 50% saturated ammonium sulphate in a small test tube.

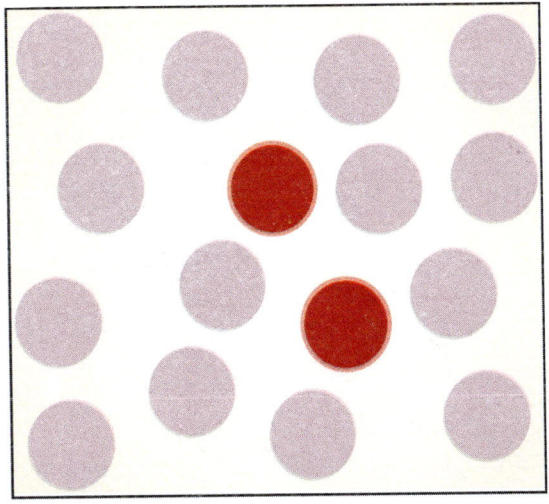

Fig. 1.34: Schematic diagram of cells with foetal Hb and normal cells as ghost cells

vi. Add 0.2 ml of haemolysate to 3.2 ml of NaOH; mix for 1 minute.
vii. After 1 minute add 6.8 ml of ammonium sulphate reagent to the above; mix by inverting.
viii. Filter, the filtrate contains undenatured HbF.
ix. Follow the same procedure for control.
x. For positive control, cord blood is used.

Interpretation

- Colourless—negative
- Pink colour—positive.

Note: KOH also can be used instead of NaOH
Acidified ammonium sulphate also can be used.

2. Acid Elution Method (Fig. 1.34)

Kleihaur, Braun and Betke in 1957 introduced this method. This method detects HbF containing cells; and their detection in maternal circulation has provided valuable information on the pathogenesis of haemolytic disease of the newborn. It must be noted that the HbF containing cells resist acid elution better than the normal cells. They appear as darkly staining cells amongst pale staining ghost cells. Occasional cells (reticulocytes) stain to an intermediate degree and are less easy to evaluate.

Fixative: 80% ethanol

Elution Solution

Solution A: 7.5 g/L haematoxylin in 96% ethanol.

Solution B: $FeCl_3$ 24 g, 25% HCl—20 ml, double distilled water to make 1 L.

For use, five volumes of solution A and one volume of solution B are mixed well. The pH is approximately 1.5. Once prepared the solution can be used for 4 weeks. If precipitate occurs, it should be filtered.

Counter stain: 1 g/L aqueous erythrocin or 25 g/L aqueous eosin.

Procedure

Air dry the smear, fix in 80% ethanol for 5 minutes in a coplin jar rapidly.

Then it should be rinsed in water and dried for 10 minutes. The slide is placed for 20 seconds in a coplin jar containing elution solution. Then the slide is washed thoroughly in water, placed for 2 minutes in eosin or erythrocin solution. Lastly, the slide is rinsed in tap water and dried.

Results: Cells with HbF—red, cells with HbA—pale pink (ghost cells)

OSMOTIC FRAGILITY (OF) (Fig. 1.35)

The rate of haemolysis is determined by the structure of the red cells. If the red cells are placed in 0.85% salt solution, the water neither enters nor leaves the cells. At lower concentrations of salt, the water enters the cells, eventually swells, ruptures and haemolyse the cells. When the rate of haemolysis is increased; the fragility of red cells is said to be increased. Similarly, when the rate of haemolysis is decreased, the fragility of the red cells is said to be decreased.

Methods: Following are the different methods to test for osmotic fragility.

Sanford method: Blood is added to graded series of 12 hypotonic salt solutions; the extent of haemolysis is noted after a period of 2 hours.

Dacie's method: Add heparinised blood to graded series of 12 hypotonic salt solutions buffered to pH of 7.4 and allow them to stand for 30 minutes. Centrifuge, read the degree of haemolysis spectrophotometrically and plot the percentage of haemolysis, against the percentage of salt concentrate.

Fragiligraph method: This method employs an electronic instrument.

Incubation method: In this method fibrinogen is removed; then incubate the defibrinated blood at 37°C for 24 hours, then follow the procedure of Dacie method.

OF increased
- Spherocytosis
- Acquired auto-immune haemolytic anaemia
- Erythroblastosis foetalis
- Burns
- Chemical poisons.

OF decreased
- Iron deficiency anaemia
- Thalassaemia major
- Sickle cell anaemia
- Obstructive jaundice
- Polycythemia vera
- Haemoglobin 'C' disease.

One set—test sample

No. of drops of 0.5% sodium chloride	25	24	23	22	21	20	19	18	17	16	15	14
No. of drops of distilled water	0	1	2	3	4	5	6	7	8	9	10	11
% of salt concentration obtained	0.5	0.48	0.46	0.44	0.42	0.4	0.38	0.36	0.34	0.32	0.30	0.28

Example:

	Haemolysis starts (Salt conc.)	Haemolysis completed (Salt conc.)	Inference
Control (normal)	0.44%	0.34%	Normal
Spherocytosis	0.48%	0.40%	OF increased
Sickle cell anaemia and thalassaemia	0.38%	0.30%	OF decreased

Haematology

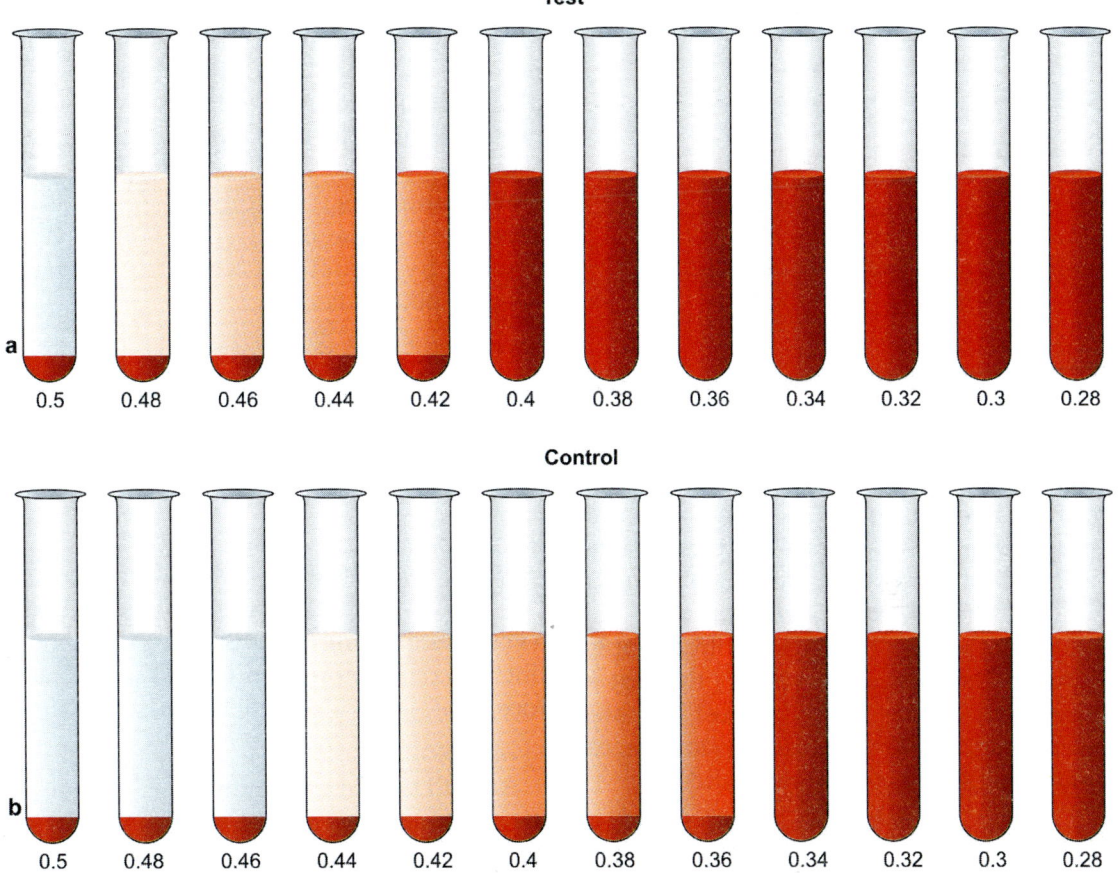

Figs 1.35a and b: Osmotic fragility

Sanford Method (Giffen and Sanford method)

The following reagents and equipment are required:
1. 0.5% sodium chloride
2. Distilled water
3. Two sets of Kahn test tubes: One set for control, and the other set for the test. One set has 12 test tubes in each row.

Procedure

Place one drop of blood in each tube.

Mix and allow to stand at room temperature for 2 hours.

Examine for the initial haemolysis and complete haemolysis.

Record the % of salt solution showing initial haemolysis and complete haemolysis.

Compare the patient's results with the control results.

In control samples the initial haemolysis occurs at 0.44% or 0.42% of saline solution and completed in 0.34% saline solution.

Microcytic hypochromic cells are more resistant to haemolysis when compared to normal RBCs. Screening test for thalassaemia trait.

NESTROF Test (Necked eye single tube red cell osmotic fragility test)[2]

NESTROF test is performed using 0.36% buffered saline solution (Fig. 1.36). 2 ml of the solution is taken in two tubes and one is used for test and other as control. A drop of blood is added to each tube and they are left

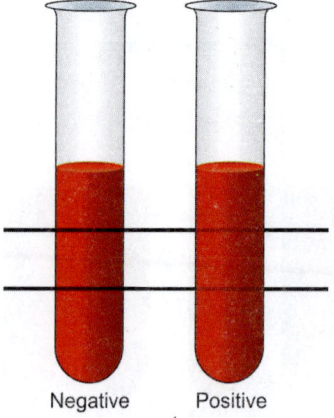

Fig.1.36: NESTROF

undisturbed for half an hour at room temperature. Both the tubes are then shaken and held against a white paper with a black line. The line is clearly visible through the contents of the tube containing control sample. If the line is not clearly visible, the test is considered positive. A positive test indicates lowered red cell osmotic fragility, and useful in detecting thalassaemia trait patients.

HAEMOGLOBIN ELECTROPHORESIS (Fig. 1.37)

1. Cellulose Acetate Electrophoresis at Alkaline pH

For routine work, electrophoresis at pH 8.4–8.6 using cellulose acetate membrane as a substrate is simple, rapid and sensitive.

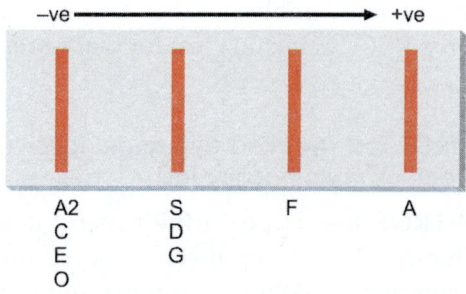

Fig. 1.37: Haemoglobin electrophoresis with separation of various haemoglobins

Principle

Electrophoresis is the movement of charged particles in an electrical field. At an alkaline pH, haemoglobin is a negatively charged protein. Therefore, the haemoglobin migrates towards the anode in an electric field. During electrophoresis, various haemoglobins separate because of differences in charges caused by structural variations of the haemoglobin molecule.

Specimen: EDTA or heparinised blood.

Equipment: Electrophoresis tank with power pack, wicks of filter or chromatography paper, blotting paper, applicators, cellulose acetate membrane, staining equipment, drying oven and pH metre.

Preparation of lysate for immediate use

Lyse one volume of washed red cells in 4 volumes of lysing agent. Such a lysate should not be kept for more than 1–2 days at 4°C as it forms gel.

Lysing agent
- 3.8 g EDTA, tetrasodium salt
- 0.7 g potassium cyanide
- Water to make 1 litre.

Note: There are different methods to prepare the lysate.

Reagents

Electrophoresis buffer: Tris/EDTA/borate (TEB) pH 8.5, Tris (hydroxymethyl) amino-methane 10.2 g, EDTA 0.6 g, boric acid 3.2 g and water to make 1 litre.

The buffer is stored at 4°C and can be used without any deterioration.

Protein stain: Ponceau S 5 g, trichloracetic acid 7.5 g and water to make 1 litre.

Destaining solution: 5% acetic acid—50 ml and water to make 1 litre.

Clearing solution: Glacial acetic acid 125 ml, methanol 375 ml and polyethylene glycol 20 ml.

Method

1. Prepare a lysate, further dilute the sample to 1 : 4 or 1 : 5 in water (to about 20 g/L).

2. Fill the electrophoresis tank with TEB buffer. Soak and position the wicks.
3. In a separate dish, soak the cellulose acetate membrane in TEB buffer for 5 minutes. Immerse the membrane slowly to avoid trapping of air bubbles.
4. Blot the membrane between two pieces of absorbent paper, but do not let it dry.
5. Place small volume (10 µl) of each diluted sample into a sample well.
6. Dip the applicator into the sample.
7. Apply the samples to the cellulose acetate approximately 3 cm from one end of membrane.
8. Place the membrane upside down across the bridge of the tank so that the cellulose acetate surface is in contact with the buffer, with the line of application at the cathode end.
9. Connect the power supply and run at 250–350 V for 20 minutes until a visible separation is obtained.
10. Disconnect the power supply, remove the membrane and stain with ponceau S for 3 to 5 minutes.
11. Remove the membrane, drain and elute the excess stain with three changes of destaining solution for 2 minutes each.
12. Dehydrate in methanol for 2 to 3 minutes.
13. Immerse in clearing solution for 4 to 6 minutes.
14. Dry at 65°C for 4 to 6 minutes.
15. Label and store the membrane in a protective plastic envelope.

Cellulose acetate electrophoresis is useful in the diagnosis of HbS and HbC haemoglobinopathies. It is also used to screen the elevated levels of HbA2 in thalassaemia trait.

Other methods

Citrate agar gel electrophoresis and acid gel method.

Globin chain synthesis rate studies: Peripheral blood incubated with radioactive labelled amino acid, which is then incorporated into the newly synthesised chains, which are separated by chromatography and their relative production is estimated by determining radioactivity.
- Reduced β to α chain ratio <0.25
- Mutation detection—PCR.

HbF estimation—alkali denaturation test

HbF resists alkali denaturation
- Washed RBCs → lysed + 1.2 N NaOH → HbA denatured, HbF resists → add ammonium sulphate → precipitation of HbA → filter → HbF left in filtrate → measure spectrophotometrically
- % HbF = HbF by alkali denaturation total Hb by cyanmethaemoglobin method
- Reference interval for adults is <2%.

Exercise 16

Leukaemias

Leukaemia is the clonal expansion of a single transformed stem cell resulting in accumulation of immature and non-functional haematopoietic cells in the bone marrow and body organs.

Aetiology and Leukaemogenesis

- Activation of proto-oncogene to oncogene—e.g. t(8;14) C-MYC to immunoglobulin, BALL, abnormal cellular proliferation
- Formation of chimeric transcription factor t(15;17) RAR/PML transcription repressors block differentiation—AML
- Formation of fusion protein with enhanced tyrosine kinase activity—t(9;22) BCR/ABL enhanced tyrosine kinase activity
- Inactivation of tumour suppressor gene pathway—RB1 p53.

Leukaemias are broadly classified as acute or chronic depending upon age of onset, course of disease and clinical presentation. Comparison between acute and chronic leukaemia is given in Table 1.5.

ACUTE LEUKAEMIAS

Definition

These are stem cell disorders characterised by malignant neoplastic proliferation of a transformed cell. Classic triad of acute leukaemia is anaemia, infections and bleeding. Two major categories are:
1. Acute myeloid leukaemia (AML) or acute non-lymphoid leukaemia.
2. Acute lymphoblastic leukaemia (ALL).

Presentation

Age: Acute leukaemia may occur at any age. ALL is common during 2–10 years of age.
Symptoms: Fatigue, pallor, fever, weight loss, bone pains.
Signs: Hepatosplenomegaly, lymphadenopathy, anaemia, neutropaenia, thrombocytopaenia

Table 1.5: Comparison of acute and chronic leukaemias

	Acute	Chronic
Age	All ages	Adults
Clinical onset	Sudden	Insidious
Course of disease	Weeks to months	Months to years
Predominant cells	Blasts and few mature forms	Mature forms
Anaemia	Mild to severe	Mild
Thrombocytopaenia	Mild to severe	Mild
WBC count	Variable	Increased

General Laboratory Findings

Peripheral smear: Leukocyte count usually increased but may be normal or decreased. There can be presence of lymphoblasts or myeloblasts in the peripheral blood. Platelets are usually reduced.

Bone marrow: Hypercellular with lymphoblasts or myeloblasts equal to or >20%.

Other Investigations of Leukaemias

- Hyperuricaemia and increased LDH (increased cell turnover)
- Impairment of renal function (leukaemic infiltration)
- CNS—frequent site for extramedullary spread, CSF should be analysed for presence of blasts
- Cytochemistry
- Flow cytometry
- Cytogenetics.

Classification of ALL (FAB classification)

L1: Small, homogenous blasts, scanty cytoplasm, indistinct nucleoli.

L2: Large, heterogeneous blasts, indented nuclei, one or more nucleoli, abundant cytoplasm, minimal cytoplasmic vacuolation.

L3: Large, homogenous blasts, abundant basophilic cytoplasm with prominent cytoplasmic vacuolations (Burkitt).

Acute Myeloid Leukaemia (Figs 1.38a to c)

The defect primarily affects the common myeloid progenitor (CMP) cell.

Myeloblasts in peripheral blood or bone marrow should be >20% (WHO, 2001).

According to the FAB classification of myeloblasts in peripheral blood or bone marrow should be >30% (Table 1.6).

Table 1.6: FAB classification acute myeloid leukaemia

	Morphology		Myeloperoxidase (MPO)	Sudan black B (SBB)
M0	Acute myeloblastic leukaemia (AML): Minimally differentiate	>30% blasts; no granules	–ve	–ve
M1	AML with no maturation	>30% blasts, few granules +/– Auer rods	+ve	+ve
M2	AML with maturation	>30% blasts, granules common, + Auer rods	+ve	+ve
M3	Acute promyelocytic leukaemia	>30% blasts, prominent granules, ++ Auer rods	++	++
M4	Acute myelomonoblastic leukaemia	>30% blasts, >20% monocytes, + Auer rods	+	+
M4eos	Acute myelomonocytic leukaemia with eosinophilia	>30% blasts, >20% monocytes, > 5% abnormal eosinophils, + Auer rods	+	+
M5 a/b	Acute monblastic leukaemia with or without maturation	>30% blasts, >80% monoblasts with or without maturation	+	+
M6	Acute erythroleukaemia	>30% myeloblasts, >50% erythroblasts, + Auer rods	+(myeloblasts)	+(myeloblasts)
M7	Acute megakaryocytic leukaemia	>30% megakaryoblasts, cytoplastic budding +	–	–

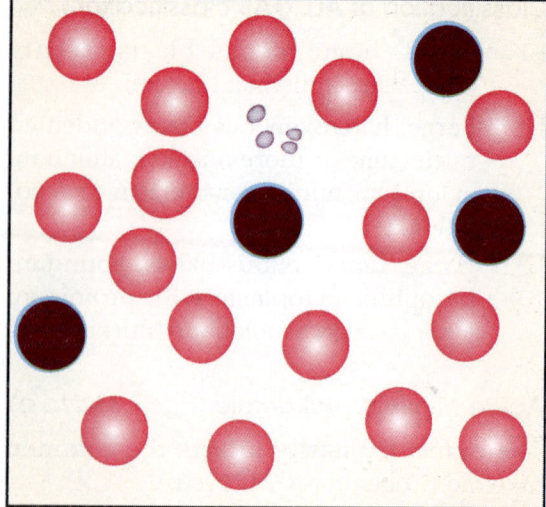

Fig. 1.38a: Peripheral smear in acute leukaemia (ALL—L1)

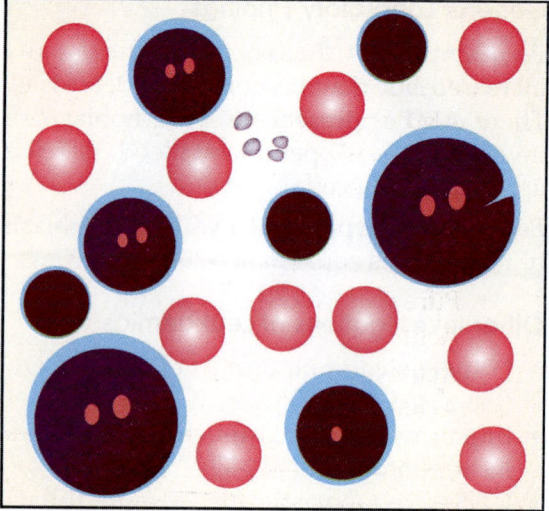

Fig. 1.38b: Peripheral smear in acute leukaemia (ALL—L2)

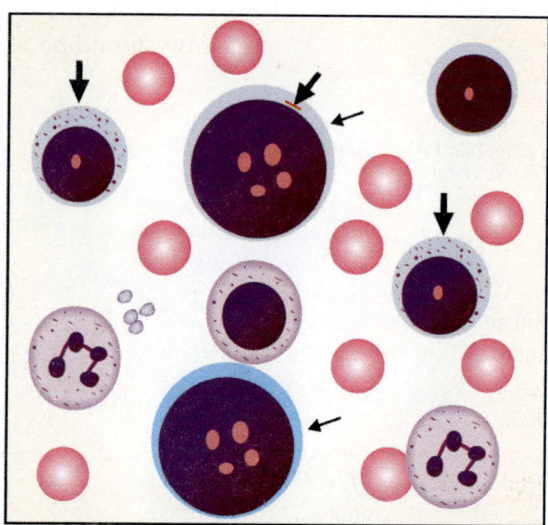

Fig. 1.38c: Peripheral smear in acute leukaemia (AML), note myeloblasts (one myeloblast with Auer rod) and promyelocytes (thin arrow—myeloblast, thick arrow—promyelocyte)

Modified 2016 WHO Classification[3]

I. *AML with Recurrent Genetic Abnormalities*
- AML with t(8;21) (q22;q22); RUNX1-RUNX1T1
- AML with inv(16)(p13;q22) or t(16;16)(p13.q22),CBFB/MYH11
- APML with t(15;17)(q22;12), PML-RARA and variants
- AML with t(9;11)(p22;q23);MLLT3-MLL
- AML with t(6;9)(p23;q34);DEK-NUP214
- AML with inv(3)(q21q26.2); RPN1-EVI1
- AML (megakaryoblastic) with t(1;22)(p13;q13); RBM15-MKL1
- AML with BCR-ABL (Provisional)
- AML with mutated NPM1
- AML with mutated CEBPA
- AML with mutated RUNX1

II. *AML with Myelodysplasia Related Changes*
III. *Therapy Related Myeloid Neoplasms*
IV. *AML-NOS*
- AML with minimal differentiation
- AML without maturation
- AML with maturation
- Acute myelo monocytic leukemia
- Acute monoblastic leukemia
- Pure erythroid leukemia
- Acute megakaryocytic leukemia
- Acute basophilic leukemia
- Acute panmyelosis with myelofibrosis

V. *Myeloid Sarcoma*
VI. *Myeloid Proliferations Related to Down Syndrome*
VII. *Blastic Plasmacytoid Dendritic Cell Neoplasms*
VIII. *Acute Leukemia of Ambiguous Lineage*
IX. *B-Lymphoblastic Leukemia/Lymphoma*
X. *T-Lymphoblastic Leukemia/Lymphoma*

General Laboratory Findings in AML

Peripheral Blood

WBCs:
Total count—elevated, may exceed 1 lakh/cmm.

50% of the cases may have normal or decreased counts at the time of presentation.

Differential count shows presence of myeloblasts (WHO > 20%).

Myeloblast in AML—typically 20 μm in diameter. Nucleus composed of dispersed chromatin and has 3–4 prominent nucleoli. Cytoplasm may show Auer rod.

RBCs: Decreased in number.

Platelets: Reduced, hypogranular and occasional giant platelets may be present.

Buffy coat smear—undertaken if strong suspicion of AML but no blasts in the peripheral smear.

Bone Marrow Examination

It is typically—hypercellular with predominance of blasts (≥20).

FAB group classified neoplastic myeloblasts as:
- Type I—Blasts without any granules
- Type II—Blasts with <20 granules
- Type III—Blasts with numerous granules.

CHRONIC MYELOID LEUKAEMIA (CML)

Definition

It is a clonal stem cell disorder characterised by the acquisition of an oncogenic BCR/ABL fusion protein [usually the result of a reciprocal translocation (9;22)(q34;q11)] and by proliferation of granulocytic elements at all stages of differentiation.

- t(9;22) is also referred to as the Philadelphia chromosome
- Average incidence of CML 45 years
- Men > women.

Three Clinical Phases

- Chronic phase
- Accelerated phase
- Blast crisis

Most patients are diagnosed while still in the chronic phase.

Chronic Phase

- <10% are myeloblasts, platelets tend to be normal or increased in number low to absent.
- Increased percentage of myelocytes
- Low leukocyte alkaline phosphatase activity (low LAP score).
- There is basophilia.

Accelerated Phase

- Myeloblasts—10–19% in PS or BM
- Basophils more than 20%
- Persistent thrombocytopaenia
- Increasing spleen size and counts in spite of therapy
- Cytogenetic evidence clonal evolution.

Blast Phase

- Blasts ≥20%
- Extramedullary blast proliferation
- Large aggregates/clusters of blasts in the bone marrow.

Clinical features indicating a more difficult-to-control marrow proliferative state are suggestive of progression. These include:
- Rapidly rising WBC count that is more refractory to treatment
- Increasing splenomegaly
- Fever, bone pain, and weight loss
- Laboratory features include more immature cells in the peripheral blood or marrow
- Increasing eosinophils or basophils
- The appearance of more chromosome anomalies, including additional Philadelphia chromosomes.

Diagnostic Approach to CML (Figs 1.39a to d)

Peripheral blood smear and marrow biopsy.

Ph+ chromosome by karyotypic analysis or the presence of the BCR-ABL translocation by Southern blot or polymerase chain reaction (PCR) assays confirms the diagnosis.

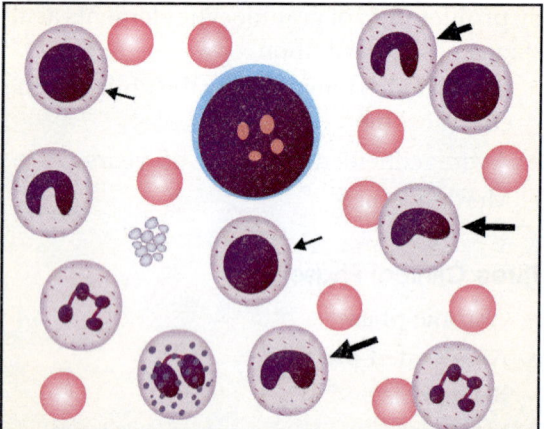

Fig. 1.39a: Schematic diagram of peripheral smear in CML (thin arrow—myelocytes, thick arrow—metamyelocytes, short arrow—band forms)

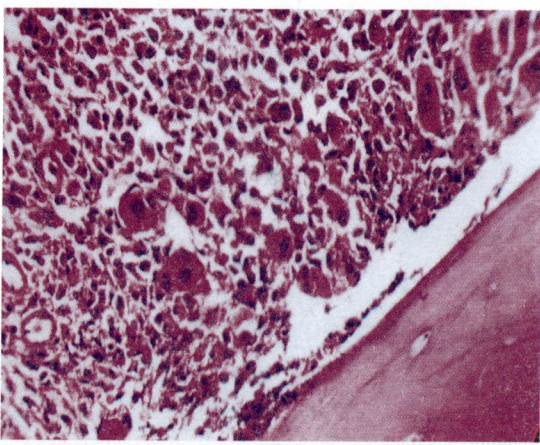

Fig. 1.39c: Trephine biopsy in CML (note plenty of megakaryocytes)

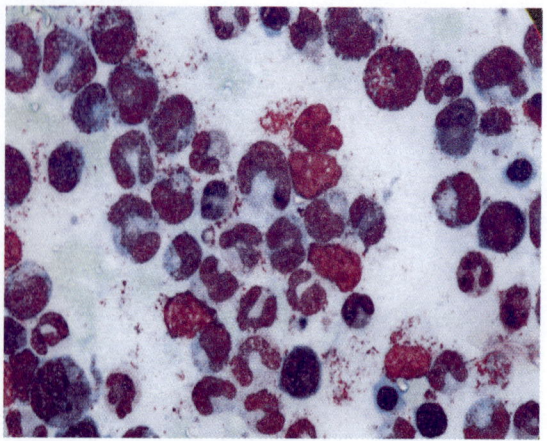

Fig. 1.39b: Bone marrow in CML

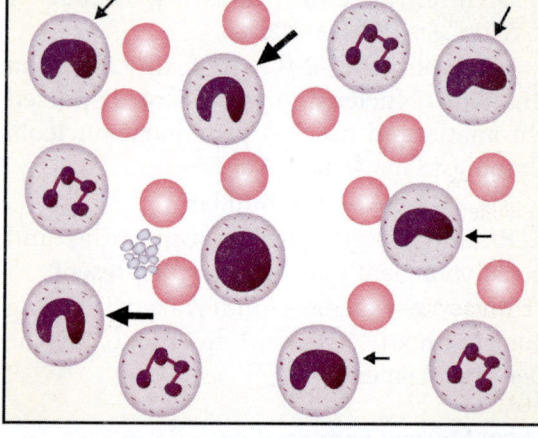

Fig. 1.39d: Schematic diagram, leukaemoid reaction (note metamyelocytes—thin arrow, band forms—thick arrow and increased neutrophils)

Peripheral Blood

1. There is a predominance of mature neutrophils.
2. Basophils are increased in number.
3. Increased percentage of myelocytes (so-called myelocyte bulge).
4. <10% are myeloblast.
5. Many patients may also demonstrate eosinophilia.
6. Platelets tend to be normal or increased in number.
7. Low to absent leukocyte alkaline phosphatase activity (low LAP score).

Differential Diagnosis (WHO 2008 classification of MDS/myeloproliferative diseases)

1. Chronic myelomonocytic leukaemia (CMML)
2. Juvenile myelomonocytic leukaemia (JMML)
3. Atypical CML
4. MDS/myeloproliferative diseases, unclassifiable.

The differences between chronic myeloid leukaemia and leukaemoid reaction are shown in Table 1.7.

CHRONIC LYMPHOCYTIC LEUKAEMIA

Chronic lymphocytic leukaemia (CLL) is characterized by the accumulation of mature-appearing lymphocytes in the blood, marrow, lymph nodes, and spleen.

The CLL cells are monoclonal B lymphocytes that express CD19, CD5, and CD23, with weak or no expression of surface immunoglobulin (Ig), CD20, CD79b, and FMC7.

Clinical Findings

1. CLL occurs in elderly people usually in more than 60 years of age.
2. About 70 to 80% of the patients are diagnosed incidentally.
3. Lymphadenopathy and or splenomegaly may be detected during a routine physical examination.
4. Less frequently, enlarged nodes or the development of infection is the initial complaint.
5. Fever and weight loss are uncommon at presentation but may occur with advanced stage.
6. Enlargement of the cervical and supraclavicular nodes occurs more frequently

Table 1.7: Differences between chronic myeloid leukaemia and leukaemoid reaction

Laboratory parameter	CML	Leukaemoid reaction
Leukocytes	Blasts and promyelocyte in peripheral blood; toxic changes usually absent; eosinophilia and basophilia; neutrophila with single lobed nuclei and hypogranular forms may be present	Toxic granulation; Dohle bodies and vacuoles present; blasts and promyelocytes rare; no absolute basophilia or eosinophilia
Platelets	Often increased with abnormal morphological forms present; occasional micromegakaryocytes	Usually normal
Erythrocytes	Anaemia usually present; variable anisocytosis; poikilocytosis; NRBC present	Anaemia may be present, but NRBC not typical
LAP	Low	Increased
Chromosome karyotype	Ph chromosome or BCR/ABL translocation present	Normal

than axillary or inguinal lymphadenopathy. The lymph nodes are usually discrete, freely movable, and non-tender.
7. Usually mild to moderate enlargement of the spleen is present.
8. Enlarged tonsils and mesenteric or retroperitoneal lymphadenopathy is less common.
9. Anaemia and thrombocytopaenia occur in later stages.
10. CLL patients may present with autoimmune hemolytic anaemia (AIHA).

Prognosis depends upon the stages of Binet and modified Rai clinical staging:
Binet Staging System for CLL

Stage	Description
A	≤2 lymphoid bearing areas enlarged
B	≥3 lymphoid bearing areas enlarged
C	Presence of anaemia (Hb <10 g/dl) or thrombocytopaenia (platelet count <100,000/L).

Five lymphoid bearing areas are cervical, axillary, inguinofemoral, spleen and liver.

Modified Rai Clinical Staging for Chronic Lymphocytic Leukaemia

Risk	Stage	Description
Low	0	Lymphocytosis in blood and bone marrow
Intermediate	I	Lymphocytosis + enlarged lymph nodes
	II	Lymphocytosis + enlarged liver or spleen with or without lymph nodes
High	III	Lymphocytosis + Anaemia (Hb <11 g/dl) with or without enlarged liver, spleen or lymph nodes
	IV	Lymphocytosis + thrombocytopaenia (platelet count <1,00,000/cu mm) with or without anaemia or enlarged liver, spleen or lymph nodes

Peripheral Blood and Bone Marrow (Figs 1.40a and b)

- In most patients, there is increased number of mature lymphocytes in the peripheral blood and bone marrow. These cells have the morphologic appearance of normal

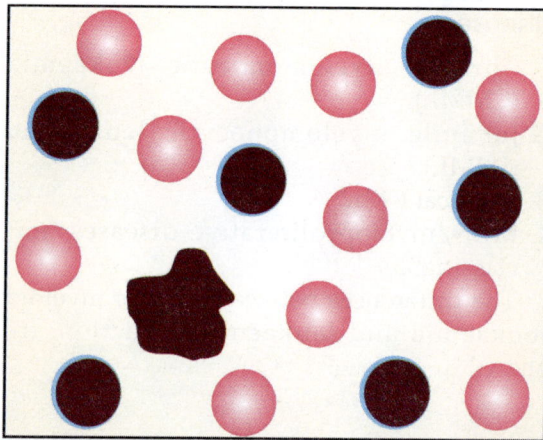

Fig.1.40a: Peripheral smear in CLL. Note increased number of mature lymphocytes and a smudge cell

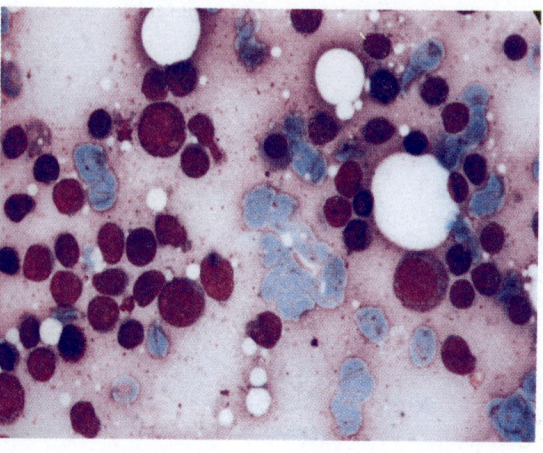

Fig. 1.40b: Bone marrow in CLL

small to medium-sized lymphocytes with clumped chromatin, inconspicuous nucleoli, and scant cytoplasm.
- Smudge cells (basket cells or shadow cells of Gumprecht) are commonly seen in the blood smear.
- In classical CLL, >90% of the cells are mature lymphocytes.

When 11 to 54% of the cells are prolymphocytes, it is termed CLL/PLL.
- If ≥55% of the cells are prolymphocytes, it is termed prolymphocytic leukaemia.

When >15% of the lymphocytes are plasmoid or cleaved and <10% are prolymphocytes, it is termed atypical CLL.

Exercise

17

Multiple Myeloma/Plasma Cell Dyscrasias

Plasma Cell Dyscrasias Constitute the Following:

Malignant proliferation
- Multiple myeloma (MM)
- Waldenström macroglobulinaemia (WM)
- Plasmacytoma
- Heavy chain disease.

Relatively benign
- Monoclonal gammopathy of undetermined significance (MGUS)
- Smoldering MM
- Primary systemic amyloidosis
- POEMS syndrome (polyneuropathy, organomegaly, endocrinopathy, monoclonal gammapathy and skin changes).

Multiple Myeloma

Definition: Multiple myeloma is a malignant disorder characterised by proliferation of a single clone of plasma cells in the bone marrow. There will be lytic lesions of bones, increased monoclonal gammaglobulins and hypercalcemia (Table 1.10).

Etiology: Radiation exposure, exposure to benzene, smoking, alcohol and obesity has increased risk while diet with cruciferous vegetables, fish and vitamin C has reduced risk.

Pathogenesis: IL-6 plays role in proliferation of plasma cells and lytic lesions of bone.

The different diagnostic criteria are given in Tables 1.8 and 1.9.

Table 1.8: International myeloma working group criteria for diagnosis

1. M Protein in serum or urine
2. Clonal bone marrow plasma cells ≥10% or plasmacytoma biopsy proven
3. Myeloma related organ dysfunction—CRAB features
    a. Calcium elevation >11.5 mg%
    b. Renal insufficiency serum creatinine >1.96 mg%
    c. Anaemia <10 g/dl
    d. Bone lesions: Lytic/osteoporosis
4. In the absence of end organ damage, clonal plasma cells ≥60%
5. In updated International myeloma working group, myeloma is considered when CRAB features are present in a patient with smouldering MM.

CRAB features of MM: Calcium (elevated), renal failure, anaemia and bone lesions

Table 1.9: Revised criteria International myeloma working group 2014[4]

In asymptomatic patients following criteria can label the patient as MM:
1. Clonal bone marrow plasma cells ≥60%.
2. Free light chain ratio more than 100.
3. MRI showing more than one focal lesion.

Haematology

Table 1.10: Clinical presentation of multiple myeloma	
Age: Old age (median age 65 years)	Elevated ESR markedly raised often >100 mm/hr
Insidious onset	Hypercalcaemia
Weakness, fatigue	BJ proteins
Pallor	Renal failure
Bone pains	Hyperviscocity: Hypergammaglobulinaemia
Pathological fractures	Amyloidosis
Recurrent infections	Marrow failure

Laboratory Evaluation

- CBC with peripheral smear
- ESR: Increased
- Bone marrow examination (Figs 1.41a and b)
- Chemistry panel (creatinine, Ca^{++}, LDH, 2M)
- Immunofixation electrophoresis
- Serum free light chain (FLC)
- Urinalysis/24 hours urine for protein
- Bence Jones protein
- Immunophenotype, cytogenetics
- Skeletal survey/CT/MRI/PET
- Plasma cell labelling index.

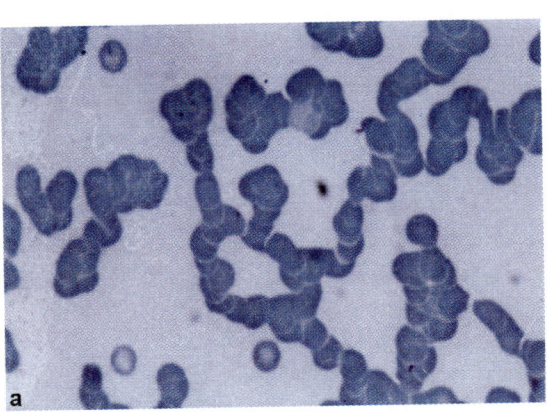 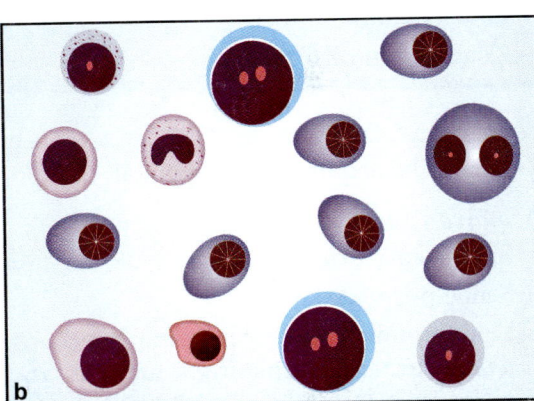

Figs 1.41a and b: (a) Peripheral smear, (b) bone marrow in multiple myeloma

Note: In peripheral smear Rouleaux formation and bone marrow with increased plasma cells.

Exercise 18

Bleeding Disorders

Bleeding disorders or haemorrhagic disorders can be due to any of the following:
- Vascular defects
- Platelet abnormalities
- Coagulation disorders.

VASCULAR CAUSES

These can be acquired or congenital

Acquired causes
- Simple easy bruising
- Senile purpura
- Non-thrombocytopenic purpura: Infections, drugs, uraemia, Cushing's disease, and adrenocorticosteroid administration
- Scurvy
- Dysproteinaemias
- *Miscellaneous disorders:* Orthostatic purpura, mechanical purpura, fat embolism, systemic disorders—collagen disease especially polyarteritis nodosa.

Congenital
Osler-Rendu-Weber disease, Ehlers-Danlos disease.

PLATELET CAUSES

These can be: Thrombocytopenia or functional defects.

Causes of thrombocytopenia: Acquired or congenital.

Acquired causes: Common causes are:
- **Idiopathic thrombocytopenic purpura** (ITP)—acute or chronic
- Drugs and chemicals
- Leukaemias
- Aplastic anaemias
- Bone marrow infiltration
- Hypersplenism
- Disseminated lupus erythematosus.

Less common causes
- HIV infection
- Megaloblastic anaemia
- Liver disease
- Alcoholism
- Massive blood transfusion
- DIC
- Food allergy.

Functional defects
- Membrane receptor defects—Glanzmann's thrombasthenia, Bernard-Soulier syndrome
- Enzyme defects
- Granule defects

COAGULATION DISORDERS

- Haemophilia A and B
- von Willebrand's disease
- Other factor deficiency disorders—Factor I (fibrinogen), Factor II (prothrombin), Factor V, Factor VII, Factor X, Factor XI, Factor XII and Factor XIII.

Exercise 19

Tests Related to Bleeding Disorders

BLEEDING TIME

The time between blood oozing out of a vessel after injury until the arrest of haemorrhage is bleeding time (BT). In case of any vessel wall defects and platelet disorders the bleeding time is increased.

Ivy's Method

Tie the blood pressure apparatus to the arm and raise the pressure to 40 mm Hg. The area below the antecubital fossa is cleaned with 70% alcohol. Two separate punctures of 2.5 × 1 mm size, 5–10 cm apart are made using disposable lancet. Blot every 30 seconds. Record the time when bleeding stops. Take average of the two.

Normal range: 2–7 minutes.

Template Method (Modified Ivy's method)

This method is similar to Ivy's method. Raise the blood pressure to 40 mm Hg. Clean the antecubital fossa with 70% alcohol. With disposable template, make two standard cuts of 11 × 1 mm (length × depth). Blot every 30 seconds until bleeding stops. Take the average of the two.

Normal range: 2–10 minutes.

Duke's Method

Ear lobe is cleaned with 70% alcohol; 2.5 × 1 mm puncture is made with a lancet, start the stopwatch. Blot every 30 seconds. The time required for bleeding to cease is recorded.

Normal range: 2–7 minutes.

Note: Not a reliable method when compared to Ivy's method.

CLOTTING TIME

Clotting time (CT) is the time taken for the fluid blood to be converted into blood clot that is solid mass of platelets and fibrin.

CT increases in coagulation factor disorders and in such patients who are on anticoagulant treatment.

Capillary Tube Method

Prick the finger after aseptic precautions and simultaneously start the stopwatch as soon as the prick is given. Allow a drop of blood to collect at the prick site. Touch one end of the capillary tube to the blood collected. Blood enters the capillary tube by capillary action. At the end of 2½ minutes the capillary tube is gently broken into two pieces in the middle. Observe for fibrin thread. Repeat this thereafter every ½ minute and record the time taken for the fibrin thread formation.

- Normal range: 4–9 minutes

Note: It is not a reliable method.

Whole Blood Coagulation Time (Lee and White's method)

Take 3 test tubes each of 13 mm × 100 mm (2 or 4 test tubes also can be used). Start the stopwatch as soon as blood enters into the syringe. In each tube 1 ml of blood is taken.

3rd test tube will be the last to receive the blood. Place all the test tubes in a water bath at 37°C.

Every 30 seconds tilt the first test tube until the blood clots. Note the time of clotting. Similarly repeat the second and followed by the third test tube. Time of clotting is noted in each of the test tubes and then the average is calculated.

Normal range: 7–15 minutes

CAPILLARY RESISTANCE TEST (HESS/TOURNIQUET TEST)

Other names: Hess test, tourniquet test, cuff test, Rumpel-Leede test, Rumpel-Leede phenomenon.

Purpose

To determine the resistance of capillaries. In health, capillaries resist pressure of 100 mm Hg.

Procedure

Blood pressure cuff is tied to the arm. Blood pressure is raised to 100 mm Hg (80–100 mm Hg). Maintain the pressure for 5 minutes. After 15 minutes observe the forearm for petechiae. Count the number of petechiae.

Following inference is drawn:

Less than 10 petechiae	Negative/Normal
10–20 petechiae	Doubtful
> 20 petechiae	Positive

The test is positive in thrombocytopaenia and in von Willebrand's factor deficiency.

CLOT RETRACTION

Volume of serum expressed by the blood, which is allowed to clot at 37°C is recorded as a percentage of the original volume of blood.

Collect 5 ml of blood in a 10 ml centrifuging graduated test tube. Place a glass rod in vertical position in the tube. Incubate the tube at 37°C for 1 hour undisturbed. Normal clot retraction is 50–60%.

CLOT LYSIS TIME

After noting the clot retraction, continue to incubate the tube until 72 hours. The fibrin clot dissolves due to fibrinolysis and the red cells sink to the bottom. Normal clot lysis time is 72 hours. It is abnormal when the clot lysis occurs within 24 hours.

PROTHROMIN TIME (PT)

Clinical Significance

- PT reflects the overall efficiency of the extrinsic system
- Most sensitive to changes in factor V, VII, X
- Lesser to factor II and I.

Principle

Thrombokinase preparation containing calcium is added to citrated plasma. In presence of factor VII, extrinsic pathway is activated leading to clot formation.

Procedure

To 0.1 ml of patient's plasma add 0.1 ml of brain thromboplastin. Then add 0.1 ml of $CaCl_2$. Start the stop watch and note the time when clot forms. Test should be done with control plasma.

Normal range: 0.8–1.2 seconds

PT international normalized ratio (PT-INR): (PT test/PT control) ISI

ISI: International Sensitivity Index for any tissue factor they manufacture (WHO-primary thromboplastin). The ISI is usually between 1.0 and 2.0.

Normal range of PT-INR: 0.9–1.3.

ACTIVATED PARTIAL THROMBOPLASTIN TIME (APTT)

Clinical Significance

- Intrinsic coagulation pathway
- Deficiency of factor VIII, IX, XI, XII
- Deficiency of common pathway

Principle

Partial thromboplastin is incubated with Kaolin and clotting time is noted after adding calcium.

Procedure

To 0.1 ml of brain extract add 0.1 ml of Kaolin, add 0.2 ml of patients plasma. Incubate at 37°C for 1 minute and add 0.1 ml $CaCl_2$. Start the stopwatch and note the time for clot formation. Test should be done with control plasma.

Normal range: 30 to 40 seconds.

THROMBIN TIME (TT)

Clinical Significance

Fibrinogen converted to fibrin.

Abnormal Values

- Decreased level of fibrinogen
- Qualitative abnormality of fibrinogen
- Presence of heparin/heparin-like substance.

Procedure

To 0.2 ml of plasma add 0.1 ml of thrombin and $CaCl_2$. Start the stopwatch and note time of clot formation. Test should be done with control plasma.

Normal range: 15 to 20 seconds.

Exercise 20

LE Cell Phenomenon

Lupus erythematosus (LE) cell phenomenon detects anti-nuclear protein antibody which occurs in serum of SLE, Sjögren's syndrome, rheumatoid arthritis, thyroiditis, myasthenia gravis, cirrhosis and discoid lupus erythematosus (Fig. 1.42).

LE factor has the property of causing *in vitro* lysis of nuclei of neutrophil and subsequent phagocytosis of lysed nuclei by other neutrophil.

LE cell has a typical amorphous pale purple body, surrounded by the nucleus of a polymorph. Rarely monocyte and eosinophil engulf LE body. The LE body may be found extracellularly also.

LE cell has to be differentiated from Tart cell (Fig. 1.43) where in monocyte or rarely a neutrophil does engulf another cell or the nucleus of another cell (most often nucleus of lymphocyte). Here the chromatin pattern of engulfed nucleus is retained without any change.

Procedure to Demonstrate LE Cell Phenomenon

1. *Blood clot method of Zimmer and Hargraves:* In this method blood is allowed to clot and is incubated. With two wooden applicator sticks, the clot is mashed into its own serum. The mixture is centrifuged and smears prepared with buffy coat.
2. *Blood clot method of Magath and Winkle:* The clot is squeezed (passed forcefully) through a wire sieve or strainer and then

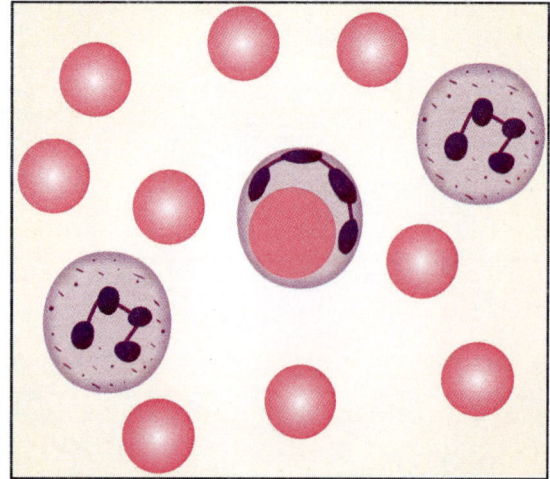

Fig. 1.42: LE cell

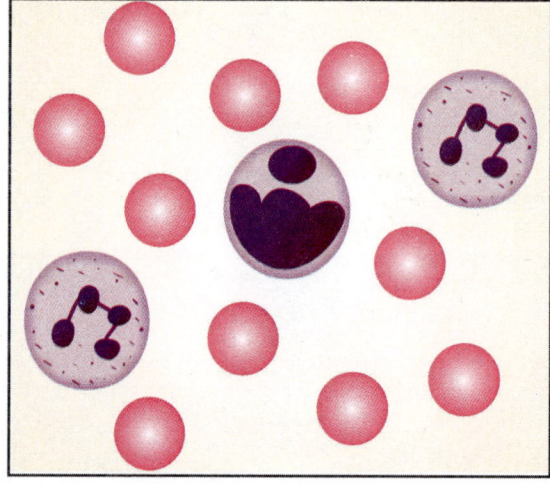

Fig. 1.43: Tart cell

the smears are prepared in a similar way as in the above procedure.

3. ***Zinkham and Conley method:*** The heparinised blood is traumatised by glass beads for 30 minutes and smears are prepared in a similar way. For demonstration of LE cell phenomenon, trauma to the leukocytes is necessary.

LE factor does not appear to act on healthy leukocytes. To achieve certain degree of trauma to the leukocytes, different methods are employed before making the smears like shaking with glass beads, mashing the blood clot with wooden applicator, passing forcefully through a wire sieve or strainer or by squeezing.

Examine the films under low power (20X) magnification and confirm under oil immersion. Slide should be examined at least for 10 minutes before a negative report is arrived at.

Exercise 21

Romanowsky Stains, Buffer, Instruments and Cleaning of the Glassware

ROMANOWSKY STAINS

Romanowsky dyes consist of a mixture of basic dye that is methylene blue and an acidic dye eosin. Methylene blue stains the acidic cell components (nucleus and cytoplasmic RNA). Eosin is red coloured, and it stains the basic components such as haemoglobin.

A number of Romanowsky stains are available which are used singly or in combination.
- Wright's stain
- Leishman stain
- Giemsa stain
- May-Grünwald Giemsa stain
- Jenner-Giemsa stain.

Wright's Stain

Actually, it is a polychromatic stain as it produces a variety of colours. It is a methyl alcoholic solution of an acidic (eosin) and a basic (methylene blue) dye. Wright's stain powder is also available commercially.

Wright's power is obtained after drying a solution containing:

Methylene blue	1 g
Sodium carbonate 0.5%	100 ml
Eosin w/s (yellowish) 0.1% aqueous solution	500 ml
Methyl alcohol (absolute)	60 ml

Preparation of Wright's Stain

Wright stain containing about 2.5 g of Wright's powder in 1 L of chemically pure absolute methyl alcohol (acetone free) is prepared. The powder is ground in a mortar by adding a few ml of methyl alcohol till 1 L have been added. This step requires 20–30 minutes. The stain is left standing for a day or two and then it will be ready for use. Few laboratories add about 30 ml of glycerin to the Wright's powder, mix it well in a mortar. Incubate this for 24 hours at 37°C and then mix with 1 L of methanol.

The dye is sensitive to water and detergents. So the bottle should be tightly stoppered to prevent entry of water vapour. Exposure to acid or alkali should be totally avoided.

Structures which are stained with basic dyes are basophilic. Structures that take up acidic dye are called acidophilic, whereas structures which are stained with both are called, neutrophilic.

Leishman Stain

0.2 g of powdered dye is taken in a conical flask of 200–250 ml capacity. 100 ml methanol is added and then warmed to 50°C for 15 minutes with occasional shaking. The solution is ready for use.

Note: The alkaline pH accentuates the methylene blue component and *vice versa* is also true. pH of 7.2 is recommended for malarial parasites in order to demonstrate Schuffner's dots.

Giemsa Stain

It is the best stain for identifying blood parasites and other protozoa.

Composition

Azur II eosin	3.0 g
Azur II	0.8 g
Glycerin (Merck CP)	250 ml
Methyl alcohol	250 ml

BUFFER

Buffer maintains the pH of the stain solution. For staining the peripheral smear, buffer of pH of 6.4–6.7 is preferred.

Buffer for Wright's stain (pH 6.4): The contents of the buffer are as follows:

Primary (monobasic) potassium phosphate (KH_2PO_4), anhydrous 6.63 g; secondary dibasic sodium phosphate Na_2HPO_4, anhydrous 2.56 g and distilled water up to 1 litre are added.

For pH of 6.7, about 5.13 g of potassium salt and 4.12 g of sodium salt are used. In case of the films stained with Wright's stain, the RBCs should stain pink and not lemon yellow or red and the nuclei of leukocytes should stain purple.

The distilled water placed in a glass bottle for at least 24 hours (aged distilled water) has the pH of 6.4–6.8 can also be used.

Different Methods for Cleaning of the Glasswares

1. Wash the slides with soap and water and then with abundant clean hot water followed by distilled water. Dry them and polish with lint free cloth. Only edges should touched and these slides can be stored in a slide box for use when required.
2. The slides, cover glasses and other glasswares can be cleaned with a mixture of dichromate and H_2SO_4. They can be dropped into the above solution and left in it for 4 to 24 hours. Later the solution is poured off and the slides are washed with multiple changes of tap water. Complete removal of acid is assessed using litmus paper. The litmus paper should show neutral pH and then the slides are washed with distilled water, dried and stored.
3. Dirty slides are put into some detergent solution; heated to 60°C for 20 minutes, washed in hot running tap water and dried with clean linen cloth.
4. The glass slides are washed in running tap water, boiled in some detergent solution, rinsed in acid and washed in hot running tap water.

Exercise 22

Automation in Haematology

Automation is the process where haematology tests are performed by humans by computerised methods. Until recently haematological tests were performed by manual methods. Both the manual and automated laboratory techniques have their own advantages and disadvantages. It is very unlikely that one method will completely replace the other.

AUTOMATED HAEMATOLOGY ANALYSER
(Figs 1.44 and 1.45)

It is of two types.
A. Semi-automated—few parameters are only performed. Few steps are performed manually by technologists requiring more time.
B. Fully automated—measures multiple parameters in less time.

Principles of Working

Automated haematology analysers work on different principles or combination of different principles.
- Electrical impedance
- Light absorption
- Light scatter
- Electrical conductivity
- Fluorescence.

Electrical Impedance

As this was first developed by Coulter electronics it is also known as Coulter principle. In an isotonic solution two electrodes are separated by a glass tube having a small aperture. Cell passes through the aperture after applying vacuum, the flow of current is impeded and a voltage pulse is generated. The height of pulse is proportional to the cell volume and the width corresponds to time taken to traverse the aperture.

Anticoagulated blood is aspirated into the system which is divided into two portions and mixed with diluents. One dilution passed through RBC aperture (for RBC and platelet counting) and the other through WBC aperture (for WBC and Hb estimation). Haemoglobin is estimated by light transmission at 535 nm (Fig. 1.45). RBCs are counted between 36 and 360 fl, platelets between 2 and 20 fl, 35 and 90 fl are lymphocytes, 90 and 160 fl are mononuclear cells, and neutrophils between 160 and 450 fl.

Light Absorption

Haemoglobin is converted to cyanmethaemoglobin or other compound and measured by absorption spectrophotometry. Leukocytes are classified by peroxidase cytochemistry. The peroxidase activity is detected by principle of absorbance.

Light Scatter

Cells flow or move in a single line. Laser device is focussed on the cell flow, the laser light beam strikes the cell and is scattered in various directions. There are two cell detectors. The forward scatter light is detected

Haematology

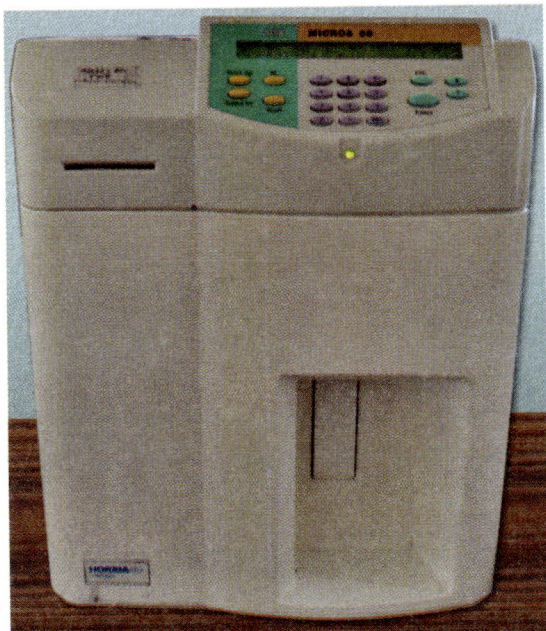

Fig. 1.44: Cell counter—3 part differential count

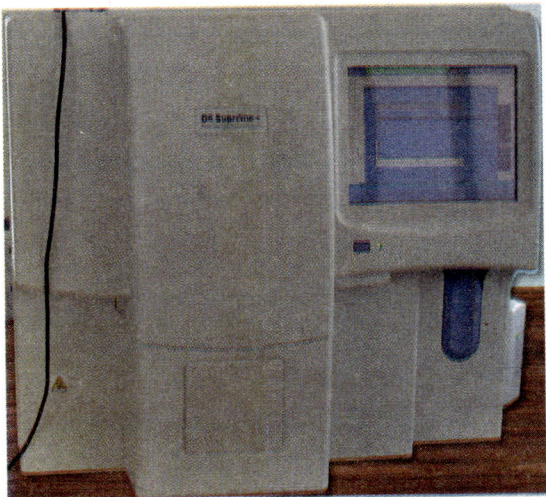

Fig. 1.45: Cell counter—5 part differential count

Electrical Conductivity

High frequency current is used to determine and classify leukocytes by their physical and chemical composition.

Fluorescence

RNA (reticulocytes), DNA (NRBCs) and cell surface antigens can be measured by cellular fluorescence.

Parameters Measured by Haematology Analysers

- Routine analysers
- Upgraded analysers
- RBC count
- Reticulocyte count
- WBC count (TC)
- Red cell distribution width
- WBC differential count (DC)
- Reticulocyte haemoglobin content
- Platelet count
- Mean platelet volume (MPV)
- Mean cell volume (MCV)
- Platelet distribution width (PDW)
- Mean cell haemoglobin (MCH)
- Reticulated platelets.

Mean Cell Haemoglobin Concentration (MCHC)

The haematology analysers produce the RBC, WBC and platelet results in the form of histograms, scattergrams.

The haematology analysers could be three part differentials where WBC differential is reported as granulocytes, lymphocytes and monocytes and it works on the principle of electrical impedance or 5 part differential where neutrophils, basophils, eosinophils, lymphocytes and monocytes are measured by using combination of different principles.

Advantages

- Accurate and precision in tests
- Can perform multiple tests on a single platform

by one detector and it is proportional to cell size. The second detector captures side scatter which assess the nucleus and granules in the cytoplasm. The simultaneous scatter in both directions helps to differentiate the granulocytes, lymphocytes and monocytes.

- Significant reduction in manpower
- Speed and efficient handling of large number of samples
- Accurate determination of red cell indices in automated haematology analyser.

Disadvantages
- Erroneous results due to interfering factors
- Expensive machine and reagents
- RBC morphology (shape and size) at times not recognised
- Hence, flags develop which have to be confirmed by manual examination
- Machine maintenance.

Flagging
These are the signals generated by the analyser when abnormal results are detected. It reduces the false-positive and false-negative results requiring manual review of the blood smear examination.

Platelet Function Analyser (PFA-100)
It is a screening test for platelet adhesion and aggregation. Anticoagulated blood is passed through small membranes coated with either collagen and epinephrine or collagen and ADP. The platelets adhere to the membranes and occlude the aperture at the centre of the membrane. Normal closure time is 1–3 minutes.

Normal PFA with collagen/epinephrine: No significant platelet function defect.

Prolonged collagen/epinephrine and normal collagen/ADP—aspirin induced platelet defect.

Prolonged collagen/epinephrine and collagen/ADP—congenital or acquired platelet function defects.

Haemoglobin Estimation (Fig. 1.46)
The HaemoCue haemoglobin photometer has been widely used for as a point-of-care device for haemoglobin estimation in mobile blood donations and critical care areas in health

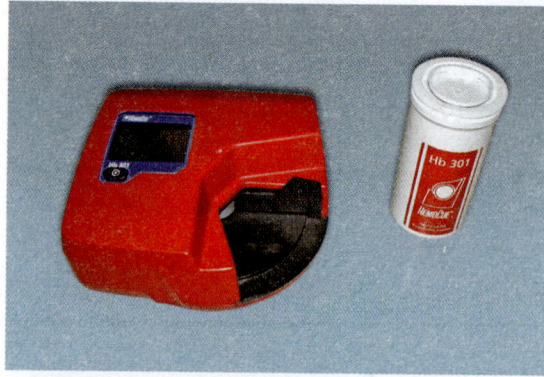

Fig. 1.46: HaemoCue for haemoglobin estimation

facilities. However, it is not recommend in general practice.

Automation to Determine Hb Variants
Inherited haemoglobin disorders, haemoglobinopathies and thalassaemias, largely originated in the tropics, but now are common worldwide due to migration. At least 5.2% of the world population (and more than 7% of pregnant women) carry a haemoglobin variant. It is also estimated that around 1.1% of couples worldwide are at risk for having children with a haemoglobin disorder, and 2.7 per 1,000 conceptions are affected.

The haemoglobinopathies, or Hb variants, are attributable to amino acid substitution(s) in either globin chain.

DETECTING Hb DISORDERS, WITH AN EMPHASIS ON CAPILLARY SEPARATION

Automated Separation Methods
Most large laboratories currently use automatic high-throughput methods, such as high-performance liquid chromatography (HPLC) and/or capillary electrophoresis (CE). With virtually 100% sensitivity, these methods easily identify elevated HbA2 in β-thalassaemia and common Hb variants.

High pressure liquid chromatography: On HPLC, haemoglobin samples are injected into a resin column and separated based on charge. Haemoglobin variants elute from the column and are detected at 415 nm, then at 690 nm to correct the baseline. The haemoglobin retention time (from injection until the maximum point of each peak) is calculated and plotted on a chromatogram. Glycosylated fractions and other post-translational adducts separate from the main peaks, making the chromatogram somewhat challenging to interpret.

HPLC has been implemented in the clinical laboratory for evaluating haemoglobin abnormalities. HPLC systems provide automation, allow for precise quantitation of HbA2 (with some exceptions), and are effective at detecting common and rare variants. Some rare variants could be missed on HPLC, where they would be detected on CE or other technique, but the opposite is also true.

Capillary Electrophoresis (CE) Separation Technology

Capillary electrophoresis separates haemoglobin variants by electro-osmotic flow and electrophoretic mobility in alkaline buffer (pH 9.4). Multiple samples (two to eight, depending on the instrument used) undergo high-resolution separation concurrently in silica glass capillaries, taking approximately eight minutes to complete the analysis. For Hb variant detection, UV at 415 nm wavelength is used. The detection methodology is similar to one used in HPLC systems. As a result, the methodology is sometimes considered a "hybrid" type of separation technique between classical zone electrophoresis and liquid chromatography.

An electrophoregram consists of 300 consecutive readings and is divided into 15 zones that are either numbered (i.e. Z1) or named according to the common variants (e.g. Z(S) for the zone where HbS migrates). Haemoglobin variants are displayed as peaks, and the zones where the variants belong are automatically marked by the system. All normal haemoglobins (HbA, HbA2 and HbF) are automatically identified. An on-board drop-down library assists with the interpretation of the results.

Significant changes have been made in the latest generation CE systems in order to provide complete automation and improve workflow in the laboratory, while maintaining separation profiles and results identical to those from previous generation instruments. Such systems run two whole-blood programmes.

Diabetes Mellitus and Haemoglobin Variants

Correct interpretation of HbA1c measurements depends on normal erythrocyte lifespan. In individuals with sickle cell, HbC, or HbD disease it is recommended that tests other than HbA1c be used for the determination of glycemic control (e.g. glycated serum albumin), since the lifespan of red blood cells is altered. If heterozygous carriers show normal erythrocyte survival, HbA1c can be used as long as the haemoglobin variant does not interfere with the assay method, nor with glucose binding to haemoglobin. There is some evidence to suggest that Hb variants may affect RBC life-span even in Hb trait patients who are asymptomatic. Thalassaemia also can affect lifespan of RBC, resulting in a markedly low HbA1c value.

Automation in Reticulocyte Count

Using an seven part automated haematology analyser, the automated absolute reticulocyte count, the reticulocyte index, or reticulocyte production index (RPI), immature reticulocyte fraction (IRF) can be obtained.

Measurement of Reticulocyte-specific Haemoglobin Content

The automated haematology analyser can also report a measurement of reticulocyte-specific haemoglobin content as mean reticulocyte haemoglobin content (CHr) or reticulocyte haemoglobin equivalent (Ret-He), depending on the type of instrument used. CHr and Ret-He, two comparable but not identical parameters, give a snapshot of the functional iron available for incorporation into haemoglobin within RBCs over the previous 3–4 days. A decreased value generally reflects reduced cellular haemoglobin content and is reliable in identifying functional iron deficiency. Furthermore, this parameter is the strongest predictor of iron deficiency anaemia in children.

Indications

The reticulocyte count is not usually a part of a standard CBC count, but is ordered and used along with CBC, as CBC with reticulocyte count, to guide anaemia workup or response to treatment. Depending on the type of automated haematology analyser used in the laboratory, reticulocyte-specific haemoglobin content and IRF may be reported along with reticulocyte count to provide additional valuable information. These parameters are useful in the following situations:

- Anaemia workup (peripheral destruction vs failure of production)
- Response to therapy (iron, vitamin B_{12}, folic acid supplementation)
- Bone marrow recovery after bone marrow transplantation or intensive chemotherapy.

Flow Cytometry

It is a procedure which measures multiple cellular and fluorescent properties of cells. The instrument is called flow cytometer.

Principle: The cells suspended pass through a single flow suspension through a laser beam. Cells of 0.2 to 150 μm are analysed by flow cytometric analysis.

It has three main components
1. *Fluidics:* It transports the cells in a stream to the laser beam for interrogation.
2. *Optics:* It consists of lasers-argon-ion laser for illumination of cells.
3. *Electronics:* The optical signals are converted to corresponding electronic signals by photodetectors.

Hence, the flow cytometer provides following information of cell.
- Cell size
- Granularity or internal complexity
- Relative fluorescence intensity.

Applications in Haematology

1. Diagnosis, prognosis and to assess minimal residual disease in leukaemias and lymphomas.
2. Diagnosis and prognosis of leukaemias, MDS, plasma cell neoplasms, mast cell neoplasms.
3. Enumeration of CD34 positive cells.
4. It is used in haemopoietic stem cell therapy, targeted therapy.
5. Protein profiling.
6. Measurement of drug uptake and multi-drug resistance proteins.
7. Identification of leukaemic stem cells/side population cells.
8. Newer application in RBC disorders—PNH, antibody detection in AIHA, feto-maternal haemorrhage, fetal RBC measurement in haemoglobinopathies and myelodysplasia, reticulocyte analysis, immature reticulocyte fraction, alloimmunisation detection, transfusion related immunologic reactions, erythrocyte phenotyping, rheology, bone marrow engraftment and regeneration evaluation, sickle cell and thalassaemia monitoring, parasite infection detection, congenital chimerism and mosaicism detection.
9. Helpful in diagnosis of primary immunodeficiency disorders.

Section II

Clinical Pathology and Basics of Cytology, Charts/Case Studies in Haematology, Clinical Pathology and Cytology

- Exercise 23. Urine Examination
- Exercise 24. Pregnancy Test
- Exercise 25. Semen Analysis
- Exercise 26. Glucose Tolerance Test (GTT)
- Exercise 27. Fractional Test Meal (FTM)
- Exercise 28. Renal Function Tests
- Exercise 29. Liver Function Tests
- Exercise 30. Thyroid Function Tests
- Exercise 31. Instruments
- Exercise 32. Malaria and Filariasis
- Exercise 33. Basics of Cytology
- Exercise 34. Haematology, Clinical Pathology and Cytology Charts/Case Studies

Exercise 23

Urine Examination

This is the oldest of the laboratory procedures for diagnostic purposes in medicine.

Purpose of Urine Analysis
1. Diagnosis and management of renal and urinary tract diseases.
2. Detection of metabolic and systemic diseases.

FORMATION OF URINE

In the body, the lungs control the concentrations of oxygen and carbon dioxide and the kidneys maintain the normal chemical composition of the body fluids. The kidneys remove metabolic wastes and perform homeostatic functions.

The regulation of the internal environment by the kidney is composite of three processes, namely:
1. Filtration of blood plasma at the glomeruli.
2. Selective reabsorption of threshold substances like sugar, fatty acids, amino acids, salts and water.
3. Secretion of certain substances like creatinine, potassium, uric acid, organic ions and hydrogen ions.

Urine is formed by summations of all these three processes. The anatomic unit which performs this function is nephron, and each kidney possesses about one million nephrons.

About 1 litre/minute blood flows through the kidneys and about 120 ml/minute glomerular filtrate is formed at the Bowman's capsule.

Glucose, amino acids, proteins, most of the water and ions are reabsorbed by the proximal convoluted tubule. In the distal portion of convoluted tubule, remainder of water and ions are reabsorbed and acidification of urine takes place, with elimination of hydrogen and ammonium ions.

About 180 litres/24 hours filtrate is formed and due to reabsorption of this filtrate only about 1200 to 1500 ml of urine is excreted per 24 hour.

Glucocorticoids control water and sodium excretion by their effect on glomerular filtration rate. Mineralocorticoids exert an influence by absorption of sodium and excretion of potassium in the distal tubules. Anti-diuretic hormone acts on the distal convoluted tubular reabsorption of water; thus kidneys maintain acid–base and water balance.

The urine formed in the kidneys passes from the collecting ducts, into renal pelvis, ureter, bladder and urethra when voided.

Clinical Conditions Related to Urine Excretion

Polyuria: Abnormal increase of urine volume more than 2000 ml/24 hours as in diabetes insipidus and diabetes mellitus is polyuria.

Oliguria: Less than 500 ml of urine volume in 24 hours is termed oliguria.

Anuria: Near complete suppression of urine formation is termed anuria.

COMPOSITION OF URINE

Urine is composed of water and solute. Major portion of the solute in the urine is urea and sodium chloride. The quantum of protein intake will affect nitrogen excretion such as urea. Other substances like uric acid, creatinine, amino acids, ammonia, traces of proteins, glycoproteins, enzymes and purine account for nitrogen excreted.

Urine contains potassium, which is ubiquitous in the diet; sulphates and other sulphur containing substances such as sulphides, cysteine and mercaptan phosphate excretion is variable and is derived chiefly from nucleic acids in food, casein and other organic and inorganic phosphates. Small amounts of sugars like pentoses will vary with dietary intake. Intermediary metabolites such as oxalic acid, citric acid and pyruvate are present. Free fatty acids and trace amounts of cholesterol are also found in urine as also are trace amounts of metals.

Hormones such as ketosteroids, oestrogens, aldosterone, pituitary gonadotrophins, catecholamines and serotonin are normally found in urine and reflect the endocrine status. Vitamins such as ascorbic acid are excreted in urine.

Types of Urine Samples for Urine Analysis

1. Random sample: This sample is convenient for the patient and suitable for screening tests.
2. The first morning urine sample: This is best for nitrates, proteins, microscopic examination and preferred for chemical examination.
3. Fasting and postprandial urine samples: These samples are preferred for diabetic patients.
4. 24 hours urine sample: This sample is best for hormones, protein and electrolytes.
5. 2–12 hours urine sample: This sample is best for urobilinogen, xylose excretion and quantitative cell count.
6. *For bacteriological purposes:* Midstream urine and collected in sterile containers.
7. 24-hour sample is preferred for parasitic diseases like onchocerca and schistosoma.
8. Other techniques
   Urethral catheterization: This is done when the patient is unable to void.
   Suprapubic aspiration: This is a procedure for anaerobic cultures and cultures in infants.

COLLECTION OF URINE SAMPLE

Urine is collected in a clean, dry container, and ideally examined within one hour of voiding. If analysis is delayed, then refrigerate or some chemical preservative is to be added.

Container for Collection

1. A wide mouthed plastic or glass container of 100–200 ml capacity is commonly used.
2. For 24 hours sample collection, 3 litres capacity rigid brown plastic container having wide mouth and a screw cap is suitable. The 24-hour urine sample is used for estimating protein, creatinine clearance and glucose.
3. Urine collectors of pliable polyethylene are available.

Preservation Methods

Refrigeration at 4°C is the best for casts, cells and chemical analysis.

Freezing is recommended for urobilinogen, bilirubin and porphobilinogen. But it must be remembered that there remains undissolvable turbidity after thawing.

Following are the different chemicals for preservation:

Toluene	2 ml/100 ml, interferes with protein test by sulphosalicylic acid method
Thymol	One crystal/100 ml, interferes with sugar, acetone and diacetic acid reactions
Formalin	3 drops/100 ml, useful for urine sediment, interferes with test for proteins as it precipitates proteins
Chloroform	5 ml/100 ml

Boric acid	1 g/dl, used for hormone assay (oestriol and oestrogen are preserved for 7 days)
Concentrated hydrochloric acid	10 ml/24 hour specimen, calcium and nitrogen content are preserved
Sodium fluoride	0.5 g/3–4 L, for glucose in 24-hour sample; preserves xylose, not used for glucose by strip method

PHYSICAL EXAMINATION

The physical examination findings to be noted are appearance, colour, odour, volume, reaction and specific gravity.

1. Appearance

Fresh urine is normally clear. It may be cloudy due to the following causes:

1. Amorphous phosphates are present in alkaline or neutral urine and cloudiness disappears on addition of dilute acetic acid.
2. Uric acids and urates are present in acidic urine and these dissolve on warming to 60°C.
3. Presence of leukocytes, cloudiness persists even after addition of acetic acid and presence of leukocytes is confirmed by microscopy.
4. Presence of bacteria causes uniform opalescence which is not removed by acidification or filtering; microscopy confirms the presence.
5. The presence of red cells produces smokiness and presence is confirmed by microscopy.
6. Spermatozoa and prostatic fluid may cause turbidity and is not cleared by acidification.
7. The presence of mucous may produce fluffy and bulky deposits.

2. Colour

Normal colour is pale yellow; this is due to the presence of urochrome in urine. Abnormal colours may be because of the following reasons:

1. Chyluria—presence of lymph in urine (obstruction or rupture of lymphatics). Colour varies with the amount of chyle present, it may be normal, opalescent or milky.
2. Fat globules in urine are seen in nephrotic syndrome, skeletal trauma and fractures of long bones and pelvis. This condition is called lipiduria.
3. Yellow colour can be due to acriflavin.
4. Yellow orange colour suggests concentrated urine and it may be due to presence of urobilin or bilirubin.
5. Yellow green/yellow brown colour suggests the presence of bilirubin/biliverdin.
6. Red/red brown colour may be because of haemoglobin, RBCs, myoglobin, porphyrin or due to consumption of beetroot or menstrual contamination. Presence of RBCs produce cloudy, smoky, pink and red or red brown colour. In haemoglobinuria, the colour may be red, red brown or dark brown. In the presence of methaemoglobin, the colour may be brown black in acidic urine.
7. Homogentisic acid (alkaptonuria)—with the presence of homogentisic acid in urine, on standing brown black colour develops.
8. Blue green colour suggests Pseudomonas infection.
9. Different drug intake can produce different colours.

Urine colour with commonly used drugs and dyes: The drugs and dyes used and colour of the urine excreted are as below.

Drugs	Colour
Alcohol	Pale
Desferal (chelates iron)	Red
Furazolidine	Brown
Indigo carmine dye (cystoscopy)	Blue
L-dopa	Red to brown
Mepacrine	Yellow

Methocarbamol—muscle relaxant	Green to brown
Methyldopa	Red to brown
Metronidazole	Reddish brown
Nitrofurantoin	Brown yellow
Rifampicin	Orange
Riboflavin	Bright yellow

3. Odour

The normal odour of urine is aromatic.
The abnormal odour is due to the following causes:

Ketone bodies	Fruity odour
Bacterial contamination	Ammoniacal, fetid
Maple syrup urine disease	Maple syrup odour

(Maple syrup urine disease is an inborn error of metabolism of valine, leucine and isoleucine. There is deficiency of α-ketoacid dehydrogenase and α-ketoacids are excreted in urine).

Phenylketonuria	Mousy odour
Trimethylaminuria	Rotten fish odour
Tyrosinemia	Rancid odour
Isovaleric acidemia and glutamic acidemia	Sweaty feet odour

4. Reaction (pH)

Normal range of pH is 4.6 to 8.

Methods

a. *Litmus paper indicator:* Change of colour from blue to red is acidic and red to blue is alkaline.
b. Reagent strip and titrable urine acidity can be used.

Acidic urine is due to high meat protein, diabetic ketoacidosis, and metabolic/respiratory acidosis.

Alkaline urine is due to consumption of vegetables, citrus fruits, metabolic/respiratory alkalosis.

Crystals found in acidic urine: Calcium oxalate, uric acid and cysteine crystals are some of the crystals found in acidic urine. All of these dissolve in alkaline urine.

For therapeutic induction of alkaline urine, sodium bicarbonate, potassium citrate and acetazolamide are used.

Crystals found in alkaline urine: Phosphates, triple phosphates, ammonium biurate and calcium carbonate are some of the crystals found in alkaline urine. Calcium carbonate and phosphates dissolve in acidic urine.

Therapeutic acidification with ammonium chloride and methenamine mandelate are used for the treatment of crystals found in alkaline urine.

Specific Gravity

The specific gravity, at a constant temperature is the weight of volume of urine to the weight of same volume of distilled water. It indicates the relative proportion of dissolved solid components to the total volume of the specimen. In other words it reflects the density of the specimen.

Several methods are available to measure the specific gravity of urine. This can be measured by using urinometer, refractometer, reagent strip and falling drop method. Normal adults with adequate fluid intake will produce urine of specific gravity 1.016 to 1.022 over a 24-hour period.

Urine of low specific gravity (hyposthenuria) is encountered in diabetes insipidus and in various renal abnormalities including pyelonephritis and glomerulonephritis. The specific gravity in these patients will be less than 1.007.

High specific gravity (hypersthenuria) can be encountered after excess water loss/dehydration, adrenal insufficiency, hepatic disease, congestive heart failure, eclampsia, proteinuria or lipoid nephrosis. When there is little or no variability between several specimens from a patient and the specific gravity is fixed at about 1.010, this is known as isosthenuric. This is indicative of severe renal damage in which there is disruption of both concentrating and diluting abilities.

To measure the specific gravity by urinometer, the urinometer vessel is filled three-fourth full with urine. The urinometer is inserted with spinning motion. The urinometer should not touch the sides of the cylinder and take the reading at the lower meniscus. As temperature influences the specific gravity, urine samples should be allowed to come to room temperature before reading is taken. A correction of 0.001 should be made for each of 3°C, above or below the calibration temperature.

CHEMICAL EXAMINATION

Tests for proteins

Heat and acetic acid test (Fig. 2.1a)
Take three-fourth full of urine in a test tube, boil upper half of urine column.
1. If white cloud appears, this may be due to the presence of phosphates, carbonates and proteins.
2. Add 3% acetic acid. If cloud disappears, it is because of phosphates and carbonates.
3. Cloud persists with proteins.
4. Add 2 drops of nitric acid, cloudiness disappears with mucin and nucleoproteins; cloud persists with albumin.

Bence Jones (BJ) proteins: These proteins consist of either kappa or lambda light chain immunoglobulins. These are filtered through the glomeruli. These were described by Henry Bence Jones in 1847. These proteins possess unusual solubility properties, precipitate when heated to 40–60°C and become soluble when boiled (100°C) and reappear on cooling. 50–80% of the multiple myeloma cases excrete BJ proteins; remaining percentage of cases can be diagnosed by serum electrophoresis.

Sulphosalicylic Acid Test (Fig. 2.1b)

Take 2 ml of urine in a test tube and add 2 ml of 3% sulphosalicylic acid, or

Take 5 ml of urine in a test tube and add 0.5 ml of 20% sulphosalicylic acid.

Observe for turbidity after adding sulphosalicylic acid. Depending upon the turbidity following is the approximate amount of proteins excreted in urine:

No turbidity	No proteins, test is negative.
Traces	Milky white/perceptible turbidity/opalescent (>20 mg/dl of proteins or corresponds to about 0.2 g to less than 0.5 g/24 hours)
+	Distinct turbidity but no distinct granules/can read print through tube (50 mg/dl of proteins or more than 0.5 g up to 1.5 g/24 hours)
++	Turbidity with granules but no floccules/can read only black lines (more than 150–200 mg/dl of proteins or more than 1.5 to 2 g/24 hours)
+++	Turbidity with granules and floccules/no visible black lines (200–500 mg/dl of proteins or 2–5 g/24 hours)
++++	Clumps of precipitated proteins or solids (>700 mg to 1 g/dl of proteins or 7 to 10 g/24 hours or greater)

Heller's ring test/nitric acid test (Fig. 2.1c): Take 0.5 ml of nitric acid in a small test tube and add equal amount of urine from the side of test tube, the resulting white ring at the interphase suggests the presence of proteins.

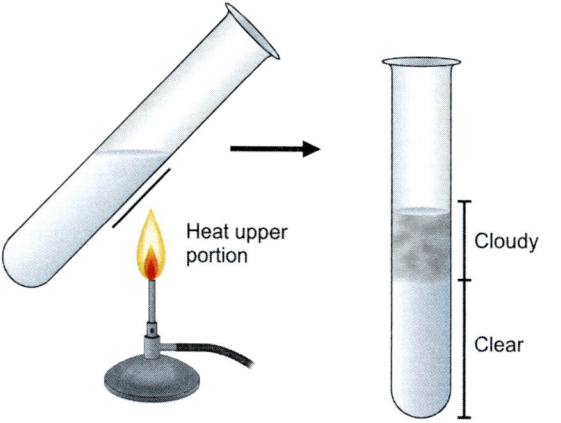

Fig. 2.1a: Heat coagulation test

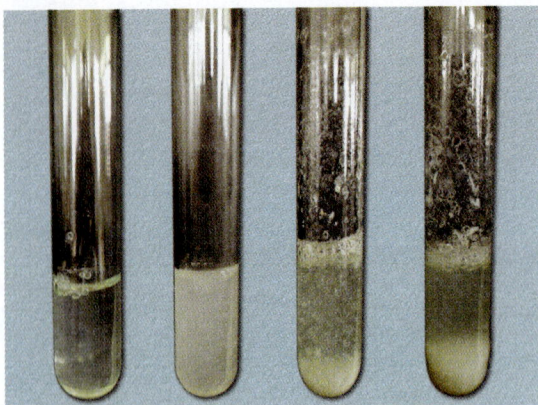

Fig. 2.1b: Sulphosalicylic acid test (presence of protein in various grades)

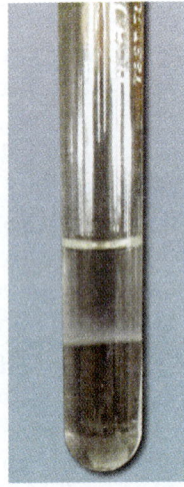

Fig. 2.1c: Heller's ring test (note white ring)

Causes of Proteinuria (according to severity of proteinuria)

Mild proteinuria: When the protein excretion is less than 1.0 g/day in urine it is mild proteinuria. Some of the causes may be chronic pyelonephritis, chronic interstitial nephritis and polycystic disease.

Moderate proteinuria: Protein excretion of 1.0 to 4.0 g/day in urine is moderate proteinuria. Some of the causes may be nephrosclerosis, multiple myeloma, toxic nephropathy and lower urinary tract diseases.

Severe proteinuria: Protein excretion more than 4.0 g/day in urine is severe proteinuria. The causes may be nephrotic syndrome and acute rapidly progressive glomerulonephritis.

Other causes are malaria, malignant hypertension, drugs (penicillamine), heavy metals, amyloidosis and primary anti-phospholipid syndrome.

Causes of Proteinuria (according to renal/prerenal/postrenal causes)

Prerenal causes: Orthostatic, exercise, exposure to cold, rich protein meal, pregnancy and premenstrual period.

Renal causes: Nephrotic syndrome, nephritic syndrome, pyelonephritis, renal transplant, renal tubular acidosis, oculocerebrorenal syndrome and cystinosis.

Postrenal causes: Lower urinary tract diseases—inflammation, malignant diseases and presence of calculi.

Microalbuminuria: This is a condition in which the protein levels would be of the range between 30 and 300 mg/L in a 24 hours sample and that indicates early excretion of proteins and possibly reversible glomerular damage.

In such a case, the presence of albumin would be higher than the normal level but below the detectable range of conventional methods.

Microalbuminuria is a potent risk factor for cardiovascular events in diabetic patients.

Test for Glucose

Benedict's Test (Fig. 2.2)

Procedure: In a test tube measure and take 5 ml of Benedict's reagent; boil it. If there is no colour change then add 8 drops of urine and boil. Cool it and observe for colour of the precipitate. The resulting observation would be as under.

Observation

Blue colour	0–100 mg/dl of glucose
Green colour	100–500 mg/dl of glucose

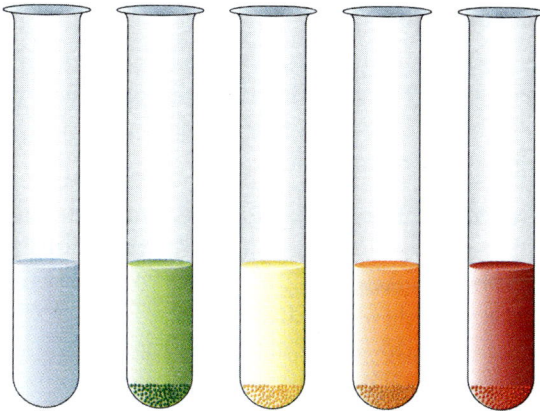

Fig. 2.2: Benedict's test

Yellow colour	More than 500–1000 mg/dl of glucose
Orange colour	More than 1000–1500 mg/dl of glucose
Brick-red colour	> 2000 mg or more of glucose

Preparation of Benedict's reagent

$CuSO_4.5H_2O$	17.3 g
Sodium citrate	173 g
Sodium carbonate (anhydrous)	100 g
Water to make	1000 ml

Procedure

i. Dissolve copper sulphate in 100 ml of hot water.
ii. Sodium citrate and sodium carbonate anhydrous are dissolved in 800 ml of water with the aid of heat. Cool and pour into the first solution and make the final volume to one litre.

Principle of Benedict's Test

The principle of the test is based on the property of sugar to reduce copper sulphate in alkaline solution into insoluble cuprous oxide.

Reducing Agents for Benedict's Test

Carbohydrates (such as glucose, fructose, lactose, pentoses) and non-carbohydrates (such as ascorbic acid, salicylates, creatinine and uric acid) are the reducing agents for Benedict's test.

Causes of Glycosuria

Diabetes mellitus

Endocrine disorders—acromegaly, Cushing's syndrome, hyperthyroidism, pancreatic tumours

CNS disorders—haemorrhage/tumours.

Asphyxia, metabolic disturbances, burns, infection

Drugs—oral contraceptives, thiazides, steroids
Renal tubular dysfunction and lead poisoning.

Other sugars in urine

Fructose

- Appears in urine in fructose intolerance, liver and kidney diseases, increased fruits intake
- Fructose can be detected by Selivanoff's test.

Galactose—appears in urine in patients with deficiency of galactokinase enzyme (galactose intolerance).

Lactose—appears in urine in lactose intolerance and also observed in pregnancy and lactational period.

Maltose

Pentose

Sucrose—This is not reduced by Benedict's test.

Lactose and maltose (osazone test): These react with phenylhydrazine hydrochloride in acidic medium and after placing in boiling water bath to form characteristic phenyl hydrazone crystals. Lactose gives lactosazone crystals which are different from crystals formed by maltose.

Galactose: Orthotoluidine test is done only if lactose and glucose are absent in urine since they also react with orthotoluidine.

Principle: Orthotoluidine reacts with oxidase enzyme in acidic medium to form green coloured compound.

Fructose: Selivanoff's test

Resorcinol (Selivanoff's) reagent: It is prepared by dissolving 50 mg of resorcinol in 33 ml of concentrated hydrochloric acid and diluted to 100 ml with distilled water.

Hydrochloric acid reacts with fructose to form furfuraldehyde which gives red coloured compound linked to resorcinol.

Procedure: Take 5 ml of Selivanoff's reagent in a test tube; add 0.5 ml of urine. Place in a boiling water bath for 5 minutes. Change of colour to red indicates presence of fructose.

Tests for Ketone Bodies (Fig. 2.3)

Due to the defect in carbohydrate metabolism, the body tends to metabolise increasing amount of free fatty acids. In this process, intermediate products of fat metabolism are formed. They are acetone (2%), acetoacetic acid (20%) and β-hydroxybutyric acid (78%). Acetone is formed non-reversibly from acetoacetic acid and β-hydroxybutyric acid reversibly from acetoacetic acid.

Acetoacetic acid $\xrightarrow{-CO_2}$ acetone

Acetoacetic acid $\xrightleftharpoons[-2H]{+2H}$ β-hydroxybutyric acid

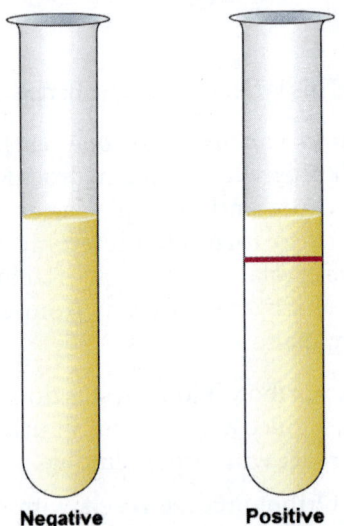

Negative   Positive

Fig. 2.3: Rothera's test

Rothera's Test

Principle: Rothera's test is based on the principle that sodium nitroprusside reacts with acetone and acetoacetic acid to produce a coloured compound.

Procedure: Take 5 ml of urine in a test tube; fully saturate the urine with ammonium sulphate. Add 1–2 crystals of sodium nitroprusside or 1–2 drops of freshly prepared solution. Add liquor ammonia by the side of the test tube. Permanganate (purple) coloured ring indicates positive test.

Gerhardt's Test

This test is positive for acetoacetic acid/β-hydroxybutyric acid. This test is done on fresh sample of urine as acetoacetic acid is converted to acetone on standing.

Add 10% $FeCl_3$ solution drop by drop to 5 ml of urine in a test tube. A precipitate of ferric phosphate usually forms but disappears when more $FeCl_3$ is added. The colour becomes brownish red if acetoacetic acid/β-hydroxybutyric acid or both are present.

Boiling of urine for 5 minutes before adding $FeCl_3$ destroys acetoacetic acid. Therefore, urine which has been boiled and still gives a positive test is not due to acetoacetic acid or β-hydroxybutyric acid.

Other tests: To demonstrate acetoacetic acid—Lindeman's test and for β-hydroxybutyric acid—Hart's test are done.

Causes of ketonuria: Some of the causes include diabetes mellitus with complications, anorexia, starvation, fasting, fever and prolonged vomiting.

Tests for Detection of Haematuria/Myoglobinuria/Haemoglobinuria

Benzidine Test (Fig. 2.4)

Principle: Peroxidase activity of haemoglobin decomposes hydrogen peroxide so as to liberate nascent oxygen which oxidises benzidine to produce a green blue compound.

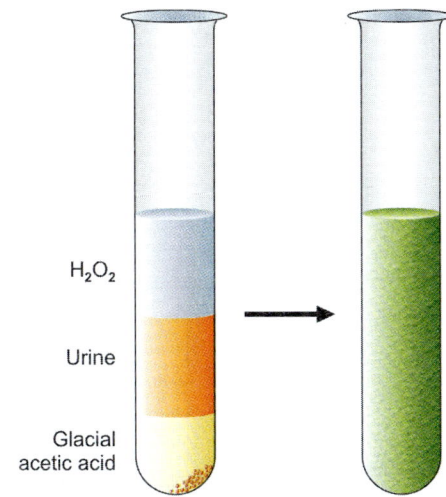

Fig. 2.4: Benzidine test

Procedure: Take pinch of benzidine powder in a test tube and add about 1 ml of glacial acetic acid; further add 2 ml of urine followed by 2 ml of hydrogen peroxide. The resulting blue or green colour indicates positive test. The test is positive for presence of RBCs as well as myoglobin and haemoglobin.

Causes of haematuria

Prerenal causes: Some of the causes include fever, hypertension and exercise.

Renal causes: Some of the causes are congenital anomalies, polycystic kidney, calculi, infections—tuberculosis, Wilms' tumour, trauma, oxaluria, radiation damage and analgesic nephropathy.

Postrenal causes

Ureter	Trauma, calculi, infection
Tumours	Papilloma, carcinoma
Prostate	Benign prostatic hyperplasia, carcinoma
Bladder	Diverticula, trauma, infection
Urethra	Calculi, tumours, ulcers
Parasites	Schistosomiasis, filariasis

Haemoglobinuria: Haemoglobinuria indicates intravascular hemolysis. Haemoglobin binds to plasma haeptoglobin and the excess free haemoglobin would pass through the glomerulus. Haemoglobin is subsequently reabsorbed by the PCT, where it can be catabolised to ferritin and haemosiderin. Haemosiderin usually will be present in urine two to three days after a haemolytic episode.

Causes: Some of the causes include haemolytic anaemia, snake venom poisoning, bacterial toxins and malaria.

Myoglobinuria: Myocardial infarction, skeletal muscle trauma/infarcts, crush injury, heat stroke, marathon running and strenuous exercise.

Determination of bile salts, bile pigments, and urobilinogen is useful in the diagnosis of jaundice.

Unconjugated bilirubin does not appear in urine, only conjugated bilirubin appears in urine. The causes of unconjugated hyperbilirubinaemia include:
- Haemolytic anaemia
- Hepatic causes due to impaired hepatic uptake of conjugation of bilirubin as in Gilbert syndrome, Crigler-Najjar syndrome, neonatal jaundice and drugs.

The causes for bilirubin in urine are:
- Obstruction to bile outflow (intra or extrahepatic)
- Hepatocellular diseases—acute viral hepatitis, drug-induced cholestasis, acute alcoholic hepatitis
- Congenital hyperbilirubinaemia as in Dubin Johnson's disease and Rotor's disease.

Note the following:
1. Bilirubin may be found in urine in liver disease and is usually found in patients who have biliary tract obstructions.
2. Bilirubinuria is seen when intracanalicular pressure rises secondary to periportal inflammation, fibrosis or hepatocyte swelling.
3. Gallstones in the common bile duct or carcinoma of the head of pancreas are possible sources of extrahepatic biliary obstruction leading to bilirubinuria.

4. Conjugated bilirubin appearing in urine generally indicates that there is excess conjugated bilirubin in bloodstream.
5. Congenital hyperbilirubinemia seen in Gilbert's disease or Crigler-Najjar disease.
6. When liver cells are damaged, excretion of urobilinogen in the bile decreased, where as its urinary excretion is increased. This may be seen in cirrhosis, hepatitis and congenital heart failure with congestion of the liver.
7. Excessive urobilinogen also may be found in the urine of those with liver disease or haemolytic disorder.

Urinary findings of bilirubin and urobilinogen in different situations are described in Table 2.1.

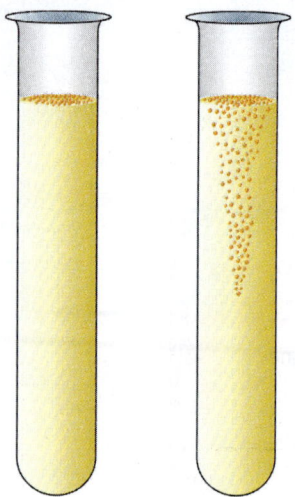

Fig. 2.5: Hay's test

Test for Bile Salts

Hay's Test (Fig. 2.5)

This test detects bile salts in urine.

Principle: The principle of the test is that bile salts reduce surface tension.

Procedure: Sprinkle some amount of sulphur powder on the surface of urine. The sulphur powder sinks to bottom when bile salts are present.

Tests for Bile Pigments

Fouchet's test: This test detects bile pigments in urine (Fig. 2.6).

Principle: The principle of the test is that barium chloride reacts with sulphates in urine to form barium sulphate precipitate. The bile pigments adhere to this precipitate. Ferric chloride in the Fouchet's reagent oxidises yellow bilirubin in presence of trichloroacetic acid to form green biliverdin.

Procedure: Take 10 ml of urine in a test tube and add 2.5 ml of 10% barium chloride. Then mix and filter, unfold and spread the filter paper on another dry filter paper. Add one to two drops of Fouchet's reagent on the precipitate; the resulting green or blue colour indicates positive test.

Fouchet's reagent
Trichloroacetic acid   25 g
10% ferric chloride   10 ml
Distilled water   100 ml

Dissolve 25 g of trichloroacetic acid in 50 ml of distilled water; and then add 10 ml of 10% ferric chloride and make it to 100 ml.

Gmelin's test: About 5 ml of urine is filtered; add a few drops of fuming nitric acid to the centre of the filter paper. Play of colours, green being prominent, suggests bile pigments (Fig. 2.7). Or

Table 2.1: Urinary findings of bilirubin and urobilinogen in different situations (prehepatic, hepatic and posthepatic conditions)

Condition	Urine bilirubin	Urine urobilinogen
Bile duct obstruction	+ + +	Negative
Liver damage	+ or −	+ +
Haemolytic disease	Negative	+ + +

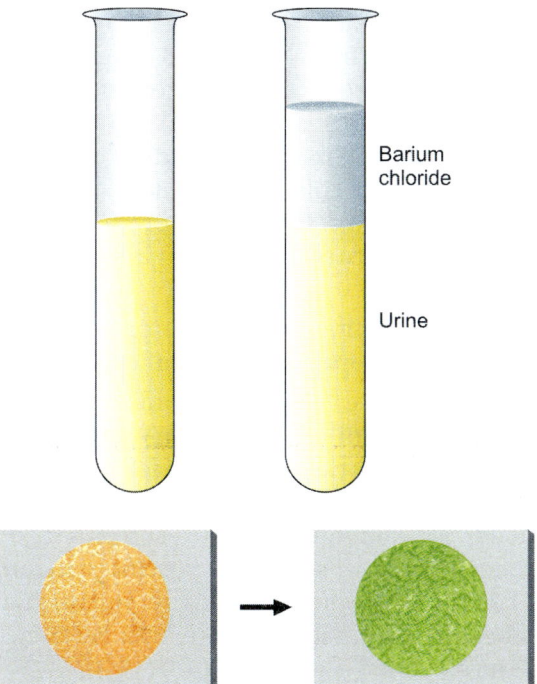

Fig. 2.6.: Fouchet's test (note change of colour after adding Fouchet's reagent to the precipitate on filter paper)

Take 3 ml of concentrated nitric acid and add equal quantity of urine to it. Shake gently; play of colours indicates positive test.

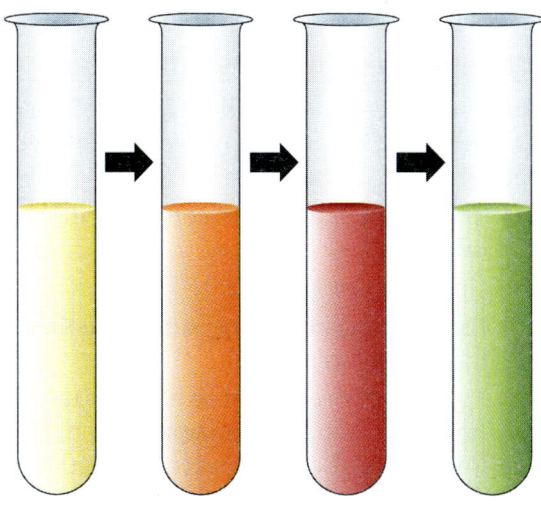

Fig. 2.7: Gmelin's test

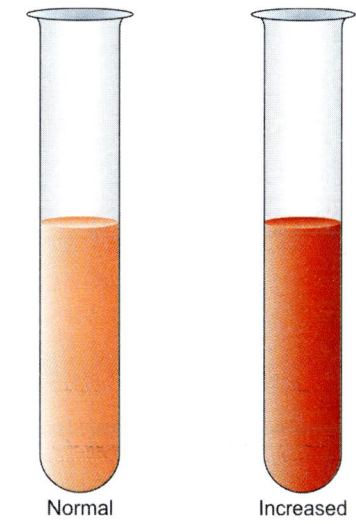

Fig. 2.8: Ehrlich's aldehyde test for urobilinogen

Test for Urobilinogen

Ehrlich's Aldehyde Test (Fig. 2.8)

This test detects urobilinogen in urine.

Principle: The principle of the test is that urobilinogen reacts with p-dimethyl aminobenzaldehyde in acidic media to form pink coloured compound.

Test is conducted on fresh sample of urine. If delayed, then urobilinogen will oxidise to urobilin.

Procedure: Add 1 ml of Ehrlich's aldehyde to 10 ml of fresh urine and mix well. Allow it to stand for 3 to 5 minutes.

Results: The normal urine gives pink colour. Distinct red colour suggests increased amounts of urobilinogen. For semiquantitative assessments, test is done in 1:10, 1:20, 1:40, 1:80 and 1:160 dilutions. Normal urine gives positive test for urobilinogen up to 1:10 dilution.

Ehrlich's reagent
p-dimethyl aminobenzaldehyde   2.0 g
50% (v/v) hydrochloric acid   100.0 ml

Dissolve the above ingredients and store in a brown coloured bottle.

Urobilinogen and porphobilinogen produce similar results (Fig. 2.9). Hence, when

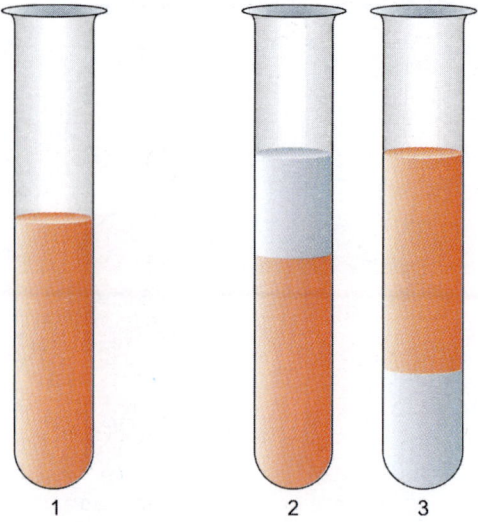

Fig. 2.9: Test for porphobilinogen (tube 2 pink colour in chloroform layer indicates urobilinogen, tube 3 extraction of pink colour in butanol indicates porphobilinogen)

Porphobilinogen is suspected in urine further testing with Watson-Schwartz test is necessary. To the above add 1–2 ml of chloroform and shake for 2 minutes and allow it to stand. Pink colour in the chloroform layer indicates Urobilinogen while pink colour in the aqueous layer indicates presence of porphobilinogen. Further the aqueous layer taken in another test tube and shaken with butanol. Extraction of pink layer into butanol layer suggests porphobilinogen.

MICROSCOPY

Microscopic examination is an important component of urine analysis which is highly informative and continues to be an undisputed discipline in urine analysis.

Alfred Donne in 1837 used microscope and observed pus cells in urine. Centrifuged sample of the urine should contain all the insoluble materials that have accumulated in the urine following glomerular filtration and during the passage of fluid through the renal tubule and lower urinary tract.

Cellular elements may be from the following sources.

The desquamated/spontaneously exfoliated epithelial cells from kidney and lower urinary tract, cells from haematogenous origin (leukocytes and erythrocytes), cellular and non-cellular elements formed in the renal tubules and the collecting tubules, organisms and neoplastic cells may be present which necessitates further investigation of the case.

Casts and crystals may be present with variable clinicopathologic significance.

The reference values of the formed elements may vary from one laboratory to another because of variation in concentration of random urine specimen and different methods used to concentrate the sediment by centrifugation. There is no specific standard procedure as such and the individual laboratories establish their own reference values.

Caution for Microscopic Urine Examination

i. Examination of fresh sample is preferred.
ii. Time of examination should not exceed 1 to 1 ½ hours after collection.
iii. If delay is expected then refrigeration is necessary for delayed examination.
iv. Midstream collection is recommended, especially for females to reduce vaginal contamination.

PREPARATION OF URINE SEDIMENT

Different procedures are adopted for sediment preparation. One of the procedures is given below:

i. Take 10 ml of urine in a conical centrifuge tube.
ii. Centrifuge at 1500–2000 RPM × 5 minutes
iii. Discard 9 ml and reconstitute the sediment in the remaining 1 ml.
iv. Put a drop of sediment on a slide, examine under 10X and 40X magnification with lowered condenser. Under subdued light casts, crystals and mucous threads are better and clearly appreciated.

To study the formed elements, crystal violet-safranin stain/methylene blue/ toluidine blue stain can be used.

a. 2% solution of methylene blue, 0.1 to 0.5% of toluidine blue can be used.
   One drop of stain is mixed with one drop of sediment on a slide and observed.
b. Crystal violet—safranin stain:

Solution I:

Crystals violet	3.0 g
Ethyl alcohol (95%)	20.0 ml
Ammonium oxalate	0.8 g

Solution II

Safranin-O	1.0 g
Ethyl alcohol (95%)	40.0 ml
Distilled water	400.0 ml

3 parts of solution I and 97 parts of solution II are mixed and filtered. Add 1 to 2 drops to 1 ml of sediment, mix well and observe under microscope.

c. Several commercially available stains can be used.

CELL COUNT

The cell count can be done by any of the two methods:
1. Semiquantitative count
2. Precise count

Semiquantitative count depends upon the number of cells in any average high power field, i.e. 40X (40 magnification).

Normal values
Red cells 0 to 2/HPF
Leukocytes 3 to 5/HPF
Epithelial cells 3 to 5/HPF

For precise count the haemocytometer is used to quantify the elements in urine. The cells and casts from undiluted and well-mixed urine are counted.

Thomas Addis' procedure to count the cellular elements can also be followed.

Normal values

Leukocytes	5 to 30/ml
Red cells	3 to 20/ml
Casts	1 to 2/ml

Microscopic Components in Urine Sediment (Fig. 2.10)

Cells

1. *Erythrocytes*
   - These cells appear as biconcave discs, about 7 μ in diameter and do not contain nuclei
   - In hypotonic urine, cells swell and lyse, and the lysed cells may appear as ghost cells. Further, these red cells crenate in hypertonic urine.

2. *Leukocytes*
   - Normal urine may contain 2–3 plus cells/HPF
   - These cells are mostly neutrophils
   - Lymphocytes, mononuclear cells and eosinophils may be found in some instances.

3. *Epithelial cells*

   Squamous epithelial cells
   - These cells are commonly found and are large, flat and polygonal in shape
   - They have abundant cytoplasm and small central nuclei.

4. *Transitional epithelial cells*

   These cells are peer/round in shape and are two to four times as large as white cells.

5. *Tubular epithelial cells*
   - These cells are larger than leukocytes and contain a large round nucleus
   - These cells may be cuboidal, flat or columnar.

CASTS

These are colourless gels, the matrix is formed by Tamm-Horsfall protein in which entrapped are the cells, cell fragments or granular material. This Tamm-Horsfall protein is secreted by the thick part of ascending loop of Henle and possibly by the distal convoluted tubule. These can be:

1. Matrix casts consisting of hyaline casts and waxy casts.
2. Inclusion casts consisting of granular casts, fatty casts and crystal casts.

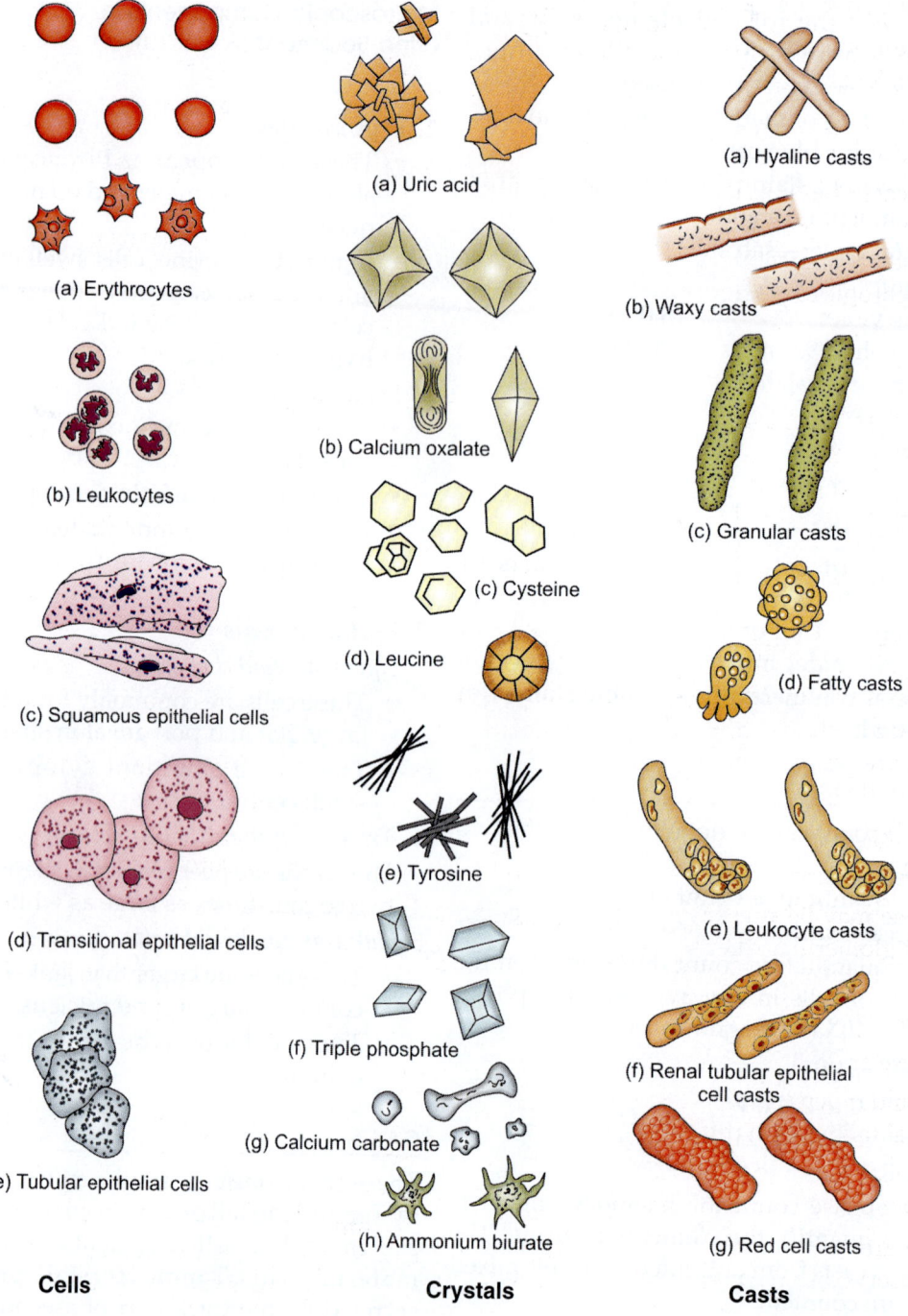

Fig. 2.10: Microscopy of urinary sediment, note different types of cells, casts, and crystals

3. Pigmented casts consisting of haemoglobin casts, myoglobin casts and bilirubin casts.

4. Cellular casts consisting of erythrocyte casts, leukocyte casts, tubular epithelial cell casts and mixed cellular casts.

Hyaline Casts

Hyaline casts are found in renal diseases, exercise, fever, CCF and even in dehydration.

Waxy Casts

Waxy casts have smooth margins and are convoluted along the lateral margins.

These are increased in tubular inflammation or chronic renal failure and graft rejection.

Granular Casts

- These casts have coagulated proteins with granules representing cells, plasma proteins and cell remnants
- These are observed in pyelonephritis, viral infections, renal papillary necrosis and chronic lead poisoning.

Fatty Casts

- In these casts, fatty material is incorporated
- They are observed in nephrotic syndrome and are positive for fat stains.

Haemoglobin Casts

- These casts are red to yellow coloured
- These may be present in tubular bleeding and glomerular diseases.

Myoglobin Casts

- These are reddish brown casts
- Found in acute muscular damage and acute renal failure.

Bilirubin Casts

These are deep yellow brown in colour and are observed in biliary obstructive diseases.

Erythrocyte Casts

- In these casts, the RBCs should be sharply defined in at least one part of the cast.
- With stasis, erythrocytes may degenerate and appear as granular haemoglobin casts.

Leukocyte Casts

- These are refractile, exhibit granules with visible nuclei.
- These are observed in pyelonephritis.

Renal Tubular Epithelial Cell Casts

These are observed in acute tubular necrosis viral disease and graft rejection

CRYSTALS

A. Crystals Present in Acidic Urine

Uric acid crystals

- These are diamond/rhombic-shaped or in rosette form, soluble in sodium hydroxide.
- Found normally.
- Encountered in pathological conditions such as gout, chronic nephritis, increased nucleoprotein turnover during chemotherapy of leukaemia/lymphoma.

Calcium oxalate crystals

- These are small, colourless, octohedran shaped and resemble envelope
- These crystals appear in urine with increased intake of cabbage and asparagus
- These are observed in pathological conditions such as chronic renal disease.

Amorphous urates

- These are urate salts of sodium, potassium, calcium and magnesium
- These are yellow red granules
- These are soluble in alkali.

Cysteine crystals

- These are colourless, refractile hexagonal plates
- These are soluble with hydrochloric acid and ammonia
- These crystals are observed in pathological condition like congenital cystinosis.

Leucine crystals

- These are oily, refractile spheroids, with radial and concentric striations
- These crystals are observed in pathological conditions such as hepatitis and maple syrup urine disease.

Tyrosine crystals
- These are fine, refractile needles and in clusters or sheaves
- These are soluble with ammonium hydroxide and are observed in pathological conditions such as tyrosinosis and severe liver diseases.

B. Crystals Found in Alkaline Urine

Triple phosphate crystals
- These are colourless prisms with 3–6 sides and are soluble in acetic acid
- These are found in normal urine and observed in pathological condition such as infections of urinary tract.

Amorphous phosphates
These are granular in appearance and dissolve with acetic acid.

Calcium carbonate crystals
These are uncommon crystals but are colourless, dumb-bell or spherical shapes and are soluble in acetic acid.

Calcium phosphate crystals
These are long, thin and colourless crystals and are soluble in acetic acid.

Ammonium biurate crystals
These are yellow brown, spherical bodies with long irregular spicules (thorn apples) and are soluble in acetic acid.

Parasites found in urine
- *Trichomonas vaginalis* trophozoites
- *Enterobius vermicularis* ova
- *Schistosoma haematobium* ova.

Use of Bright Field Microscopy, Phase Contrast Microscopy and Polarised Microscopy

Bright field microscopy is performed up to a limited extent on unstained urine preparations. Identification of leukocytes, epithelial cells and cellular casts may be difficult; under subdued light hyaline casts, crystals and mucous threads can be well-delineated.

Phase contrast microscopy is beneficial in detection of translucent formed elements, notably casts.

Polarised microscopy is used to identify crystals.

EXAMINATION BY REAGENT STRIPS

These are plastic strips on which cellulose areas are impregnated with some specific testing chemicals according to the test to be conducted. The advantages of chemical examination of urine by strip method are as follows:
- Gives quick screening of the tests
- The method is fast
- The method is reliable and sensitive
- The procedure avoids corrosive reagents, glass and other materials required for chemical testing
- The procedure can be performed on uncentrifuged urine.

Reagent Strip for Glucose

Glucose of about 100 mg/dl is detected by strip method. Glucose oxidase acts on glucose, removes 2 H ions and forms glucuronolactone which is later hydrated to gluconic acid. The removed hydrogen ions combine with atmospheric oxygen and form hydrogen peroxide. The resulting hydrogen peroxide in the presence of peroxidase, oxidize ortho-toluidine (clinistix) which in oxidized state turns blue.

$$\text{Glucose} + O_2 \xrightarrow{\text{Glucose oxidase}} \text{Gluconic acid} + H_2O_2$$

$$H_2O_2 + \text{Chromogen} \xrightarrow{\text{Peroxidase}} \text{Oxidised chromogen} + H_2O$$

Multistix strips utilise potassium iodide chromogen and the colour changes from blue to a brown colour after 30 seconds.

Chemstrip utilises aminopropyl carbazol chromogen and the colour changes from yellow to orange brown after 60 seconds.

Reagent Strip for Proteins

Proteins are tested on the basis of protein-error of pH indicators. In the presence of proteins there is colour reaction.

The reagent strip is impregnated with tetrabromophenol blue buffered to an acid pH of 3 or with tetrachlorophenol-tetrabromo-sulphophthalein.

In the absence of protein, the strip is yellow. As a result of urine application, in 30–60 seconds variable shades of green or blue colour develop depending on the type and concentration of proteins present and results can be read as negative, trace, 1+ to 4+.

Most methods detect 5 to 20 mg of albumin per decilitre. Trace amounts may be observed with physiological normal excretion of protein in concentrated urine specimens from any healthy individuals.

High salt content will lower the results. Alkaline and highly buffered urine samples may yield a positive result in the absence of significant proteinuria.

Reagent Strip for Ketone Bodies

Chem strips containing sodium nitroferricyanide and glycine react with acetoacetic acid and acetone in alkaline medium to form violet dye. The change of colour is from beige to violet, read after 60 seconds.

This method detects 10 mg/dl of acetoacetic acid and 70 mg/dl of acetone.

Multistix contains buffers and sodium ferricyanide which react with acetoacetic acid producing pink colour in 15 seconds. This detects 5–10 mg/dl of acetoacetic acid but does not detect acetone.

Strip for Haemoglobin and Myoglobin

The principle in this case is based on the liberation of oxygen from hydrogen peroxide in the reagent strip by peroxidase like activity of haem in free haemoglobin, lysed RBCs or myoglobin. The reagent strip is impregnated with buffered mixture of peroxide and the chromogen tetramethylbenzidine.

$$H_2O_2 + \text{Chromogen} \underset{\text{Peroxidase activity}}{\overset{\text{Haem}}{\rightleftarrows}} \text{Oxidized chromogen} + H_2O_2$$

Multistix and chemstrip detect 0.05 to 0.3 mg haemoglobin/dl.

Haemoglobin 0.3 mg/dl is equivalent to 10 lysed erythrocytes.

Strip for Bilirubin and Urobilinogen

Bilirubin: In this case, urine should be fresh as urine quickly hydrolyses to less reactive free bilirubin. However, it is pertinent to remember that oxidisation of bilirubin in specimens that stood long-time or exposed to sunlight result in false negative results.

False positivity is observed with drugs such as phenazopyridine because it renders reddish colour to the strip; rifampicin and chlorpromazine metabolites also cause false positivity. Urobilinogen does not affect the test.

Strip test utilises the coupling reaction of bilirubin with diazonium salt in an acid medium. Multistix uses diazotinised 2,4, dichloroaniline as the diazo salt with a colour change from cream buff to tan after 20 seconds. The test detects 0.8 mg bilirubin/dl urine.

Chem strip utilises 2, 6 dichlorobenzene diazonium tetrafluoroborate and the colour change is from pink to violet after 30–60 seconds. The test detects 0.5 mg bilirubin/dl urine.

Urobilinogen: Acid buffer and p-dimethyl-amino benzaldehyde used in this test produces reddish brown colour with urobilinogen.

Exercise 24

Pregnancy Test

Purpose: To detect human chorionic gonadotropin (HCG).

HCG is a glycoprotein produced by the trophoblastic cells. In pregnancy, HCG is produced from these cells by about 10 days of conception.

Methods: There are two methods: Bioassays and Immunoassays.

Bioassays

1. *Ascheim and Zondek test (1928):* In this test, five immature mice of 21 days old and 5 to 7 g in weight are injected with patient's urine for 2 days. Four days after the first injection, animal is sacrificed and the ovaries are inspected for haemorrhagic follicles and corpus luteum.
2. *Friedman test (1931):* In this test mature female rabbit is injected intravenously with patient's urine. After 48 hours, the animal is sacrificed and ovaries are inspected for corpus luteum and haemorrhagic follicles.
3. *Toad test (1934, Bellarby):* In this test, toads deposit eggs within 24 hours after injection with HCG containing urine.
4. *Galli Mainini test (1948):* In this test, in 4 to 6 hours after injection with HCG, male frogs release sperms.

Disadvantages

1. Animals are relatively insensitive and need higher concentration of HCG.
2. HCG expressed in animals is difficult to compare with humans.

Immunoassays (Fig. 2.11)

One drop of patient's urine and one drop of anti-HCG are mixed for one minute. Then add one drop of latex particles coated with HCG. Read the results after 2 minutes. The test is based on latex agglutination inhibition test.

If urine contains HCG, it is neutralized by anti-HCG. No anti-HCG is available for binding with latex particles coated with HCG. Hence, no agglutination is visible.

If there is no HCG in urine, anti-HCG remains unused. HCG coated on latex particles combines with anti-HCG producing agglutination.

Results: Agglutination present—no HCG in urine

Agglutination absent—HCG is present in urine

For immunoassays, the first morning urine sample in a clean, dry and detergent free bottle is needed. Drug excretion in urine, proteinuria and haematuria may give false positive test.

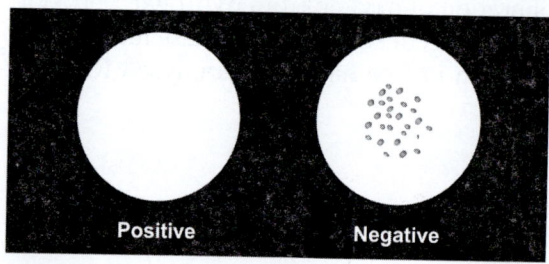

Fig. 2.11: Pregnancy test: Slide method (immunological)

Exercise 25

Semen Analysis

Indications
1. Infertility.
2. To know the effectiveness of vasectomy.

Composition of Seminal Fluid
1. Spermatozoa from testis contribute less than 5% to the seminal volume (Fig. 2.12).
2. Fluid from seminal vesicles forms 60% of the seminal volume. It is alkaline or neutral in reaction, semisolid or viscid. It is a major source of fructose.
3. Prostatic fluid forms 20% of the seminal fluid which is milky coloured and slightly acidic; it is rich in acid phosphatases and proteolytic enzymes (responsible for coagulation and liquefaction of semen).
4. 10–15% of the seminal fluid is contributed by bulbourethral and urethral glands.

During ejaculation all these fluids enter the urethra separately in rapid succession.

First fraction—constitutes fluid from urethra and bulbourethral glands.

Second fraction—constitutes fluid from prostate and spermatozoa from testis.

Third fraction—constitutes fluid from seminal vesicles.

Collection of Semen
Abstinence for 3 days is required for collecting the specimen. It is preferably collected by masturbation/coitus interruptus. It is collected in a clean, detergent free, wide mouthed jar. The time of collection is noted, sample should reach the laboratory within half an hour of collection.

Examination of Semen
Gross examination: When fresh, semen is viscid, opaque and milky white in colour. In 10–20 minutes it liquefies. The time taken for liquefaction should be noted. Reaction is alkaline. Normal quantity of semen is about 1.5 to 5 ml.

Counting of sperms
Reagents and equipment
- Seminal diluting fluid
- Counting chamber and WBC pipette.

Composition of seminal diluting fluid
Sodium bicarbonate   5 g
Formalin   1 ml
Distilled water   100 ml

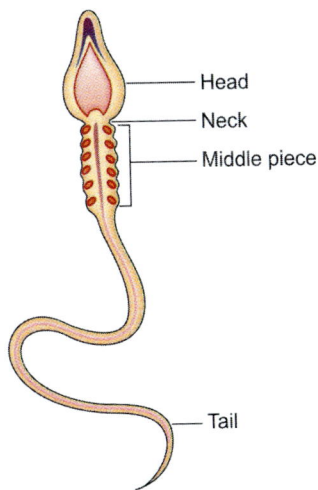

Fig. 2.12: Sperm structure

Procedure

Take semen up to '0.5' mark of the WBC pipette, seminal diluting fluid up to '11' mark and charge the counting chamber. Count the sperms in the corner 4 large squares.

Calculations = $\dfrac{n \times \text{dilution factor}}{\text{Volume of chambers counted}}$

= $n \times 20/0.4 \times 1000$ cells/ml
= $n \times 50{,}000$ cells/ml

(n— no. of sperms counted)

Motility

Take a drop of semen on a clean slide, put a coverslip and observe for motility under microscope.

In fresh sample, about 70–80% of the sperms are actively motile. With the lapse of time gradually motility reduces. Following is the motility with lapse of time.

In 2–4 hours	62% of the sperms are motile
In 6–7 hours	46% of the sperms are motile
In 12 hours	27% of the sperms are motile
In 24 hours	8% of the sperms are motile

Morphology of Sperms (Fig. 2.13)

Make smears with the seminal fluid directly or after saline washing. Stain the smears with Giemsa or Pap stain. Look for the morphology. In normal individuals about 70–80% of the sperms have normal morphology and about 20% of the sperms have abnormal morphology.

Fructose Test (Fig. 2.14)

Take 5 ml of resorcinol reagent and 0.5 ml of semen in test tube. Place in a boiling water bath for 5 minutes or heat on a spirit lamp. Red colour indicates presence of fructose. No change of colour indicates fructose is absent.

Preparation of resorcinol: Dissolve 50 mg of resorcinol in 33 ml of concentrated HCl and dilute to 100 ml with distilled water.

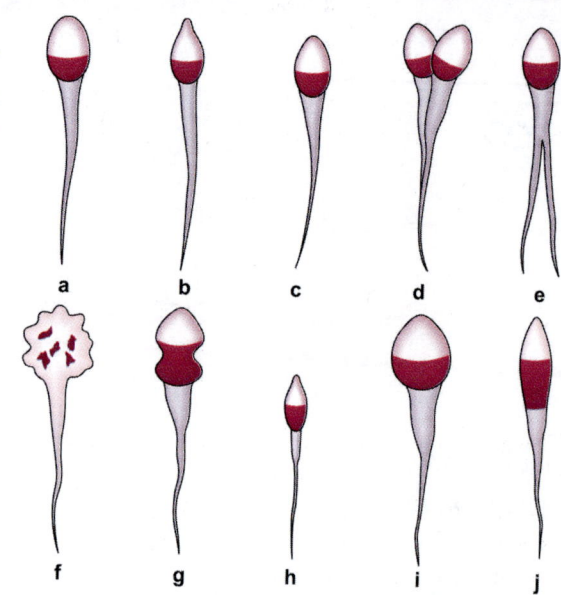

Fig. 2.13: Diagram to show morphology of sperms. a. Normal sperm, face view; b. normal sperm, lateral view; c. spermatid; d. sperm with two heads; e. sperm with two tails; f. amorphous form; g. sperm with constricted neck; h. pin-headed sperm; i. giant-headed sperm; j. acute tapering form

Note: Various procedures are being employed to demonstrate the presence of fructose in semen qualitatively and quantitatively.

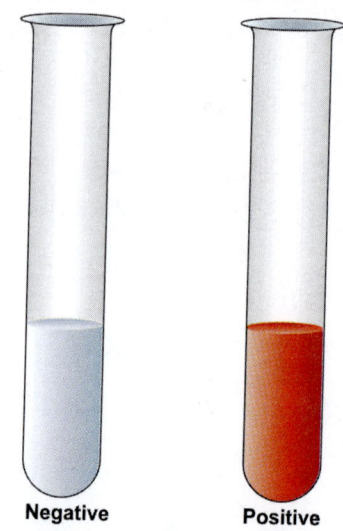

Fig. 2.14: Fructose test

Exercise 26

Glucose Tolerance Test (GTT)

The procedure requires fasting of 12 hours. Stress, emotions and exercise are to be avoided and fasting urine and blood are collected. The patient is given 75 g (75–100 g) of glucose in 200 ml of water. For children 1.75 g/kg body weight (minimum of 10 g and maximum of 50 g) of glucose is given. Blood and urine are collected every half an hour for subsequent 3 hours. Blood glucose and urine sugar are estimated and graph is plotted.

In normal individuals, peak level of blood sugar is reached by 30–60 minutes and reaches the baseline after 2½ hours. In severe diabetics, even after 2–2½ hours the levels remain high.

Preparation of Patient for GTT

For the earlier three days, the patient is kept on adequate carbohydrate diet. On bedridden and operated patients, GTT is not performed. The medication is stopped for one day prior to the day of test. Oral contraceptives are stopped for one cycle.

Indications
- Patients with family history of diabetes
- Obese individuals
- Unexplained weakness and fatigue
- Non-healing ulcers
- Pyoderma.

Renal glycosuria: Blood sugar is normal, there is low renal threshold and glucose appears in urine.

Alimentary glycosuria: After large quantities of carbohydrate diet, sugar appears in urine.

Diabetes of pregnancy

Other causes: Thyrotoxicosis, Cushing's syndrome, pheochromocytoma.

Exercise

27

Fractional Test Meal (FTM)

With the use of fibreoptic instruments, FTM is not routinely done in recent years.

The following procedure is followed:
Minimum of twelve hours fast is required. Introduce the Ryle's tube and collect the fasting gastric juice. Give gruel test meal, start aspirating 10 ml of gastric juice every 15 minutes for 3 hours.

Specimens are labelled and examined for mucous, starch, bile and blood. Free, total and combined acidity are estimated.

Other stimulant test meals
- Riegel meal—200 ml of beef broth
- Alcohol meal—100 ml of 7% alcohol
- Ewald's test meal—two pieces of toast and 8 ounces of tea.

Exercise 28

Renal Function Tests

The renal function tests may be divided into four groups.

A. Clearance Tests

Clearance is measured to assess quantitatively the rate of excretion of any given substance by the kidneys. This constitutes the volume of blood or plasma that contains the amount of substance which is excreted in one minute. The clearance of a substance may be defined as the volume of blood or plasma cleared of the amount of substance found in one minute excretion of urine. The following are the tests to measure the glomerular filtration rate. The different methods are:
- Inulin clearance
- Endogenous creatinine clearance
- Urea clearance.

Inulin Clearance

1. Inulin is a polysaccharide which is filtered at the glomerulus but not secreted or absorbed by the tubule. This is a measure of glomerular filtration rate. Mannitol also can be used for this purpose.
2. These clearances vary with body size.
3. To measure the inulin clearance, maintain a constant plasma level of the test substance during the period of urine collection. The clearance is measured according to the following formula:

$$C_{in} = \frac{U \times V}{P}$$

C_{in} = Clearance of inulin (ml/min)

U = Urinary inulin (mg/100 ml)
V = Volume of urine (ml/min)
P = Plasma inulin (mg/100 ml)

Normal values

Urinary inulin = 35 mg/ml
Blood inulin = 0.25 mg/ml
Volume of urine = 0.9 ml/minute

Inulin clearance = $\frac{35 \times 0.9}{0.25}$ = 125 ml/min

Normal inulin clearance is 120–125 ml/minute for a male of 1.73 m² surface area.

Endogenous Creatinine Clearance

1. Creatinine is filtered at the glomerulus; only marginally secreted by the tubules and its clearance is measured to get the GFR.
2. This method can estimate the GFR without estimation of a test substance.
3. Normal value for creatinine clearance is 95–105 ml/minute.

Urea Clearance

This test is used to appraise the renal function clinically. The subject is given two glasses of water. One hour later, collect a specimen of urine and also a blood sample. Second sample of urine and blood are collected after one more hour and analysed for urea. The normal value of urea clearance is 75 ml/min; it is usually reported as % of normal (75 ml/min). The normal range is 75–120%.

Urea clearance is less than that of inulin and it indicates that some of the filtered urea is reabsorbed by the tubules. With any renal damage, the clearance may fall to 50% or even less.

B. Tests to Measure Tubular Function

    i. Dilution test
   ii. Urine concentration test
  iii. Vasopressin (ADH) test
  iv. Urine acidification test
   v. Phenolsulphonephthalein test (PSP) test.

Dilution Test

Empty the bladder after overnight fast at 7 am in the morning and ask the patient to drink 1200 ml of water in 30 minutes. During the next four hours, urine is collected hourly. The specific gravity should be about 1.003 in at least one of the specimens. In normal individuals, in cold climate almost all the water drank is excreted in 4 hours, whereas some amount of it is lost due to perspiration in hot climate.

With impaired renal function, the amount of water eliminated in four hours will be less than the normal.

Urine Concentration Test

It is carried out as follows: At 7 pm, a meal with good protein content is given to the patient. Fluid given should not be more than 200 ml. No more fluid is given afterwards. Bladder is emptied while going to the bed. On the following day, two samples of urine are collected at 8 am and 9 am and specific gravity is determined. In normal individuals, the specific gravity has to be between 1.018 and 1.022.

If the specific gravity is less than 1.018, it means that the concentrating power of the tubules is impaired. If the volume of urine is large and specific gravity is less, vasopressin test is to be carried out.

Note: There are several concentration tests, e.g. concentration test of Fishberg, Addis test, etc.

Vasopressin Test

Patient is not given any food or water after 6 pm and vasopressin (5 units) is injected intramuscularly/subcutaneously at 7 pm. Next day morning, the urine is collected at 7 am and 8 am and the specific gravity is determined. If the specific gravity is 1.022, the patient is suffering from diabetes insipidus. Vasopressin (ADH) injection is effective in controlling it.

Urine Acidification

This test should not be conducted on patients with acidosis or with poor liver function.

No diet or water restriction is needed. Bladder is emptied at 8 am. Thereafter, hourly sample of urine is collected until 6 pm. At 10 am, ammonium chloride in a dose of 0.1 g/kg body weight is given. Specimen of urine collected is noted for pH immediately.

In normal patients, all samples collected after 2 hours of ammonium chloride administration should have pH of 4.6 to 5.

The Phenolsulphonephthalein (PSP) Test

This is a dye that is completely eliminated within 2 hours. If the dye is retained, then it indicates impairment in kidney function. The test mainly gives measure of secretory capacity of the tubules as well as renal blood flow.

C. Blood or Serum Analysis

Blood non-protein nitrogen (NPN), urea, creatinine, serum total proteins, albumin, globulin and serum cholesterol are often useful to assess renal function.

In acute nephritis NPN values are increased and range from mild increase to very high values. With mild increase, NPN value is 45 mg/dl; urea nitrogen is 25 mg/dl and creatinine 2 mg/dl. With severe increase, NPN rises to as high as 200 mg/dl, urea nitrogen to 60 mg/dl and creatinine 25 mg/dl.

Mild/moderate/severe loss of proteins and raised serum cholesterol are observed in cases of nephritis.

D. Urine Examination

Examination of urine for proteins, cells and casts gives an idea of the disease process.

Exercise 29

Liver Function Tests

The liver has multiple and diverse functions essential for functioning of the whole body. Some of the important functions are:

a. Synthesis of plasma proteins including albumin, globulins, clotting factors and transport proteins. Clotting factors II, VII, IX and X are synthesised in the liver and these need vitamin K for their activation.

b. Synthesis of bile acids from cholesterol; this achieves two purposes.
   1. Cholesterol metabolism is regulated.
   2. Bile acids help in the absorption of dietary fat.

c. Liver is the site for detoxification of many noxious substances.

d. Liver is the site for catabolism of many hormones like thyroid hormones, steroid hormones and some of the polypeptide hormones.

e. It is a site for storage of energy, iron, copper, and vitamin A, D and B_{12}.

f. Liver has metabolic functions of carbohydrates, proteins and fats.

Tests for Liver Function

I. Tests for Bile Secretory Capacity

a. Serum bilirubin

Bilirubin reacts with diazotinised sulphanilic acid to give a red-violet reaction product measured at 540 nm. To obtain a complete reaction use of accelerants such as caffeine, methanol or alcohol is necessary.

Normal values

Total bilirubin	0.1–1.3 mg/dl
Direct bilirubin	0.1–0.4 mg/dl
Indirect bilirubin	0.2–0.8 mg/dl
In haemolytic anaemia	Indirect bilirubin is increased
In obstructive jaundice	Direct bilirubin is increased
In hepatic jaundice	Direct and indirect bilirubin are increased

b. Urobilinogen in urine and in faeces

Urinary and faecal urobilinogen
- Increased in haemolytic anaemia
- Normal or low in obstructive jaundice.

II. Tests for Synthetic Function of Liver

i. Serum or plasma albumin estimation:

Normal value of serum albumin is 3.5 to 5 g/100 ml.

Hepatic failure is associated with low values of serum albumin.

ii. Serum albumin and globulin ratio:

Normal A : G ratio is 1.5 : 1.

In case of liver failure, the proportion of globulin increases.

iii. Electrophoresis of serum proteins reveals that there is relative hypergammaglobulinaemia as gammaglobulins are synthesised by the reticuloendothelial cells, i.e. extrahepatically.

iv. *Clotting factors:* Synthetic function of liver is assessed with coagulation factors already mentioned. A simple test is to determine prothrombin time which is increased in liver failure. Improvement in prothrombin time does not occur even with vitamin K injection.

III. Metabolic Tests

a. *Serum lipids:* Liver failure is associated with decreased values of total serum cholesterol.
b. *Carbohydrate metabolism:* Galactose tolerance test can be done. Ingested galactose is absorbed and reaches the liver via portal venous blood where it is broken down and glucose is released into blood. Normally galactose concentration of blood does not rise after oral ingestion of galactose.

IV. Tests for Detoxification Function of Liver

Hippuric acid test: A dose of sodium benzoate is given and an amount of hippuric acid formed by the reaction of benzoic acid and glycine is determined. 6 g of sodium benzoate is dissolved in 250 ml of water and given orally.

About 3 to 3.5 g of hippuric acid should be excreted in urine in 4 hours duration.

About 1.77 g of sodium benzoate in 20 ml of distilled water is slowly injected intravenously for 5 minutes. Bladder is emptied after one hour. Urine that is excreted should contain 0.7–1.6 g of hippuric acid in one hour duration.

V. Test for Excretory Function of Liver

Bromosulphalein (BSP) test: BSP is a phenolphthalein derivative, about 5 mg/kg body of the dye BSP is given intravenously, it is taken up by the liver and excreted into bile. Normally, after 45 minutes of injection of BSP, there is less than 5% of the original concentration in blood.

In obstructive and hepatic jaundice, the excretion of the dye BSP into bile is unsatisfactory.

VI. Changes in Certain Enzymes

When damage is caused to the liver cells, it would be observed that the enzymes serum aspartate aminotransferase (AST) and alanine aminotransferase (ALT) are increased. Alkaline phosphatase along with gamma glutamyl transferase is increased in biliary obstruction/injury. AST is also called serum glutamate oxaloacetate transaminase (SGOT). Similarly ALT is called serum glutamate pyruvate transaminase (SGPT).

Normal levels

SGOT (AST)	5–45 IU/L
SGPT (ALT)	5–40 IU/L
Alkaline phosphatase	20–80 IU/L (adults)

VII. Other Specific Tests

Alpha fetoproteins	Indicate hepatocellular carcinoma
Serum metals	Elevated iron and decreased iron binding capacity indicate haemosiderosis
	Elevated copper indicates Wilson's disease
	Decreased zinc and magnesium are observed in alcoholic cirrhosis
Vitamins	Decreased vitamin A suggests parenchymal hepatic diseases

Exercise 30

Thyroid Function Tests

The thyroid gland makes two thyroid hormones, triiodothyronine (T_3) and thyroxine (T_4), which circulate in the bloodstream and act on virtually every tissue and cell in the body.

Thyroid hormones affect metabolic rate of the body, brain development, breathing, CVS and CNS functions, body temperature, muscle strength, skin dryness, menstrual cycle, weight, cholesterol levels, and so on. It plays an important role in the development of foetus and growth in the children.

Thyroid hormone production in the thyroid is regulated by another hormone called thyroid-stimulating hormone (TSH). TSH is made by the pituitary gland, which is located in the brain. From the pituitary gland, TSH initiates proteolysis of thyroglobulin and releases T_3 and T_4 into the bloodstream. About 93% of the hormone is T_4 and only 7% is T_3. In tissues T_4 is converted to T_3 and this T_3 hormone is active than T_4. The conditions and variations of these hormones are given in Table 2.2.

TSH

Blood levels of TSH is sensitive to evaluate thyroid function.

The normal range for TSH is between 0.3 and 4 mIU/L.

In people whose thyroid produces too much T_3 and T_4, the pituitary shuts down TSH production, leading to low or even undetectable TSH levels in the blood. An abnormally low TSH level suggests hyperthyroidism.

In people whose thyroid is not functioning normally and produces too little thyroid hormones (T_3 and T_4), the thyroid cannot respond normally to TSH by producing thyroid hormone. As a result, the pituitary keeps making TSH, trying to get the thyroid to respond. An abnormally high TSH level suggests hypothyroidism.

Occasionally, a low TSH level and Low T_4 can indicate a type of hypothyroidism called secondary hypothyroidism. This type of hypothyroidism is due to an abnormality in the pituitary that prevents it from making enough TSH to stimulate thyroid hormone production.

T_4

T_4 is the principal thyroid hormone and exists in two forms—T_4 that is bound to proteins in the blood and kept in reserve until the body needs it, and a small amount of unbound or "free" T_4 (FT_4), which is the active form of the hormone and is available to body tissues.

The normal range for total T_4 bound and free together is usually about 5.1–14.1 µg/dl. The normal FT_4 range is about 0.7 to 1.8 nanograms per deciliter (ng/dL).

Elevated total T_4 or FT_4 suggests hyperthyroidism, and low total T_4 or FT_4 suggests hypothyroidism.

Table 2.2: TSH, T_3, T_4 and the conditions

TSH	T_4	T_3	Condition
High	Normal	Normal	Subclinical hypothyroidism
High	Low	Low/normal	Hypothyroidism
Low	Normal	Normal	Subclinical hyperthyroidism
Low	High	High	Hyperthyroidism
Low	Low/normal	Low/normal	Pituitary disorder (secondary hypothyroidism)

Elevated TSH levels with normal T_4 levels indicate primary hypothyroidism.

T_3

T_3 is far more active than T_4 and, like T_4, exists in both bound and free states. In some cases of hyperthyroidism, FT_4 is normal but free T_3 (FT_3) is elevated, so measuring both forms is useful if hyperthyroidism is suspected.

The normal range of total T_3 bound and free together is 85–202 µg/dl.

The normal FT_3 range is about 0.2 to 0.5 ng/dL. In severe hypothyroidism T_3 is the last one to become abnormal. Thus, high TSH, low T_4 and normal T_3 can be expected in some hypothyroid states.

In pregnancy and patients on oral pills, high T_3 and T_4 levels can exist as oestrogen increases the levels of binding proteins. In such situations ask for TSH and free T_4 levels.

Thyroid-stimulating Immunoglobulin (TSI)

TSI is an autoantibody present in Graves' disease, the most common cause of hyperthyroidism. TSI mimics TSH by stimulating the thyroid cells, causing the thyroid gland to secrete excess hormone. The TSI circulating in the blood and is usually measured in specific instances in people with Graves' disease or when the diagnosis is obscure or during pregnancy.

Antithyroid Antibodies

Various antithyroid antibodies are present in Hashimoto's disease, the most common cause of hypothyroidism.

Antithyroid antibodies are markers in the blood, and their presence is extremely helpful in diagnosing Hashimoto's disease. Two main types of antithyroid antibodies are:

1. Anti-thyroglobulin antibodies, which attack a protein in the thyroid called thyroglobulin.
2. Anti-thyroperoxidase, or anti-TPO, antibodies, which attack an enzyme in thyroid cells called thyroperoxidase.

Exercise 31

Instruments

Bone Marrow Aspiration Needle (Fig. 2.15)

There are different types of bone marrow needles, e.g. Osgood's needle, Jamshidi needle and so on. The bone marrow needle is a short and stout needle with well-fitted stylet and an adjustable guard. The needle edge is bevelled. Total length of the needle is about 5 cm. The guard is adjustable and useful in adjusting the depth of the piercing portion of the needle. The length has to be more in obese patients and less in thin individuals. The needle is sterilised by autoclaving or by dry sterilisation in hot air oven. Sites of bone marrow aspiration depend upon the age of the patients and the presence of red marrow in those areas. The preferred sites are:

a. In infants—tibial tuberosity.
b. Older children and adults—anterior surface of sternum, manubrium, anterior and posterior iliac spines.
c. In old age people—spinous processes of vertebrae.

In infants, red marrow will be in all the bones and safer will be the tibial tuberosity.

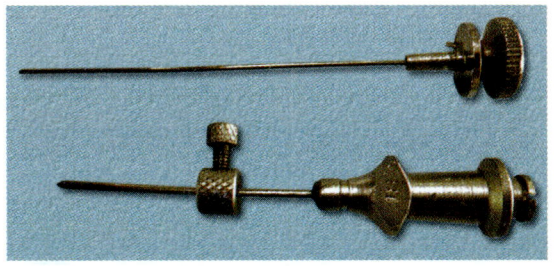

Fig. 2.15: Bone marrow aspiration needle

In older children and adults tibial tuberosity will be more thickened and hence sternum, manubrium, anterior and posterior iliac spines are preferred.

Indications
- Anaemias: Megaloblastic anaemia, aplastic anaemia and sideroblastic anaemia
- Leukaemia: Aleukaemic leukaemia
- Leukaemoid reaction
- Metastatic lesion
- Multiple myeloma
- Thrombocytopaenia
- Unexplained leukopaenia
- Unexplained fever
- Parasitic infections.

Contraindications
- Haemophilia
- Local sepsis
- In patient's with aortic aneurysm, marrow aspiration of sternum is contraindicated.

Procedure
Place the patient in the required position. If the site of aspiration is sternum, anterior iliac crest or upper end of tibia, the patient has to be in supine position. For posterior iliac crest or spinous process, the patient has to be in the lateral position.

The area of aspiration is shaved and cleaned with suitable antiseptics and draped. The bone marrow needle should be sterilised and kept ready. For sterilisation, autoclaving or hot air sterilisation could be used.

The skin, subcutaneous tissue and periosteum are infiltrated with 2% xylocaine as local anaesthesia. While injecting local anaesthesia, the depth of the piercing portion of the needle is approximately estimated. Another 0.2 to 0.4 mm is added (to pierce the cortical bone) for the above evaluated depth and then the guard is adjusted. It is roughly about 1 cm in adults and 0.2 to 0.6 cm in children.

With screwing movements, the needle is pierced and when the needle is in the marrow cavity a 'give way' sensation is felt.

Remove the stylet and aspirate about 0.3 to 0.5 ml of marrow material. If one tries to aspirate more marrow material, it may get contaminated with blood. Check for the marrow particles and if the marrow particles are present put the stylet back and take out the needle proper along with the stylet.

Preparation of Marrow Smears

Various methods as mentioned below are followed for the preparation of marrow smears.

1. Place the cleaned slides in a slant position. On these slides, place a drop of marrow material. If any blood is present it has to be drained off so that only marrow particles would remain behind. Then take one more slide and press slowly on the marrow material and take them apart.
2. Blow out the marrow material in a watch glass containing normal saline, then decant the supernatant and prepare the smears with the sediment particles similar to the earlier mentioned procedure.
3. Place a drop of marrow on a clean glass slide and make smears similar to the peripheral smears.

To conclude that the marrow aspirate is satisfactory:
a. The marrow should not be blood contaminated.
b. All the marrow elements should be present and should have been distributed in a single layer.
c. The cells should not be damaged during the preparation of the smears.

At the hands of any experienced person, if the marrow material cannot be aspirated, it is concluded as 'dry tap'. The reasons for dry tap can be:
a. Marrow is highly cellular as in leukaemia or
b. Marrow is replaced by fibrosis or it could be a case of
c. Aplastic anaemia

In such cases, trephine biopsy is recommended.

The complications of bone marrow aspiration are almost nil. However, infection in the form of osteomyelitis and injury to the skin and subcutaneous tissue are the rare possibilities.

Lumbar Puncture Needle (Fig. 2.16)

The instrument used for lumbar puncture is a long, flexible needle, 10 to 12 cm in length and of 17 to 20 gauge. It has two components, the hollow needle and the stylet. Both of these have bevelled edges. The stylet has a hub/pin which fits into the notch at the head portion of the hollow needle. The needle is made of platinum or German alloy. The needle is sterilised by autoclaving.

Sites of Lumbar Puncture

In adults: Intervertebral space between L3 and L4

In children: Intervertebral space between L4 and L5

Cerebrospinal fluid can be also obtained by other procedures:
  i. Cisternal puncture

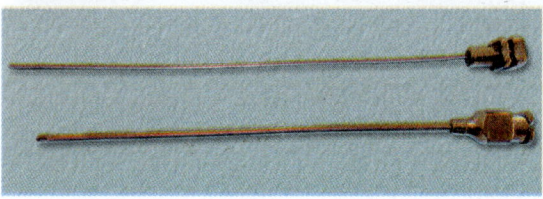

Fig. 2.16: Lumbar puncture needle

ii. Shunt drainage
iii. Directly from the ventricles

Indications
1. *Diagnostic purposes*
   - *Absolute*
     Meningitis
     Subarachnoid haemorrhage
   - *Relative*
     Neurosyphilis
     Unexplained coma
     GB syndrome
     Multiple sclerosis.
2. *Radiological purposes*
   Myelography
   Pneumoencephalography.
3. *Therapeutic purposes*
   To introduce drugs
   i. Methotrexate in leukaemia
   ii. Gentamycin in gram-negative meningitis
   iii. Crystalline penicillin in pyogenic meningitis.
   To reduce raised intracranial pressure in hypertensive encephalopathy.
4. *Anaesthetic purposes*

Procedure: The patient is put in lateral position with knees drawn up and the head flexed. It can also be done in sitting with bending position. The site of lumbar puncture is identified.

About 5 ml of 2% lignocaine as local anaesthetic agent is infiltrated up to ligamentum flava. After 2 to 3 minutes a sterile lumbar puncture needle with stylet in position is introduced. When the needle is in the subarachnoid space a 'give way' sensation is felt.

The stylet is then withdrawn and about 1 to 2 ml of cerebrospinal fluid (CSF) is collected slowly in three different bulbs for cytological, microbiological and biochemical examination.

The needle is withdrawn and puncture site is sealed with tincture benzoin seal. The patient is advised to take plenty of oral fluids; headlow position is insisted upon to prevent headache.

Other uses of needle
i. For obtaining aspirates from deep seated masses and organs under ultrasonographic guidance
ii. For carotid angiography
iii. For splenoportogram
iv. For tapping fluids from serous cavities, e.g. ascitic fluid, pleural fluid.

Fundoscopy should be necessarily done prior to lumbar puncture to rule out raised intracranial tension.

Contraindications
i. Raised intracranial pressure with papilloedema has risk of herniation of brain through foramen magnum and this could damage to medullary centres causing death.
ii. Skin infection at the site of lumbar puncture.
iii. Bony deformities at the site of puncture.
iv. Suspected cord compression.

Complications
i. Meningitis
ii. Headache and backache
iii. Paraplegia due to trauma to the spinal cord
iv. Medullary herniation leading to death.

Normal composition of CSF, its findings in different types of meningitis and for other details refer to CSF cytology.

Liver Biopsy Needle (vim Silverman's needle)

The instrument consists of three parts (Fig. 2.17): They are:
1. An outer cannula
2. A trocar
3. A bifid needle

The liver biopsy needle is a stout needle of 16 gauge. The cannula and trocar have bevelled edges. The bifid needle is longer than the other two parts. The trocar and outer cannula are of the same length. The bifid needle cuts the biopsy and holds it by the bifid end. The bifid needle is introduced after removing the trocar.

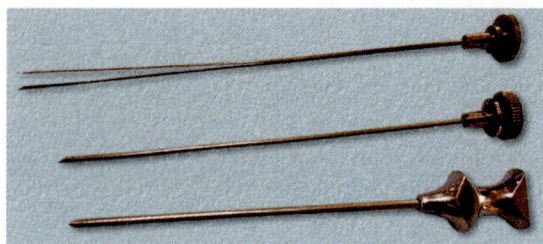

Fig. 2.17: Liver biopsy needle

The instrument is sterilised by autoclaving or hot air oven. The liver biopsy is done in 8th, 9th and 10th intercostal spaces in the right mid-axillary line. If the liver is enlarged, the biopsy can be done subcostally.

Indications

Liver biopsy is safe, simple and provides valuable information for the diagnostic evaluation of the liver diseases. It is done in suspected cases of:

i. Cirrhosis
ii. Primary neoplasms of liver
iii. Secondary neoplasms of liver
iv. Leukaemia
v. General disorders affecting liver like tuberculosis, sarcoidosis and amyloidosis
vi. Fever of unknown origin
vii. Unexplained hepatomegaly or hepatosplenomegaly
viii. Abnormal liver function tests
ix. Metabolic or storage diseases like Wilson's disease
x. Jaundice due to chronic hepatitis

Contraindications

a. Bleeding disorders
b. Congestive cardiac failure
c. Haemangioma of liver
d. Surgical jaundice
e. Tense ascites
f. Infections of peritoneum, biliary tract, base of right lung and subphrenic abscess
g. Hydatid cyst of liver.

Complications of liver biopsy are rare; however, it is likely that the following problems may be encountered.

a. Pleurisy and perihepatitis
b. Haemorrhage
c. Biliary peritonitis
d. Puncture of other viscera
e. Anaphylactic shock due to rupture of hydatid cyst.

The liver biopsy needle can also be used for obtaining biopsy from kidney, spleen, etc.

The other kinds of needles by which liver biopsy could be obtained are Menghini needle and Trucut needle.

Procedure of liver biopsy: Preanaesthetic medications such as injection atropine 0.6 mg and injection for sedation (phenobarbitone 50 mg) could be given half an hour before the procedure or this step could as well be omitted.

The patient is made to lie on the back and the liver biopsy site is located in the mid-axillary line of 8th, 9th or 10th intercostal space. The area chosen is sterilised with antiseptics. Local anaesthesia with 2% xylocaine is infiltrated into skin, subcutaneous tissue up to the capsule of liver or this step can omitted.

Sterilised vim Silverman's needle is taken and trocar with cannula is introduced into the liver substance. Let the patient hold the breath till the procedure is completed. Trocar is removed and the bifid needle is introduced. The bifid needle cuts the liver tissue; the cannula with the bifid needle is rotated, only the cannula is pushed ahead into the liver substance so as to cover the liver biopsy in the bifid needle and withdrawn together. The biopsy sample is collected in Bouin's fluid which acts as a fixative.

Ryle's Tube (Fig. 2.18)

This instrument is a long flexible rubber or plastic tube of 75 cm long. One end of this is blind and the other end is funnel-shaped. The blind end has lead shots which gives bulbous appearance and has three perforations at different levels.

The Ryle's tube has 4 markings at intervals. The first mark represents lower end of oesophagus, while the second mark represents

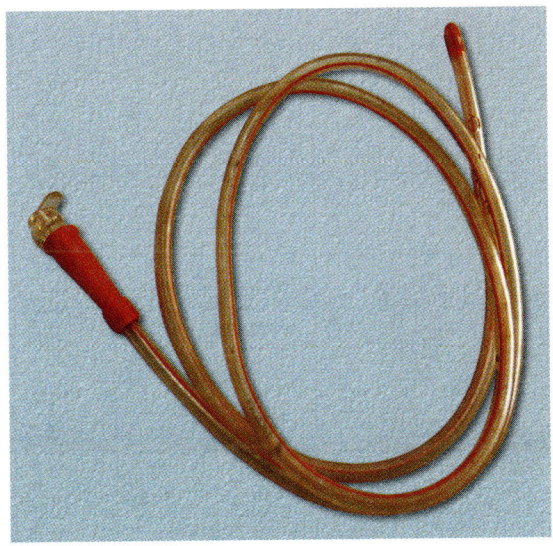

Fig. 2.18: Ryle's tube

cardiac end of the stomach, the third mark represents pylorus and the fourth mark represents duodenum.

Such Ryle's tubes are of different sizes. The lead shot is radio-opaque and helps in locating the tip of the Ryle's tube when under fluoroscopy. It also gives gravity and facilitates the swallowing of the tube.

The holes at the tip region are necessary because even if one is clogged by mucous, the other openings would serve the purpose for aspirating or introducing. The holes are at different levels. If the holes are at one level, then this part of the tube would be weak and there is likelihood of breaking.

The Ryle's tube should not be boiled before introducing, as boiling would soften the tube and then it becomes difficult to insert the tube. The Ryle's tube can be washed and sterilised by antiseptics.

Uses of Ryle's Tube

i. To aspirate gastric juice for gastric analysis.
ii. For feeding purpose in infants and unconscious patients.
iii. To administer drugs like mepacrine.
iv. To aspirate sputum in paediatric patients when tuberculosis is suspected.

Contraindications

i. In cases of corrosive poisoning, the tube should not be passed as it may perforate the oesophagus.
ii. In suspected cases of oesophageal varices, the tube should not be passed as it may rupture the varices and produce severe haemorrhage.

Procedure

The tube is lubricated with sterile liquid paraffin or glycerin. Then the patient is given water and asked to hold water in the mouth. The bulbous end of the tube is gently pushed along the floor of the nose.

As the tip reaches the throat, the patient is asked to swallow water. Along with water the tube also reaches the oesophagus and later the tube is pushed up to stomach/duodenum.

Different markings on the tube enable us to locate the level of the tip. The outer part of tube is plastered to the side of the neck. The part of the tube in the nose should be smeared with antiseptics and withdrawn for a few inches/cm and again replaced. Ryle's tube should not be left for more than 48 hours.

Esbach's Albuminometer (Fig. 2.19)

The instrument consists of a glass tube, measuring 15 cm in length. There are 'U' and 'R' marks on it.

Procedure: Acidify the urine with dilute hydrochloric acid. If any turbidity or precipitation is present, the urine has to be filtered.

Fill the acidified urine up to 'U' mark and then Esbach's reagent up to 'R' mark. The urine and the reagent are thoroughly mixed by inverting the tube several times after plugging the open end with a rubber cork. Avoid air bubbles and keep the tube in its stand for 24 hours. After 24 hours, the

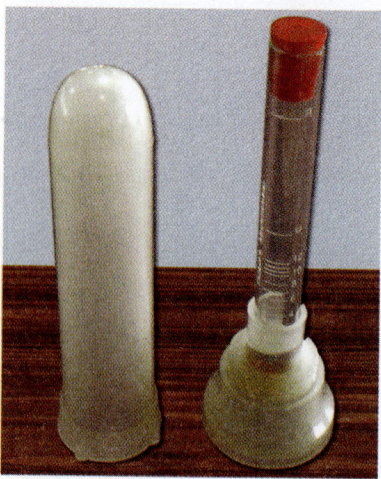

Fig. 2.19: Esbach's albuminometer

precipitated protein level is recorded and expressed in grams/litre.

Conditions for proteinuria

For proteinuria, the conditions can be categorised into mild, moderate and severe proteinuria. Severe proteinuria is observed in nephrotic syndrome, amyloidosis, etc. For details refer to urine analysis.

Composition of Esbach's reagent

1 g of picric acid to precipitate proteins
2 g of citric acid to dissolve phosphates
100 ml of water as a solvent.

Exercise 32

Malaria and Filariasis

MALARIA

It is a protozoal disease transmitted by the bite of an infected female anopheles mosquito.

Species: The species of malaria are: *P. vivax, P. falciparum, P. ovale, P. malariae.*

Malaria is endemic in tropics (40°S to 60°N). Malarial parasites infect the RBCs after passing through a development phase in the parenchymal cells of liver and then carried to all the organs (Fig. 2.20a).

Life Cycle

Among humans, these parasites reside in the liver cells and the red cells. The sexual forms originate inside the human host.

In female anopheles mosquito, the female and male sexual forms are transferred to their insect host and develop further and are transformed into sporozoites. These sporozoites are infective to man. The mosquito acts as a definitive host.

Among humans there are different stages (Figs 2.20b1 and b2). They are:

Pre-erythrocytic schizogony: This occurs in the liver (6 to 8 days) and releases the merozoites.

Erythrocytic schizogony: The merozoites enter the red cells and undergo stages—trophozoites, schizonts and merozoites.

Erythrocytic schizogony lasts for 48 to 72 hours in *P. vivax* and *P. ovale:* but in *P. falciparum* it lasts for 48 hours and in *P. malariae* for 72 hours.

Some of the merozoites develop into sexual forms into red cells. Only mature gametocytes are found in the peripheral blood. The

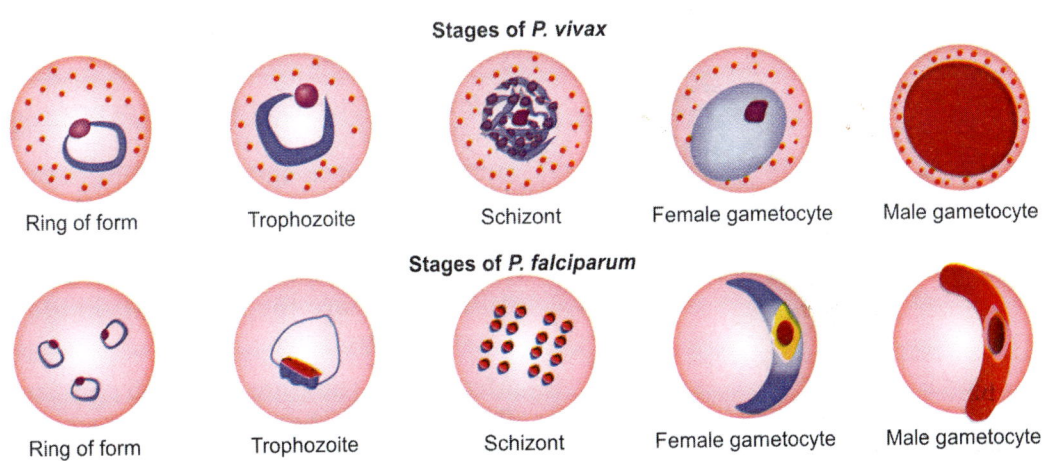

Fig. 2.20a: Stages of development of *P. vivax* and *P. falciparum*

Table 2.3: Points to differentiate *P. falciparum* and *P. vivax* in peripheral smear

P. falciparum	P. vivax
In a single RBC multiple ring forms may be seen	Single ring form
Ring forms are smaller, have double chromatin dots	
Accole (marginal form) forms are present	
Schüffner's dots not present	Schüffner's dots present
Normal red cell size	Red cell size enlarged
Ring forms and crescentic gametocytes only seen	Ring forms, schizonts, gametocytes all together can be seen
Other stages rarely seen	
Red cells of all ages affected	Younger red cells and reticulocytes often affected

individual who harbours the gametocytes is called a carrier. The sexual forms are demonstrated in thick smears after 3 to 4 days of pre-erythrocytic schizogony. The features which differentiate *P. falciparum* and *P. vivax* are given in Table 2.3.

After the red cell infection, the initial tissue phase (pre-erythrocytic phase) disappears completely in *P. falciparum*, whereas in others, it persists (exo-erythrocytic phase) and thus causes relapse.

When parasites reach a density of 50/µl of blood, symptomatic stage begins.

P. vivax invades younger red cells as well as reticulocytes and it is observed that one parasite invades one red cell only. *P. falciparum* invades younger cells and cells of all ages and 2 to 6 parasites invade one red cell. *P. ovale* invades only reticulocytes and *P. malariae* invades older red cells.

About 1 to 2% of red cells are infected by the parasites.

Trophozoites: These have blue cytoplasmic ring with red nuclear mass and an unstained area of vacuole. The ring is 2.5 to 3 µ; and one side of the ring is thicker than the other side; further the nucleus is on the thinner part of the ring. The trophozoites have amoeboid movement. After a growth of 10 hours, some yellow-brown pigment appears in the cytoplasm.

Schizonts: After 36 to 40 hours of growth, the trophozoites become round in shape, lose their amoeboid movement; the vacuole disappears, the pigment granules are scattered throughout the cytoplasm, the nucleus is large and situated at the periphery; it measures 9 to 10 µ. These are the ones that divide and produce merozoites.

Merozoites: These are 1.5 to 1.75 µ in size and 0.5 µ in-depth. The merozoites can attack new erythrocytes or enter the exo-erythrocytic schizogony.

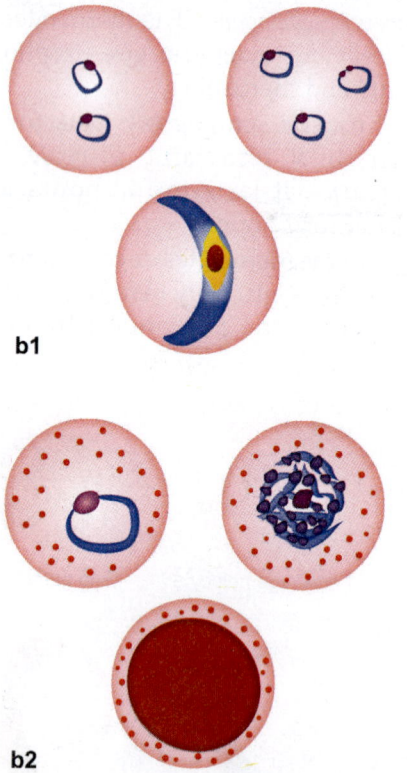

Fig. 2.20b1 and b2: Differentiating features in (b1) *P. falcifarum* and (b2) *P. vivax*

Gametocytes: In *P. vivax*, the size of the erythrocyte is increased; whereas in *P. falciparum* the erythrocytes are normal sized and the cytoplasm shows Maurer's dots. In *P. ovale*, the erythrocytes are irregular with Jane's dots.

Methods for Diagnosis of Malaria

i. *Thick and thin smears:* Thick smears are dehaemoglobinised by using mixture of glacial acetic acid and tartaric acid. Stain with Wright, Giemsa, fields or JSB. Examine 100 to 200 fields before reporting as negative.

Collection of blood for peripheral smear: Should be 2–6 hours from the febrile paroxysm as number of parasites will be more during this period.

Parasite load: Following is the parasite load depending upon the number of parasites observed in the peripheral smear.

+ 1 to 10 parasites/100 thick film field
+ + 11 to 100 parasites/100 thick film field
+ + + 1 to 10 parasites/each thick field
+ + + + more than 10 parasites/each thick field

For Romanowsky stains, pH of 7.2 is preferred for malarial parasites.

ii. *QBC test/microtube concentration method with acridine orange staining:* Blood is collected in a tube with acridine orange, anticoagulant and a float. Centrifuge leads to concentration of parasitised cells around the float and the parasites are detected with fluorescent microscopy.

iii. *Pf HRP$_2$ dipstick/card test:* Put a drop of blood on a card which is immersed then in washing solution. Monoclonal antibodies capture parasite antigens and read out as coloured band. It is rapid and sensitive.

Disadvantage: In this method, the disadvantage is that it detects only *P. falciparum* and remains positive for weeks together after the infection.

FILARIASIS (*WUCHERERIA BANCROFTI*)

Filariasis is a parasitic disease that is caused by thread-like worms belonging to the filariodea family inhibiting mainly in lymphatics, blood vessels and connective tissues. The life-cycle is passed in two hosts. *Microfilaria bancrofti* completes its development in insect host, giving rise to infective forms (microfilaria). Infection is transmitted to humans by the bite of the insect mosquito (Aedes, Anopheles). Adult worms are found in lymphatics and lymph nodes in definitive host. Species identification is made by the identification of larval forms.

Signs and Symptoms

Most common—elephantiasis

Diagnosis

Filariasis is usually diagnosed by identifying microfilariae on Wright or Leishman stained, thin and thick blood film smears (Fig. 2.21a).

Microfilaria bancrofti measures 290 µ in length, and 6 to 7 µ in width. It sheathed, somatic cells or nuclei extend from head to the tail end. The granules do not extend up to the tail end which is distinguishing feature. The cephalic end is devoid of granules (Figs 2.21b and c1).

The other sheathed microfilaria found in blood are:
- *Microfilaria malayi:* The granules are up to tail end (Fig. 2.21c2)
- *Microfilaria loa:* The granules are up to tail end (Fig. 2.21c3).

The unsheathed microfilaria are:
- *Microfilaria perstans*
- *Microfilaria ozzardi*
- *Microfilaria streptocerca*
- *Microfilaria volvulus.*

Blood must be drawn at appropriate times, which reflect the feeding activities of the

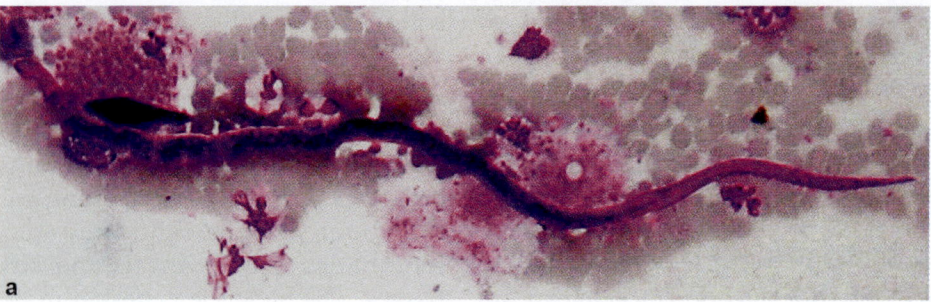
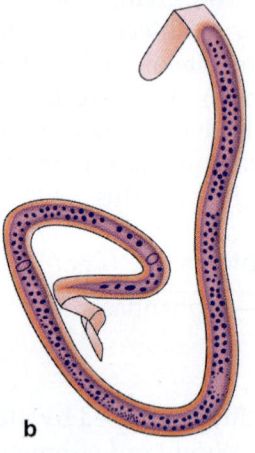
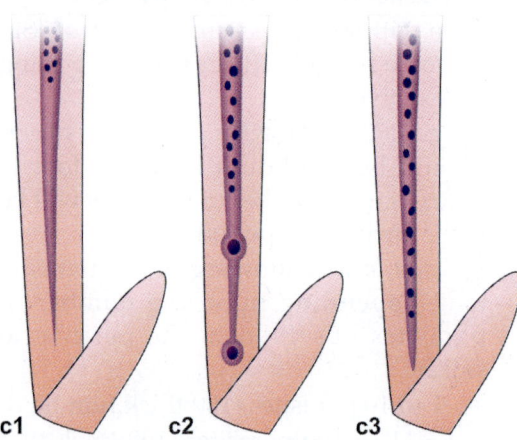

Figs 2.21a to c3: (a) Microfilaria in peripheral smear; (b) schematic diagram: *Microfilaria bancrofti*; (c1 to c3) sheathed microfilarias (tail ends c1—*M. bancrofti*, c2—*M. malayi*, c3—*M. loa*)

vector insects. *W. bancrofti*, whose vector is a mosquito; night is the preferred time for blood collection. Various concentration methods are applied. They can be also diagnosed by the following methods:

- PCR and antigenic assays
- Lymph node aspirate and chylus fluid may also yield microfilariae
- Medical imaging, such as CT or MRI, may reveal "filarial dance sign" in chylus fluid
- X-ray can show calcified adult worms in lymphatics.

Exercise 33

Basics of Cytology

The various body fluids are looked for gross features, cell counts and the following different cytopreparatory techniques for microscopy are used.
a. Toluidine blue stained wet film
b. Permanent smears
   - Wet fixed smear, stained with Pap stain
   - Air dried smears stained with MGG/Diff-quick stain
c. Cell block sections
   - Stained with H & E
   - Used for IHC/special stains.

For cervical smears Pap stain is used.

The superficial and deep seated masses. Fine needle aspiration cytology is done.

For details refer to Part V cytology techniques.

Exercise 34

Haematology, Clinical Pathology and Cytology Charts/Case Studies

Haematology Charts

1. Female aged 40 years presented with soreness of tongue, numbness and burning sensation of feet.
   Hb—9 g/dl
   Peripheral smear is provided.

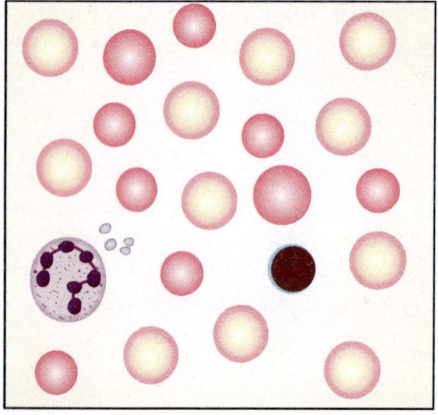

2. Female aged 25 years presented with menorrhagia.
   Peripheral smear is provided.

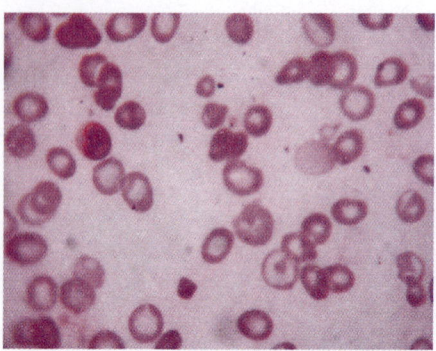

3. Farmer aged 40 years, presented with generalised weakness, easy fatigability, cough with expectoration and wheezing. Peripheral smear is provided.

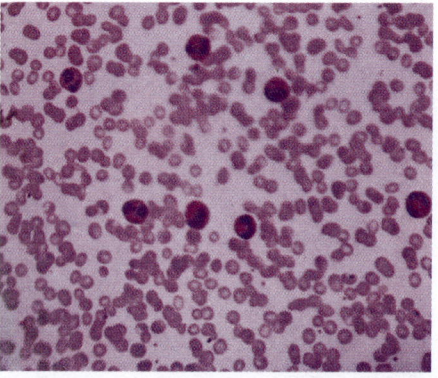

4. A 6-year-old girl presented with pain abdomen, joint pains, on and off pain in the fingers and toes since 5 years.

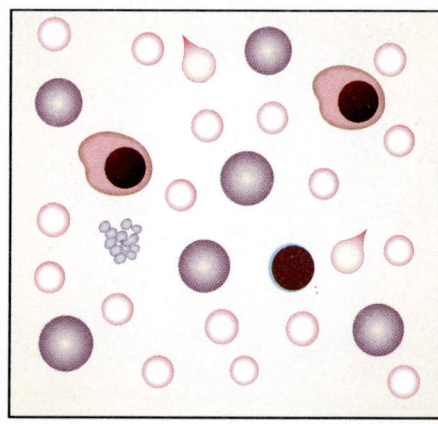

Past history of jaundice +
Hepatosplenomegaly +
O/E mild pallor is seen. No icterus. hepatosplenomegaly +
Investigations done are:
Hb—8 g/dl
Reticulocytes—20%
Peripheral smear is provided.

5. 10-year-old boy presented with fever and generalised lymphadenopathy of 3 months duration.
Investigations done are:
Hb—6 g/dl
TLC—1,60,000 cells/cmm
Platelet count—50000 cells/cmm
Peripheral smear is provided.

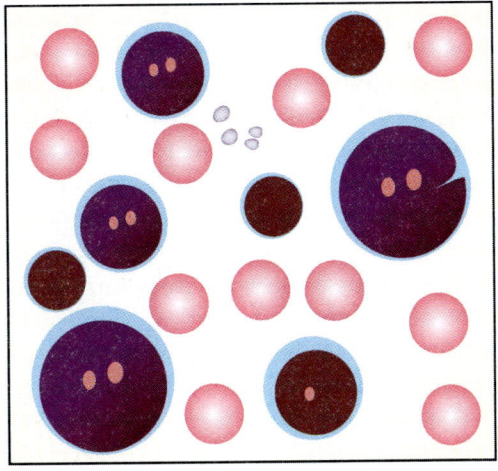

6. 32 years female presented with fever, weight loss, bleeding gums and hepatosplenomegaly since 6 months

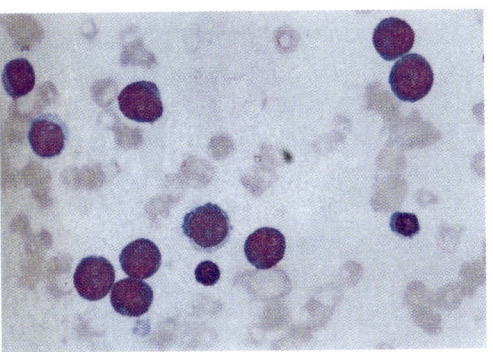

Investigations done are:
Hb—6.8 g/dl
TLC—1,72,000 cells/cmm
Peripheral smear is provided.

7. 40 years male presented with weakness, dyspnoea, pallor, weight loss and massive splenomegaly
Investigations done are:
Hb—9.4 g/dl
TLC—1,02,000 cells/cmm
Peripheral smear is provided.

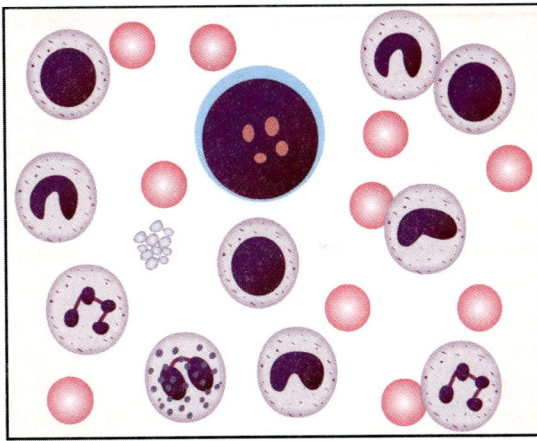

8. 70 years male presented with fever, weight loss, generalised lymphadenopathy and mild splenomegaly
Investigations done are:
Hb—10 g/dl
TLC—1,20,000 cells/cmm
Bone marrow is provided.

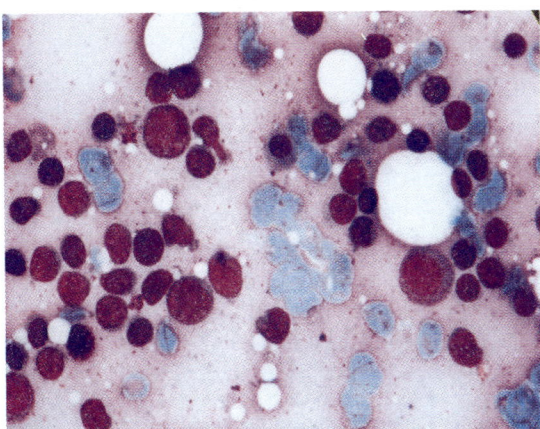

9. 65 years male presented with fatigue, weakness, weight loss, and low backache
   Investigations done are:
   Hb—9.6 g/dl
   ESR—120 mm at the end of one hour
   Peripheral smear is provided.

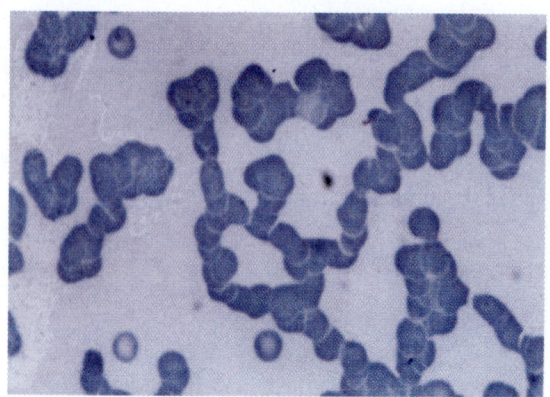

10. 30 years male presented with episodes of abdominal pain, yellowish discolouration of eyes, pale stools and passing dark yellow urine—2 months
    O/E icterus ++, tender splenomegaly +
    Investigations done are:
    Hb—6 g/dl
    ESR—raised
    Reticulocyte—20%
    Serum bilirubin—4.0 mg
    Direct antiglobulin test—positive

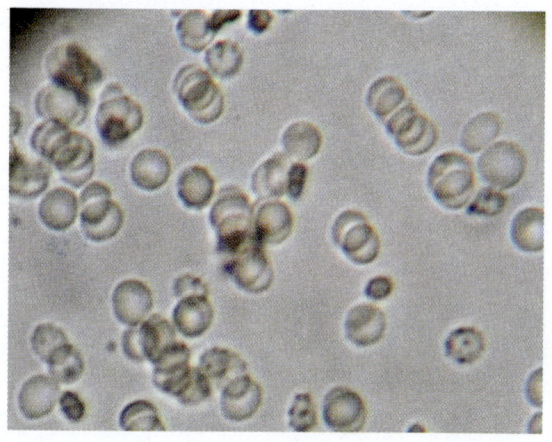

Cytology Charts

1. Synovial fluid from a 30-year-old female
   Gross—yellow
   Mucin clot test—fair
   Cell count—1,000 cells/cmm
   Microscopy—rheumatoid arthritis cells are seen.
2. Synovial fluid from a 50-year-old male
   Gross—yellow
   Mucin clot test—fair
   Cell count—7,000 cells/cmm
   Microscopy needle-shaped birefringent crystals seen.
3. 25 years male history of joint pains. Synovial fluid for analysis
   Gross—gray purulent
   Mucin clot test—negative
   Cell count—2,00,000 cells/cmm
   Microscopy—sheets of neutrophils seen.
4. 55 years female, blood-stained discharge
   Pap stain: Cervical smear revealed good number of squamous epithelial cells with large hyperchromatic irregular nuclei. Many tadpole cells are also seen. Background showed neutrophils and necrotic debris.
5. 15 years male, fever, vomiting and headache.
   CSF analysis
   Colurless, turbid
   Cell count: 5,000 cells/cmm
   Biochemistry
   Sugar: 30 mg%
   Proteins: 70 mg%
   Chlorides : 600 mg%
   Wet preparation: Shows good number of neutrophils.
6. 30 years female, history of fever, cough with expectoration, headache and altered sensorium.
   CSF analysis
   Gross: Colourless, opalescent with cobweb formation
   Cell count: 800 cells/cmm
   Biochemistry

Sugar: 20 mg%
Proteins: 90 mg%
Chlorides: 800 mg%
Wet preparation: Shows good number of lymphocytes.

7. 40 years male, history of hypertension and altered sensorium
   CSF analysis
   Gross
   Reddish, opalescent, xanthochromia +
   Cell count: Contaminated with RBCs
   Biochemistry
   Sugar: 70 mg%
   Proteins: 70 mg%
   Chlorides: 750 mg%
   Wet preparation: Shows sheets of RBCs and occasional lymphocytes.

8. 25 years male, history of fever—3 months, loss of weight.
   FNAC from cervical lymph node
   Pap and MGG stains: Smear shows moderately cellular aspirate comprising of good number of oval cells with vesicular elongated nuclei in small clumps. Background shows lymphocytes and granular necrotic debris.
   ZN stain for AFB—positive.

9. 50 years male, ascitic fluid for analysis
   Ascitic fluid analysis
   Gross: Reddish, opalescent cells/cmm
   Cell count: RBCs—2000 cells/cmm
   WBCs—35 cells/cmm
   Wet preparation: Shows good number of RBCs and a few lymphocytes and atypical cells.
   Pap stain: Smear shows atypical cells arranged in clumps. These cells are round to oval with moderate amount of cytoplasm and large irregular hyperchromatic nuclei. Few of these cells show nucleoli.

10. 60 years male, history of cough with expectoration, blood tinged, loss of weight and appetite. Sputum for examination.
    Gross: Reddish, mucoid—2 ml
    Pap stain: Smears show good number of squamous epithelial cells scattered singly. They have moderate amount of cytoplasm and large irregular hyperchromatic nuclei. The cells show nuclear pleomorphism. Few of these cells show nucleoli. Background shows neutrophils, RBCs and macrophages.

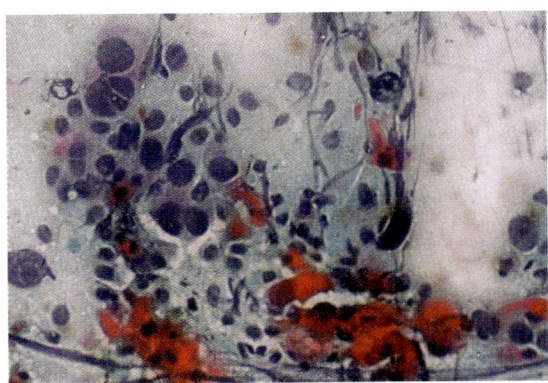

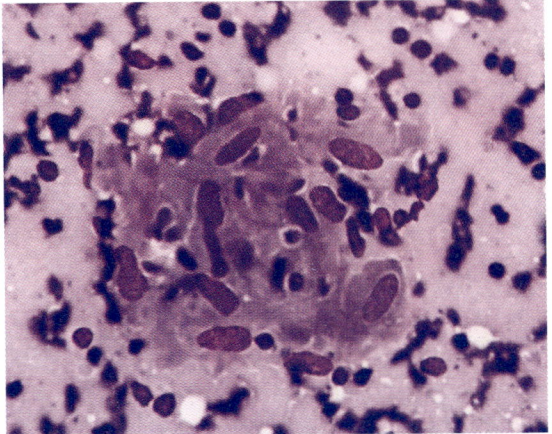

Clinical Pathology Charts

1. 40 years male C/O polyurea, polyphagia and polydipsia for 4 years. There is tingling and numbness for 1 year.
   Investigations done

   Urine examination
   Physical findings
   Colour—colourless
   Quantity—500 ml
   Reaction—acidic
   Appearance—clear

Chemical examination
Albumin—absent
Sugar—orange ppt
Microscopy—NAD

2. 56 years female C/O polyurea, polyphagia and polydipsia burning micturition, generalised weakness and loss of weight—3 years.
Investigations done

Urine examination
Physical findings
Colour—Yellow
Quantity—500 ml
Reaction—acidic
Appearance—turbid
Odour—aromatic

Chemical examination
Albumin—trace
Sugar—brick red ppt
Ketone bodies—present
Microscopy—sheets of pus cells present
Bacteria ++

3. 25 years female C/O fever, chills, nausea, pain in abdomen, frequent burning micturition—3 days. H/O delivery—10 days.
Investigations done

Urine examination
Physical findings
Colour—colourless
Quantity—100 ml
Reaction—acidic
Appearance—turbid

Chemical examination
Albumin—present +++
Sugar—absent
Blood—present
Microscopy—sheets of pus cells present
60–80 RBCs/HPF
No cast or crystal seen.

4. 16 years male C/O fever, joint pains, swelling on the face—8 days.
Investigations done

Urine examination
Physical findings
Colour—reddish smoky
Quantity—50 ml
Reaction—acidic
Appearance—slight turbid

Chemical examination
Albumin—present (+++)
Sugar—absent
Blood—present
Microscopy
100–200 RBCs/HPF
Hyaline and granular casts ++/HPF

5. 30 years male C/O shooting pain in the loin, painful micturition—1 day, no fever.
Investigations done

Urine examination
Physical findings
Colour—reddish
Quantity—150 ml
Reaction—alkaline
Appearance—turbid

Chemical examination
Albumin—trace
Sugar—absent
Blood—present (+++)
Microscopy—sheets of RBCs seen, plenty of oxalate crystals, no pus cells.

6. 25 years male H/O fever, vomiting, pain in abdomen, loss of appetite, and passing high coloured urine—6 days
Investigations done

Urine examination
Physical findings
Colour—high coloured—yellowish brown
Quantity—100 ml
Reaction—acidic
Appearance—clear

Chemical examination
Albumin—absent
Sugar—absent
Bile salt—present

Bile pigment—present
Urobilinogen—present (1 : 10 ratio)
Microscopy—NAD

7. 50 years male C/O pain in the back—1 year, loss of appetite, generalised weakness—1 month.
High coloured urine—15 days
Investigations done

Urine examination
Physical findings
Colour—reddish brown
Quantity—50 ml
Reaction—acidic

Chemical examination
Albumin—trace
Sugar—absent
Blood—present
Microscopy—50–100 RBCs/HPF
Wet preparation—Large atypical polygonal cells seen in clumps.
Pap stain confirmed malignancy.

8. 23 years female C/O amenorrhoea—45 days. H/O nausea and vomiting—15 days.
Investigation done
Pregnancy test (latex agglutination inhibition test)
Observation—no agglutination seen

9. 2 years male C/O no issues. Married life—7 years
Investigations done
Semen analysis—2 ml semen sample, liquefied within 30 minutes
Reaction—alkaline
Fructose test—positive
Cell count—30 millions/ml
Motility—70% actively motile, 20% sluggishly motile, 10% dead
Morphology—most are of normal morphology.
No pus cells seen

10. Child of 10 years, repeated transfusions, jaundice on and off
Investigations done:
Hb%–6.2 g%
Bilirubin—total—2 mg%, indirect—1.8 mg%, direct—0.2 g%
Urine routine—NAD, urobilinogen—increased, bile salts and pigments—absent

Diagnosis of Haematology Charts

Chart 1: Megaloblastic anaemia
Chart 2: Iron deficiency anaemia
Chart 3: Eosinophilia
Chart 4: Haemolytic anaemia
Chart 5: ALL-L2
Chart 6: AML
Chart 7: CML
Chart 8: CLL
Chart 9: Multiple myeloma
Chart 10: Autoimmune haemolytic anaemia

Diagnosis of Cytology Charts

Chart 1: Rheumatoid arthritis
Chart 2: Gout
Chart 3: Septic arthritis
Chart 4: Carcinoma cervix
Chart 5: Pyogenic meningitis
Chart 6: Tubercular meningitis
Chart 7: Subarachnoid haemorrhage
Chart 8: TB lymphadenitis
Chart 9: Metastatic adenocarcinoma
Chart 10: Squamous cell carcinoma—lung

Diagnosis of Clinical Pathology Charts

Chart 1: Glycosuria
Chart 2: Diabetes mellitus with complications
Chart 3: Acute urinary tract infection
Chart 4: Acute glomerulonephritis
Chart 5: Haematuria—renal calculi
Chart 6: Infective hepatitis
Chart 7: Renal carcinoma
Chart 8: Pregnancy test—positive
Chart 9: Oligospermia
Chart 10: Pre-hepatic jaundice due to haemolytic anaemia

Section III

General Pathology and Systemic Pathology

Exercise 35. Fixation and Processing for Paraffin Section and Frozen Section
Exercise 36. Cell Injury
Exercise 37. Fatty Change (Liver, Heart) and Amyloidosis
Exercise 38. Inflammation (Acute and Chronic) and Granulation Tissue
Exercise 39. Chronic Venous Congestion, Thrombosis, Infarction, Myocardial Infarction (MI) and Lung Infarction Oedema and Shock
Exercise 40. Neoplasia
Exercise 41. Some Common Tumours
Exercise 42. Atherosclerosis and Vascular Pathology in Hypertension
Exercise 43. Heart Lesions
Exercise 44. Lesions of Respiratory Tract
Exercise 45. Salivary Gland Tumours
Exercise 46. Lesions of Gastrointestinal Tract
Exercise 47. Common Lesions of Liver
Exercise 48. Neoplasms of Breast
Exercise 49. Kidney Lesions
Exercise 50. Neoplasms Arising from Stratified Squamous Epithelium
Exercise 51. Tumours of Melanocytes
Exercise 52. Endometrium and Uterus, Trophoblastic Diseases and Cervix the Normal Endometrium
Exercise 53. Common Ovarian Tumours
Exercise 54. Common Testicular Lesions
Exercise 55. Lesions of Prostate
Exercise 56. Common Bone Lesions
Exercise 57. Lesions of Thyroid
Exercise 58. Lesions of Lymph Node
Exercise 59. Lesions of Brain

Exercise 35

Fixation and Processing for Paraffin Section and Frozen Section

FIXATION

Fixation is employed to the tissues that are removed from the body or from the dead bodies for investigation.

Aims of Fixation

Main aims

1. To prevent autolysis and putrefaction.

Autolysis: Literally autolysis means self-inflicted death or destruction. It is caused by action of intracellular enzymes released by ruptured lysosomes. The enzymes are cathepsin, proteinase, carboxypeptidase and aminopeptidases. The practical outcome is that the nuclei may become condensed or even break up, cytoplasm may become swollen and eventually entire architecture is lost. In case of epithelium, it gets split off from the basement membrane.

Putrefaction: The tissues like gastrointestinal tract with high bacterial content will rapidly breakdown after death or removal from the body by the action of organisms with production of gas.

2. Preserves various cell constituents in life like manner.

Other aims

3. Soft tissues become firm in consistency so that the tissues can be easily handled.
4. Semifluid consistency is changed to semisolid consistency.
5. Aids in visual differentiation of the structure of the tissues by application of dyes and chemicals.

Commonly 10% formalin, i.e. formaldehyde (HCHO) is used for routine fixation and preparation is given below.

Preparation of 10% formalin (4% formaldehyde):
40% formaldehyde   100 ml
Distilled/tap water   900 ml

Duration of fixation

Duration of fixation varies according to the fixative used. With formalin 2 to 6 hours is needed for small tissues and 6 to 12 hours for big tissues. Big tissue specimens have to be cut at definite intervals for proper fixation.

PROCESSING

The aim of processing is to get thin sections by embedding the tissue in paraffin wax. To embed the tissue in wax, the water content of tissue has to be removed slowly in such a way that there is no tissue shrinkage. This step is called dehydration. The dehydrating agents are not miscible with wax. So, clearing agents are to be applied after dehydration which are miscible with both dehydrating agents and paraffin.

Steps of processing
- Fixation
- Dehydration
- Clearing
- Impregnation with molten wax
- Embedding or block making.

Fixation

The tissues are generally fixed for 6 to 12 hours. 10% formalin is the routinely used fixative. For further details, refer to the topic on fixatives.

Dehydration

Dehydration involves removal of water from the tissues. Different solutions can be used to dehydrate and most commonly, upgraded alcohol solutions are used for effective dehydration. By using upgraded alcohols, water is removed slowly and gradually, in such a way that there is no much shrinkage of the tissue.

In the last jar of alcohol, a layer of anhydrous copper sulphate of about 0.5 to 2.5 cm is usually placed. When the water content of the alcohol increases, the colourless anhydrous copper sulphate absorbs water and becomes bluish in colour. At this stage, alcohol has to be changed.

Clearing

The term 'clearing' relates to the appearance of the tissues after they have been treated by the fluid chosen to remove dehydrating agent.

These clearing solutions have refractive index similar to proteins which consequently renders the tissue translucent.

Clearing agent is necessary because the dehydrating agent is not miscible with paraffin. The clearing agent is miscible with both dehydrating agent as well as paraffin.

Clearing agents commonly used are:
  i. Chloroform
  ii. Xylene

Chloroform

This is mainly used in automatic tissue processor (Histokinette). Moreover, it is not flammable but toxic because it releases toxic gas called phosgene. The tissue can be left in chloroform overnight without rendering the tissue brittle.

The disadvantage in use of chloroform is that it does not alter the refractive index; so the endpoint of clearing is difficult to determine.

Xylene

This is a fast acting clearing agent. When this agent is used as a clearing agent, the small tissue pieces are cleared in 1/2–1 hour; 5 mm thickness tissue pieces are cleared in 2–4 hours. As the solution replaces alcohol, the tissue becomes clear due to the difference in the refractive index; thus it is possible to determine the endpoint of clearing with better accuracy and one can avoid over exposure of the tissue to the hardening effect of the solution. But on keeping for longer time tissue becomes brittle. Further it is flammable and toxic too.

Impregnation

Paraffin wax with low melting point (MP) of 56–58°C is used for impregnation.

Embedding and Block Making

Wax of slightly higher melting point 58–60°C is used for embedding and block making.

Block making needs moulds and such required moulds are prepared using Leuckhart's L pieces and metal plates. By adjusting the L pieces, the size and shape of the mould can be decided. At first, the moulds are filled with molten wax after which the tissue is placed at the bottom and pressed with a rod. When the wax gets solidified, the block can be easily separated from L pieces and metal plate and then the block is labelled.

Processing Steps used in Automatic Tissue Processor (Histokinette, Riechart Jung Ltd.)

Alcohol and acetone are the dehydrating agents, chloroform is a clearing agent and paraffin wax is used for impregnation. Following are the steps of automatic tissue processing.

Jar with processing agent	Timing (hours)
1. 70% alcohol	1
2. 80% alcohol	1
3. 90% alcohol	1
4. 95% alcohol	1
5. 95% alcohol	1
6. Absolute alcohol	1
7. Absolute alcohol	1
8. Acetone	1
9. Chloroform	2
10. Chloroform	2
11. Paraffin wax	2
12. Paraffin wax	2
Total	18

There are 12 jars each containing the above reagents and it takes about 18 hours to complete one rotation. In this case, the advantages are: (i) there is no need of manpower, (ii) there is continuous agitation because of which the solutions penetrate and come out evenly at faster rate. There are some disadvantages and one of the disadvantages is that the machine depends on electricity.

Manual processing: In this processing, alcohol and acetone are the dehydrating agents, xylene is a clearing agent and liquid paraffin is used for impregnation. Following are the steps of manual processing.

Jar with processing agent	Timing (hours)
1. 70% alcohol	1
2. 80% alcohol	1
3. 90% alcohol	1
4. 95% alcohol	1
5. Absolute alcohol	1
6. Acetone	1
7. Xylene	1
8. Paraffin wax	1
9. Paraffin wax	2
Total	10

Note: Timing varies from one laboratory to another laboratory. Each laboratory may select its own convenient and suitable timings. A technical personnel is required to monitor the processing.

Refer to Section IV, Histopathology techniques for details.

FROZEN SECTION

This method is to produce sections without the use of either the dehydrating agents or clearing agents.

Principle: When the tissue is frozen, the water in it turns into ice, making the tissue firm and the ice itself acts as an embedding medium.

The uses of frozen section are
1. Demonstration of fats and lipids.
2. Enzyme histochemistry.
3. Early reporting of biopsy specimens particularly during emergency.

To get frozen sections, following methods or instruments can be employed:
- Freezing microtome
- Cryostat
- Freeze drying
- Freeze substitution.

Freezing microtome is attached to a cylinder of liquid CO_2 or a thermo-module unit. The CO_2 is fed to the microtome block stage, so that it maintains the tissue in a frozen state. In thermo-module, the Peltier effect is observed, i.e. heat generated across one surface is lost at the opposite surface, when direct current passes through two dissimilar metals. With thermo-module, $-30°C$ temperature can be obtained.

Cryostat is a refrigerated cabinet in which rotary microtome is fitted. The temperature can be adjusted between -5 and $-30°C$. Usually $-16°C$ is preferred. Freon 22, a gas is used for its cooling effect. An anti-roll plate placed parallel to the knife blade is a glass device coated with perspex. This plate is meant to prevent any possible curling of the tissue.

Freezing can be also achieved by liquid nitrogen ($-190°C$), isopentane cooled by liquid nitrogen ($-150°C$), solid carbon dioxide also called dry ice or cardice ($-70°C$), carbon dioxide gas under pressure and aerosol sprays ($-50°C$). The tissue has to be held between two pieces of dry ice.

Normally, wedge knife is used for taking frozen sections.

The sections have to be 5–10 μ thick. Thinner sections are difficult to cut. The sections are cut and with the help of a brush, the sections are floated on a water bath and the necessary stains are applied. After staining, again these sections are floated on water bath and collected on albuminised slides and spread properly. A drop of glycerol is put followed by a coverslip; and observed under microscope.

Stains applied routinely are

1. For study of malignant cells—methylene blue or H & E stain is employed.
2. For fat demonstration oil red 'O' stain is employed.

Exercise 36

Cell Injury

The cells have efficient mechanisms to sustain the effects of injurious agent to some extent. The effects of injury are evident, only when the cell can no more able to maintain the normal homeostasis because of sustained exposure to injurious agent.

Causes of Cell Injury Include (Fig. 3.0)

1. Oxygen deprivation (Ischemia)
2. Chemical agents
3. Physical agents
4. Infectious agents
5. Immunological mechanisms
6. Genetic defects
7. Nutritional imbalance
8. Ageing

The Injury can be of Following Types

- Reversible cell injury
- Irreversible cell injury.

Reversible Cell Injury

If the injurious agent is removed in time, or if the cell can withstand the assault with mild forms of injury, the changes can be reversed and complete structural and functional integrity can be restored. If the cell is exposed for sublethal injury for a prolonged period, the cell has time to adapt to reversible injury. For example, exposure of bronchial mucosa to tobacco smoke, the metaplasia of respiratory epithelium to stratified squamous epithelium occurs.

Irreversible Cell Injury

If the injurious agent is of severe nature and not taken off and the damage continues, the cell undergoes irreversible injury, the cell cannot recover and its death occurs. The death can be of two types: Necrosis and apoptosis.

Mechanism of Cell Injury

Cell injury results in functional and biochemical changes. They are mentioned below:

- ATP depletion
- Damage to mitochondria
- Defects in cell membrane permeability
- Influx of calcium
- Accumulation of oxygen free radicals/Reactive oxygen species (ROS)
- Damage to DNA and proteins.

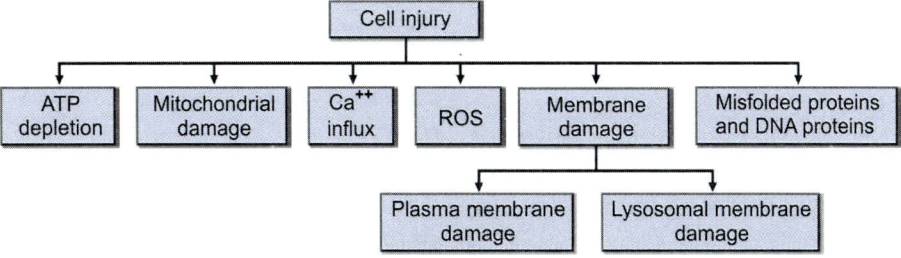

Fig. 3.0: Cell injury: Various effects on cell

CELLULAR ADAPTATIONS

Cellular adaptations refer to reversible changes in size, number, phenotype, appearance and metabolic and functional activity of cells due to adverse environmental changes. It can be reversible if the causative factor is taken off. The cell adapts to the new environment in different ways due to adverse environment.

The basic types of cellular adaptation are:
1. *Hyperplasia:* Increase in number of cells.
2. *Hypertrophy:* Increase in size of cells.
3. *Atrophy:* Decrease in size of cells.
4. *Metaplasia:* Change from one adult type to other (epithelial or mesenchymal).

Examples of Hyperplasia

Breast during puberty and pregnancy, uterus in pregnancy, benign prostatic hyperplasia (BPH) or nodular prostatic hyperplasia (NPH), islet cells in infants born to diabetic mothers, thyroid follicular hyperplasia due to increased TSH, compensatory hyperplasia (liver, lung and kidney), endometrial hyperplasia, squamous cell papilloma, etc.

Examples of Hypertrophy

Uterus during pregnancy, skeletal muscle of limbs in athletes, heart muscles in hypertension or aortic incompetence or stenosis, hypertrophy of smooth muscle in pyloric stenosis, etc.

Examples of Atrophy

Involution of branchial cleft, thyroglossal duct and notochord, involution of wolffian duct and mullerian duct in females and males respectively, Atrophy of ovary, endometrium after menopause and atrophy of other tissues in old age, senile atrophy, disuse atrophy of limb, loss of innervation, loss of blood supply, pressure atrophy, lack of nutrients, reduced hormones, loss of endocrine stimulation, etc.

Examples of Metaplasia

Epithelial metaplasia—respiratory epithelium in smokers, endocervical epithelium, ducts of various glands, transitional epithelium of bladder and pelvis of kidney changes to stratified squamous epithelium, endometrial metaplasia, Barrett's oesophagus, etc.

Mesenchymal metaplasia—osseous metaplasia in old scars, necrotic areas, myositis ossificans, walls of diseased arteries, laryngeal and bronchial cartilage of old people, etc. and uterine leiomyoma with osseous and mesenchymal metaplasia.

DEGENERATIONS

Definition: These are retrogressive changes in the cells due to direct action of the injurious agents.

The term reversible cell injury or degeneration is used to denote changes in the cell due to sublethal injury. There is no death of the cells. The cell has time to adapt to reversible injury in many ways. If the injury is severe, it leads to cell death.

Types of Degenerations Include

- Cloudy degeneration
- Hydropic degeneration/vacuolar change
- Hyaline change
- Mucoid degeneration
- Fatty degeneration
- Amyloid degeneration.

Hyaline degeneration is glassy, amorphous and homogenous material which stains pink/eosinophilic with H & E stain.

Physiological conditions with hyaline degeneration are: Arteries of atrophic uterus, colloid in multinodular goiter, *Corpora amylacea* in prostate and *Corpora albicans* in ovary.

Extracellular hyaline: Collagen in: Old scar tissue and keloid, fibroma, vessel wall in diabetes mellitus and hypertension, KW lesions of kidney in diabetes mellitus and hyalinzation of islets of langerhans in diabetes mellitus.

Intracellular hyaline: Mallory hyaline, Councilman bodies, Russel bodies, epithelial hyaline and Zenker's degeneration.

APOPTOSIS

Definition: Apoptosis is a process that helps to eliminate unwanted cells, by an internally programmed series of events, the process is tightly regulated and the cells are destined to die.

The physiological causes of apoptosis include:
1. During development, removal of excess cells during embryogenesis including implantation, organogenesis, involution and metamorphosis, e.g.
   a. During limb formation separate digits evolve by involution of unwanted cells.
   b. Ablation of cells which are no longer needed (tadpole).
2. To maintain cell population in tissues with high turnover of cells, such as skin and intestinal crypt epithelium, so as to maintain constant number.
3. To eliminate autoreactive T-cells.
4. Hormone-dependent involution in tissues such as endometrium while shedding during menstrual cycle, ovary during post-menopausal period, regression of breasts after weaning period, etc.

The pathological causes include:
1. Apoptosis mechanism tries to eliminate potentially harmful cells.
2. It helps in deletion of damaged/dangerous cells.
3. It removes cells damaged by viruses.
4. It eliminates cells with damaged DNA by radiation, cytotoxic agents, genetically altered cells (mutated cells), etc.
5. It causes cell death in tumours.
6. Pathological atrophy after duct obstruction as in pancreas, parotid gland and kidney.

Mechanism of Apoptosis

Extrinsic Pathway (Death Receptor Pathway)

1. The activated T lymphocytes having FasL recognise Fas expressing targets. The Fas molecule as it cross links with FasL or TNFR on cell membrane binds to TNF expressing cells, adaptor proteins and cytosolic part of death domain gets activated.
2. This activates initiator caspase 8. This further activates other caspases 9, 10, 12.
3. Executioner caspases like caspase 2, 3, 6, 7 are activated.
4. Cytoplasmic and nuclear proteins are broken down by executioner caspases.
5. The apoptotic bodies are engulfed by the macrophages.
6. Undergo degradation.

Intrinsic Pathway (Mitochondrial Pathway)

Mitochondria contain several proteins capable of inducing apoptosis which include cytochrome C and inhibitors of apoptosis.

Steps

1. Following cellular stress the pro-apoptotic proteins from cytosol relocate to the surface of the mitochondria where the anti-apoptotic proteins are located.
2. This interaction between pro- and anti-apoptotic proteins disrupts the normal function of the anti-apoptotic Bcl-2 proteins and can lead to the formation of pores in the mitochondria and the release of cytochrome C and other pro-apoptotic molecules from the intermembrane space.
3. The release of cytochrome C from the mitochondria is a particularly important event in the induction of apoptosis. Once cytochrome C has been released into the cytosol, it is able to interact with apoptosome protein activating factor 1 (Apaf-1), procaspase 9 and dATP, together form an apoptosome.
4. Apoptosome formation leads to activation of initiator pro-caspase 9, blocks the action of caspase inhibitors.

5. Further activates executioner caspases 3 and 7 which breakdown cytoskeleton and nuclear proteins.
6. The apoptotic bodies are engulfed by the macrophages.
7. Undergo degradation.

Morphology of Cells in Apoptosis

1. Shrinkage of cells.
2. Condensation of nuclear chromatin peripherally under nuclear membrane.
3. Formation of apoptotic bodies by fragmentation of the cells and nuclei. The fragments remain membrane bound and contain cell organelles with or without nuclear fragments.
4. Phagocytises of apoptotic bodies by phagocytes.
5. Unlike necrosis, apoptosis is not accompanied by inflammatory reaction.

NECROSIS

Definition: Spectrum of morphological changes that follow cell death in a living tissue, largely resulting from progressive degradative action of enzymes on lethally injured cells is necrosis. The damage caused is irreversible.

Mechanism

1. Enzymic digestion of the cell.
2. Denaturation of the proteins.

Necrotic cells show the following changes:
1. *Cytoplasmic changes:*
   i. Increased eosinophilia: This is due to loss of RNA material and accumulation of lactic acid due to anaerobic respiration.
   ii. Glassy homogenous appearance: This is due to loss of glycogen.
   iii. Cytoplasmic vacuolations: This is because of digestion of organelles and cytoplasm appears "moth eaten".
   iv. Calcification of dead cells—this is due to dystrophic calcification.
2. *Nuclear changes indicating cell death are of three patterns and these are:*
   i. Karyolysis
   ii. Pyknosis
   iii. Karyorrhexis.

Differences between necrosis and apoptosis are given in Table 3.1.

Types of Necrosis

1. Coagulative necrosis
2. Liquefactive necrosis
3. Caseous necrosis
4. Fibrinoid necrosis
5. Fat necrosis

Table 3.1: Differences between necrosis and apoptosis

Necrosis	Apoptosis
Detrimental	Beneficial
Pathological	Physiological/pathological
Groups of cells affected	Single cells affected
Effects	**Effects**
Cellular swelling	Cellular condensation, reduced (shrinkage)
Membranes are broken	Membranes remain intact, membrane blebs formed, membrane bound bodies formed
Leakage of lysozymes	No leakage of lysozymes
ATP is depleted	Requires ATP
Specific proteases not activated	Specific proteases activated
Cell lysis, eliciting an inflammatory reaction	Cell is phagocytosed by macrophage, no tissue reaction
DNA fragmentation is random	Chromatin condensation and ladder-like DNA fragmentation
In vivo, whole area of the tissue are affected	*In vivo*, individual cells appear affected

Coagulative Necrosis

The outlines of the cells and architecture of the tissue is well-preserved. There is denaturation of structural proteins and enzymatic proteins. Examples are myocardial infarction and kidney infarct. The cytoplasm of necrotic cells is deeply eosinophilic than usual. The nuclear chromatin may show: Pyknosis, karyorrhexis and karyolysis.

Liquefactive Necrosis

This type of necrosis is seen in infarction of brain, fungal and bacterial infections. There will be complete digestion of dead cells by the hydrolytic enzymes, e.g. brain infarct and abscess

The end result is transformation of tissue into a liquid viscous mass or abscess cavity. The solid tissue is converted into a cavity filled with liquid material.

Caseous Necrosis

This is encountered in tuberculosis. This type of necrosis is due to the toxic effects of mycobacterial cell wall which has mycolic acid and glycolipids. The necrotic cells fail to retain their cellular outlines as in coagulative necrosis or do not disappear. The dead cells persist as granular eosinophilic debri. It is a combination coagulative and liquefactive necrosis.

Gross: The necrotic area is soft, gray white and cheesy.

Microscopy: The tissue architecture is destroyed. Necrotic focus appears as amorphous granular debris composed of fragmented cells enclosed within a distinctive inflammatory granulomatous reaction.

Fibrinoid Necrosis

It is a special form of necrosis seen in immune mediated reaction. It is mainly seen in the wall of the blood vessels, e.g. vessel walls in polyarteritis nodosa (PAN).

There is deposition of antigen antibody complexes along with fibrin material which has been leaked from the lumen of the vessel giving the appearance of pink/eosinophilic amorphous material on H & E stain.

Fat Necrosis

Fat necrosis of abdominal mesentry and omental fat is commonly associated with pancreatic injuries or acute pancreatitis. It can be also observed in trauma to breast fat tissue or subcutaneous fat tissue due to inflammatory response.

Gross: Pancreas and affected mesenteric and peritoneal fat is swollen, indurated, oedematous and shows haemorrhagic/necrotic areas, bright yellow areas of saponification and chalky white areas of calcification.

Microscopy: Shows shadowy outline of necrotic fat cells with basophilic calcium deposits, surrounded by an inflammatory reaction.

GANGRENE

Definition: Gangrene is a form of death of tissue which results from severe hypoxic injury along with necrosis and may be associated with superadded putrefaction.

Dry gangrene: The tissue undergoes basically coagulative necrosis.

Cause for dry gangrene: Arteriosclerosis, TAO, Raynaud's disease, trauma and ergot alkaloids, e.g. gangrene of extremities and toes and fingers.

Gross: The affected part is dry, shrunken, mummified, and skin is wrinkled. The colour of the affected organ changes to dark brown or black due to formation of iron sulfide. Hydrogen sulfide combines with iron from haemoglobin of broken RBCs and forms iron sulfide which is brown in colour. The spread of dry gangrene is slow. There is clear line of demarcation between the affected tissue and normal tissue.

Microscopy: Affected tissue shows coagulative necrosis. The vessels show atherosclerosis, arteriosclerosis and thrombosis of the vessels and normal appearing tissue above the line of separation.

Differences between dry and wet gangrene are given in Table 3.2.

Table 3.2: Differences between dry and wet gangrene

Features	Dry gangrene	Wet gangrene
Site	Common in limbs	Common in bowel and tissue affected with Clostridia organisms
Mechanism	Thrombus or emboli are arterial origin	Thrombus or emboli are venous origin and toxins produce necrosis
Type of necrosis	Mainly coagulative	Mainly liquefactive necrosis
Gross	Dry, shrunken and black due to formation of iron sulfide	Moist, soft, swollen, crepitent and dark
Putrefaction	Limited	Marked
Line of demarcation	Present	Absent
Bacteria	Absent	Present
Prognosis	Good	Poor, toxaemia

Moist Gangrene/Wet Gangrene

There is liquefactive necrosis. Along with ischaemia, bacterial infection supervenes as secondary complication. Thus, in wet gangrene, the organisms are present. The infection spreads proximally, there is no clear line of demarcation between the affected and normal tissue. This type of gangrene develops rapidly.

Causes

1. Veins with thrombosis or embolism
2. Blockage of vessels in diabetes mellitus, e.g. diabetic foot, bedsores, gangrene occurring in tissues like bowel, lung, etc.

Gross: Organ is soft, swollen, putrid, rotten, dark and pulseless.

Microscopy: Tissue is congested, intense inflammatory infiltration and shows liquefactive necrosis. The outlines of the cells affected cannot be made out.

Gas gangrene: This is a form of wet gangrene seen with soil contaminated wounds during road traffic accidents, with compound fractures or trauma with external soft tissue injury infected with bacteria like *Cl. perfringens* or *Cl. welchii*. The toxins produce profound systemic effects along with extensive necrosis and oedema.

Gross morphology: Affected part is swollen, oedematous, painful, crepitant, later becomes dark and foul smelling. There is formation hydrogen sulfide gas which is responsible for formation of blebs and crepitus in the parenchyma of these affected organs.

Microscopically: Muscle fibres undergo coagulative necrosis with liquefaction. Capillary and venous thrombi are common.

Exercise

37

Fatty Change (Liver, Heart) and Amyloidosis

FATTY CHANGE LIVER

Abnormal accumulation of triglycerides within the parenchymal cells is referred to as fatty change. It is also called steatosis. Terms like fatty degeneration, fatty phanerosis and fatty metamorphosis were used earlier. It is most commonly seen in liver as it is a major organ of fat metabolism. It is also seen in heart, skeletal muscle, kidney and other organs.

Causes (Aetiology)

- Diabetes mellitus
- Congenital hyperlipidaemia
- Alcohol
- Starvation
- Protein calorie malnutrition
- Chronic illness
- Pregnancy
- Hypoxia
- Hepatotoxins—CCl_4
- Drugs
- Reye's syndrome.

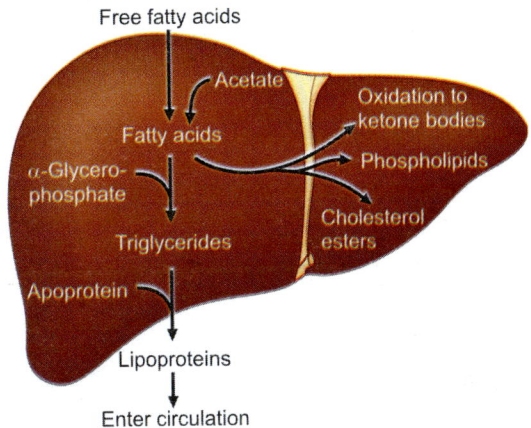

Fig. 3.1a: Mechanism of fatty change

Mechanism of Fatty Change (Fig. 3.1a)

Free fatty acids from fat depots or diet are transported to hepatocytes. In the liver they are esterified to triglycerides, converted into cholesterol or phospholipids or oxidised to ketone bodies. Some fatty acids are synthesised from acetate also. In association with apoproteins, triglycerides form lipoproteins which enter the circulation. Excess accumulation of triglycerides within the liver may occur from defects in anyone of the events from entry as fatty acids to exit as lipoproteins.

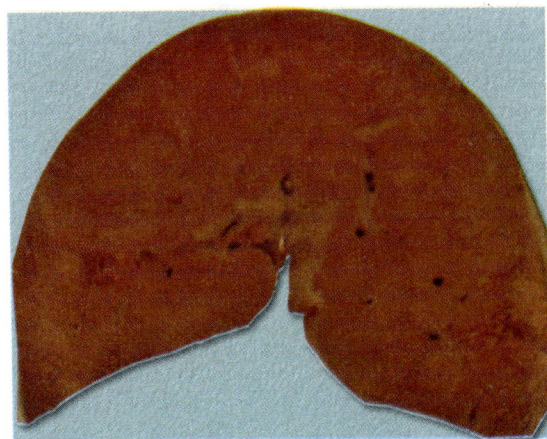

Fig. 3.1b: Gross picture of fatty change liver

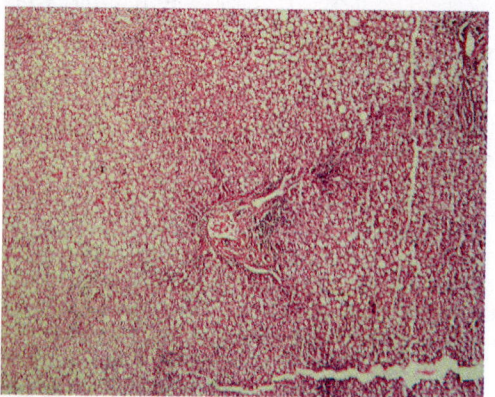

Fig. 3.1c: Photomicrograph of fatty change liver, note severe fatty change (low magnification)

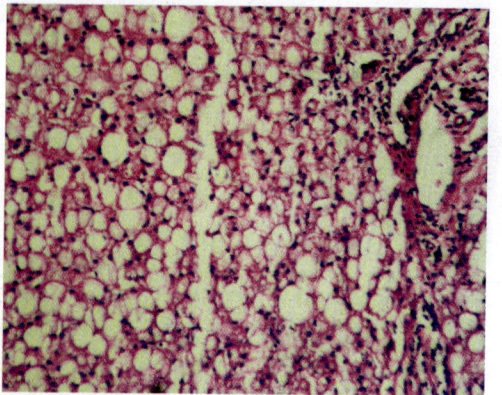

Fig. 3.1d: Photomicrograph of fatty change liver, note severe fatty change (high magnification)

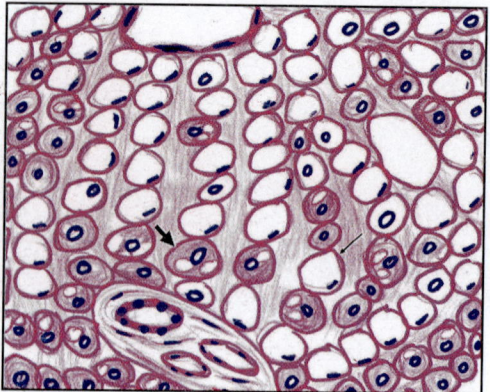

Fig. 3.1e: Schematic diagram of fatty liver, note microvesicular (thick arrow) and macrovesicular fatty change (thin arrow)

Gross: The liver is enlarged (mild/moderate/severe enlargement) depending upon the accumulation of fat. The capsule is tense and glistening. The margin are rounded. It is yellowish in colour, greasy to touch, soft in consistency, C/S bulges slightly and weight is increased. In severe fatty change, the liver may weigh 3 to 6 kg.

Microscopy: The normal liver architecture is maintained. The characteristic feature is presence of numerous lipid vacuoles in the cytoplasm of hepatocytes. In mild fatty change, small sized fat vacuoles/liposomes are present around the nuclei (microvesicular); later they coalesce and displace the nucleus to the periphery (macrovesicular). The contiguous cells rupture and form fatty cysts.

The demonstration of fat can be done by using frozen sections. Some of the fat stains which can be applied are:

i. Oil red 'O'—fat stains red.
ii. Sudan III/IV—fat stains orange to red.
iii. Osmium tetroxide—with alpha naphthylamine reaction phospholipids are stain orange red; cholesterol and triglycerides are stained black.
iv. Neutral fat is stained black with 1% osmic acid in saturated bichlorides or mercury.

FATTY CHANGE HEART

Fatty change heart occurs in two patterns:

1. Prolonged moderate hypoxia as seen in severe anaemia results in focal intracellular fat deposits, grossly, this gives yellowish appearance to the affected myocardial fibres and the normal fibres remain darker and red brown. This pattern is referred as 'tigered' or 'thrush breast' effect. It may also occur in myocarditis, coronary arteriosclerosis, starvation, fever, etc.

2. The other pattern is myocardial fibres are uniformly and diffusely affected due to some toxins, e.g. diphtheria. The anaemia is more severe and profound.

AMYLOIDOSIS

Amyloidosis refers to extracellular protein deposits that have:
1. Common morphological types.
2. Affinity for special dyes.
3. Characteristic appearance under polarised light.

Amyloid is an abnormal proteinaceous substance deposited extracellularly in various organs. It is eosinophilic and hyaline like with H & E stain. The accumulation encroaches and produces pressure atrophy of adjacent cells.

Amyloidosis was first described by Rokitansky in 1842. Virchow named it as amyloid after its starch or cellulose like nature after staining with iodine and sulphuric acid which turned violet coloured. Mechanism of amyloidosis is shown in Flow Chart (Fig. 3.1).

Physicochemical Nature

Amyloid is fibrillar in nature.

Ultrastructurally, it is comprised of non-branching fibrils, polypeptide chains, and these are 7.5 to 10 nm in diameter. These are arranged in beta pleated sheets.

All amyloids have a "*p* component" (10% of amyloid) which is pentagonal, doughnut-shaped and has complex carbohydrates (glycoproteins) which have given its name amyloid.

Classification of Amyloidosis (Table 3.3)

Amyloidosis can be classified as:
1. Primary amyloidosis
2. Secondary amyloidosis

They can be also classified as:
1. Systemic
2. Localised

More than 20 biochemically known distinct forms of amyloid proteins are identified. The most common are:

1. AL (amyloid light chains) protein is produced by plasma cells and is comprised immunoglobulin light chains and seen in monoclonal B cell proliferations like:
   - Multiple myeloma
   - Waldenström's macroglobulinaemia
   - Lymphomas.
2. *AA (amyloid associated) protein:* It is a non-immunoglobulin protein derived from serum precursor protein—SAA (serum amyloid associated) which is synthesised in the liver and defective proteolysis leads to the deposition in conditions like:
   - Tuberculosis
   - Rheumatoid arthritis
   - Carcinomas
   - Bronchiectasis
   - Other causes like:
     – Dermatomyopathies
     – Crohn's disease
     – Ankylosing spondylitis and
     – Lepromatous leprosy.

Table 3.3: Classification amyloidosis with precursor proteins and clinical setting

Amyloid protein	Protein precursor	Clinical setting
Systemic/generalized		
AL	Kappa or Lamda chains	Multiple myeoloma, plasma cell dyscrasiasis
AA	ApoSAA	chronic inflammations, certain neoplasia, hereditary conditions, familial Mediterranean fever
Localised		
Beta amyloid	Abeta protein	Alzheimer's disease and blood vessels
Mutant transthyretin (ATTR)	Transthyretin	Familial amyloid polyneuropathies and heart in aged people
Beta2 microglobulin	Beta2 microglobulin	Renal dialysis
ACal	(Pro)calcitonin	Medullary carcinoma
PrPs	Plasma membrane protein	Prion disease

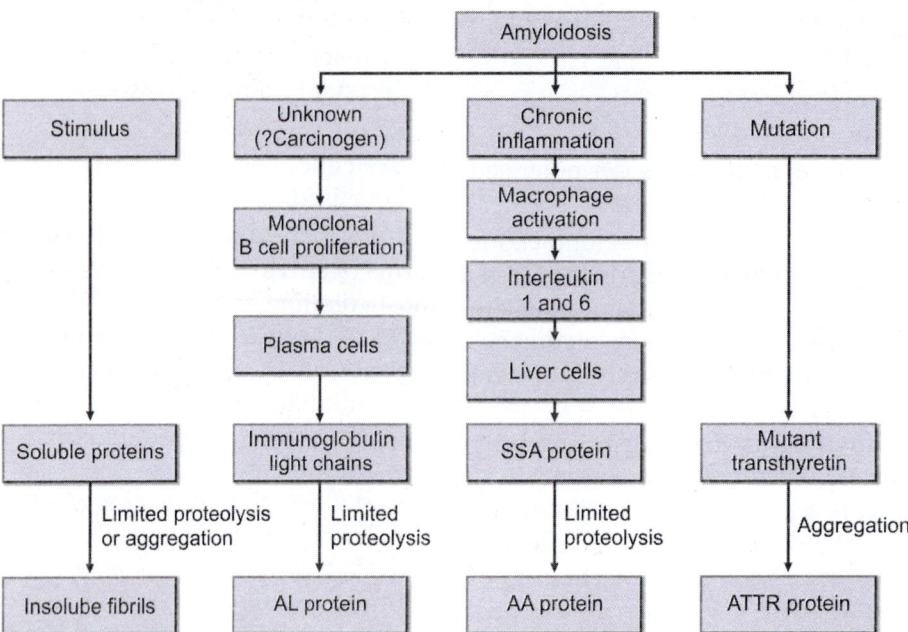

Flow Chart 3.1: Mechanism of amyloidosis

3. A β-amyloid protein is found in cerebral lesions in Alzheimer's disease in cerebral plaques and blood vessels.
4. Mutant transthyretin, the mutations of transthyretin that transports thyroxin and retinol aggregates in the form of amyloid deposits. This results in familial amyloid polyneuropathies. It can also develop in the heart in aged people.
5. β_2 microglobulin, this protein is present in the serum of patients with renal disease which is retained in circulation as it is not filtered through dialysis membranes.

Amyloidosis of liver (Figs 3.2a and b)

Gross: The amyloid deposits may be grossly inapparent or may show moderate to marked hepatomegaly. The cut section is waxy.

Microscopy: The amyloid gets deposited in the space of Disse and progressively encroaches on the adjacent hepatocytes and sinusoids. In advanced stages, it has pressure atrophy features with disappearance of hepatocytes. Vascular involvement is frequent.

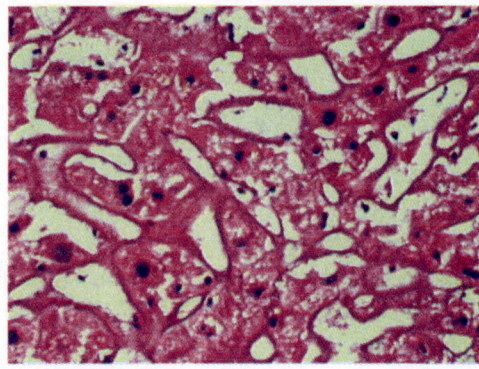

Fig. 3.2a: Photomicrograph of amyloidosis liver

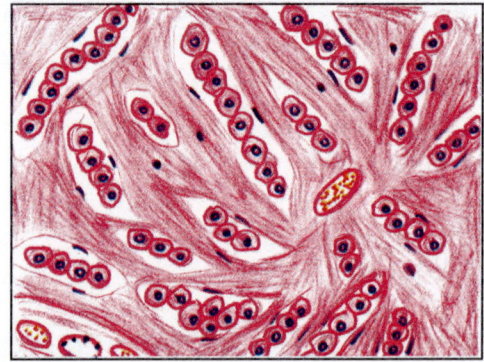

Fig. 3.2b: Schematic diagram of microscopy in amyloidosis liver

Amyloidosis of Spleen

Gross: The amyloid deposits may be grossly inapparent or may show moderate to marked splenomegaly. Deposits in malpighian corpuscle may present as sago spleen (tapioca like granules) and deposits in red pulp (sinusoids) give the appearance of lardaceous spleen (large map like areas). The cut section is waxy.

Microscopy

Sago spleen: The amyloid deposits are limited to the splenic follicles (in the vessel and may replace the follicle) (Fig. 3.2c).

Lardaceous spleen: The amyloid spares the follicles but involves the walls of the splenic sinusoids and connective tissue framework of the red pulp.

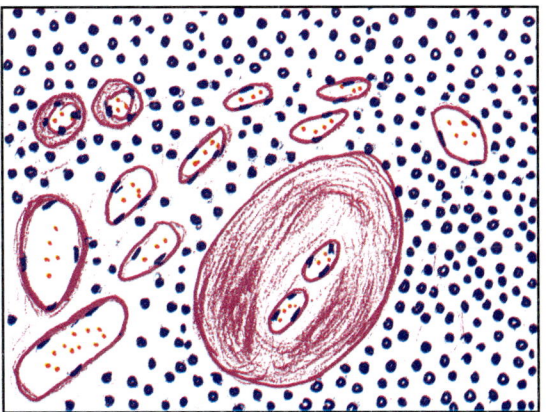

Fig. 3.2c: Schematic diagram of microscopy of amyloidosis spleen (sago spleen)

Amyloidosis of Kidney

This is the serious form of organ involvement. The renal amyloidosis is the major cause of death.

Gross: The kidney may appear normal in size and colour. It may be enlarged and waxy. In advanced cases, it may be shrunken and contracted owing to the vascular narrowing induced by amyloid deposits within the arterial and arteriolar walls.

Microscopy: The amyloid gets deposited in the glomeruli, interstitium, peritubular tissue, arteries and arterioles. In the glomeruli, the amyloid is deposited in the glomerular basement membrane and in the mesangial matrix (Fig. 3.2d).

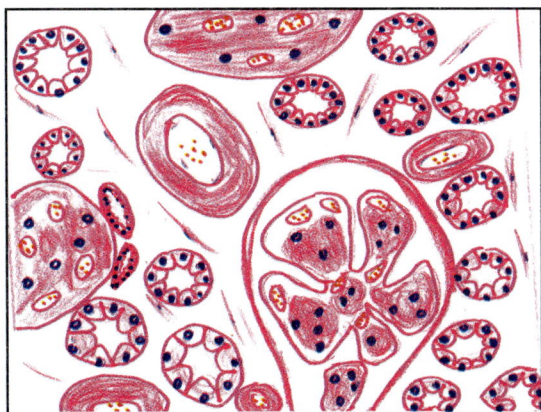

Fig. 3.2d: Schematic diagram of microscopy in amyloidosis kidney

Stains for Amyloid

1. H & E stain—amyloid stains homogenous and pale pink.
2. PAS stain—amyloid stains magenta pink.
3. van Gieson—amyloid stains yellow to yellow brown.
4. Iodine (Gram's or Lugol's)—amyloid stains mahagony brown turning to blue or violet with application of dilute sulphuric acid.
5. Metachromatic stains (e.g. 1% methyl violet, 1% toluidine blue)—amyloid stains pink, other tissues violet.
6. Congo red—amyloid stains orange.
7. Congo red with polarisation—apple green birefringence.
8. X-ray diffraction—cross beta pleat structure.
9. Fluorescence with thioflavin T and S.

Exercise

38

Inflammation (Acute and Chronic) and Granulation Tissue

INFLAMMATION

Inflammation is defined as the local response of a living mammalian tissues to injury due to any agent. It is body's defence reaction in order to eliminate or limit the spread of injurious agent as well as to remove the damaged or necrosed cells and tissues. It may be acute or chronic. The different chemical mediators and the differences between the two are given in Tables 3.4 and 3.5.

Cardinal signs: The cardinal signs were named by the Roman scientist Celsus. They are:
- Rubor (redness)
- Tumour (swelling)
- Calor (heat)
- Dolor (pain)
- Virchow added the 5th cardinal sign which is functio laesa (loss of function).

Redness is due to vasodilatation, swelling is due to oedema because of increased vascular permeability, calor is due to vasodilatation and increased vascular flow, dolor is because of prostaglandins, neuropeptide and other chemical mediators which stimulate nerve endings and loss of function is due to inability to move the affected region due to pain.

Causative Agents

- Infections: Bacteria, viruses, fungi, parasites
- Trauma
- Physical agents: Heat, cold, pressure effects, radiation, mechanical injury
- Chemical: Drugs, toxins, alkali and acids
- Immunological disorders: Hypersensitivity reactions, autoimmunity, immuno deficiency states, etc.
- Genetic and metabolic disorders: Gout, diabetes, etc.
- Tissue necrosis
- Foreign bodies

Inflammation can be acute or chronic. The changes taking place are classically evident in acute inflammation. The differences between the two have been listed later of this topic.

Table 3.4: Different inflammatory findings and mediators responsible

Inflammatory findings	Mediators responsible
Fever	IL-1, IL-8, TNF, prostaglandins
Pain	Prostaglandins, bradykinins, histamine, serotonin neuropeptide
Vasoconstriction	TXA2, LT4, D4, E4
Vasodilatation	Histamine, prostaglandins, NO
Increased vascular permeability	Histamine, serotonin, C3a, C5a, LTB4, D4, E4, PAF, substance P
Recognition	C3b, Fc portion of IgG
Opsonisation	Mannose receptors, scavenger receptors, TLRs
Chemotaxis	C5a, LTB4, IL-8, PAF, 5-HETE

Table 3.5: Differences between acute and chronic inflammation

	Acute inflammation	Chronic inflammation
Duration of inflammation	Short duration	Prolonged duration—weeks to months to years
Type of inflammatory cells including giant cells	Neutrophils are the main inflammatory cells. Giant cells are not seen	Lymphocytes and plasma cells are the main inflammatory cells. Giant cells are seen, e.g. Foreign body giant cells, Langhan's giant cells, Touton giant cells
Cause	It is caused by trauma, infectious agents with organisms of high virulence, injury caused may be severe	It is caused by irritant substances and granulomatous infections. Occurs due to persistent and less virulent microbes (as seen in TB, leprosy, etc.), autoimmune or allergic diseases
Signs of inflammation	Classical signs of inflammation are seen—pain, redness, heat and swelling	Classical signs of inflammation are not seen
Lewis response	Lewis triple response is seen	Lewis triple response is not seen
Vascular changes and cellular changes	Consists of haemodynamic changes, increased vascular permeability, exudation of leucocytes and phagocytosis	Infiltration with mononuclear cells and formation of granulomas oedema and vascular changes less predominant
Inflammation, tissue injury and healing process	Inflammation and tissue injury only occur	Inflammation, tissue injury and healing occur simultaneously
Systemic effects	Systemic manifestations are fever, leukocytosis, shock, DIC, metabolic abnormalities	Systemic manifestations are less pronounced

During inflammation initially there will be vascular changes followed by cellular changes.

I. Vascular Changes

1. The changes in vascular flow and caliber.
2. Increased vascular permeability.

Changes in Vascular Flow and Caliber

Soon after the injury, there is transient vasoconstriction lasting for a few seconds, after this there is arteriolar vasodilatation, resulting in engorgement of the arterioles, capillaries and venules. There is increased blood flow which is responsible for redness (rubor), and warmth (calor or erythema).

Increased Vascular Permeability

Increased vascular permeability begins in early phase of inflammation. Arterioles, capillaries and venules show dilatation. There is increased vascular flow which leads to increased hydrostatic pressure and with increased vascular permeability, protein rich fluid moves out into extracellular space causing oedema (Tumour or swelling is a cardinal sign due to oedema fluid). Initially this is transudate, later it becomes exudate as white blood cells move out of the vessel. Several chemical mediators and mechanisms will contribute to the increased vascular permeability. Because of loss of fluid, thus there is slowing of blood flow and stasis occurs.

Chemical Mediators of Increased Permeability

Acting immediately and transiently are: histamine, bradykinin, serotonin, NO, leucotriene B4 and Platelet Activating Factor (PAF).

Causes: Heat, cold, UV rays, X-rays, bacterial toxins, chemicals, etc. Some of these bring about delayed and prolonged vascular permeability.

II. Cellular Phenomenon in Inflammation

Early phase of inflammation, for the first 24 hours neutrophils are the cells which try to eliminate the injurious agent.

The cellular events in inflammation are as below:
- Margination, rolling, pavementation, adhesion and transmigration
- Chemotaxis
- Recognition and attachment
- Phagocytosis/engulfment
- Killing and degradation.

Margination, rolling, pavementation, adhesion and transmigration: Following are the events:

Margination: Leukocytes from axial flow move towards plasmatic flow due to stasis. Margination is peripheral positioning of leukocytes on the endothelial cells from the axial flow.

Rolling and Pavementation

Subsequently rows of leukocytes tumble along the endothelium in a process called rolling. Leukocytes adhere to the vascular endothelium and become activated. For rolling selectin family of adhesion molecules play a role. These are weak and cause transient adhesion and this makes them roll.

Selectin family: This family of adhesion molecules includes:
- P-selectins on platelets and endothelial cells
- E-selectins on endothelial cells
- L-selectins on leukocytes

In time, the white blood cells are lined up on the endothelial cells and this appearance is called pavementation.

Adhesion

Firm adhesion of leukocytes is brought about by adhesion molecules mediated by integrins. These are normally expressed on leukocyte plasma membrane in a low affinity form. When leukocytes are activated by chemokines, the integrins undergo conformational changes and get converted into high affinity form. At the same time, TNF, IL-1 and endotoxins activate ligands on endothelial cells (LFA1 and VLA4) for integrins. These are:

1. Intercellular adhesion molecule 1 (ICAM 1) which binds to lymphocyte function associated molecule 1 (LFA 1).
2. Membrane attack complex 1 (Mac 1) which binds to very late activation molecule 4 (VLA 4).
3. Vascular cell adhesion molecule 1 (VCAM 1) which binds to VLA4.

Transmigration

After firm adhesion, leukocytes escape from the vessels in between the endothelial cells, by active movement and their extending pseudopodia helps them to come out of the vessels. Platelet/endothelial cell adhesion molecule 1 (PECAM 1) also called CD31 is an adhesion molecule expressed both on leukocytes and endothelial cells, helps in traversing through the endothelium. After traversing the endothelium, the leukocytes cross the basement membrane by focally degrading with the help of collagenases secreted by the leukocytes. Along with leukocytes, RBCs also come out passively.

Chemotaxis

The movement of leukocytes along a chemical gradient is called chemotaxis. This is unidirectional movement of leukocytes from vascular channels towards the site of inflammation.

The chemotactic factors for leukocytes are:
a. Components of complement system C5a.
b. Bacterial products particularly peptides with N-formyl methionine terminal amino acids and some lipids.
c. Chemokines: Cytokines especially from chemokine family (IL-8).
d. Products of the lipoxygenase family particularly leukotriene B4 (LTB4).

After the step of chemotaxis, the pathogen has to be phagocytosed. Phagocytosis involves three different, but interrelated steps. These are:
- Recognition and attachment
- Engulfment
- Killing and degradation.

Recognition and Attachment

Recognition of the injurious agent by the leukocytes is through the following:
- Mannose receptors present on leukocytes recongise mannose molecules on microbes
- Scavenger receptors present on macrophages recognize bacteria
- Macrophage integrins
- Opsonins
- Toll receptors recognize toll proteins on microbes

For leukocytes to attach to the injurious agent, it has to be coated with certain plasma proteins called opsonins. The important opsonins are:
- Fc portion of immunoglobulin G class.
- Complement C3b, is an important complement molecule, when bound to the antigen on the pathogen, is recognised by the phagocytes. These are present in the blood or produced as a reaction to microbes.
- Lectins are carbohydrate binding proteins, which are present in the plasma membrane. These bind to the cell wall of pathogen and act as opsonins.

The leukocytes have surface receptors for these opsonins.

Engulfment

Binding of opsonised particles triggers the process of engulfment. During this process extension of cytoplasm flow around the object engulfed, eventually resulting in complete closure of the particle by the cytoplasm. This is phagosome; the organism is covered by cytoplasmic membrane. For degradative action by the leukocyte, the phagosome has to combine with lysosomes, thus forming phago-lysosome, in which degradative enzymes are present.

Killing and Degradation

The steps in killing and degradation are production of microbicidal substances which are present within the lysosomes and fusion of these lysosomes with phagosome. Thus, the ingested particle is exposed to destructive mechanism of leukocytes.

The microbicidal activity may be produced by:
1. *Myeloperoxidase independent mechanisms:* These mechanisms do not require the myeloperoxidase enzyme. The two important mechanisms in this are:
   a. The phagocytosis stimulates an oxidative burst with increase reactive oxygen species (ROS) and these are superoxide anion (O_2^-), hydrogen peroxide (H_2O_2) and hydroxyl radical (OH). The ROS can destroy the microbes. After the action is over, ROS are degraded.
   b. The dead microbes are degraded by the action of lysosomal acid hydrolases, the most important being elastase.
   c. The leukocyte granules have bactericidal permeability increasing protein causing damage to cell membrane, lysozymes degrade bacterial wall oligosaccharides and major basic protein present in the granules of the eosinophils is cytotoxic to parasites.
2. *Myeloperoxidase dependent mechanisms:* Lysosomes contain myeloperoxidase enzyme (MPO) which converts H_2O_2 in presence of Cl^- ions to HCLO (hypochlorous acid). The H_2O_2-MPO-halide system is the most powerful oxidant and an anti-microbial agent. This is the major bactericidal agent. HCLO also activates collagenase and other enzymes released by neutrophils and inactivates α-1 antitrypsin.

CHEMICAL MEDIATORS

These originate from the cells or plasma. They are in precursor form and later get activated. They are synthesized *de novo*. Chemical mediator production is triggered by microbial products or host proteins. They perform their activity by binding to the receptors on the target cells. One mediator can stimulate release of other mediators by target cells with opposing activities. The mediators can act on few or one target cell types, having different cell types. Once activated or released, they are short-lived. They get decayed/inactivated/scavenged/inhibited. There are checks and balances to control their synthesis, function and time of action.

The chemical mediators are as below:

Cell derived
- Vasoactive amines—histamine, serotonin
- Lysosomal component
- Platelet activating factor
- Cytokines
- NO and O_2 metabolites
- Arachidonic acid metabolites.

Plasma derived
- The kinin system
- The clotting system
- The fibrinolytic system
- The complement system.

Morphological Patterns of Inflammation

The vascular changes, leukocyte infiltrate, severity of reaction, its specific causes, particular tissue and site involved introduce morphological variations in the basic pattern. Many patterns are recognised which vary in morphology and clinical condition.

Serous inflammation: This is characterised by outpouring of thin fluid which may be derived from plasma or epithelial secretions particularly involves epithelial cells, mesothelial cells and skin. This type of inflammation is seen in:
- Skin in burns and viral infections
- Pericardial, pleural and peritoneal effusions.

Fibrinous inflammation: With severe injuries, there is increased vascular permeability and fibrinogen passes through the vessels. The fibrin is deposited into extravascular spaces. In H & E sections fibrin appears as eosinophilic mesh. This inflammation is characteristic in inflammations lining body cavities like meninges, pericardium and pleura. This may be resolved by fibrinolysis and clearing by macrophages, resolve completely assuming original features or undergoes fibrosis. Conversion to scar tissue is called organisation which leads to thickening and adhesions.

Suppurative or purulent inflammation: This is characterised by production of large amounts of pus or purulent exudate consisting of neutrophils, necrotic debris, and oedema fluid. Certain bacteria are responsible for this type of inflammation, e.g. Staphylococci. The classic features can be appreciated in acute suppurative appendicitis and acute pyogenic meningitis.

Abscess: It is a localised collection of pus within a part of tissue because of an inflammatory process, e.g. liver abscess and lung abscess.

Gangrene: Gangrene is localised death, necrosis or decomposition of body tissue resulting because of obstruction to circulatory system or due to bacterial infection.

Ulcer: There is a local defect or breach in the continuity or excavation of the surface epithelium or organ which is produced by sloughing of the cells. This is seen in:
1. Ulcers of mouth, stomach, intestine and genitourinary tract.
2. In older people, subcutaneous inflammation of lower extremities occur because of circulatory disturbances.

Granulomatous Inflammation

Granulomatous inflammation is a distinctive type of chronic inflammation characterised by focal collection of epithelioid cells (modified macrophages), giant cells and mantle of lymphocytes (Table 3.6).

Pathogenesis: Refer to the topic on tuberculous lymphadenitis.

Causes: These are as shown in Table 3.6 and some are described.

Table 3.6: Causes of granulomatous diseases

Bacterial infections—Mycobacteria	*Mycobacterium tuberculosis*
	Atypical mycobacteria
	Leprosy
Gram-negative/positive bacillus	Cat-scratch disease
	Brucellosis, actinomycosis, nocardiosis
Fungi	Cryptococcosis, histoplasmosis, aspergillosis, sporotrichosis, etc.
Parasites	Schistosomiasis, leishmaniasis (worms, larvae, eggs)
Spirochaetes	Syphilis, pinta, yaws
Viruses	Measles, mumps, etc.
Materials that do not get digested	Endogenous like keratin, necrotic bone, cholesterol, sodium urate
	Exogenous—talc, silica, suture material, oils
Specific chemicals	Berylliosis
Unknown mechanism	Crohn's
	Sarcoidosis
	Wegener's granulomatosis
	Chronic granulomatous disease of childhood
Drugs	Hepatic granulomas due to allopurinol, phenylbutazone, sulfonamides

Tuberculous granuloma: There can be initially non-caseating granulomas and later caseating granulomas develop.

The classical microscopic picture is that the granulomas have central area of caseation necrosis surrounded by epithelioid cells, Langhan's type of giant cells and surrounding this is a mantle of lymphocytes.

Leprosy: In tuberculoid leprosy there will be non-caseating granulomas.

Syphilis: There is a gumma with good number of plasma cells, histiocytes and lymphocytes. The centre may be necrotic.

Cat scratch disease: There will be stellate granulomas, containing central granular debris, neutrophils, and giant cells.

DIFFERENT TYPES OF GIANT CELLS

- Langhans' type of giant cell (tuberculosis)
- Foreign body giant cell (foreign body with chronic infection)
- RS cell (Hodgkin's disease)
- Touton giant cell (xanthogranuloma)
- Osteoclastic giant cell (bone, giant cell tumour of bone)
- Tumour giant cell (malignant tumours)
- Warthin-Finkeldey giant cell (measles and viral infection.

Acute and Chronic Appendicitis

Appendiceal inflammation is associated with obstruction, usually by faecolith and less commonly by a gallstone or ball of *E. vermicularis* worms. Continued secretion of mucinous material in the obstructed appendix presumably leads to increased intraluminal pressure and ischaemia which favours bacterial growth and inflammation.

In early acute appendicitis, wall is oedematous; serosa shows fibrinopurulent exudate with congested vessels.

In acute suppurative appendicitis, mucosa is ulcerated. The wall is oedematous. It is infiltrated by acute inflammatory cells and foci of necrosis are present. Serosa is covered with purulent exudate. Further vascular compromise leads to gangrenous changes creating acute gangrenous appendicitis.

Gross: Appendix is swollen, oedematous and covered with exudate, the serosal vessels are congested. Cut section, lumen shows exudate (Fig. 3.3a).

Microscopy: Mucosa is ulcerated, wall is oedematous and lymphoid follicles are hyperplastic. Neutrophilic infiltrate is present in all the layers. Serosa is inflamed and the blood vessels are congested (Fig. 3.3b).

Chronic Appendicitis

The symptoms and signs of chronic appendicitis are vague. There may be collection of lymphocytes in the muscular wall of the appendix. Plasma cells or eosinophils may be seen in the mucosa.

Residual changes of acute appendicitis that subsided in the past may be seen.

- If gangrene has occurred, only a stump of the appendix may remain.
- When inflammatory process has destroyed the muscle, fibrous replacement is present.
- If the original process was superficial and confined to the mucosa and submucosa, no residual changes will be found.
- Many cases diagnosed as chronic appendicitis represent recurrent acute appendicitis, the pathologic findings depending on whether the appendicectomy was performed during an acute attack or between bouts. Significant increase in neural fibres, Schwann cells and enlarged ganglia in cases of clinically acute appendicitis may be indicative of repeated bouts of inflammation.

Gross: Appendix is shrunken in size, it is thin and cord-like.

Microscopy: The mucosa may be ulcerated or shows regenerative changes. It may sometimes show obliteration of lumen with fibrosis. There is submucosal and subserosal fibrosis. The wall shows chronic inflammatory cell infiltration.

Complications of Acute Appendicitis

Perforation: It can lead to diffuse peritonitis and periappendiceal abscess which may perforate into the caecum, ileum or rectum or even open onto the skin surface.

Spread of inflammation: This is via the ileocolic, upper mesenteric and portal veins to the liver with formation of 'pyelophlebitic abscess' and it is a serious complication.

Periappendicitis: It is the acute or chronic inflammation of the appendiceal serosa. It is invariably present in the advanced stages of appendicitis, but it can also be seen in the absence of a primary inflammation of this

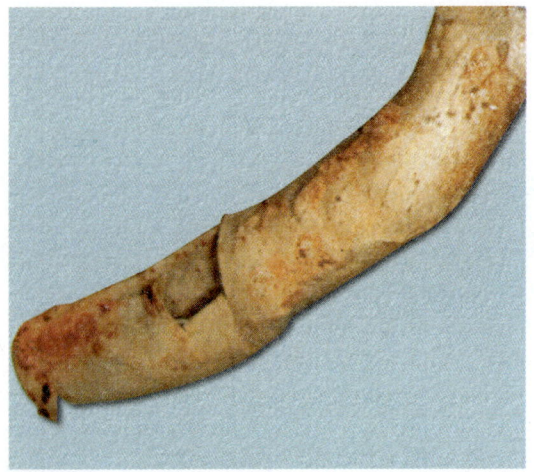

Fig. 3.3a: Gross picture of acute appendicitis, note oedema and exudate

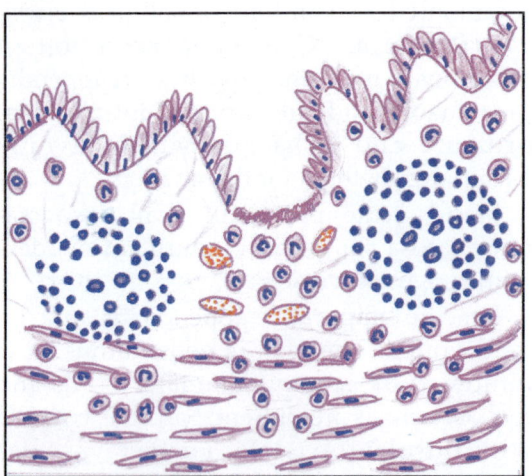

Fig. 3.3b: Schematic diagram of microscopy in acute appendicitis

organ, as a result of spread of an inflammatory process from another site, such as infection from pelvic organs in females.

Appendicular abscess: This is due to rupture of an appendix giving rise to localised abscess in the right iliac fossa. The abscess may spread between the liver and the diaphragm (subphrenic abscess), into the pelvis between the urinary bladder and rectum and in females may involve the uterus and fallopian tubes.

Adhesions: Late complications of acute appendicitis are fibrous adhesions to the greater omentum, small intestine and other abdominal structures.

Mucocele: Distension of distal appendix by mucus following recovery from an attack of acute appendicitis is referred to as mucocele. It occurs generally due to proximal obstruction but sometimes may be due to a benign or malignant neoplasm in the appendix. Rupture of mucocele can give rise to "*Pseudomyxoma peritonei*". An infected mucocele may result in formation of empyema of the appendix.

Sialoadenitis

Inflammation of salivary glands may be viral, bacterial, traumatic or autoimmune origin.

Bacterial inflammation by *Staphylococcus aureus* and *Streptococcus viridans* causes acute sialoadenitis possibly secondary to obstruction by stones (sialolithiasis) or strictures of salivary ducts. The stagnant secretions act as medium for bacterial overgrowth. It may occur due to retrograde entry of oral cavity bacteria during severe dehydration such as postoperative state. Persons with chronic, debilitating illness, immunocompromised states or medications contributing to acute dehydration increases the risk of infection. The sialoadenitis is mainly interstitial, may cause focal areas of suppurative necrosis or abscess formation.

Chronic inflammation occurs due to reduced production of saliva with subsequent inflammation, the common cause is autoimmune sialadenitis or of viral origin. This is almost always bilateral. All the major salivary glands and minor salivary glands are affected. Sjögren's syndrome is of autoimmune origin and is associated with xerostomia, keratoconjunctivitis sicca and sialoadenitis. There is enlargement of lacrimal gland and salivary gland due to inflammation. These are painless. Dryness of mouth, and dryness of eyes are present due to less or no secretion of saliva and tears. This is referred to as Mikulicz syndrome.

Mumps caused by viral infection leads to acute enlargement of salivary glands. It usually produces interstitial inflammation showing oedema and mononuclear cell infiltration, sometimes necrosis. Mumps in childhood is self-limited. In adults, it may be accompanied by pancreatitis and orchitis. The later is the cause of permanent sterility in these patients.

Microscopy: In acute sialoadenitis parenchyma shows suppurative necrosis and abscess formation. There is neutrophilic infiltration in the interlobular and intralobular connective tissue (Fig. 3.4).

Pneumonia (Figs 3.5a to e)

Pneumonia is a bacterial infection of lung parenchyma.

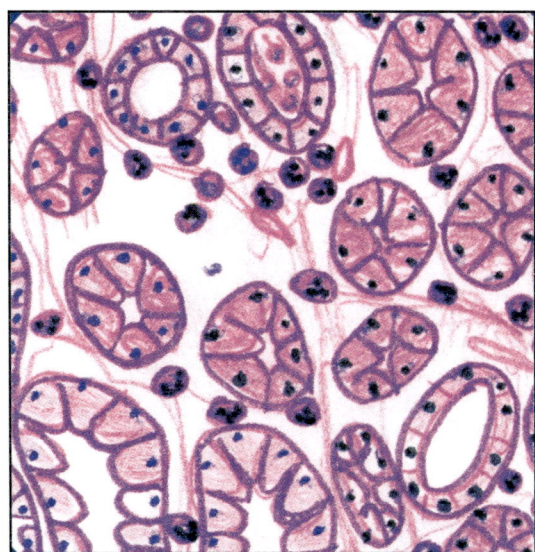

Fig. 3.4: Schematic diagram of microscopy in acute sialoadenitis

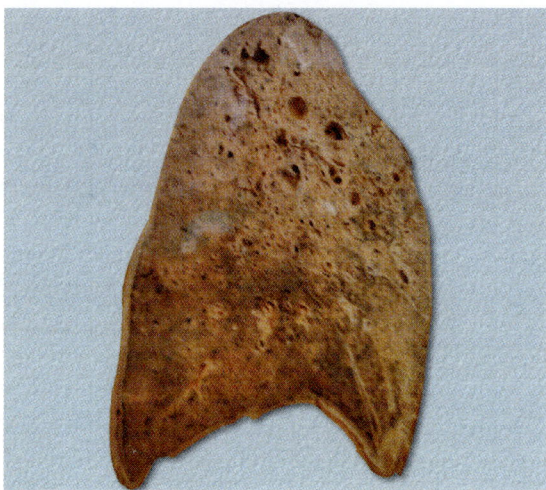

Fig. 3.5a: Gross picture of lung in lobar pneumonia

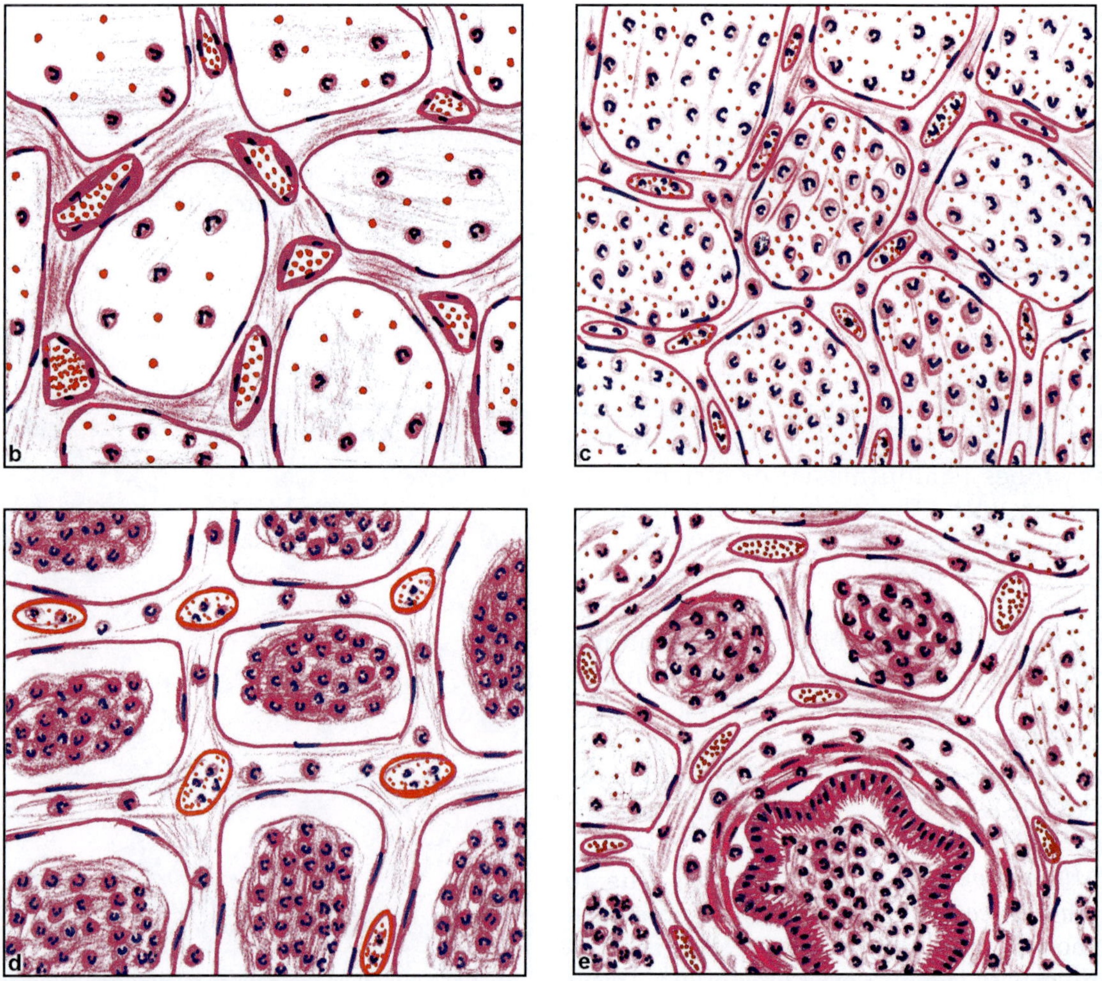

Figs 3.5b to e: (b) Schematic diagram of microscopy in lobar pneumonia congestion stage; (c) red hepatisation stage; (d) grey hepatisation stage; (e) bronchopneumonia

Lobar pneumonia: Classical lobar pneumonia now is infrequent. In 90–95% of the cases *Streptococcus pneumoniae* types 1, 3, 7 and 2 cause the infection. Occasionally *Klebsiella pneumoniae*, Streptococcus, Staphylococcus, H. influenzae, Pseudomonas and Proteus may also cause pneumonia.

The organisms reach the lungs by four ways:
a. Inhalation
b. Aspiration
c. Hematogenous
d. Direct spread from contiguous infection.

Normally lung has defense mechanisms. When defence mechanisms (mucociliary function, alveolar macrophages, phagocytosis, humoral and cellular immunity) fail, infection spreads. Infection spreads through pores of Kohn.

Clinical Features

Sudden onset of fever, chills, and rigors. There is cough, breathlessness, hemoptysis (rusty sputum), and chest pain due to pleuritis. Loss of appetite, bodyache and headache are present. Patient is dyspnoeic, has trachycardia, high grade fever.

Investigation

- Total count increased
- Pulmonary opacities on X-ray/CT establishes diagnosis
- Pleural tap for microscopy and culture
- Blood gas analysis impaired.

Gross

Stage of congestion: Lung is heavy, boggy and red.

Stage of red hepatisation: Lung is dry, solid, granular and reddish coloured.

Stage of grey hepatisation: Affected lobe is solid, dry and grey white. Pleural surface is covered with exudate.

Microscopy

Stage of congestion: The lung parenchyma shows vascular engorgement, intra-alveolar fluid with a few neutrophils and numerous bacteria.

Stage of red hepatisation: Alveoli show marked fibrinous exudate with polymorphs and RBCs.

Stage of grey hepatisation: Alveoli show exudate with contracted fibrin; the RBCs are lysed. The septal capillaries are congested.

Stage of resolution: Exudate undergoes progressive enzymatic digestion to produce granular debris that is reabsorbed.

Bronchopneumonia: This occurs during extremes of age groups (children and old age people), debilitating illness, pre-existing lung diseases and local obstruction to the upward flow of mucus. The organisms which can cause bronchopneumonia are: *Staph. aureus,* streptococci, Klebsiella. *E. coli,* Proteus, Pseudomonas.

Unlike in lobar pneumonia, the inflammation is distributed in patches around the bronchioles with intervening uninvolved normal lung tissue. These patches may become confluent. Pleural involvement is less common than lobar pneumonia. The suppurative inflammation fills the bronchi, bronchiole and surrounding alveoli. Some of the alveoli are filled with oedema fluid, others may show fibrinous exudate while some alveoli are collapsed, thus giving the microscopic appearance different from that of lobar pneumonia, all alveoli not being in one stage.

Sequelae or Complications

With appropriate therapy, the lung can resume normal state in both types of pneumonias, but occasionally following complications can occur:

- Organisation—fibrous tissue formation
- Lung abscess due to tissue destruction and necrosis
- Empyema—accumulation of exudate in the pleural cavity
- Meningitis
- Septic arthritis
- Infective endocarditis.

Differences between lobar pneumonia and bronchopneumonia are given in Table 3.7.

Table 3.7: Differences between lobar pneumonia and bronchopneumonia

Lobar pneumonia	Bronchopneumonia
Caused by pneumococci in 90% of cases, a few cases are caused by Klebsiella, *Staph aureus*	Caused by Staphylococci, Streptococci, *H. influenzae*, Proteus and Pseudomonas
Occurs in healthy individuals between 30 and 50 years of age	Occurs in infants, old age people and those suffering from chronic debilitating illness or immunosuppression
Onset is sudden with high grade fever, chills and rusty sputum	Onset is insidious with low grade fever and productive cough of purulent sputum
Causes consolidation of whole lobe	Causes patchy consolidation
Complications: Bacteremia, meningitis, endocarditis, septic arthritis	Complications: Fibrosis, bronchiectasis, lung abscess

Pyogenic Meningitis

Different organisms are responsible in various age groups.

In neonates—*E. coli* and group B streptococci

Infants and children—*H. influenzae*

Adolescents and young adults—*N. meningitidis*

Elderly—*Streptococcus pneumoniae* and *Listeria monocytogenes*.

Gross: Meningeal vessels are engorged. There is exudate in the subarachnoid space; in *H. influenzae* meningitis exudates predominantly at the base of brain and in *N. meningitidis* infection over the cerebral convexities. Exudate is present along the vessels in early stages.

It may be seen in the ventricles also.

Microscopy: Neutrophils fill the subarachnoid space. The vessels are congested. Cerebritis may be present. Phlebitis may lead to venous obstruction and subsequent infarction (Fig. 3.6a to c).

Complications: If not treated, fibrous adhesions with hydrocephalus is known to occur.

Tuberculous Lymphadenitis

M. tuberculosis is responsible for most of the cases of tuberculosis. *M. bovis* is rare but still present in countries which have tuberculous dairy cows and where consumption of pasteurised milk is not practiced.

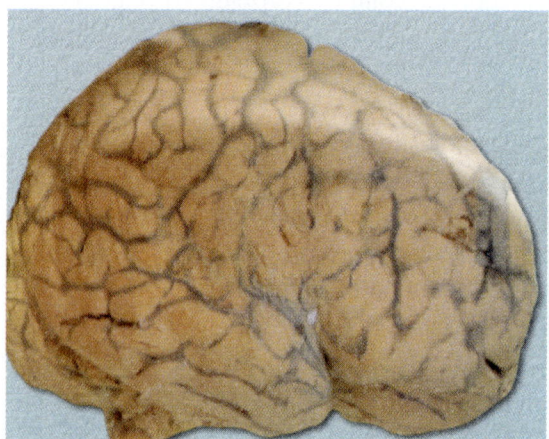

Fig. 3.6a: Gross picture of pyogenic meningitis

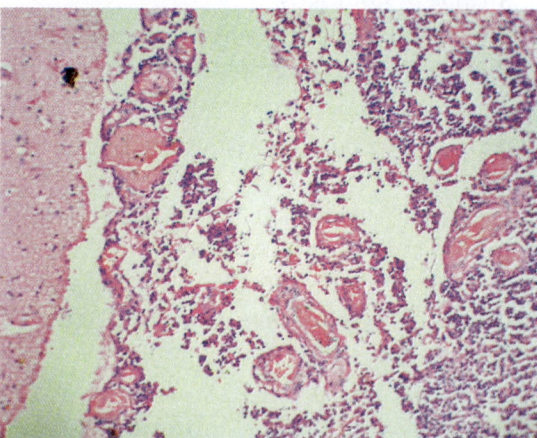

Fig. 3.6b Photomicrograph of pyogenic meningitis, note exudate in subarachnoid space

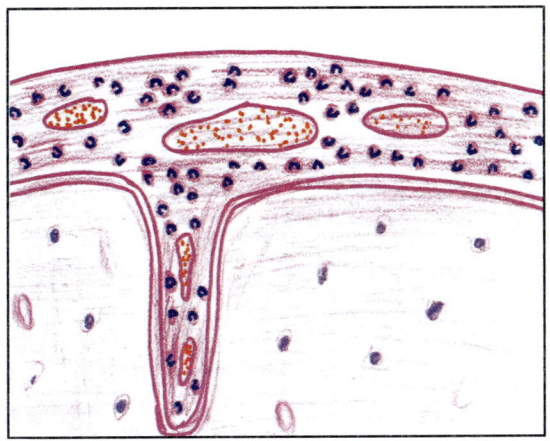

Fig. 3.6c Schematic diagram of microscopy in pyogenic meningitis

M. tuberculosis typically leads to the development of delayed hypersensitivity to mycobacterial antigens (Fig. 3.7). The antigen presenting cells (macrophages) produce IL-12 and stimulate the T lymphocytes by about 3 weeks. These T cells release IFN-γ which creates an inhospitable acidic environment for the bacteria; also stimulates production of NO and free O_2 radicals and cause oxidative destruction of the bacilli. IFN-γ also in turn activates the macrophages with release of TNF and IL-1 which leads to formation of epithelioid cells and granuloma formation.

Gross: The lymph nodes are enlarged, matted and soft in consistency. Cut section shows areas of caseation necrosis (Fig. 3.8a).

Microscopy: The normal lymphnode architecture is effaced and replaced by granulomas which are comprised of central necrosis surrounded by epithelioid cells and Langhan's type of giant cells with a mantle of lymphocytes. Fibrosis is present surrounding these cells (Figs 3.8b and c).

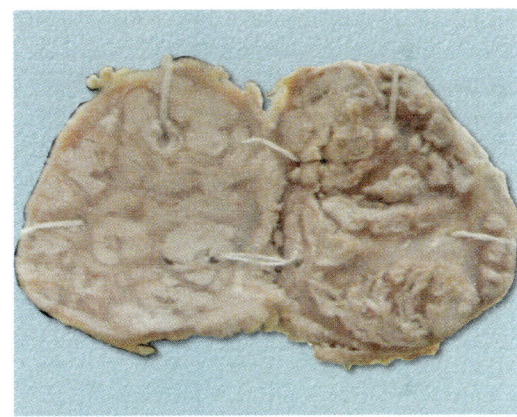

Fig. 3.8a Gross picture of lymph node with areas of caseation necrosis

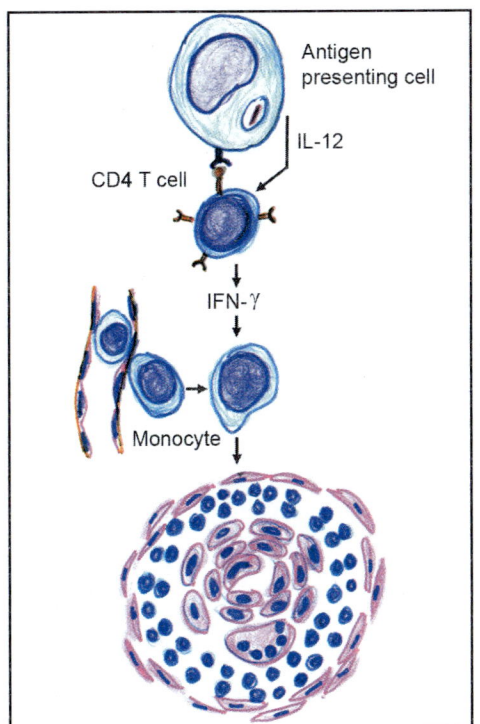

Fig. 3.7: Mechanism of granuloma formation

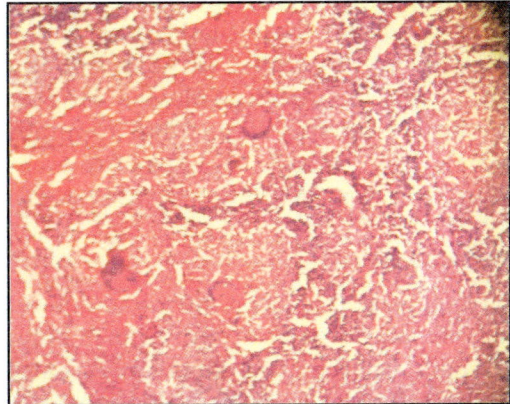

Fig. 3.8b Photomicrograph of granuloma in tuberculosis. Note: Necrosis, epithelioid cells and giant cells

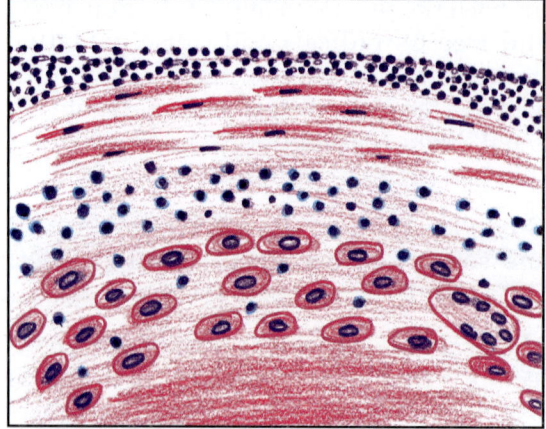

Fig. 3.8c: Schematic diagram of microscopy in tuberculosis

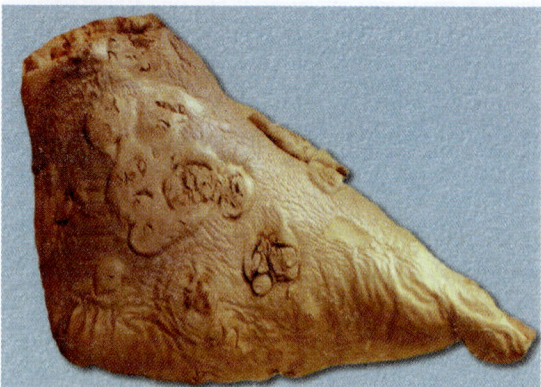

Fig. 3.9a: Gross picture of actinomycosis, note sinus openings

Actinomycosis

It is a type of chronic suppurative inflammation. The classical forms are cervicofacial, abdominal and thoracic actinomycosis. The infection is caused by *A. israeli*; other species such as *A. viscosus, A. odontolyticus* and *A. naeslundi* rarely produce the disease (Figs 3.9a to c).

Gross: The infection produces microabscesses with formation of sinus tracts. The colonies of organisms appear as sulphur granules on gross inspection (Fig. 3.9a).

Microscopy: There are microabscesses with central suppurative necrosis. The centre of the microabscess has the colony of organisms. The organisms show intertwined radial filaments; the periphery of these filaments is capped by eosinophilic clubs. Good number of neutrophils, histiocytes, plasma cells and lymphocytes are seen around the suppurative necrosis (Figs 3.9b and c). Adjacent to this area, granulation tissue and fibrosis are present.

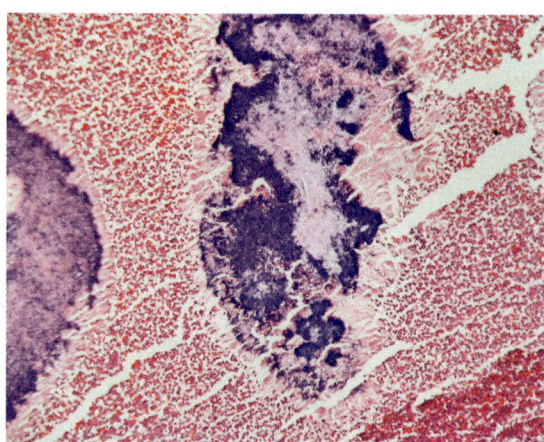

Fig. 3.9b: Photomicrograph of actinomycosis

Rhinosporidiosis

Rhinosporidiosis is a chronic granulomatous disease characterised by production of polyps or hyperplasia of mucous membrane surfaces. The aetiological agent is rhinosporidium seeberi. The commonest sites involved are mucosa of nose, nasopharynx and soft palate.

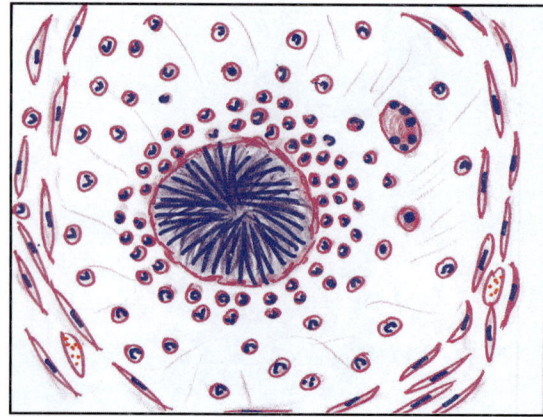

Fig. 3.9c: Schematic diagram of actinomycosis, note colony of organisms

Seeber (1900) first described this infection. It was first grouped under protozoa and later into fungus. It has neither been grown in culture nor transmitted experimentally.

The mature spore (8–12 µ) present in the sporangia can infect the human beings. The source of infection is water. Swimmers in swimming pools or those who work in stagnant water pools can get the infection. The spore undergoes different stages of maturation like: Early trophocyte has central nucleus with distinct nucleolus. The cell wall is laminated and consists of chitinous membrane incorporating neutral polysaccharides. In later stages the cell undergoes nuclear divisions, can have numerous nuclei surrounded by cytoplasm and develops into sporangia (350 µ). The chitinous wall ruptures releasing spores and the cycle continues.

Gross: Rhinosporidiosis usually presents as friable, highly vascular, sessile or pedunculated polyps on the mucosal surfaces.

Microscopy: There are good number of sporangia in varying stages of maturation. As these mature, they have spores. Some of the sporangia may rupture and there is a chronic inflammation at the rupture site (Fig. 3.10).

RHINOSCLEROMA

Rhinoscleroma affects the upper respiratory tract. It is a chronic granulomatous disease caused by bacteria Klebsiella rhinoscleromaticus. It is a gram-negative, encapsulated rod-shaped diplococci. It is a tropical disease, endemic in Africa and central Asia.

- Nose is involved in 95 to 100% of the cases. It also affects nasopharynx, larynx, trachea, and bronchi.
- Females are more commonly affected than the males.
- Three stages:
  a. Catarrhal/atrophic stage
  b. Granulomatous stage
  c. Sclerotic stage
    – *Catarrhal/atrophic stage:* There is non-specific rhinitis which progresses to purulent fetid rhinorrhoea and crusting. This lasts for weeks to months.
    – *Granulomatous stage:* Mucosa becomes bluish red with development of nodules and polyps. Epistaxis, nasal deformity and destruction of nasal cartilage are noted. There may be obstruction of various degrees.
    – *Sclerotic stage:* There is sclerosis and fibrosis.
- *Microscopy in rhinoscleroma:* Shows pseudoepithelial hyperplasia. Subepithelial tissue has chronic inflammatory cells, vacuolated histiocytes containing organisms (Mikulicz cells), plasma cells, plasma cells with Russel bodies and lymphocytes (Figs. 3.11a and b).
- Tetracyclin and ciprofloxacin are effective.

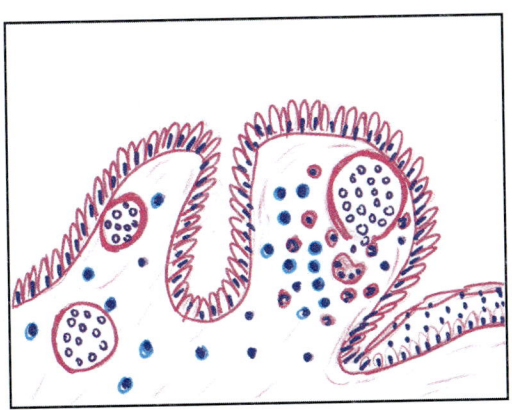

Fig. 3.10: Schematic diagram of microscopy in rhinosporidiosis. Stroma shows chronic inflammation

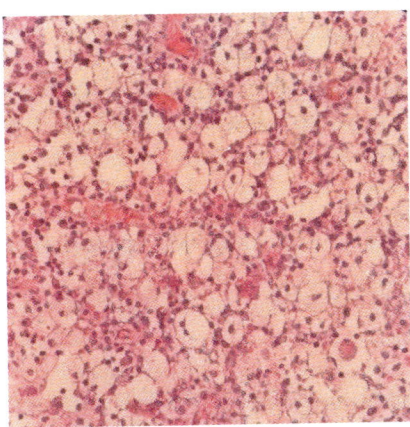

Fig. 3.11a: Microscopy, rhinoscleroma, note Mikulicz cells

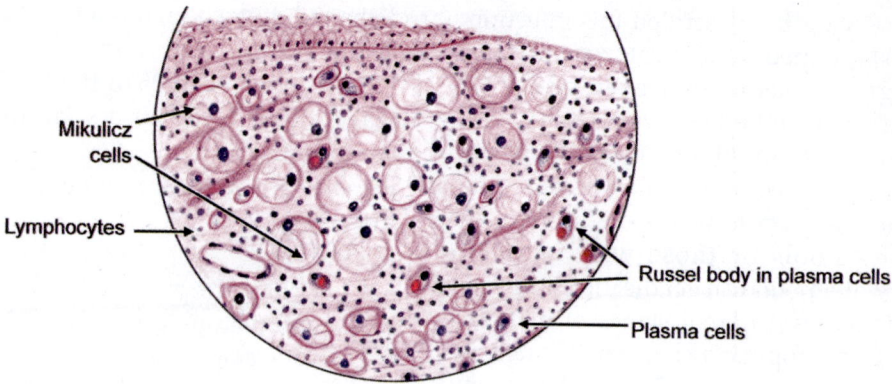

Fig. 3.11b: Schematic diagram, microscopy of rhinoscleroma. Note Mikulicz cells, plasma cells and plasma cells with Russel body

Leprosy (Figs 3.12a to d)

Leprosy is a slowly progressive chronic inflammatory disease caused by *M. leprae* affecting the skin and the peripheral nerves.

There are various classifications. According to the classification by Ridley and Jopling there are five types of leprosy. They are:
- Tuberculoid leprosy (TT)
- Borderline tuberculoid leprosy (BT)
- Borderline borderline leprosy (BB)
- Borderline lepromatous leprosy (BL)
- Lepromatous leprosy (LL).

Madrid (1953) classification:
- Lepromatous leprosy
- Tuberculoid leprosy
- Dimorphous leprosy
- Indeterminate leprosy(I).

WHO classifies based on bacterial load as
- Paucibacillary (includes I, TT, BT types)
- Multibacillary (includes BB, BL, LL types)

Indian classification by Dharmendra (1955) and Job and Chacko (1981) is given below.

Dharmendra	Job and Chacko
Lepromatous leprosy	Lepromatous leprosy
Tuberculoid leprosy	Tuberculoid leprosy
Maculoanaesthetic	Borderline tuberculoid
Borderline	Borderline lepromatous
Polyneuritic	Polyneuritic
Indeterminate	Indeterminate

Tuberculoid leprosy has asymmetrical patches with loss of sensation (hypoaesthetic or anaesthetic). The patches are flat and red initially and later have pigmented margins with pale centres (depigmented). Because of the destruction of nerve, there may be skin ulcers, paralysis of eyelids, keratitis, corneal ulceration, etc.

Lepromatous leprosy patients have symmetrical hypoaesthetic patches with plenty of bacilli in the tissues such as skin, Schwann cells, endoneural and perineural macrophages.

Differences between tuberculoid leprosy and lepromatous leprosy are given in Table 3.8. *Microscopy:* In tuberculoid leprosy, the epithelium is within normal limits: the dermis shows granulomas around the skin appendages, nerves and vessels. The granulomas closely resemble those granulomas found in tuberculosis except for necrosis. The absence of bacteria suggests T cell immunity.

In case of lepromatous leprosy, the epidermis is thinned out. The dermis shows sheets of foamy macrophages which are lipid laden macrophages with masses of acid-fast bacilli in their cytoplasm.

The bacilli can be demonstrated with special stains like Wade-Fite or Fite-Faraco stain on tissues or Ziehl-Neelsen technique on smears.

Bacterial index (BI) is the numerical index of density of bacilli in a smear or biopsy and the below table shows BI and average number of bacilli in oil immersion field.

General Pathology and Systemic Pathology

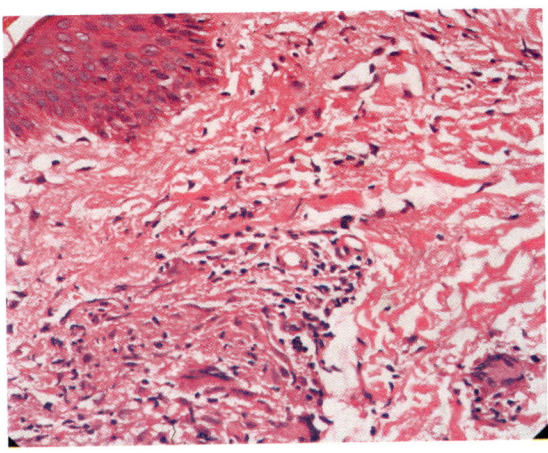

Fig. 3.12a: Photomicrograph of tuberculoid leprosy

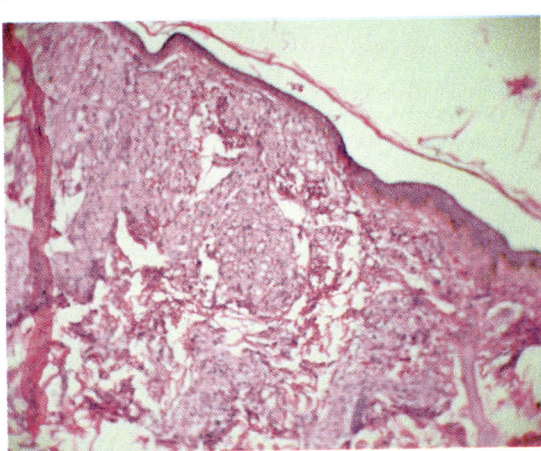

Fig. 3.12c: Photomicrograph of lepromatous leprosy

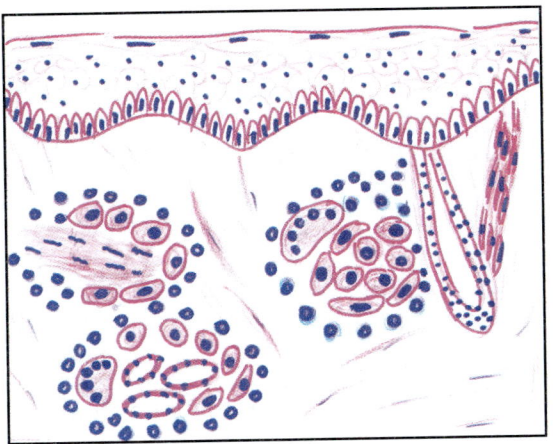

Fig. 3.12b Schematic diagram of microscopy in tuberculoid leprosy

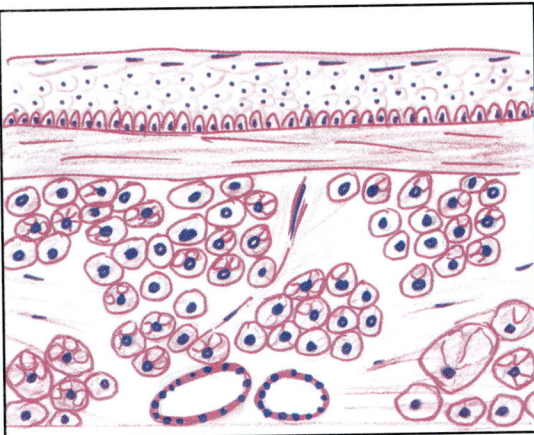

Fig. 3.12d: Schematic diagram of microscopy in lepromatous leprosy

BI	Average no. of Lepra bacilli in oil immersion field
0	0/100 fields
1+	1–10/100 fields
2+	1–10/10 fields
3+	1–10/ field
4+	10–100/field
5+	100–1000/field
6+	> 1000/field

Lepromin test is done to know the level of immunity and it has two reactions:
1. Fernandez reaction
2. Mitsuda reaction.

About 0.1 ml of lepromin reagent (obtained from experimentally inoculated armadillos) is injected intradermally, on the forearm and the Fernandez reaction is read after 48–72 hours. It is positive in tuberculoid leprosy (TL) with increased reaction of skin and nerve lesion. It is negative in LL and BL types.

Mitsuda reaction is read after 3–4 weeks and it is positive in TT and BT and negative in LL patients.

Granulation Tissue

Granulation tissue is formed as a result of repair process. It is fragile and prone to injury. Granulation tissue is pinkish to velvety red and granular in appearance when it is healthy; when inadequate blood flow exists, granulation tissue may be pale in colour. The

Table 3.8: Differences between tuberculoid leprosy and lepromatous leprosy

		Tuberculoid leprosy	Lepromatous leprosy
1	Cell mediated Immunity	Good	Poor
2	Cell response	Good Th1 cell response with production of IL2 and interferon gamma	Th1 response weak
3	Microbial burden (Bacillary index)	Less or absent (Paucibacillary)	Plenty (Multibacillary)
4	Histology	Granulomas with plenty of lymphocytes	No or less lymphocytes with lipid laden foamy macrophages with globi of bacteria
5	Nerve involvement	Asymmetric involvement of peripheral nerves	Symmetrical involvement

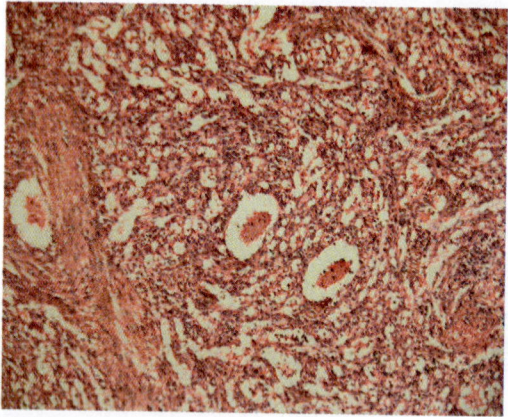

Fig. 3.13a: Photomicrograph of granulation tissue

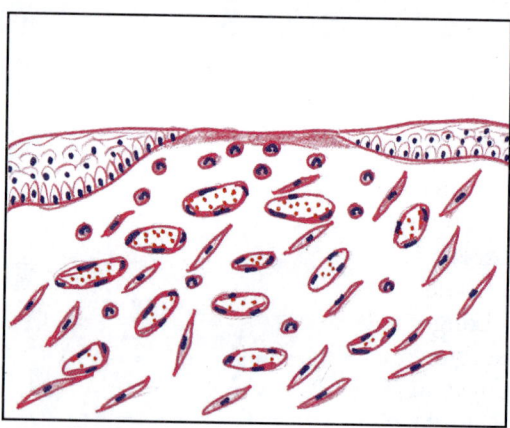

Fig. 3.13b: Schematic diagram of microscopy of granulation tissue

granulation tissue provides the scaffold for healing from the edges of the wound. Granulation tissue is eventually covered by a layer of epidermal tissue. Granulation tissue can be injured by wound dressing and excessive pressure.

Gross: Granulation tissue is pinkish in colour, soft and granular. Healthy granulation tissue bleeds on touch.

Microscopy: There is proliferation of new capillaries and fibroblasts (Figs 3.13a and b). The new blood vessels have leaky inter-endothelial junctions with passage of red cells and proteins and hence the granulation tissue is oedematous.

Keloids develop due to overgrowth of dense fibrous tissue, usually seen after healing of a skin injury, extends beyond the borders of the original wound (claw-like outline of a keloid) and tends to recur after excision. Keloids have the clinical appearance of a raised amorphous growth and are frequently associated with pruritis and pain.

Hypertrophic scars are erythematous, pruritic, raised fibrous lesions that do not extend beyond the boundaries of the wound and may undergo spontaneous resolution. Hypertrophic scars are common with thermal injuries and injuries of deep dermis. Hypertrophic scar reaches certain size and subsequently stabilises or regresses. Similar to keloids, hypertrophic scars are associated with adverse wound healing factors.

In normal scars and hypertrophic scars, the collagen bundles are arranged parallel to the skin surface. Keloid scar shows haphazard arrangement of fairly acellular collagen with decreased myofibroblasts.

Exercise 39

Chronic Venous Congestion, Thrombosis, Infarction, Myocardial Infarction (MI) and Lung Infarction Oedema and Shock

Chronic Venous Congestion

Hyperaemia and congestion indicates local increase of volume of blood in a particular tissue.
- Hyperaemia is an active tissue process
- Congestion is a passive process resulting from impaired venous return from the tissue.

Long-standing congestion is called chronic passive congestion (CPC) or chronic venous congestion (CVC).

The stasis of poorly oxygenated blood causes chronic hypoxia, which causes:
- Degeneration
- Death of parenchymal cells.

Rupture of dilated and congested capillaries can cause haemorrhage, haemosiderin laden macrophages followed by fibrosis and in some organs calcification occurs as seen in spleen producing Gamna-Gandy bodies (siderofibrotic calcific nodules).

Chronic Venous Congestion of Lung

Chronic venous congestion of lung is encountered whenever there is elevated left atrial pressure and consequent elevated pulmonary venous pressure. Long-standing chronic venous congestion can lead to fibrosis and haemosiderin laden macrophages giving rise to "Brown Induration Lung". The common conditions include:
1. Congestive cardiac failure
2. Left-sided heart failure
3. Mitral stenosis.

Gross: The lungs are heavy and reddish brown coloured. The vessels are engorged. In long-standing cases, the lungs are firm in consistency, brownish and reduced in size (Fig. 3.14a).

Microscopy: The septae are widened and the vessels are tortuous and congested. The alveolar spaces contain numerous haemosiderin laden macrophages (heart failure cells) (Fig. 3.14b). In late stages, the septae are thickened, fibrotic with deposition of haemosiderin pigment (brown induration).

Chronic Venous Congestion of Liver

Chronic venous congestion of liver is usually seen in patients with
- Right-sided heart failure
- Obstruction to the inferior vena cava
- Obstruction to hepatic vein as in cirrhosis.

Long-standing chronic venous congestion of liver can progress to hepatic fibrosis followed by cirrhotic changes termed "Cardiac Cirrhosis".

Gross: The liver is congested and enlarged. The cut section shows pale and dark areas (Nutmeg appearance). The red/dark areas are the regions around the central vein and the surrounding sinusoids. The pale areas represent the cells with fatty change around the portal triad (Fig. 3.15a).

Microscopy: The normal liver architecture is maintained. The central vein and the surrounding sinusoids are congested and dilated.

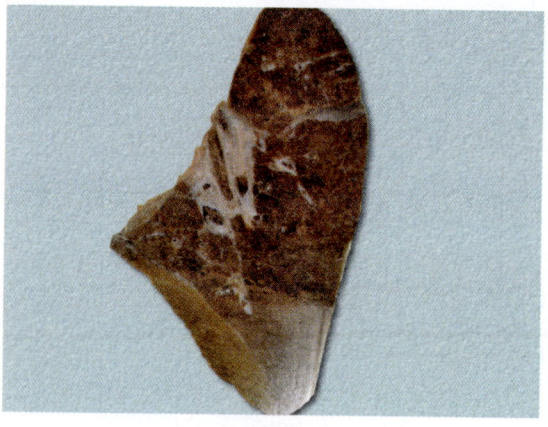

Fig. 3.14a: Gross picture, CVC lung

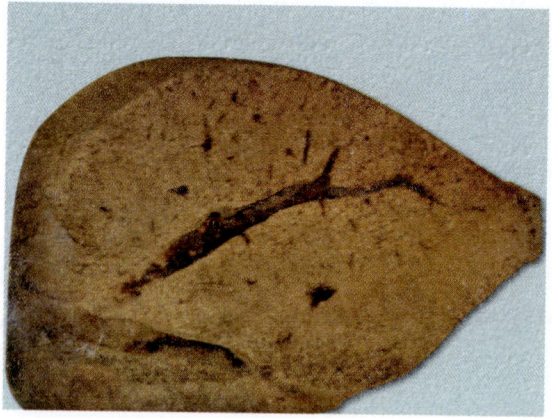

Fig. 3.15a: Gross picture, CVC liver

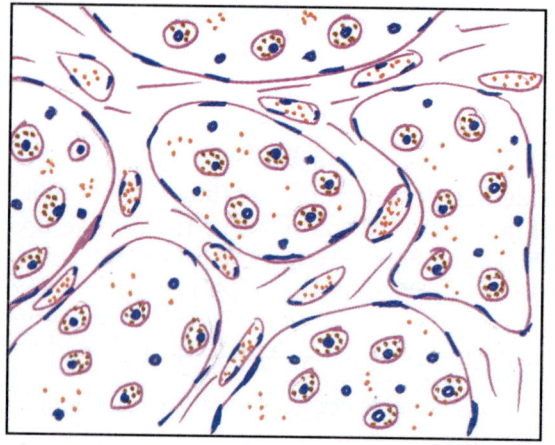

Fig. 3.14b: Schematic diagram of microscopy of CVC lung

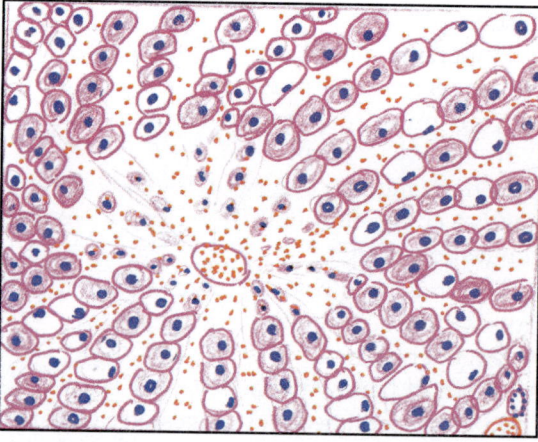

Fig. 3.15b: Schematic diagram of microscopy of CVC liver

There is evidence of centrilobular necrosis showing loss of hepatocytes with areas of haemorrhage (Fig. 3.15b). In late stages, there may be hepatic fibrosis and cardiac cirrhosis.

Chronic Venous Congestion of Spleen (Figs 3.16a to c)

The causes for chronic venous congestion of spleen are:
- Right-sided heart failure as in cor pulmonale, tricuspid/pulmonary valvular disease
- Following left-sided heart failure
- Portal vein and splenic vein thrombosis
- Cirrhosis
- It can also occur secondary to obstruction of intrahepatic or extrahepatic disorders those impinge on portal vein and splenic vein.

Gross: In passive congestion, the spleen is enlarged, weighs more and may show fibro-siderotic calcified areas (Gamna-Gandy bodies).

Microscopy: The sinusoids of the red pulp are dilated with areas of haemorrhage. The white pulp is reduced. In late stages, there is fibrosis

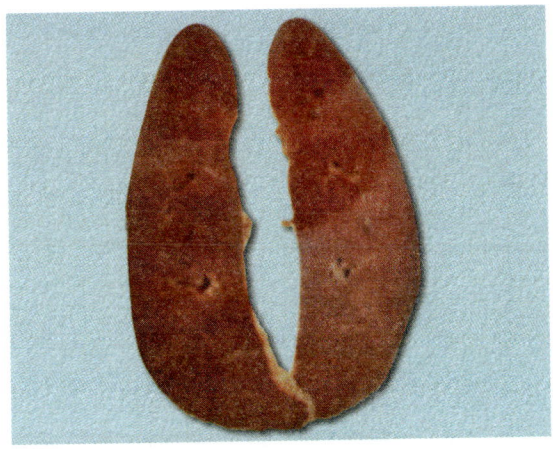

Fig. 3.16a: Gross picture, CVC spleen

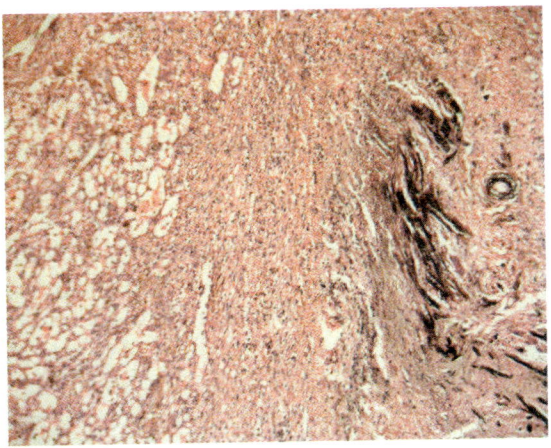

Fig. 3.16b: Photomicrograph of CVC spleen, note congestion with Gamna-Gandy bodies

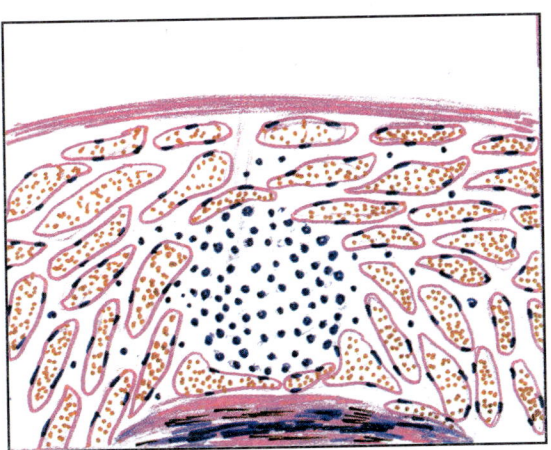

Fig. 3.16c: Schematic diagram of microphotograph of CVC spleen

with haemosiderin laden macrophages and calcification.

THROMBOSIS

Thrombosis is formation of a thrombus which is a solid mass formed from the constituents of blood within a vascular system during life.

Predisposing factors (Virchow's triad)
1. Abnormalities of the vessel wall
2. Abnormalities of the blood flow
3. *Abnormalities in blood coagulation (hypercoagulable states):* Thrombosis due to antiphospholipid antibody syndrome, SLE, mutation of Factor V Leiden, antithrombin III deficiency or secondary to bedrest, tissue damage, malignancy, and many other causes.

Anyone of these may lead to thrombus with turbulence (e.g. as in atheroma) and stasis/hyperviscosity of flow of blood. There is loss of endothelial cells and subendothelial collagen is exposed leading to platelet aggregation. The coagulation cascade sets in with fibrin meshwork formation in which RBCs and WBCs are trapped. The platelets, followed by fibrin with entrapped WBCs and RBCs form alternate layers, this is called 'lines of Zahn'.

Gross: Thrombus is firmly attached to the vessel, occluding or non-occluding, with lines of Zahn which are alternating pale and dark areas (pale areas representing platelets, dark areas representing RBC rich layer with fibrin and WBCs). These are arterial thrombi, which develop in flowing blood. Venous thrombi form in a sluggish flow and are red due to more trapping of RBCs.

Microscopy shows platelet aggregates and RBCs and WBCs caught in fibrin (Fig. 3.17).

Venous thrombosis is usually due to damaged valves (trauma, stasis and occlusion). Immobilized patients are at higher risk of deep vein thrombosis.

Clinical effects
- Infarction
- Stroke

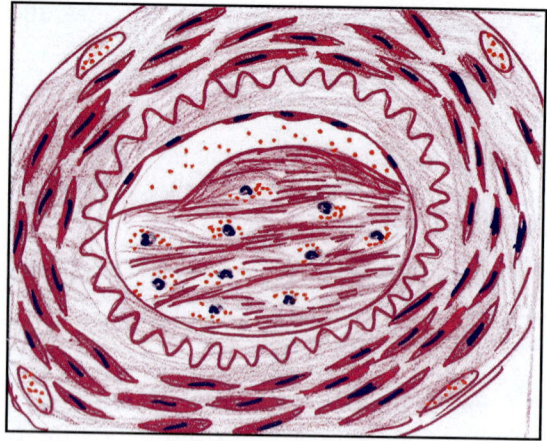

Fig. 3.17: Schematic diagram of microscopy of thrombus

- Thrombophlebitis migrans occurs in a previously normal vessel. Thrombosis appears and disappears with changing sites.

Fate of thrombus
1. *Propagation:* Eventually causes vessel block.
2. *Embolisation:* Thrombus dislodges a fragment and causes infarcts elsewhere.
3. *Dissolution:* Removed by fibrinolytic mechanism and blood circulation is re-established.
4. *Organisation and recanalisation:* Induce inflammation and fibrosis (organisation) or may recanalise or re-establish some degree of flow of blood.

Paradoxical embolus: This is also called as 'crossed embolus' passed from vein to artery or right side of heart to left side of heart as in patent foramen ovale, atrial septal defect and ventriculoseptal defect.

Once the embolism is in systemic circulation, it can cause stroke (cerebrovascular accidents). Thus, even a small defect in the heart has to be closed in these patients.

Saddle embolus: Saddle embolus is a embolus impacted across bifurcation of pulmonary artery. It may cause sudden death.

Following are the differences between ante-mortem clot and postmortem clot.

	Thrombus (ante-mortem clot)	Post-mortem clot
Colour	Pale	Gelatinous, lower portion is dark red (currant jelly) and upper portion Chicken fat
Cause	Endothelial injury	Stagnation
Attachment	Firmly attached to the vessel wall	Not attached
Consistency	Dry	Moist
Surface	Granular, rough	Smooth, glistening
Endothelial surface	Damaged, rough	Smooth, intact
Organisation	Partially organised	Not organised
Lines of Zahn	Laminated	Absent, homogenous

NORMAL HAEMOSTASIS

The blood in our body is maintained in fluid state by tightly regulated processes. This is normal haemostasis. The endothelial cells, platelets and coagulation factors play role in this event. The endothelium modulates normal haemostasis. It has prothrombotic and antithrombotic properties which are given in Table 3.9. With balance between the two, the blood is maintained in fluid state.

The sequence of events in haemostasis:
- Vasoconstriction followed by vasodilatation
- Endothelial injury
- Platelet adhesion to subendothelial ECM/collagen and activation
- Aggregation of platelets: Primary haemostatic plug
- Secondary haemostatic plug.

After injury to the endothelium, there is vasoconstriction followed by vasodilatation. The platelets adhere to the subendothelial collagen (ECM) by GpIb receptors present on the platelets, vWF acts as a bridge between the two. The platelets undergo release reaction

Table 3.9: To show prothrombotic and antithrombotic properties of endothelium

Antithrombotic properties	Prothrombotic properties

1. Anti-platelet effect:
   a. Non-activated platelets do not adhere to endothelium, endothelium acts as barrier
   b. PGI$_2$, NO and ADPase (produced by endothelium) prevent platelet activation, aggregation and adhesion
2. Anticoagulant properties:
   a. Heparin-like molecules activate anti-thrombin III which bind thrombin and inactivates enzymes of coagulation system
   b. Thrombomodulin binds thrombin which activates protein C which is a anticoagulant (potent inhibitor of Va and VIIIa)
   c. Tissue factor pathway inhibitors
3. Fibrinolytic properties:
Endothelium synthesizes t-PA which lysis fibrin
	1. von Willebrand factor produced by endothelium enhances binding of platelets to ECM
	2. ADP is potent platelet aggregator
	3. Tissue factor produced by endothelium, it activates extrinsic clotting pathway
	3. Plasminogen activator inhibitors (PAI)

with degranulation releasing calcium and ADP from dense granules. ADP is a potent platelet aggregator. ADP and Thromboxane A$_2$ released by the platelets help in platelet aggregation and thus primary platelet plug is formed.

ADP and thromboxane A$_2$ released from the platelets activates platelet aggregation. PGI$_2$ released from the endothelium has vasodilator effect and inhibits platelet aggregation.

Tissue factor released by the endothelial cells activates of coagulation system with generation of thrombin. This is followed by conversion of fibrinogen to fibrin which later gets polymerised and stabilises the platelet plug, this is secondary platelet plug. Erythrocytes and WBCs are caught in the haemostatic plug. Fibrin and platelets adhere to each other by cross linkage via GpIIb/IIIa receptors on the platelets which binds to fibrin.

PATHOGENESIS OF THROMBOSIS

The defects in any of the factors can cause thrombosis like endothelial injury, alterations in blood flow or hypercoagulability of blood. These three factors are discussed below.

(a) Endothelial injury: This is the major cause of thrombosis. Endothelial cells are activated by injury, infection, plasma mediators and cytokines. The prothrombotic properties are activated and anti-thrombotic functions are reduced (Table 3.9). This is particularly important in thrombosis occurring in heart and arteries.

The slowing of blood reduces the inflow of dilution of coagulation factors and stasis brings about adhesion of platelets to the endothelium. Thus, thrombosis is more common in chambers of heart after myocardial infarction, in blood vessels with ulcerated atherosclerotic plaques and in vasculitis.

With injury (dysfunction) to endothelium or loss of endothelial cells, there is release of greater amounts of procoagulant factors and reduced anti-thrombotic factors.
1. The ECM is exposed to which platelets adhere via VWF.
2. There is adhesion of platelets by thromboxane A$_2$.
3. There is downregulation of thrombomodulin with sustained activation of thrombin.
4. There is depletion of PGI$_2$ and plasminogen activation inhibitors released by endothelium.
5. There is release of tissue factor.

Significant endothelial dysfunction can be seen with hypertension, turbulent flow over damaged or scarred valves or by action of endotoxins. Radiation, smoking, homocysteinaemia and hypercholesterolaemia may play role in endothelial dysfunction.

(b) Alterations in normal blood flow (stasis and turbulence): Turbulence causes endothelial injury and endothelial dysfunction. Turbulence also causes stasis.

The examples which cause turbulence and stasis are:
- Ulcerated atherosclerotic plaque
- Aneurysms
- Valve defects.

Turbulence and stasis bring about the following changes:
- Disrupts the laminar flow, brings platelets in contact with endothelium.
- Prevents dilution of activated clotting factors by preventing flow of fresh blood.
- Prevents inflow of inhibitors and permits building of thrombus.
- Promotes endothelial cell activation resulting in thrombosis and leukocyte adhesion.

With turbulence (e.g. as in atheroma) and stasis/hyperviscosity of flow of blood, there is loss of endothelial cells and subendothelial collagen is exposed leading to platelet aggregation. The coagulation cascade sets in with fibrin meshwork formation in which RBCs and WBCs are trapped. The platelets, followed by fibrin with entrapped WBCs and RBCs form alternate layers, this is called 'lines of Zahn'.

(c) Hypercoagulability of blood: Hypercoagulability is a less frequent cause of thrombosis. Table 3.10 shows hypercoagulable states.

The common causes are:
1. In Leiden mutation, the activated factor V (Va) cannot be cleaved by protein C.
2. Mutations of prothromin, antithrombin III, protein C and S are the common causes in hypercoagulability.

Table 3.10: Hypercoagulable states

Primary (Genetic)
Common
  Mutation in factor V gene (factor V Leiden)
  Mutation in prothrombin gene
  Mutation in methyltetrahydrofolate gene
Rare
  Antithrombin III deficiency
  Protein C deficiency
  Protein S deficiency
Very rare
  Fibrinolysis defects
  Most common causes thrombosis
  Prolonged bedrest or immobilization
  Myocardial infarction
  Atrial fibrillation
  Tissue damage (surgery, fracture, burns)
  Cancer
  Prosthetic cardiac valves
  Disseminated intravascular coagulation
  Heparin-induced thrombocytopaenia
  Antiphospholipid antibody syndrome (Lupus anticoagulant syndrome)
Less common causes for thrombosis
  Cardiomyopathy
  Nephrotic syndrome
  Hyperestrogenic states (pregnancy)
  Oral contraceptive use
  Sickle cell anaemia
  Smoking

Infarction

Infarct is an area of ischaemic necrosis due to occlusion of arterial supply or venous drainage of a tissue.

Causes
- About 99% of the infarcts are due to thrombotic or embolic events of arterial occlusion
- Complication of atheroma or intraplaque haemorrhage
- Occasionally it can be because vasospasm
- Compression of vessel due to tumour or tumour like lesion, oedema or entrapment as in hernial sac
- Twisting of pedicle having vessels (testicular and ovarian torsion) and bowel volvulus
- Traumatic vessel rupture.

Infarcts are classified as red and white infarcts.

Red infarcts are seen in:
- Venous obstruction (ovarian or testicular torsion)
- Loose tissues such as lung which allows collection of blood
- Tissues with dual circulation (lung and small intestine)
- Tissues with sluggish venous outflow
- Arterial occlusion followed by re-established flow.

White infarcts occur in:
Solid organs like heart, spleen, kidney due to arterial obstruction with limitation of haemorrhage that can seep into areas of necrosis.

Infarctions can be:
Septic infarcts: Bacterial vegetations which are embolised and bacteria seed into area of infarction.

Bland infarcts: These infarcts do not have bacteria in the occluded thrombus or emboli.

Infarcts are wedge/fan-shaped, the occluded vessel is at the apex and periphery of the organ forms the base. The base with serosal surface can have fibrinous exudate. Initially infarcted zone is poorly defined and with time it becomes well-defined by narrow rim of congestion and inflammation at the edge of the infarction adjacent to normal tissue.

The histopathological characters of infarct vary with tissue involved, such as:
- Solid organs like heart, lung, spleen have coagulative necrosis
- Brain, etc. have colliquative necrosis.

Factors which influence development of infarct are:
- Nature of vascular supply
- Rate of development of occlusion
- Vulnerability to hypoxia
- Oxygen content of blood.

The histological findings
1. An inflammatory response at the margins of infarct, starts within a few hours and well-defined by 1–2 days.
2. This is followed by reparative phenomenon with formation of granulation tissue which is later replaced by scar.

MYOCARDIAL INFARCTION (MI) (Figs 3.18a to c)

Gross: The gross findings depending upon the duration of infarct are as follows:

0–4 hours: There are no gross changes during this time. To detect the infarct during this time, immerse a piece of heart tissue in a solution of TTC (triphenyl tetrazolium chloride). The necrosed area will be pale as dehydrogenase enzyme is depleted, while the normal myocardium stains brick red.

4–12 hours: There is a dark mottling of necrosed tissue (due to stagnated/trapped blood).

1–3 days: The necrosed area has yellow-tan coloured centre with mottling.

3–7 days: The necrosed area is yellow-tan coloured with soft consistency and has hyperaemic border. The hyperaemic border is due to the formation of granulation tissue.

7–10 days: The necrosed area is yellow-tan coloured with soft centre with reddish margins.

10–14 days: The necrosed area has red grey margins as granulation tissue is replaced by collagen.

2–8 weeks: During this period, the necrosed tissue is replaced by grey scar.

More than 2 months: The necrosed area is completely replaced scar tissue.

Microscopy: The microscopic findings depending upon the duration of infarct are as follows:

4–12 hours: There is oedema and haemorrhage. There are wavy fibers at the periphery, because of the forceful systolic tugs by viable fibres, adjacent to non-contractile necrosed fibres. There is vacuolar degeneration at the margins of the infarct.

12–24 hours: During this time, there is ongoing necrosis, pyknosis of the nuclei and contractile

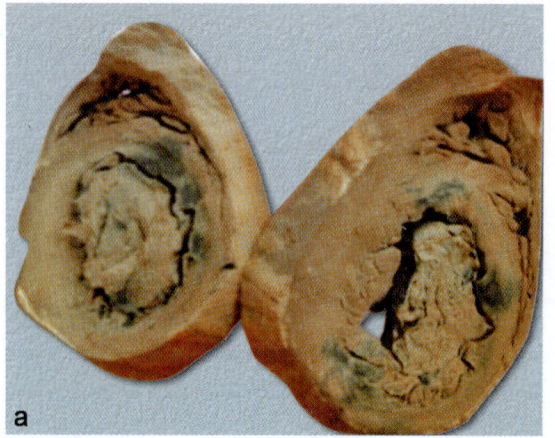
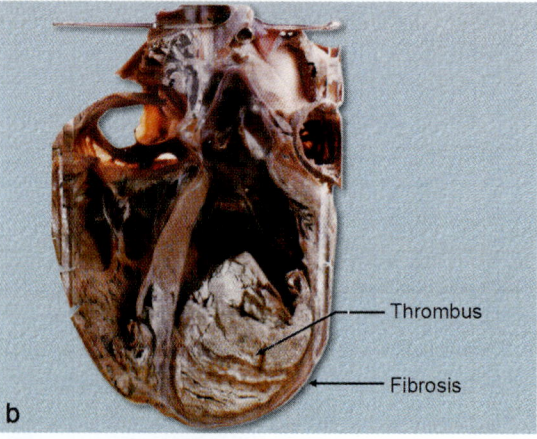
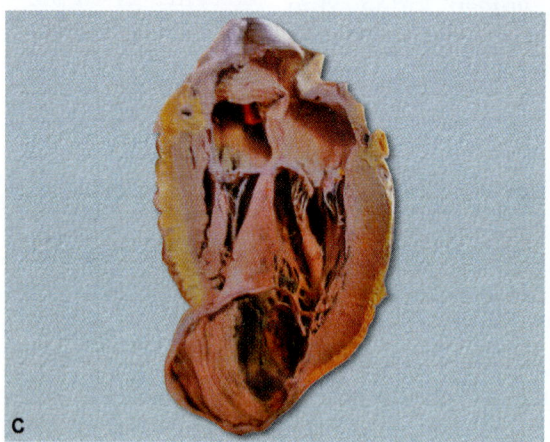

Figs 3.18a to c: (a) Gross pictures of myocardial infarction, recent, (b) healed, (c) healed with aneurysm formation

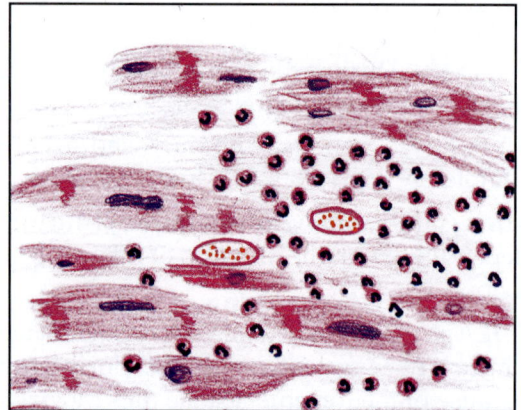

Fig. 3.18d: Schematic diagram of microscopy of myocardial infarct

band necrosis. There will be myocyte hypereosinophilia. The neutrophils start appearing in the infarcted zone.

1–3 days: During this period, the neutrophils increase in number. The myocardial fibres show coagulative necrosis with loss of nuclei and striations.

3–7 days: The neutrophils decrease in number and the other inflammatory cells make their appearance.

7–10 days: There is phagocytosis of dead cells with formation of granulation tissue at the margins.

10–14 days: Granulation tissue formation continues with laying down of collagen.

2–8 weeks: There is collagen tissue with decreased cellularity.

More than 2 months: The infarcted area is replaced by scar.

Laboratory investigations in a case of myocardial infarction are as follows:

i. *Cardiac troponin T and I:* These are normally not detected. In acute MI, the levels of both troponin T and I rise by 2–4 hours and peak levels are reached by 12–16 hours and remain elevated for 7–10 days and later return to normal.

ii. *Creatinine kinase (CK):* This is an enzyme concentrated in brain, myocardium and skeletal muscle. It is composed of M and B dimers. The isoenzyme CK-MM is predominantly localized to skeletal muscle and heart; CK-BB is localized to lungs, brain and many other tissues. However CK-MB is principally from myocardium although variable amounts are found in skeletal muscle. In myocardial infarction, the levels of CK-MB rise by 2–4 hours, peak levels are reached by 24 hours and return to normal by 72 hours. The ratio of CK-MB2 to CK-MB1 more than 1.7 is suggestive of acute myocardial infarction.

iii. *The plasma myoglobin* is increased in 2 hours and remains increased for 7–12 hours (levels are more than 85 ng/ml).

iv. *The LDH levels* are increased; LDH1 peaks by 48–72 hours and remains elevated for 10–14 days. The level of LDH1 more than LDH2 predicts the risk of myocardial infarction.

v. *The C-reactive protein (CRP)* more than 3 mg/L is associated with higher risk of myocardial infarction in angina patients.

vi. Transient leukocytosis in first 1–3 days.

vii. Plasma levels of B type natriuretic peptide (BNP) and N terminal fragment of its prohormone (NT-pro-BNP) increase according to the size of infarct.

Complications
- Contractile dysfunction
- Arrhythmias
  - Sinus bradycardia
  - Heart block
  - Tachycardia
  - Ventricular premature contraction or ventricular tachycardia
  - Ventricular fibrillation.
- Myocardial rupture may occur during 3–7 days of infarction
  - Rupture of ventricular free wall with haemopericardium and cardiac temponade
  - Rupture of ventricular septum with new ventriculoseptal defect and left to right shunts
  - Papillary muscle rupture with mitral regurgitation.
- Pericarditis
- Infarct expansion
- Mural thrombus and thromboembolism
- Ventricular aneurysm
- Papillary muscle dysfunction.

PULMONARY/LUNG INFARCTION (Figs 3.19a and b)

Pulmonary infarct occurs mainly due to venous thrombi. 95% of venous thrombi are from leg veins and pelvic veins and occur with bedrest.

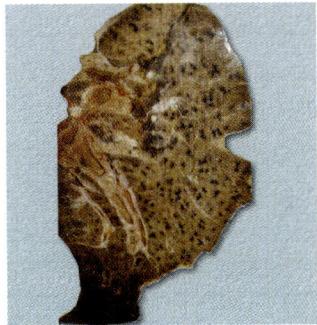

Fig. 3.19a: Gross picture of infarction lung

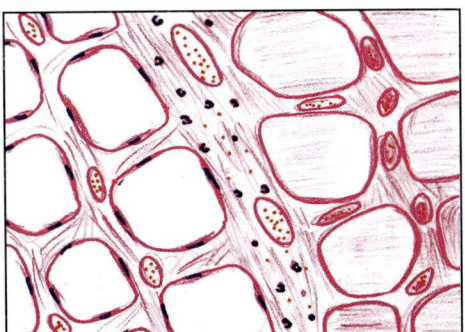

Fig. 3.19b: Schematic diagram of microscopy of lung infarct

Table 3.11: Differences between transudate and exudate

Feature	Transudate	Exudate
Definition	Filtrate of blood plasma without changes in endothelial permeability	Oedema of inflamed tissue associated with increased vascular permeability
Character	Non-inflammatory oedema	Inflammatory oedema
Protein content	Low (less than 1 gm/dl); mainly albumin, low fibrinogen; hence no tendency to coagulate	High (2.5–3.5 gm/dl), readily coagulates due to high content of fibrinogen and other coagulation factors
Glucose	Same as in plasma	Low (less than 60 mg/dl)
Specific gravity	Low (less than 1.015)	High (more than 1.018)
pH	> 7.3	<7.3
LDH	Low	High
Effusion LDH/Serum LDH ratio	< 0.6	>0.6
Cells	Few cells, mainly mesothelial cells	Many cells, inflammatory as well as parenchymal
Examples	Oedema in congestive cardiac failure	Purulent exudate such as pus

OEDEMA

The term oedema refers to increased fluid accumulation in the interstitial tissue or intercellular compartment (extracellular or extravascular).

Cardiac Oedema

Generalised oedema develops in heart failure due to right-sided or with congestive cardiac failure.

Mechanism of Cardiac Oedema

1. There is reduced cardiac output and hypoperfusion stimulates renin-angiotensin-aldosterone mechanism which initiates ADH release resulting in sodium and water retention and oedema formation (Flow Chart 3.2).
2. The other mechanism for oedema formation in cardiac oedema is increased hydrostatic pressure leading to passive congestion in the veins and capillaries as heart is not able to function.
3. Retention of tissue metabolites increases tissue osmotic pressure and causes oedema.

Renal Oedema

Generalised oedema occurs when kidney function is affected.

Mechanism of Renal Oedema

1. Renal hypoperfusion stimulates renin-angiotensin-aldosterone response and ADH release which conserves water and absorbs sodium and water, thus oedema develops (Flow Chart 3.3).
2. Increased glomerular capillary permeability to proteins, protein loss leading to hypoalbuminaemia.

   Decreased colloidal pressure, decreased blood volume and stimulation of renin-angiotensin-aldosterone response and ADH release which conserves water and absorbs sodium and thus causing oedema.

Pathophysiology of Oedema

The formation and retention of fluid depends on filtration and resorption of fluid at the level of capillaries (Starling's law).

The following factors play role in formation of oedema:
- Hydrostatic pressure
- Oncotic pressure
- Lymphatic drainage.

Apart from these three factors, the other factors which play role in oedema formation are:
- Malnutrition (kwashiorkor)
- Increased capillary permeability
- Sodium and water retention

General Pathology and Systemic Pathology

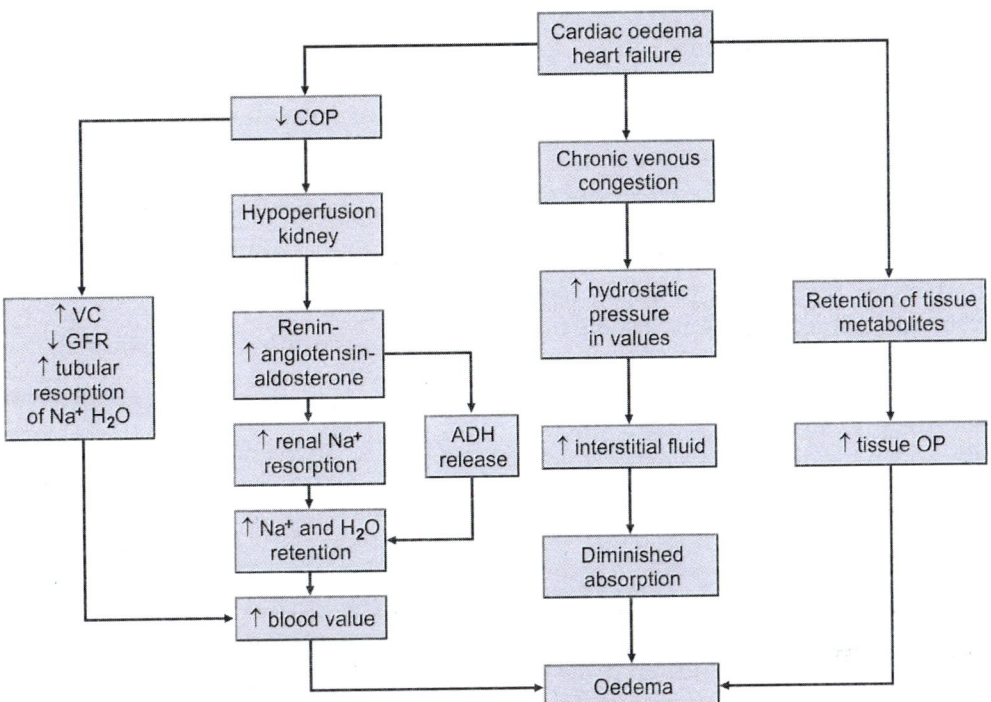

Flow Chart 3.2: Mechanism of cardiac oedema

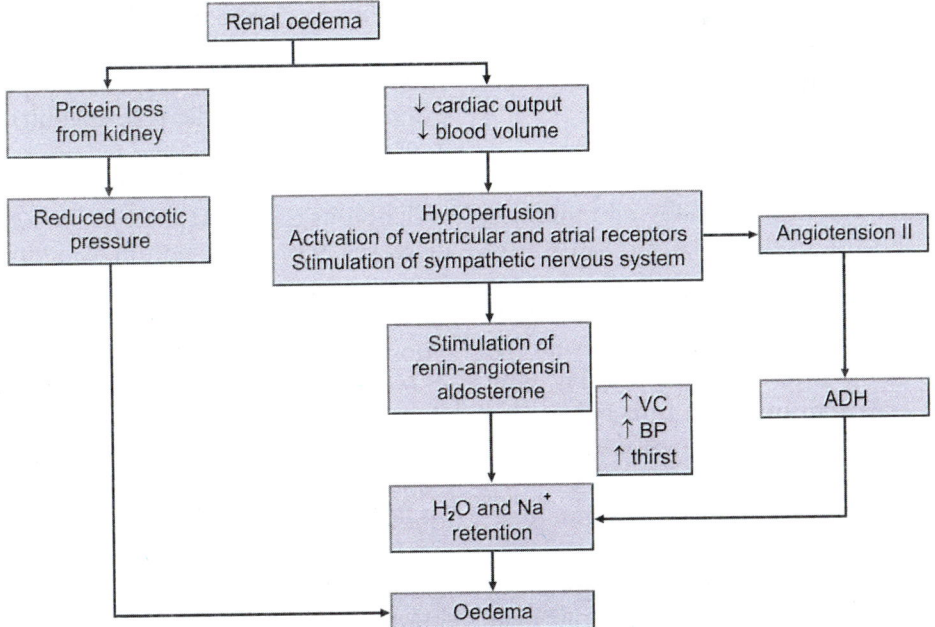

Flow Chart 3.3: Mechanism of renal oedema

- Tissue factors
- Atrial natriuretic peptide
- Renin angiotensin system
- Aldosterone
- Antidiuretic hormone (ADH).

In normal health, at arteriolar end hydrostatic pressure is more than the oncotic pressure, hence the fluid passes into interstitium. At venular end the oncotic pressure is more than the hydrostatic pressure, hence fluid returns to capillary bed. Still some fluid remains in the interstitium which is carried by lymph vessels. Thus, increased capillary hydrostatic pressure, decreased oncotic pressure and lymphatics play major role in formation of oedema.

Hydrostatic Pressure

The normal hydrostatic pressure is 32 mm Hg at the arteriolar end of the capillary, and 12 mm Hg at the venular end. Hydrostatic pressure (capillary pressure) forces the fluid from blood, pass into the tissues through the capillary wall. Some of the examples due to increased hydrostatic pressure are given below:
- Cardiac oedema (congestive heart failure)
- Ascites in portal vein obstruction
- Pregnancy
- Deep vein thrombosis
- Pulmonary oedema.

Oncotic Pressure

The plasma proteins (especially albumin) are responsible for the oncotic pressure and oncotic pressure tries to keep the fluid in the capillary and tend to draw fluid inside the vessel from the interstitial tissue. The oncotic pressure of the capillary is 28 mm Hg with albumin contributing to 22 mm Hg of this oncotic pressure. The examples due to reduced oncotic pressure are given below.
- *Protein energy malnutrition:* Hypoalbuminaemia
- *Liver disorders:* Common liver causes include cirrhosis of liver and alcoholic liver disease. It is usually seen with ascites. There is decreased albumin synthesis in liver in alcoholic liver disease
- *Protein loosing kidney diseases:* Protein loss in glomerular diseases
- *Protein loosing enteropathies:* Protein loss in intestinal diseases
- *Starvation:* Proteins are broken down.

Lymphatic Drainage

With blockage or iatrogenic causes, oedema develops. Some of the examples are as mentioned below:
- Postmastectomy lymphoedema
- Peau d' orange appearance in breast carcinoma
- Filariasis
- Radiation
- Infections
- Milroy's disease
- Other causes.

Other factors which play in oedema formation are:

Increased capillary permeability: Toxins, anoxia, smoking, certain drugs, release of chemical mediators like in infections and allergic conditions, endothelium is leaky and protein rich fluid escapes forming oedema.

Tissue factors: The oncotic pressure in the tissue is very negligible, hence with loose subcutaneous tissues such as eyelid and external genitalia oedema formation is earliest to occur.

Atrial natriuretic peptide: Causes vasodilatation and inhibits renin and angiotensin release and increases water and sodium excretion.

Renin angiotensin aldosterone system: Angiotensin II inhibits renin release and stimulates aldosterone with sodium and water retention.

Aldosterone: This is the mineralocorticoid hormone produced by zona glomerulosa of adrenal cortex, acts on kidney. It increases reabsorption of sodium by distal convoluted tubule.

Antidiuretic hormone (ADH): Increases reabsorption of water by distal and collecting tubule.

SHOCK

Shock is a state of life-threatening systemic hypoperfusion, with inadequate or impaired tissue perfusion and cellular hypoxia caused either by reduced cardiac output or by reduced effective circulatory blood volume. The important types of shock are:
- Cardiogenic shock
- Hypovolaemic shock
- Septic shock
- Neurogenic shock
- Anaphylactic shock.

Stages of Shock

1. An initial non-progressive stage (compensated stage) during which the body's compensatory mechanisms are able to maintain some degree of tissue perfusion.
2. A progressive stage (de-compensated stage) in which the body's compensatory mechanisms fail to maintain tissue perfusion with onset of worsening circulatory and metabolic imbalances.
3. An irreversible stage where body has tissue and cellular damage, which is so massive that even if the haemodynamic defects are corrected, the survival is not possible.

In non-progressive stage, various neurohumoral mechanisms maintain cardiac output and blood pressure which are as below:
- Baroreceptor reflexes
- Release of catecholamines
- Activation of renin-angiotensin axis
- Antidiuretic hormone release
- Generalised sympathetic stimulation.

As a result, the following effects are seen:
- Tachycardia
- Peripheral vasoconstriction
- Renal conservation of fluid
- Cold and pale skin due to vasoconstriction of skin vessels.

Septic shock may initially show vasodilatation of cutaneous vessels, thus the skin appears warm and flushed.

Coronary and cerebral vessels are less sensitive to the sympathetic stimuli and thus the vital functions of heart and brain are still unaffected.

In progressive phase, the following changes are seen:
1. The tissues suffer hypoxia.
2. Persistence of oxygen deficiency causes stoppage of aerobic respiration.
3. Anaerobic glycolysis sets in with excessive production of lactic acid.
4. The metabolic lactic acidosis lowers tissue pH and slows down vasomotor response.
5. The arterioles dilate and blood pools in microcirculation. With these effects, cardiac output is reduced.
6. The endothelial cells undergo anoxic injury and subsequently disseminated intravascular coagulation develops.

Irreversible stage, the cellular and tissue injury are so severe, the changes cannot be reversed and survival is not possible even if haemodynamic effects are corrected. The changes seen with irreversible stage are:
1. There is widespread cell injury with lysosomal enzyme leakage which further aggravates the shock stage.
2. Myocardial contractile function worsens because of nitric oxide release.
3. Ischaemic bowel may allow intestinal flora to enter circulation, and endotoxic shock may be superimposed.
4. The kidney suffers ischemic acute tubular necrosis
5. Death supervenes.

CARDIOGENIC SHOCK

This results from failure of cardiac function. The heart cannot pump enough blood to meet the metabolic demands of the body due to inadequate tissue perfusion.

Pathogenesis of Cardiogenic Shock

Whatever the aetiology, the following mechanisms will contribute to cardiogenic shock.
1. There is decreased cardiac output (COP) and decreased stroke volume. This causes hypotension and decreased coronary pressure leading to myocardial ischaemia.

2. Reduced COP stimulates catecholamine release which increases contractility and peripheral blood flow, but also increases myocardial oxygen demand which further reduces cardiac output and causes tissue hypoperfusion.
3. With reduced COP, renin-angiotensin-ADH axis is stimulated which causes vasoconstriction and conserves sodium and water from kidneys. This increases cardiac volume, COP, and atrial pressure. These mechanism increases load on the heart and again adds to tissue hypoperfusion.
4. Reduced COP stimulates systemic inflammatory response syndrome (SIRS) causing GI tract ischaemia and intestinal bacteria proliferate and cytokines like IL-6 and TNF α, NO, and O_2 free radicals are released. This adds to tissue hypoperfusion and pulmonary oedema and other organ injury.
5. Decreased tissue perfusion leads to:
   i. Heart failure.
   ii. Anaerobic glycolysis releasing pyruvate and lactate leading to metabolic acidosis.
   iii. Renal failure adds to metabolic acidosis.
   iv. Metabolic acidosis causes peripheral pooling of blood.
   v. Vasodilatation, peripheral pooling of blood which further adds to decreased cardiac output and hypoperfusion.
   vi. End result is metabolic acidosis, heart failure, pulmonary oedema and renal failure.

HYPOVOLAEMIC SHOCK

This results from loss of blood or plasma volume. The causes of this can be:
- Haemorrhage
- Fluid loss from severe burns, trauma, vomiting, diarrhoea.

Pathogenesis of Hypovolaemic Shock

In hypovolaemic shock which is also called haemorrhagic shock, there is decreased blood volume, due to fluid loss; there is decreased cardiac output and arterial pressure. The compensatory mechanisms are activated to restore the arterial pressure and blood volume back to normal.

The compensatory mechanisms include:
1. *Baroreceptor stimulation:* Arterial and cardiopulmonary baroreceptors sense fall in blood pressure, activate sympathetic system to stimulate heart and constrict blood vessels.
2. *Chemoreceptor stimulation with systemic acidosis:* This mechanism tries to increase blood pressure and regulate respiratory rate.
3. *Sympathetic adrenergic system stimulated with release of catecholamines:* Cause vasoconstriction and heart is stimulated to increase COP. Heart and brain get sufficient blood as it is redistributed from GIT, renal and musculoskeletal and other tissues.
4. *Renin-angiotensin ADH mechanism activated:* Vasoconstriction and conserve sodium and water.
5. *Activation of thirst centres.*

The de-compensatory mechanisms include:
As arterial pressure cannot be restored and cannot perfuse vital organs, irreversible shock and death occurs and following factors contribute.
1. Impaired coronary flow resulting from hypotension leads to myocardial ischaemia, acidosis and depress cardiac function and cause arrhythmias.
2. Sympathetic escape with accumulation of metabolic vasodilator substances, impair sympathetic mediated vasoconstriction which leads to loss of vascular tone, hypotension and organ hypoperfusion. Loss of capillary tone increases hydrostatic pressure and reduces plasma volume.
3. Cerebral ischaemia: Causes loss of sympathetic outflow from ischaemic adrenal medulla causes VD which reduces arterial pressure and induce cerebral ischaemia.
4. Metabolic acidosis depresses cardiac muscles and vascular tone which further reduce arterial pressure.

5. Systemic inflammatory response syndrome (SIRS) causing GI tract ischaemia may play role in vasodilatation, cardiac depression and organ injury.

SEPTIC SHOCK

Septic shock most commonly occurs in gram-negative bacterial infections (endotoxic shock). Gram-positive organisms and fungal infections may also cause septic shock.

Pathogenesis of Septic Shock

Septic shock ranks the first amongst causes of death due to shock. The causes of septic syndromes are increasing, and can be attributed to:

- Improved life support for high-risk patients
- Increased invasive procedures
- Increased number of immunocompromised hosts possibly secondary to chemotherapy, immunosuppression and HIV infection.

Most cases of septic shock are due to endotoxin producing gram-negative organisms and hence termed endotoxic shock. The events in septic shock are summarised below:

1. The cell wall of gram-negative bacilli have lipopolysaccharides (LPS) consisting of toxic fatty acid core. The free fatty acids released by these bacteria attaches to LPS binding protein and this complex binds to specific receptor (CD14) on monocytes, macrophages, neutrophils and vascular endothelial cells.
2. The LPS now gets recognised by TLR-4, which results in release of IL-1 and TNF. These cytokines in turn release IL-6, IL-8, and IL-10 from other inflammatory cells and endothelium.
3. LPS directly activate complement system.
4. There is release of NO and PAF.
5. Widespread endothelial injury and activation of endothelial cells leads to leukocyte adhesion and diffuse alveolar capillary damage in lung.
6. Systemic effects of TNF and IL-1 are responsible for fever, acute phase reactants and increase number of neutrophils.
7. Procoagulant activity of endothelium is stimulated and these also produce vasodilatation, increased vascular permeability and hypoperfusion.
8. Myocardial pump failure and DIC induces further hypotension.
9. Hypoperfusion resulting from combined effect of widespread vasodilatation, myocardial pump failure and DIC causes multi-organ failure which affects liver, kidneys, CNS and other organs.

ORGAN CHANGES IN SHOCK

The changes in tissues are mainly by hypoxic injury due to hypoperfusion and microvascular thrombosis. As shock is characterised by failure of many organs, the cellular changes may appear in any tissues. The changes are particularly evident in brain, heart, kidneys, adrenal glands and GI tract.

Adrenal gland shows changes seen in stress, such as cortical cell lipid depletion. The cells are metabolically active which use stored lipids for synthesis of steroid hormones. There may be focal or massive haemorrhage.

Kidneys show acute tubular necrosis. Fibrin thrombi are evident in any tissue, but readily visualised in glomeruli.

GIT may show acute stress ulcers (Curling's ulcer), focal mucosal haemorrhage and necrosis.

Lungs are less commonly affected in hypovolaemic shock as they are resistant to hypoxic shock. It may show interstitial pneumonitis and oedema. Septic shock may show diffuse alveolar damage (shock lung).

Heart may show subendocardial hemorrhage, patchy myocardial necrosis, and contractile band necrosis.

Brain may show neuronal damage and haemorrhage.

Exercise 40

Neoplasia

Neoplasia literally means "new growth", i.e. "Neo" meaning new and "plasia" is proliferation. Willis defines neoplasm as "an abnormal mass of tissue, the growth of which exceeds and is uncoordinated with that of the normal tissues and persists in the same excessive manner after the cessation of the stimuli which evoked the change".

Fundamental to the origin of all neoplasms are the genetic changes that allow excessive and unregulated proliferation that is independent of physiologic growth-regulatory stimuli. The nomenclature of tumours are given in Table 3.12.

A tumour is said to be benign when its microscopic and gross characteristics are considered to be:

- Relatively innocent
- Localized to its site of origin
- Cannot spread to other sites
- It can be surgically excised
- Not harmful to the patient generally
- However, benign tumours on occasions are responsible for serious problems, e.g. benign tumours of pancreas arising from beta cells can produce marked hypoglycaemia.

Malignant tumours referred to as cancers, are derived from the Latin word for crab that is, they adhere to any part that they seize in an obstinate manner, similar to a crab's behaviour.

Malignant tumours can
- **Invade and destroy** adjacent structures and spread to distant sites (metastasis).
- Histologically they may resemble the cell of origin or may not
- Their progression depends on the surgical stage and histological grade of the tumour. Early stages they can be treated successfully. Thus, detection of malignant tumours in early stages and proper treatment at right time gives longlife to the patients.

Differences between benign and malignant tumours are given in Table 3.13.

Aetiology of Cancer

Radiation: Such as UV rays, ionising radiation like electromagnetic: X-ray, γ-ray. Particulate like α and β.

Oncogenic Viruses

1. **DNA viruses** like:
   Human papillomavirus (HPV)
   Hepatitis B virus (HBV)
   Epstein-Barr virus (EBV)
   Human herpesvirus 8 (HHV8) and Adenovirus
2. **RNA viruses** like:
   HTLV
   HCV

Viruses and Cancer Association

HPV: Ca cervix
EBV: Nasopharyngeal carcinoma and Burkitt's lymphoma

Table 3.12: Nomenclature of tumours

Tissue of origin	Benign	Malignant
Tumours arising from one parenchymal cell type		
Connective tissue origin	Fibroma	Fibrosarcoma
	Lipoma	Liposarcoma
	Chondroma	Chondrosarcoma
	Osteoma	Osteosarcoma
Endothelial and related tissues		
Blood vessels	Haemangioma	Angiosarcoma
Lymph vessels	Lymphangioma	Lymphangiosarcoma
Mesothelium		Mesothelioma
Meninges	Meningioma	Invasive meningioma
Muscle		
Smooth muscle	Leiomyoma	Leiomyosarcoma
Striated	Rhabdomyoma	Rhabdomyosarcoma
Blood cells and related tissues		Leukaemia, malignant lymphoma
		Multiple myeloma
Epithelia		
Stratified squamous epithelium	Squamous cell papilloma	Squamous cell carcinoma
Basal cells of skin and adnexa		Basal cell carcinoma
Glandular/ductal epithelia	Adenoma	Adenocarcinoma
Renal	Renal cell adenoma	Renal cell carcinoma
Urinary tract	Transitional cell papilloma	Transitional cell carcinoma
Respiratory tract	Adenoma/papilloma	Bronchogenic carcinoma
		Carcinoid
Melanocytes	Neavus	Malignant melanoma
Liver cells	Liver cell adenoma	HCC
		Cholangiocarcinoma
Placental tissue	Hydatidiform mole	Choriocarcinoma
Germ cells—ovary, testis		Dysgerminoma
		Seminoma
Ovary surface epithelia	Adenoma/cystadenoma	Adenocarcinoma
More than one parenchymal cell origin-mixed tumours derived from one germ layer		
Salivary glands	Pleomorphic adenoma	Malignant mixed tumour
Breast	Fibroadenoma	Malignant cystosarcoma phyllodes
Renal		Wilms
More than one parenchymal cell origin-mixed tumours derived from more than one germ layer		
Totipotential cells of ovary, testis, midline germ cell tumours	Mature teratoma	Immature teratoma teratocarcinoma

Table 3.13: Differences between benign and malignant tumours

Characteristics	Benign	Malignant
Rate of growth	Slow growing	Fast growing
Capsule	Usually present	Absent/lacking
Localisation	Localised to site of origin, may compress underlying tissue	Not localised
Differentiation and anaplasia	Well-differentiated, resemble cell of origin	Well/moderate/poorly differentiated, may or may not resemble cell of origin
Microscopic findings cell cohesiveness	Cohesive clusters and sheets	Non-cohesive or dis-cohesive with loss of polarity, seen singly and small groups
Pleomorphism	Absent, uniform in size and shape	May show variation in size and shape
		Hyperchromatic
Nuclear features		
N : C ratio	1 : 4 to 1 : 6	1:1
Bizarre cells	Absent	Present
Tumour giant cells	Absent	Present
Increased mitosis	Absent	Present
Abnormal mitoses	Absent	Present
Local invasion	Absent	Present, invade surrounding tissues
Metastasis	Absent	Present, spread by lymphatic/haematogenous or body cavities

HBV and HCV: Hepatocellular carcinoma
HIV and HHV8: Kaposi's sarcoma.

Bacteria and Cancer
H. pylori: Gastric carcinoma

Chemical Carcinogens
Direct-acting carcinogens
Alkylating agents
- β-propiolactone
- Dimethyl sulphate
- Diepoxybutane
- Anticancer drugs (cyclophosphamide, chlorambucil, nitrosoureas, and others).

Acylating agents
- 1-acetyl-imidazole
- Dimethylcarbamyl chloride.

Procarcinogens that require metabolic activation
Polycyclic and heterocyclic aromatic hydrocarbons
- Benz(a)anthracene
- Benzo(a)pyrene
- Dibenz(a,h)anthracene
- 3-Methylcholanthrene
- 7,12-dimethylbenz(a)anthracene.

Aromatic amines, amides, azo dyes
- 2-Naphthylamine (β-naphthylamine)
- Benzidine
- 2-acetylaminofluorene
- Dimethylaminoazobenzene (butter yellow).

Natural plant and microbial products
- Aflatoxin B_1
- Griseofulvin
- Cycasin

- Safrole
- Betel nuts.

Others
- Nitrosamine and amides
- Vinyl chloride, nickel, chromium
- Insecticides, fungicides
- Polychlorinated biphenyls.

Chemical carcinogens produce mutations and is a multistep process which include the following steps:
1. Initiation
2. Promotion
3. Progression
4. Cancer.

Alkylating agents: Mainly, the chemotherapeutic drugs like cyclophosphamide, cisplatin, busulphan and these have significant risk for solid and haematological malignancies.

Polycyclic hydrocarbons derived from coal tar are benzo(a)pyrene, dibenz(a,h) anthracene and 3-methylcholanthrene. These need metabolic activation by cytochrome p450 dependent oxidase to electrophilic epoxides which inturn react with proteins and nucleic acids.

Aromatic amines and azo dyes: Produce **bladder and liver tumors.**

Aflatoxin B_1, a natural product of fungus Aspergillus flavus is metabolised to epoxide which can bind to DNA is known to produce hepatocellular carcinoma.

Nitrosamines: Nitrites commonly added as preservatives along with other dietary compounds are converted to nitrosamines, and these can produce carcinoma stomach.

Vinyl chloride used in plastics can produce hepatic angiosarcomas.

Metals: Nickel, lead, cadmium, cobalt, beryllium are electrophilic and can cause cancers.

UV rays: Have high-risk for basal cell carcinoma, squamous cell carcinoma and malignant melanoma.

Xeroderma pigmentosum an AR disease with inability to repair DNA after UV radiation has greater risk of cancers.

Asbestos: Produces malignant mesothelioma and lung carcinoma. Crocidolite fibres have greater risk than shorter and thicker amosite and flexible chrysotile fibres.

Preneoplastic Lesions

Preneoplastic conditions include disorders that are associated with a significantly increased risk of cancer, some of them are enumerated here.
- Chronic atrophic gastritis of pernicious anaemia
- Solar keratosis
- Oral lichen planus
- Oral submucous fibrosis
- Cirrhosis
- Endometrial hyperplasia
- Chronic gastritis
- Ulcerative colitis
- Polyps of colon
- Xeroderma pigmentosum
- Epidermolysis bullosa hereditaria.

The WHO specifies seven diseases with increased risk of oral squamous cell carcinoma:
- *Sideropenic dysphagia (in case of chronic iron deficiency:* Plummer-Vinson syndrome, or Paterson-Kelly syndrome)
- Oral lichen planus
- Syphilis
- Oral submucous fibrosis
- Discoid lupus erythematosus
- Xeroderma pigmentosum
- Epidermolysis bullosa hereditaria.

Tables 3.14 to 3.16 enumerate the AD and AR disorders, AD and AR diseases associated with cancer and X-linked dominant and X-linked recessive disorders.

Table 3.14: Autosomal dominant and recessive disorders

Autosomal dominant	Autosomal recessive
Hereditary spherocytosis and elliptocytosis	Phenylketonuria
Marfan's syndrome	Galactosaemia
Ehlers-Danlos syndrome	Homocystinuria
Osteogenesis imperfecta	Alkaptonuria
Achondroplasia	Lysosomal storage disorder
Familial hypercholesterolemia	α_1-antitrypsin deficiencies
Acute intermittent porphyrias	Wilson disease
Tuberous sclerosis	Haemochromatosis
Huntington's disease	Cystic fibrosis
Myotonic dystrophy	Sickle cell disease
von Willebrand's disease	Thalassaemia
Adult polycystic kidney disease	Congenital adrenal hyperplasia
Wilms' tumour	

Table 3.15: AD and AR diseases associated with cancer

AD diseases associated with cancer	AR diseases associated with cancer
Inherited retinoblastoma	Xeroderma pigmentosum
Neurofibromatosis	Friedreich's ataxia
Breast carcinoma	Bloom's syndrome
Ovarian cancer	Fanconi's anaemia
Familial polyposis coli	Ataxia-telangiectasia
MEN1 and 2	
NHPCC	
Li-Fraumeni syndrome	

Table 3.16: X-linked disorders

X-linked dominant	X-linked recessive
Vitamin D resistant rickets	Duchenne muscular dystrophy
RET syndrome	Haemophilia
Alport's incontinentia pigmenti	Chronic granulomatous disease
	G6PD
	Agammaglobulinemia
	Wiskott-Aldrich syndrome
	Diabetes insipidus
	Lesch-Nyhan syndrome

Diagnosis of Malignancy (Cancer)

- Proper clinical history
- Relevant examination findings
- Relevant tumour markers/tumour antigens, e.g. PSA—prostatic carcinoma CEA—colorectal cancers and other cancers Alpha fetoprotein—hepatocellular carcinoma, yolk sac tumour
- USG/X-ray
- FNAC/core biopsy for palpable or deep seated masses
- Exfoliation cytology—Pap smears for cervical cancer
- Cytology for malignant cells—sputum and body fluids and BAL samples, etc.
- Biopsy
- Frozen section—for rapid diagnosis of cancers when the patient is on the operation table
- Excision of tumour
- By suitable molecular diagnostic modality like: PCR, FISH, for prognosis and behaviour—HER-2/neu, N-myc for treatment purposes: ER, PR, Her-2/neu hereditary predisposition—BRCA 1 and 2 as in breast and ovarian cancers
- Immunohistochemistry (suitable markers)
- Immunofluorescence
- Cytogenetics
- *Recognition of paraneoplastic syndromes:* These may be early symptoms in some cancers.

Table 3.17: Paraneoplastic syndromes with clinical symptoms, underlying malignancy and mechanism

Clinical syndromes	Major forms of underlying cancer	Causal mechanism
Endocrinopathies		
Cushing's syndrome	Small cell carcinoma of lung Pancreatic carcinoma Neural tumours	ACTH or ACTH-like substance
Syndrome of inappropriate antidiuretic hormone secretion	Small cell carcinoma of lung; intracranial neoplasms	Antidiuretic hormone or atrial natriuretic hormones
Hypercalcaemia	Squamous cell carcinoma of lung Breast carcinoma Renal carcinoma Adult T cell leukaemia/lymphoma Ovarian carcinoma	Parathyroid hormone-related protein (PTHRP), TGF-α, TNF, IL-1
Hypoglycaemia	Hepatocellular carcinoma Fibrosarcoma Other mesenchymal sarcomas	Insulin or insulin-like substance
Carcinoid syndrome	Gastric carcinoma Bronchial adenoma (carcinoid) Pancreatic carcinoma	Serotonin, bradykinin
Polycythaemia	Renal carcinoma Cerebellar haemangioma Hepatocellular carcinoma	Erythropoietin
Nerve and muscle syndromes		
Myasthenia	Bronchogenic carcinoma	Immunological
Disorders of the central and peripheral nervous system	Breast carcinoma	
Dermatologic disorders		
Acanthosis nigricans	Gastric carcinoma Lung carcinoma Uterine carcinoma	Immunological; secretion of epidermal growth factor
Dermatomyositis	Bronchogenic, breast carcinoma	Immunological
Osseous, articular, and soft-tissue changes		
Hypertrophic osteoarthropathy and clubbing of the fingers	Bronchogenic carcinoma	Unknown
Vascular and haematologic changes		
Venous thrombosis (Trousseau phenomenon)	Pancreatic carcinoma Bronchogenic carcinoma Other cancers	Tumour products (mucins that activate clotting)
Nonbacterial thrombotic endocarditis	Advanced cancers	Hypercoagulability
Red cell aplasia	Thymic neoplasms	Unknown
Others		
Nephrotic syndrome	Various cancers	Tumour antigens, immune complexes

ACTH: adrenocorticotrophic hormone; IL: interleukin; TGF: transforming growth factor; TNF: tumour necrosis factor.

Paraneoplastic Syndromes

These are symptom complexes that occur in patients with cancer and these symptoms cannot be readily explained by local or distant spread of tumour or by elaboration of hormones indigenous to the tissue of origin of tumour (Table 3.17).

These may be
- Earliest manifestation of cancer
- May have significant clinical problems and even fatal
- May mimic metastatic disease.

The most common syndromes are associated with lung and breast cancers and haematological malignancies and these can be due to:

Mucin secreting adenocarcinomas of pancreas, lung and GIT can have:
- Non-bacterial thrombotic endocarditis (Marantic endocarditis)
- Hypercoagulability leading to venous thrombosis
- Trousseau's syndrome (migratory thrombosis in superficial veins and uncommon site).

Syndromes which can occur in Lung Carcinoma are:
- Hypercalcaemia (non-small cell carcinoma/sqamous cell carcinoma)
- SIADH (non-small cell carcinoma/squamous cell carcinoma)
- Carcinoid (small cell carcinoma)
- Venous thrombosis (Trousseau phenomenon)
- Hypertrophic osteoarthropathy and clubbing of the fingers
- Dermatomyositis
- Myasthenia gravis
- Acanthosis nigricans
- Hypoglycaemia

Paraneoplastic syndromes which can occur in breast carcinoma are:
1. Hypercalcaemia
2. CNS and nerve disorders.

Paraneoplastic syndromes which can occur in renal cell carcinoma are:
1. Polycythemia
2. Hypercalcaemia.

Exercise

41

Some Common Tumours

HAEMANGIOMAS

Haemangiomas lie in a grey zone between hamartomatous lesions and true neoplasms.

Some syndromes associated with haemangiomas:

1. **Kasabach-Merritt syndrome** has giant haemangioma with thrombocytopenic purpura and coagulopathy.
2. **Maffucci's syndrome** is rare non-hereditary syndrome characterised by multiple haemangiomas and enchondromas, less commonly with lymphangiomas.
3. **von Hippel-Lindau syndrome** has cavernous haemangiomas or haemangioblastomas which occur in cerebellum or brainstem and retina. It is an inherited multisystem disorder. The gene is on chromosome 3 and inherited dominantly.
4. **Sturge-Weber syndrome** occurs in brain and skin with haemangiomas and neurological abnormalities.

Capillary Haemangioma (Fig. 3.20)

These commonly involve the skin, subcutaneous tissue, mucous membranes of oral cavity and lips; and they also occur in the internal viscera such as liver, spleen and kidneys. They frequently occur on the skin of newborn children and fade away, when the child is of 1 to 3 years of age.

The strawberry type or juvenile haemangioma is very common in newborn.

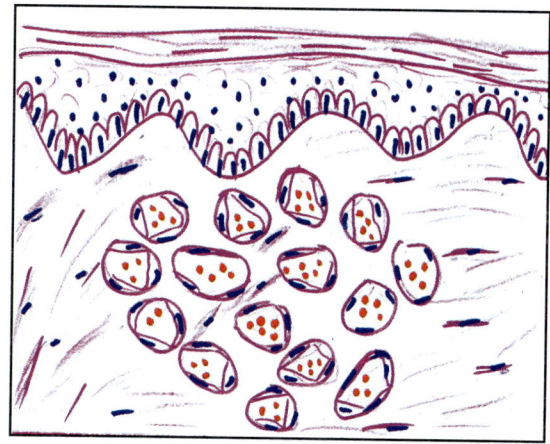

Fig. 3.20: Schematic diagram of microscopy of capillary haemangioma

Gross: These are few mm to several cm, bright red to blue coloured, slightly elevated or strawberry-shaped.

Microscopy: These show blood-filled capillary-sized vascular channels lined by endothelial cells separated by scant connective tissue. The lumen of these vascular channels may be partially or completely thrombosed.

Cavernous Haemangioma (Figs 3.21a and b)

These are less common than capillary haemangiomas. They are larger and less circumscribed.

Grossly, cavernous haemangioma can occur in skin, mucosal surfaces, and visceral organs including spleen, liver and pancreas

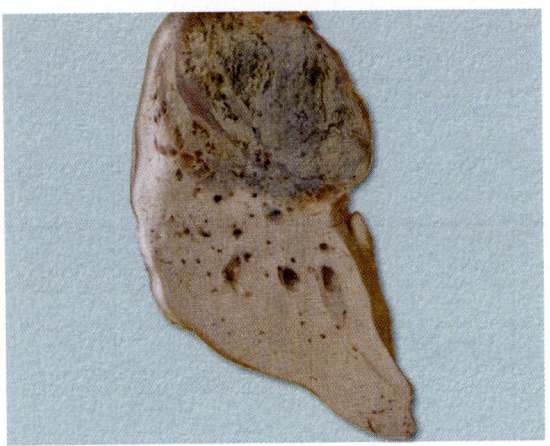

Fig. 3.21a: Gross picture of cavernous haemangioma liver

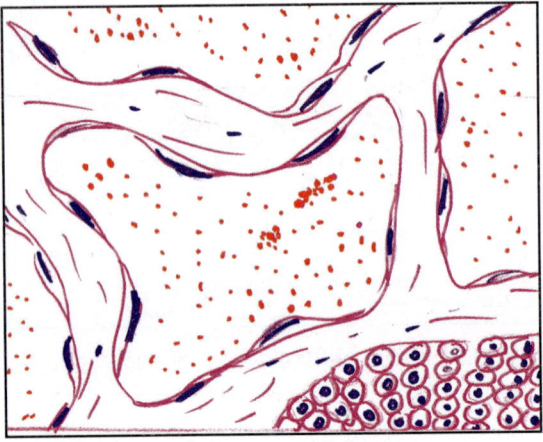

Fig. 3.21b: Schematic diagram of microscopy of cavernous haemangioma

(Fig. 3.21a). May occur in brain, when enlarges produce neurological symptoms.

Cavernous haemangioma of skin has portwine stains, in organs it may be red blue, soft spongy mass with diameter of several centimetres. These are not encapsulated; usually do not regress as that of capillary haemangioma. They may undergo thrombosis, fibrosis, cystic cavitation or haemorrhage. Rarely giant forms occur as in Kasabach-Merritt syndrome.

Microscopy: The lesion is sharply defined and not well-encapsulated. It has cavernous vascular spaces filled with blood and separated by connective tissue stroma. Intravascular thrombosis with associated dystrophic calcification is common.

Lipoma

It is a benign tumour of fat cells. The subcutaneous lipomas are common and occur in regions like arms, shoulder and buttocks.

Deep lipomas may be detected late and have larger size and are found in the omentum, mesentery, retroperitoneum, intramuscular location, juxta-articular regions, periosteum, thorax, mediastinum, paratesticular region and so on.

Apart from subcutaneous plane, they can occur in planes like intramuscular, intermuscular, myelolipoma (in bone marrow), tendon sheath, joints, intraneural, perineural, etc.

They are most common in 5th or 6th decade.

They are single or multiple.

These are soft, mobile, painless and well-circumscribed masses and slip under the palpating fingers.

Angiomyolipoma is common in kidney.

Histological variants like pleomorphic lipoma, spindle cell lipoma, fibrolipoma, chondroid lipoma, myolipoma, angiolipoma etc. are rare.

Areas of infarct, necrosis and calcification may be present.

Malignant form is called liposarcoma and these are usually deep seated.

Gross: These tumours are well-circumscribed thinly capsulated and measure several cm in dimension. They are rounded yellow coloured masses (Fig. 3.22a).

Microscopy: The neoplasm shows lobules of mature adipocytes separated by thin fibrous septae.

The amount of connective tissue and blood vessels may vary (Figs 3.22b and c).

Schwannoma

These tumours arise from the neural crest derived Schwann cells. These are usually

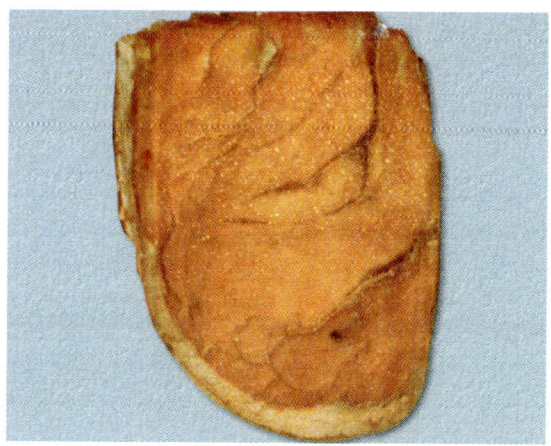

Fig. 3.22a: Gross picture of lipoma

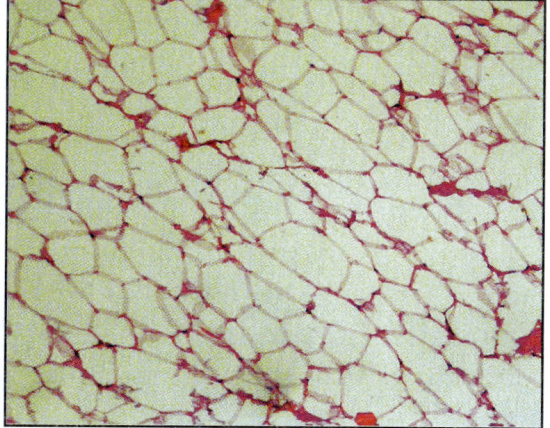

Fig. 3.22b: Microphotograph, microscopy of lipoma

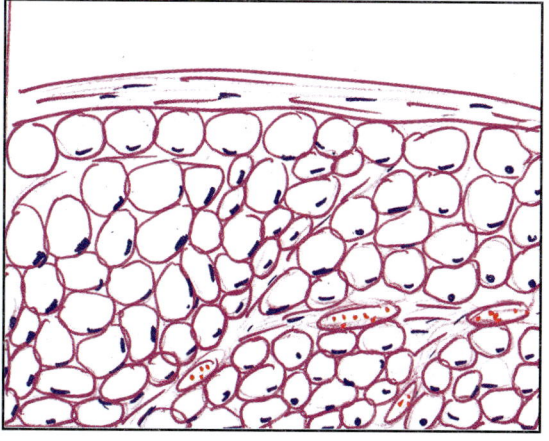

Fig. 3.22c: Schematic diagram of microscopy of lipoma

solitary. Most common locations are flexor aspects of extremities, neck, mediastinum, retroperitoneum, posterior spinal roots, and cerebellopontine angle. The commonest location is cerebellopontine angle; the vestibular branch of 8th cranial nerve is affected. Cranial nerves III, IV, or VI nerve may be affected.

Other cranial nerves and sensory nerves also can be affected. Schwannoma usually involve sensory rather than motor nerves.

Local recurrence with incomplete resection is known. Malignant change is extremely rare in contrast to neurofibroma.

Schwannomas can have 'Antoni A' with cellular areas and in 'Antoni B' schwannomas areas of degenerative changes and cystic spaces are found. Occasionally isolated cells with bizarre hyperchromatic nuclei are seen. They are common in long-standing or ancient schwannoma. Mitoses are usually absent. Blood vessels are prominent with large vascular spaces which may be confused with vascular neoplasm. Haemosiderin laden macrophages may be present.

The tumour is positive for S-100, Leu-7 and myelin basic protein.

Schwannomas are composed of proliferated Schwann cells in a background of collagenous tissue.

Initially, the tumour is fusiform, but later the nerve bundle is compressed and displaces it eccentrically. While excision, the nerve can be restored.

Gross: The tumour is well-circumscribed and encapsulated. It is attached to the nerve and can be separated from it. It is firm, grey to yellow and areas of cystic degeneration are present.

Microscopy: The elongated spindle-shaped Schwann cells are arranged in fascicles with high cellularity. There is palisading of nuclei of these cells and these cells at places form verocay bodies (Antoni A pattern). The less cellular areas may show myxoid and cystic degeneration. Areas of haemorrhage are

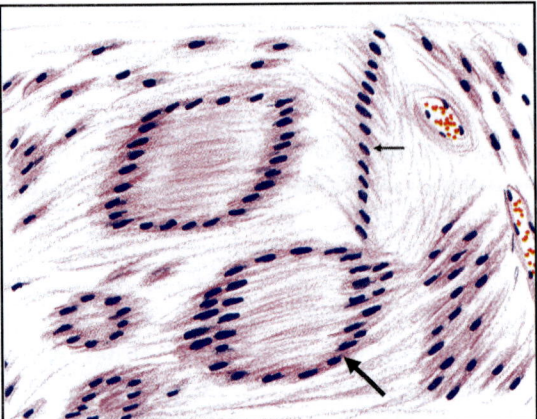

Fig. 3.23: Schematic diagram of microscopy of neurilemmoma. Note densely cellular areas (Antoni A pattern) with nuclear palisading (thick arrow verocay body, thin arrow palisading of nuclei)

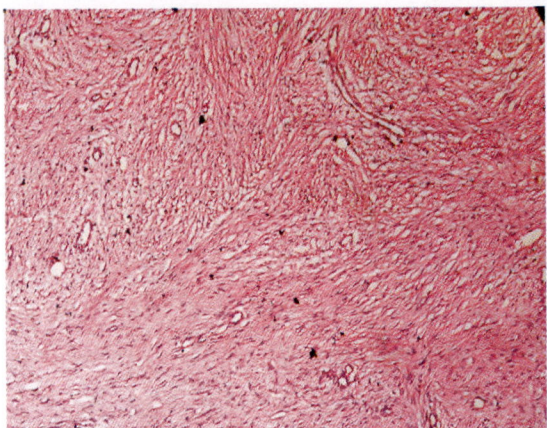

Fig. 3.24a: Photomicrograph of neurofibroma

sometimes encountered (Antoni B pattern) (Fig. 3.23).

Neurofibroma

Neurofibromas are different from schwannomas. They are superficial, small, soft and pedunculated. They are not capsulated. Sometimes these tumours, especially deeper ones grow into larger masses and may produce tortuous enlargement of peripheral nerves and are designated as plexiform neurofibromas.

Multiple neurofibromas represent important component of genetically determined disorder known as neurofibromatosis or Recklinghausen's disease type 1 which is autosomal dominant disease. The NF gene is on chromosome 17. This is also associated with café au lait spots. Type 2 Recklinghausen's disease is genetically different and the gene is located at chromosome 22.

Gross: The tumour is fusiform, grey white, soft tissue mass, and may be solitary or multiple.

Microscopy: Composed of nerve cells which are spindle-shaped with varying amounts of reticulin and collagen. No areas of myxoid or cystic degeneration seen (Figs 3.24a and b).

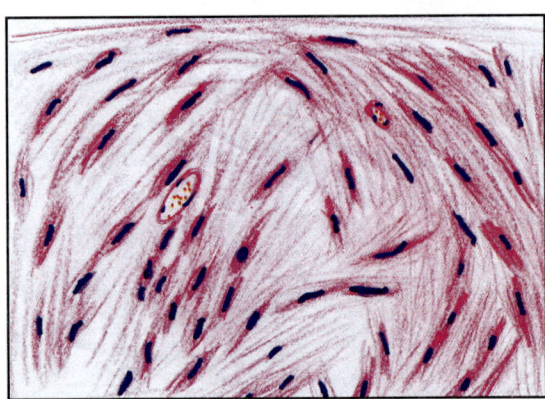

Fig. 3.24b: Schematic diagram of microscopy of neurofibroma

Differences between Schwannoma and Neurofibroma

Schwannoma	Neurofibroma
Arises from Schwann cells	Arises from nerve cells
Initially fusiform, but later nerve is compressed and is displaced eccentrically	Fusiform, involves/infiltrates nerve
Well-circumscribed, capsulated	Soft, well-circumscribed, non-encapsulated
Nerve can be restored during surgery	As nerve is involved needs to be cut
Cystic degeneration, haemorrhage, xanthomatous changes are common	Not seen

Exercise 42

Atherosclerosis and Vascular Pathology in Hypertension

ATHEROSCLEROSIS

Atherosclerosis has been derived from Greek words gruel and hardening. It is an intimal disorder of vessels with formation of atherosclerotic plaque that protrude into the vascular lamina. This plaque consists of a soft, yellow grumous core which is covered by a fibrous cap. These atherosclerotic plaques can:
- Obstruct the blood flow
- Weaken the underlying media
- May rupture and bleed
- Invite formation of thrombus

The risk factors for atherosclerosis are listed in Table 3.18.

In non-modifiable major risk factors:
1. Family history is an independent risk factor. Hypertension, diabetes mellitus run in families.
2. Increasing age has dominant influence, although atherosclerosis starts in early age and progresses to manifest with clinical features in later age. The effects are common between the age groups of 40 to 60 years.
3. Premenopausal females are protected because of estrogen, but postmenopausal females and other males have the risk.

The potentially controllable or modifiable risk factors can control atherosclerosis if the levels or severity is less.
1. HT is a major risk factor. Both systolic and diastolic levels are important. Chronic HT increases the risk of CV accidents.
2. Smoking is a well-established risk factor. Years of smoking and number of cigarettes has effect on vessel wall injury and atherosclerosis.
3. Hypercholesterolemia is major risk factor. High HDL and low levels of LDL and VLDL are to be monitored. Omega 3 fatty acids and exercise will help to keep the HDL levels high, whereas unsaturated fatty acids have adverse effects with high levels of bad cholesterol (LDL).
4. Uncontrolled DM has direct correlation with atherosclerosis and its effects.

Pathogenesis

There are many hypotheses for atherosclerosis. These are as follows:
- Thrombogenic theory
- Incorporation theory
- Imbibation theory
- Monoclonal theory
- Reaction to injury hypothesis.

Table 3.18: Risk factors for atherosclerosis

Major	Minor/lesser
Non-modifiable	Obesity
Increasing age	C-reactive protein
Male gender	Physical inactivity
Family history	Stress (Type A personality)
Genetic abnormality	High carbohydrate diet
Potentially controllable	Postmenopausal
Hyperlipidaemia	Oestrogen deficiency
Hyperhomocysteinuria	Unsaturated fat intake
Hypertension	Higher levels or defects
Cigarette smoking	in apolipoprotein [Lp(a)]
Diabetes mellitus	

The atherosclerosis is well-explained by "reaction to injury hypothesis". Endothelial injury or loss of endothelial cells of any cause, e.g. denudation, haemodynamic forces, hypercholesterolemia, immune complexes, irradiation, chemicals, toxins, smoking, homocysteine, infectious agents all can induce atherosclerosis.

The most important two factors which contribute to atherosclerosis are:
1. Haemodynamic disorders
2. Hypercholesterolemia

The haemodynamic stress can injure endothelial cells and the effect is more at the region where vessels branch and also on the parts of the vessel which lie on the bony parts. This is the reason, atherosclerosis more prominent at the ostia and on the posterior surface of the abdominal aorta.

Lipids: Lipids play a pivotal role in atherogenesis. The lipids are transported in the blood, bound to specific apoproteins after forming lipoprotein complexes. The important lipids found in atherosclerosis are cholesterol and cholesterol esters. About 70% of the cholesterol found in blood is bound to LDL followed by VLDL and IDL. The cholesterol can be increased due to:
1. Homozygous FH due to defective LDLR and inadequate uptake of lipoproteins by hepatocytes.
2. There can be deficiency of LDLR and apolipoproteins which can lead to early onset of atherosclerosis.
3. Other causes include:
   - Diabetes mellitus
   - Hypothyroidism
   - Nephrotic syndrome
   - Alcoholism.

In these patients, there is increased LDL, decreased HDL and increased levels of Lp (a). Lowering of cholesterol either by diet or drugs that inhibit synthesis of cholesterol (HMG CoA) can slow the process of atherosclerosis and reduce the risk of cardiovascular events.

Reaction to Injury Hypothesis: Mechanism of Atherosclerosis

1. Endothelial injury: Multiple factors and hyperlipidaemia cause endothelial injury and with this there is adhesion of platelets and monocytes and allows lipids to enter into intima due to increased permeability.
2. There is inflammation of the wall which is responsible for initiation, progression and complications of atherosclerosis.
3. There is accumulation of lipoproteins mainly LDL and oxidised forms of LDL due to ROS in the intimal layer of the vessel wall. T cells and monocytes gain entry into intima and these monocytes transform into macrophages and foam cells as they ingest LDL and thus become foamy macrophages. There is platelet adhesion and activation.
4. Oxidised LDL is also toxic to endothelial cells and smooth muscle cells (SMCs).
5. Growth factors released from activated platelets, macrophages (e.g. PGDF, FGDF, TGF-α) induce extracellular matrix deposition and SMCs recruitment from media. Thus, there are smooth cells and deposition of collagen and proteoglycans.
6. Lipid accumulation: Lipid accumulates extracellularly and within the cells (macrophages and SMCs).
7. Thus, central core of lipids, necrotic debris, lipid laden macrophages and smooth muscle cells and fibrous cap are components of atherosclerosis. Lipid and necrotic debris can get calcified in due course of time. Disruption of the fibrous cap with superimposed thrombus leads to complications.

Morphologically atherosclerotic lesions can be (Fig. 3.25a):
1. Streaks—earliest lesions, followed by
2. *Plaque which has:*

   Fibrous cap which has cells—SMCs, macrophages and T cells and extracellular matrix having dense collagen, elastic fibres and proteoglycans and core has intracellular and extracellular lipids mainly cholesterol and cholesterol esters.

3. Complicated atherosclerotic plaque
   - Calcification
   - Rupture
   - Ulceration
   - Erosion
   - Thrombosis
   - Haemorrhage
   - Occlusion/stenosis
   - Atheroemboli
   - Aneurysmal dilatation.

American Heart Association (AHA)[7] Classification of Atherosclerotic Plaques for Histologic Diagnosis

Type	Nature of histology
Type I	Initial lesion; isolated macrophages and foam cells (fatty dot)
Type II	Fatty streaks; foam cells, intracellular lipid
Type III	Preatheroma; raised fatty streak, small extracellular lipid core, foam cells contain lipid droplets, increasing number of smooth muscle cells
Type IV	Atheroma; covered by a proteoglycan-rich layer infiltrated with foam cells and smooth muscle cells, extracellular lipid
Type V	Fibroatheroma; lipid core, fibrotic layer, or mainly calcific or mainly fibrotic
Type VI	Complications—surface defect, haemorrhage, thrombus.

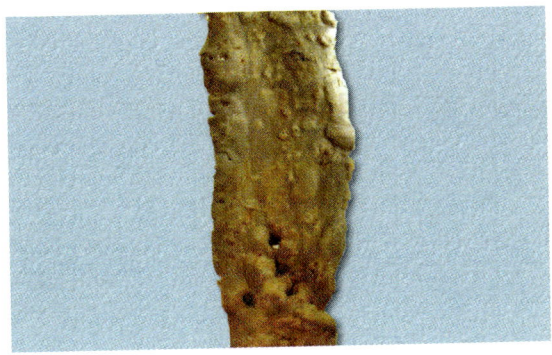

Fig. 3.25a: Gross picture of atherosclerosis

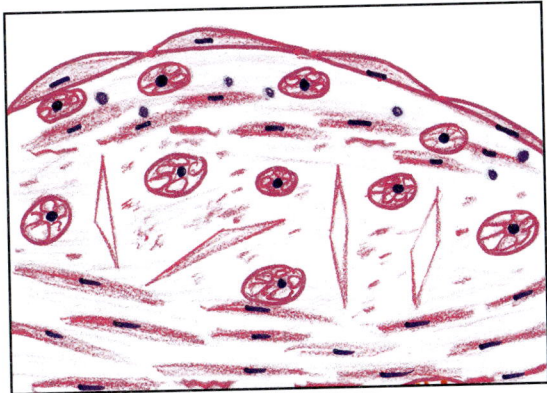

Fig. 3.25b: Schematic diagram of microscopy of atherosclerosis

VASCULAR PATHOLOGY IN HYPERTENSION

Hypertension is associated with atherosclerosis and degenerative changes of the large and medium-sized vessels. Small blood vessels in hypertension show hyaline arteriolosclerosis and hyperplastic arteriolosclerosis.

Hyaline Arteriolosclerosis

There is accumulation of homogenous pink hyaline material in the walls of arterioles with loss of underlying structures and narrowing of lumen. This type of hyaline arteriolosclerosis is commonly encountered in elderly people (normotensive and hypertensive patients). It is more generalised and severe in patients with hypertension. It is encountered in patients with diabetes mellitus and benign nephrosclerosis.

Hyperplastic Arteriolosclerosis

This type of vessel pathology is common with malignant hypertension, wherein the diastolic blood pressure is more than 120 mm Hg and associated with acute renal or cerebral injury. Hyperplastic arteriosclerosis is associated with onion skin concentric laminated thickening of the walls of the arterioles with luminal narrowing.

The laminations consist of smooth muscle cells and thickened and duplicated basement membrane. There is deposition of fibrinoid material and vessel wall necrosis (necrotising arteriolitis). This is more pronounced in vessels of kidneys.

HT usually remains asymptomatic until late in its course. Hypertension can cause the following.

- Cardiac hypertrophy
- Heart failure
- Aortic dissection
- Renal failure
- Cardiovascular accidents.

Exercise 43

Heart Lesions

CONGENITAL HEART DISEASES

Congenital heart diseases (CHDs) are abnormalities of the heart or great vessels that are present at birth.

Most such disorders arise from faulty embryogenesis during gestational weeks of 3 through 8, when major cardiovascular structures develop.

Pathogenesis

1. Cause is unknown in almost 90% of cases.
   Some causes can be:
2. Environmental factors, such as congenital rubella infection.
3. Genetic with certain chromosomal abnormalities (e.g. trisomies 13, 15, 18, and 21 and Turner syndrome).

Congenital Heart Diseases can be Subdivided into three Groups

Right-to-left shunt	Tetralogy of Fallot, transposition of great arteries, tricuspid atresia, total anomalous pulmonary venous connection, persistent truncus arteriosus
Left-to-right shunt	VSD, ASD, PDA, atrioventricular septal defect
Malformations causing obstruction	Coarctation of aorta, aortic valvular stenosis, pulmonary stenosis

Some of the important congenital heart diseases are mentioned.

CHDs causing left-to-right shunt

1. **Atrial septal defect (ASD):** An abnormal opening in the atrial septum that allows communication of blood between the left and right atria. ASDs are usually asymptomatic until adulthood (until the age of 30 years).

Three major types of ASDs
a. Secundum ASDs (90%)—single, multiple or fenestrated oval fossa near the centre of the atrial septum (mid-septum).
b. Primum anomalies (5%) adjacent to the AV valves associated with cleft in the anterior mitral leaflet.
c. Sinus venosus defects (5%) located near the entrance of the superior vena cava and may be associated with anomalous pulmonary venous return to the right atrium.

Effects of ASD
- Increased pulmonary flow (2 to 4 times than normal) with pulmonary hypertension
- Right ventricular hypertrophy.

2. **Ventricular septal defect (VSD):** There is incomplete closure of the ventricular septum, with free communication of blood between the left to right ventricles. This is the most common form of congenital cardiac anomaly.

Most VSDs are associated with other congenital cardiac anomalies such as tetralogy of Fallot.

About 90%, involve the membranous interventricular septum (membranous VSD).

The remainder lie below the pulmonary valve (infundibular VSD) or within the muscular septum.

Although most VSDs are single, those in the muscular septum may be multiple (so-called "Swiss-cheese" septum).

50% close spontaneously and remainder are tolerated.

Large defects produce left to right shunts.

Effects of VSD
- Increased pulmonary flow with pulmonary hypertension
- Right ventricle hypertrophy.

3. Patent ductus arteriosus (PDA)

PDA results when the ductus arteriosus, an essential fetal structure that normally spontaneously closes. May remain open after birth and shunts blood from the aorta to pulmonary artery. 90% occur as isolated anomalies. Remainder occur with VSD and coarctation of aorta.

Coarctation with PDA presents early in life, murmur is present. Initially no cyanosis as the shunt is left to right. When there is obstructive pulmonary vascular disease flow reverses.

Effects of PDA
Increased volume on left side of ventricle, later with increased pulmonary flow left atrium and left ventricle show volume hypertrophy.

CHDs causing right to left shunts: These patients have cyanosis with diminished pulmonary flow and poorly oxygenated blood enters the systemic circulation.

Moreover, bland or septic emboli arising from peripheral vein can bypass pulmonary circulation and can enter systemic circulation (paradoxical emboli).

1. Tetralogy of Fallot (TOF)

Four cardinal features of TOF (Fig. 3.26a) are:
1. VSD
2. Obstruction of the right ventricular outflow tract (subpulmonary stenosis)
3. An aorta that overrides the VSD
4. Right ventricular hypertrophy.

Results from anterosuperior displacement of the infundibular septum.

Heart is often enlarged and "boot-shaped" due to marked right ventricular hypertrophy, particularly of the apical region.

The VSD is usually large, aortic valve forms the superior border and override the defect VSD.

There is obstruction to the right ventricular outflow due to narrowing of infundibulum/complete atresia of pulmonary valve.

If the subpulmonary stenosis is mild, the abnormality resembles an isolated VSD, and the shunt may be left-to-right, without cyanosis (so-called pink tetralogy).

As the obstruction increases in severity, there is greater resistance to right ventricular outflow—right-sided pressure exceeds that of left-sided pressure and right-to-left shunt develops with cyanosis (classic TOF).

Most infants with TOF are cyanotic from birth or soon thereafter.

2. Transposition of the Great Arteries (TGA)

TGA is a discordant connection of the ventricles to their vascular outflow.

The embryologic defect is an abnormal formation of the truncal and aortopulmonary septa, so that the aorta arises from the right ventricle and the pulmonary artery from the left ventricle.

The atrium-to-ventricle connections, however, are normal (concordant). The functional outcome is separation of the systemic and pulmonary circulations. TGA is incompatible with life unless shunts exists.

Obstructive Lesions (Figs 3.26b and c)

Coarctation of aorta: It is narrowing or constriction of aorta.

M : F = 2 : 1, although females with Turner's syndrome frequently have aortic coarctation.

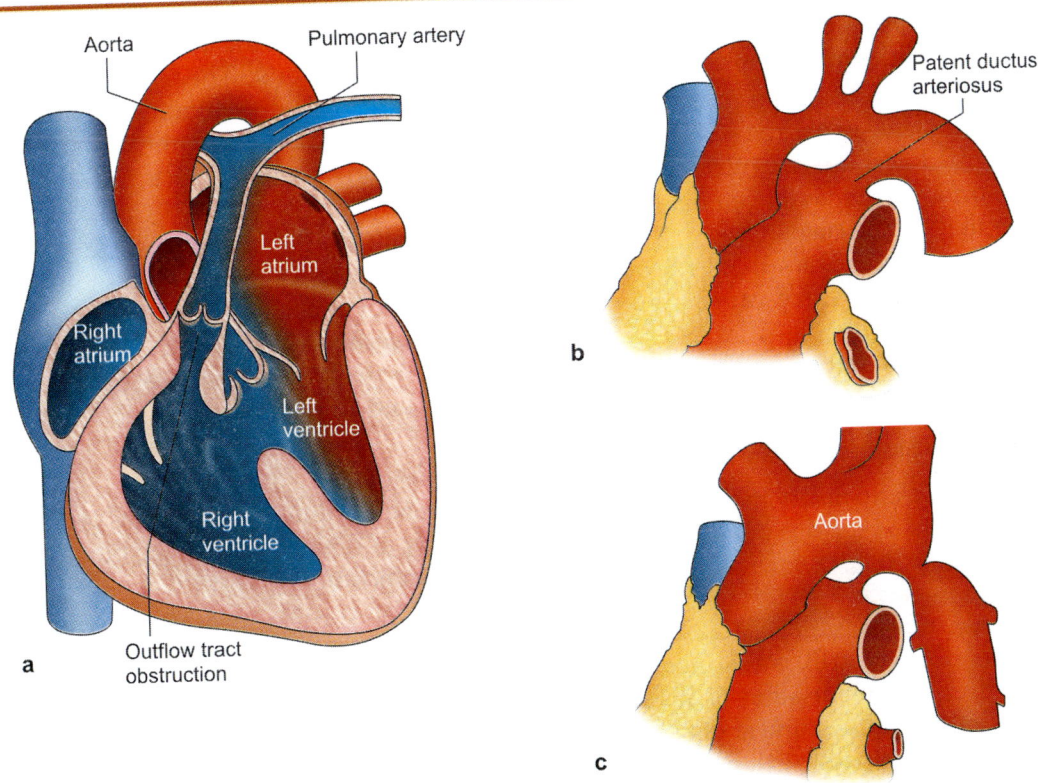

Figs 3.26a to c: Congenital heart diseases, (a) Fallot's tetralogy, (b) coarctation of aorta with PDA, (c) coarctation of aorta. Burford TH. Symposium on clinical surgery. Coarctation of aorta and its treatment. *Source: Surg Clin North Am* 1950;30:1249–58

Two classic forms
- Infantile (preductal) form
- Adult (postductal) form.

Infantile (preductal) form
Hypoplasia and tubular narrowing of the aortic arch between the left subclavian artery and the ductus arteriosus.

Ductus arteriosus is usually patent.

Right ventricle is hypertrophied and dilated.

Manifests immediately after birth.

Cyanosis localised to the lower half of the body.

Femoral pulses are almost always weaker than those of the upper extremities.

Adult (postductal) form
Aorta is sharply constricted by a ridge of tissue at or just distal to the ligamentum arteriosum; the ductus arteriosus is closed.

Proximal to the coarctation, the aortic arch and its branch vessels are dilated

Left ventricle is hypertrophic.

Usually asymptomatic.

Upper extremity hypertension, but weak pulse and lower blood pressure in the lower extremities, claudication and coldness of the lower extremities are common.

Adults show exuberant collateral circulation "around" the coarctation involving markedly enlarged intercostal and internal mammary arteries and radiographically visible "notching" of the ribs.

Aortic Stenosis and Atresia

Most common congenital anomaly of aorta is bicuspid aortic valve.

Congenital aortic atresia—incompatible with life.

Acquired aortic stenosis—rheumatic heart disease, calcified aortic stenosis.

Congenital aortic stenosis is of three types:
1. Valvular stenosis—aortic valve cusps are malformed and are irregularly thickened. The aortic valve may have one, two or all three malformed cusps.
2. Subvalvular stenosis—thick fibrous ring under the aortic valve causing subaortic stenosis.
3. Supravalvular stenosis—there is fibrous constriction above sinuses of Valsalva.

Effects Aortic Stenosis and Atresia
- Left atrium and left ventricle—volume hypertrophy
- Aortic root—dilated.

INFECTIVE ENDOCARDITIS

Infective endocarditis (IE) is a serious infection characterised by colonisation or invasion of the heart valves or the mural endocardium by microbes often with destruction of underlying cardiac tissues. There is formation of bulky, friable vegetations composed of necrotic debris, thrombus and organisms.

Causes
- *Bacterial infections (bacterial endocarditis)*: Alpha haemolytic streptococci (*Strptococcus viridans*) is the causative organism—affects 50–60% of the cases usually in damaged or abnormal valves.
  Staph aureus: 10–20% in normal or deformed valves, common in IV drug abusers.
- Other microorganisms
  - Enterococci
  - Fungi
  - Rickettsiae
  - Chlamydiae.

IE has been classified on clinical grounds into
- Acute
- Subacute forms.

Acute infective endocarditis is typically caused by infection of a previously normal heart valve by a highly virulent organism that produces necrotising and ulcerative and destructive lesions. These infections are difficult to cure with antibiotics and usually require surgery. Death occurs within days to weeks in many patients with acute IE, despite of treatment.

Subacute IE, the organisms are of lower virulence. These organisms cause insidious infections of deformed valves that are less destructive. In such cases the disease may pursue a protracted course of weeks to months, and cure is expected with antibiotics.

Etiopathogenesis
Prior to endocarditis, the organisms proliferate. The entry of organisms into the bloodstream may be infection elsewhere like:
- Dental or surgical procedure which can cause transient bacteremia
- Injection of contaminated material by IV drug abusers
- Occult source of infection from GIT—oral cavity/intestine
- Trivial injuries.

IE is common in: Rheumatic heart disease

Others
- Mitral valve prolapse
- Degenerative calcific valvular stenosis
- Bicuspid aortic valve (whether calcified or not)
- Artificial (prosthetic) valves, and unrepaired, and
- Repaired congenital defects.

Clinical features
1. Fever, chills and weakness: Fever is the most common sign, however in subacute cases fever may be absent and may have only non-specific features like fatigue, loss of weight and flu-like symptoms. Splenomegaly is common in subacute IE. Acute IE can have rapidly developing features like fever, chills, weakness and lassitude.

2. Murmurs are present in 90% of the patients with left-sided lesions.
3. Petechiae and subungual haemorrhages.
4. Janeway lesions on palms and soles, these are often haemorrhagic and non-tender.
5. Osler's nodes are red purple, raised tender lesions found on fingers and toes.
6. Roth's spots in eye are white centered retinal haemorrhages.

These haemorrhagic lesions (petechiae, subungual lesions, Janeway lesions, Osler's nodes, Roth's spots) are possibly due to immune complex mediated vasculitis or due to septic emboli.

Diagnosis is made on
- Positive blood cultures
- ECG findings
- Clinical history
- Laboratory findings.

Diagnostic criteria for infective endocarditis pathologic criteria
- Microorganisms demonstrated by culture or on histologic examination in a vegetation, embolus from a vegetation or intracardiac abscess
- Histologic confirmation of active endocarditis in vegetation or intracardiac abscess.

Clinical criteria

Major
1. Blood culture(s) positive for a characteristic organism or persistently positive for an unusual organism.
2. Echocardiographic identification of a valve-related or implant-related mass or abscess, or partial separation of artificial valve.
3. New valvular regurgitation.

Minor
1. Predisposing heart lesion or intravenous drug use
2. Fever
3. Vascular lesions including petechiae, subungual/splinter haemorrhages, emboli, septic infarcts, mycotic aneurysm, intracranial haemorrhage, Janeway lesions.
4. Immunological phenomena, including glomerulonephritis, Osler nodes, Roth's spots and rheumatoid factor.
5. Microbiologic evidence including a single culture positive for an unusual organism.
6. Echocardiographic findings consistent with but not diagnostic of endocarditis, including worsening or changing of a pre-existent murmur.

Gross: The hallmark of IE is the presence of:
- Friable, bulky, potentially destructive vegetations containing fibrin, inflammatory cells, and bacteria or other organisms.
- The vegetations may be single or multiple and may involve more than one valve.
- The aortic and mitral valves are the most common sites of infection, although the valves of the right heart may also be involved, particularly in intravenous drug abusers.
- Vegetations sometimes erode into the underlying myocardium and produce an abscess (ring abscess).
- Emboli may be shed from the vegetations at any time; because the embolic fragments may contain large numbers of virulent organisms, abscesses often develop at the sites where the emboli lodge, leading to sequelae such as septic infarcts or mycotic aneurysms.
- The vegetations of subacute endocarditis are associated with less valvular destruction than those of acute endocarditis.

Microscopy (Fig. 3.27a)
- The vegetation has platelets, fibrin, and organisms.
- The underlying valve is inflamed, vascularised and shows plenty of polymorphs along with macrophages, giant cells and areas of necrosis.
- The vegetations of typical subacute IE often have granulation tissue indicative of healing at their base. With time, fibrosis, calcification, and a chronic inflammatory infiltrate can develop.

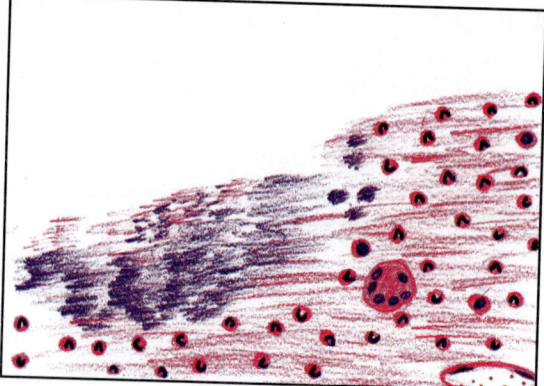

Fig. 3.27a: Schematic diagram of microscopy of vegetation in bacterial endocarditis

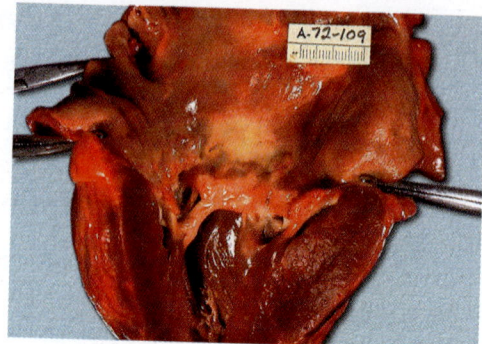

Fig. 3.27b: Gross picture of RHD, note MacCallum's patch, thickened mitral valve, chordae tendinae and hypertrophied left ventricular wall. From Public Heart Image Library (PHIL) ID 847

Complications

1. *Cardiac complications*
   - Valvular insufficiency/stenosis/cardiac failure
   - Myocardial ring abscess
   - Perforation of aorta, interventricular septum, etc.
   - Suppurative pericarditis.
2. *Embolic complications*
   - *Left-sided lesions:* Brain abscess, meningitis, spleen and kidney abscess.
   - *Right-sided lesions:* Lung abscess, pneumonia.
3. *Renal complications*
   - Embolic infarct
   - Focal/glomerulonephritis
   - Diffuse or multiple abscesses.
4. Osteomyelitis
5. Myocardial infarction
6. Mycotic aneurysms

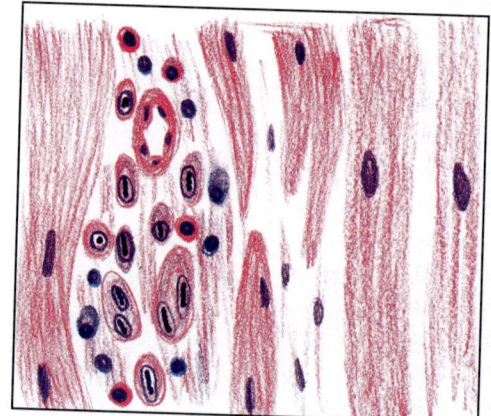

Fig. 3.27c: Schematic diagram of microscopy in RHD

RHEUMATIC FEVER AND RHEUMATIC HEART DISEASE (Figs 3.27b to d)

Rheumatic fever (RF) is an acute, immunologically mediated, multisystem inflammatory disease that occurs a few weeks after an episode of group A streptococcal pharyngitis. Acute rheumatic carditis is a frequent manifestation during the active phase of RF.

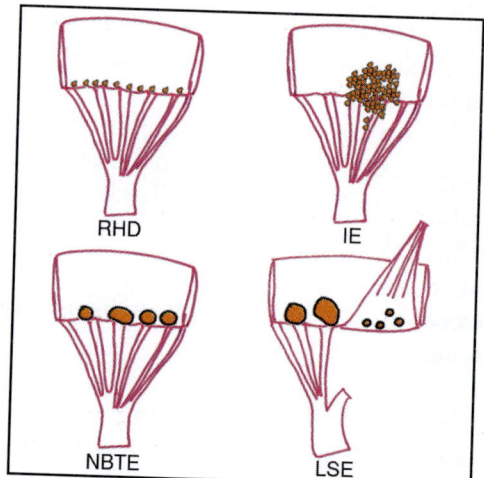

Fig. 3.27d: Verrucae—differential diagnosis

Epidemiology

This is a disease of poverty. Crowded housing, unhygienic conditions result in spread of streptococcal infection. The disease is less common in industrialised countries. Improved living condition and better hygiene and antibiotics have reduced the incidence of rheumatic heart disease (RHD) in developed and developing nations. Children between ages 5 and 15 years are commonly affected. Recurrent episodes of acute RF are known in adolescents and adults.

Pathogenesis

- Acute rheumatic fever results from immune responses to group A streptococci, which happen to cross-react with host tissues.
- Antibodies directed against the M proteins of streptococci have been shown to cross-react with self antigens in the heart.
- Antibodies and CD4+ T cells specific for streptococcal peptides react with self proteins in the heart. The antibodies can activate complement and Fc receptor bearing cells and CD4 T cells produce cytokines that activate macrophages (such as those found in Aschoff bodies).
- Damage to heart tissue may thus be caused by a combination of antibody- and T cell-mediated reactions.
- Genetic susceptibility.

Evidence for Preceeding Group A Streptococci

1. The serological evidence with raised or rising Anti-streptolysin O (ASLO) titres, hyaluronidase or Anti-DNAase titres
2. Positive throat swab
3. Rapid antigen test for Group A streptococcus
4. Recent scarlet fever

Pathology of Heart in RHD

The connective tissue or collagen tissue of heart is primarily affected. The heart changes can be divided into:

- Acute rheumatic heart disease
  - Early exudative phase
  - Proliferative phase or granulomatous phase
  - Late phase
- Chronic rheumatic heart disease.

In Acute Rheumatic Heart Disease

Early Acute/Exudative Phase

This phase persists up to four weeks.

Early exudative lesion has following features.
- Oedema
- ↑ mucopolysacharides
- Ground substance and collagen
  - Altered
- Fibrinoid necrosis

Proliferative Phase

In acute RF, the pathognomonic lesions are Aschoff bodies (Ascoff nodules). The initial lesions show perivascular focus of fibrinoid degeneration of collagen surrounded by lymphocytes, plasma cells and macrophages. With time, the classical granulomatous lesion, the Ascoff bodies or Ascoff nodules develop. Ascoff bodies have central area of fibrinoid necrosis, surrounded by T lymphocytes, macrophages, occasional plasma cells, plump histiocytes, i.e. Anitschkow cells. Some altered histiocytes are multinucleated and these are called Ascoff giant cells. These Anitschkow cells have amphophilic cytoplasm, round to oval nuclei, chromatin is disposed in a central slender wavy ribbon giving the appearance of caterpillar. On cross section this appears as owl eye appearance.

Late Phase

With time the Ascoff bodies are replaced by scar tissue and merges with chronic phase (chronic rheumatic heart disease).

These lesions are found in perivascular location and are present in all three layers of the heart, causing pericarditis, myocarditis, or endocarditis (pancarditis). Inflammation of the endocardium and the left-sided valves typically results in fibrinoid necrosis within the cusps or along the chordae tendinae.

The gross findings of heart in RHD are the following:

Acute Rheumatic Heart Disease

1. The heart shows pancarditis.
2. **Pericardium:** Shows fibrinous pericarditis (Bread and butter appearance)
3. **Myocardium:** There is myocarditis
4. **Endocardium:** Shows verrucae and MacCallum's patch.

Verrucae: These develop on the valves. These are small (1–2 mm) vegetations, present on the focus of fibrinoid necrosis and are present along the line of closure. In RHD, the mitral valve is affected alone in 65% to 70% of cases, and along with the aortic valve in another 25% of cases.

MacCallum's patch: Subendocardial lesions, perhaps exacerbated by regurgitant jets, may induce irregular thickening and **MacCallum plaque,** usually in the left atrium.

Chronic Rheumatic Heart Disease

- Leaflet thickening
- Commissural fusion
- Shortening, thickening and fusion of chordae tendinae
- The thickening and commissural fusion of the valves gives rise to stenosis (fish mouth appearance) and incompetency (regurgitation) of the valves.

Clinical Features and Diagnosis

Guidelines for Diagnosis (Jones criteria)

Major criteria
1. Migratory polyarthritis of the large joints
2. Pancarditis
3. Subcutaneous nodules
4. Erythema marginatum of the skin
5. Sydenham chorea.

Minor criteria
1. Fever
2. Arthralgia
3. Elevated blood levels of acute-phase reactants (E.g. CRP, ASLO, etc.) or elevated ESR or WBC count
4. ECG findings: Prolonged PR interval.

The diagnosis is established by evidence of a preceding group A streptococcal infection, with the presence of:
a. Two of the major criteria
b. One major and two minor manifestations.

Other causes of vegetations

Vegetations are found in bacterial endocarditis and rheumatic heart disease. Apart from these two the other causes are:

1. *Non-bacterial thrombotic endocarditis (NBTE, Marantic):*

NBTE occurs in hypercoagulable states, like in sepsis with DIC, hyperoestrogenic states, underlying malignancy; particularly mucinous carcinoma. NBTE is a part of Trousseau syndrome. Endocardial trauma due to indwelling catheter is also predisposing factor.

These vegetations have following features.
1. Small, sterile masses of fibrin and other blood elements—on valve leaflets which are previously normal values
2. No organisms
3. Non-destructive
4. Small (1–5 mm)
5. Single/multiple
6. No inflammation, thrombus
7. No valve damage.

2. *Libman sacks endocrditis:* These vegetations develop on the valves in Systemic lupus erythematosis. These occur presumably because of immune complex deposition and thus associated with inflammation. These vegetations have following features.
- Small (1–4 mm) and sterile
- Single/multiple
- Vegetations are on valvular endocardium and undersurface and on chordae tendinae.
- There is valvulitis, fibrosis and deformity.

CARDIOMYOPATHY

Cardiomyopathies (CMPs) are cardiac diseases primarily due to intrinsic myocardial dysfunction (according to 1995 WHO/International Society of Federation of Cardiology (ISFC). In 1980, WHO defined cardiomyopathies as diseases of unknown cause to distinguish cardiomyopathy from cardiac dysfunction due to hypertension, ischaemic heart diseases and valvular heart diseases.

American Heart Society 2006 classifies cardiomyopathies as:
1. Primary
2. Secondary

On clinical and functional basis, cardiomyopathies can be classified as:
1. Dilated cardiomyopathy
2. Hypertrophic cardiomyopathy
3. Restrictive cardiomyopathy

Among these three types, dilated cardiomyopathy is most common and restrictive is least common.

Dilated Cardiomyopathy

Dilated cardiomyopathy (DCM), has progressive cardiac dilatation and contractile dysfunction.

Pathogenesis

The causes include:
- Familial/Genetic
- Toxins
- Thiamine deficiency
- Viruses
- Peripartum
- Unknown.

Viruses: Coxsackie virus B and other enteroviruses are blamed for causing myocarditis and with end result of DCM.

Toxins and thiamine deficiency: Alcohol and its metabolites (especially aldehyde) have direct toxic effect on heart. Chronic alcoholism can be associated with thiamine deficiency too. Other toxins include: chemotherapeutic agents (cobalt and adriamycin).

Familial/genetic causes: Mutation of dystrophin gene, alpha cardiac actin, desmin and nuclear lamins A and C. Mitochondrial gene deletions, and mutations in genes encoding enzymes involved in fatty acid beta-oxidation can be also responsible for causation of DCM.

Peripartum period: Occurs during late gestation or several weeks or months after delivery. Cause could be pregnancy induced hypertension, volume overload, nutritional deficiency, metabolic derangement, etc.

Pathology

Gross: Following are the features
- Heart is enlarged 2 to 3 times of the normal size
- Flabby
- Dilatation of all the four chambers
- Mural thrombi are common
- No valve pathology
- Coronaries: No atherosclerosis.

Microscopy: Following changes may be encountered:
- Non-specific changes
- Myocardial fibres hypertrophied with enlarged nuclei
- Some myocardial fibres attenuated, stretched or irregular and may show empty spaces
- There is presence of focal myocyte necrosis
- There is variable interstitial or endocardial fibrosis, scar formation may be present.

Clinical Features

- DCM can occur at any age. Most commonly occurs between the age range of 20–50 years.
- It presents with slowly progressive chronic heart failure with shortness of breath, orthopnoea, dyspnoea on exertion, fatigue and dry mouth.
- There is ineffective contraction and cardiac ejection fraction is less than 25%.
- Mitral incompetence and abnormal cardiac rhythms are most common.
- Mural thrombi are frequent.

- Death is due to progressive cardiac failure or arrhythmias.
- About 50% of the patients die within 2 years and another 25% die within 5 years.

Hypertrophic Cardiomyopathy

Hypertrophic cardiomyopathy is also called by other synonyms like idiopathic hypertrophic sub-aortic stenosis. This is characterised by myocardial hypertrophy, abnormal diastolic filling and in some cases with ventricular outflow obstruction. Heart is thick walled. It is hypercontracting and is stiff and non-compliant. Systolic function is preserved, but does not relax in diastole, thus the diastolic filling defect.

Pathogenesis

Missense point mutations of sarcomeric proteins, most commonly beta-myosin heavy chains, myocin binding protein C and troponin T are commonly affected. It has AD inheritance pattern.

There is a proposal that myocyte contraction triggers growth factor release with intense hypertrophy causing myocyte disarray and fibroblast proliferation causing interstitial fibrosis.

Pathology

Gross: Following are the features:
1. Massive myocardial hypertrophy without ventricular dilatation.
2. Disproportionate thickening of the septum relative to left ventricular free wall (asymmetrical septal hypertrophy).
3. In longitudinal section of heart, left ventricular cavity appears banana-shaped.
4. There is formation of endocardial plaque in the outflow tract of left ventricle.
5. The anterior mitral leaflet is thickened.

Microscopy: Shows following features:
1. Severe myocyte hypertrophy.
2. Myofibre disarray: The myocardial fibre are arranged criss-cross.
3. Interstitial fibrosis.

Clinical Features

- There is breathlessness on exertion, dizziness, fainting and precordial pain.
- There is massive hypertrophy of left ventricle with reduced stroke volume.
- The left ventricular chamber size is small and hence impaired diastolic filling.
- About one-fourth of the patients have outflow tract obstruction. There is systolic motion of anterior leaflet of mitral valve towards the interventricular septum. This raises the pressure in left atrium.
- In these patients, there is reduced cardiac output and increase in pulmonary venous pressure which causes exertional dyspnoea and systolic ejection murmur.
- There is frequent myocardial ischaemia, atrial fibrillation, arrhythmias, mural thrombus formation, infective endocarditis and sudden death may occur.

Restrictive Cardiomyopathy

This is characterised by decrease in ventricular compliance, with impaired diastolic filling. The systolic function is normal.

Restrictive cardiomyopathy can be due to following causes:
- Idiopathic
- Radiation
- Amyloidosis
- Hemochromatosis
- Sarcoidosis
- In patients with in-born-errors of metabolism.

Gross: The following are the features:
- The ventricles are normal in size or slightly enlarged
- Myocardium is firm
- Bi-atrial dilatation is commonly observed.

Microscopy: Shows following features.

Interstitial fibrosis: This can be focal or diffuse, minimal or extensive. Endomyocardial biopsy may show amyloidosis, hemochromatosis or sarcoidosis.

The important types of restrictive cardiomyopathy are the following:

Endomyocardial fibrosis: This is a type of restrictive cardiomyopathy occurs in children and young adults in tropical countries. There is ventricular endocardial fibrosis extending from apex to the mitral and tricuspid valves. The fibrosis restricts the volume and compliance of the affected chambers.

Loeffler endomyocarditis: This causes restrictive cardiomyopathy with endocardial fibrosis. There is associated eosinophilia, the contents of the granules, especially the major basic protein initiates endocardial damage with necrosis followed by fibrosis.

PERICARDITIS

The most common causes of pericarditis include:
- Infections: Viral, bacterial, fungi
- Myocardial infarction
- Cardiac surgery
- Irradiation to the mediastinum
- Uremia.

Less common causes include:
- RHD
- SLE

Pericarditis can cause:
- Haemodymic complications
- May resolve without leaving any sequelae
- May progress to chronic process.

Morphological Types with Causes

- *Fibrinous pericarditis (Shaggy or Bread and Butter appearance):* RHD, uraemia and viral infections
- *Fibrino-purulent pericarditis:* Pyogenic bacteria
- *Pericarditis with caseation necrosis:* Tuberculosis
- *Fibrinous with bloody effusion:* Malignancy.

With suppuration or caseation, fibrosis occurs resulting in chronic pericarditis. The fibrotic scars obliterates the pericardial sac. In severe cases pericardial cavity may have dense fibrosis, and heart may not expand during diastole, this is termed constrictive pericarditis.

Clinical features in pericarditis: Pericarditis classically presents with chest pain, and a friction rub. When significant amount of fluid collects causes cardiac temponade.

PERICARDIAL EFFUSION

Normally about 30–50 ml of thin clear, straw coloured fluid is present in the pericardial cavity.

The common causes of pericardial effusion include:
- *Serous:* CHF, hypoalbuminaemia
- *Serosanguinous:* Blunt chest trauma, malignancy, ruptured MI or aortic stenosis
- *Chylous effusion as in:* Lymphatic obstruction.

In slowly collecting (chronic) effusions with fluid of 100 ml may remain asymptomatic. In rapidly (acute) developing causes such as ruptured MI, ruptured aortic dissection, effusion of even 250 ml is dangerous. This can restrict diastolic filling with cardiac temponade.

Exercise 44

Lesions of Respiratory Tract

PULMONARY TUBERCULOSIS

Tuberculosis is a chronic granulomatous inflammation. The causative organism is *Mycobacterium tuberculosis*/Koch's bacillus. The organism is a strict aerobe and thrives in tissues with high oxygen tension (Fig. 3.28).

It can be demonstrated by the following methods:

- Ziehl-Neelson/acid-fast staining
- Fluorescent dye methods
- Culture of the organism in LJ medium for 6 weeks
- Guinea pig inoculation method.

Occasionally, human tuberculosis may be caused by atypical mycobacteria which are non-pathogenic to guinea pigs and resistant to the usual antitubercular drugs. There are four groups of atypical mycobacteria: Photo-chromogens (group 1), scotochromogens (group 2), non-chromogens (group 3), rapid growers (group 4).

Mode of Transmission of Tuberculosis
- Inhalation
- Ingestion
- Inoculation
- Transplacental route.

Spread of Tuberculosis in the Body
- Local spread
- Lymphatic spread
- Haematogenous spread

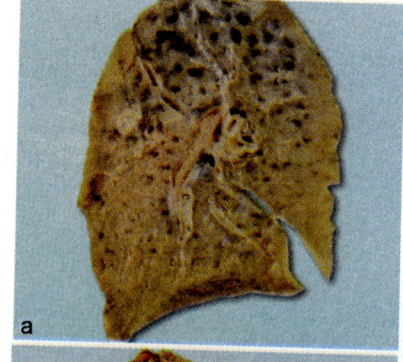
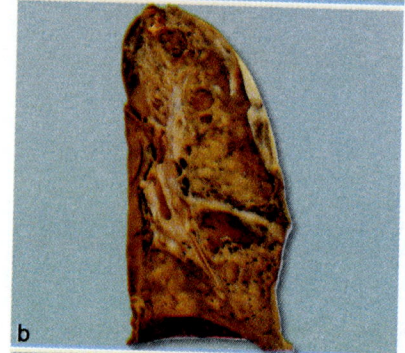
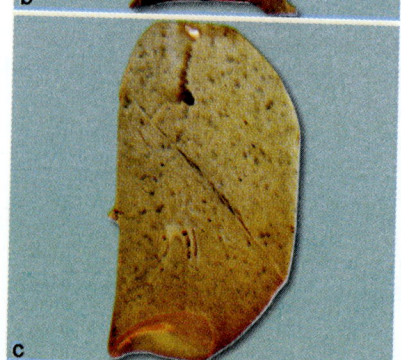

Figs 3.28a to c: Gross pictures of tuberculosis lung: (a) Ghon's focus, (b) fibrocaseous cavitary tuberculosis, (c) miliary tuberculosis

General Pathology and Systemic Pathology

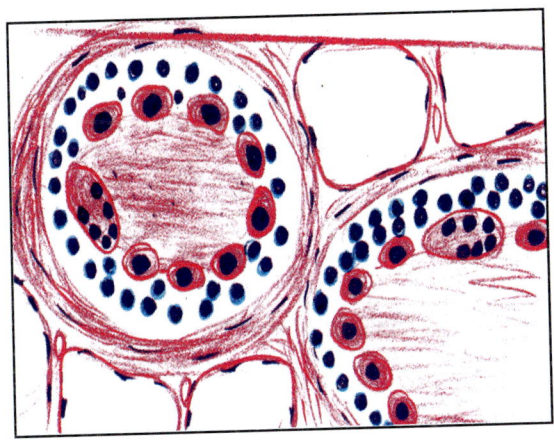

Fig. 3.28d: Schematic diagram of microscopy of tuberculosis lung

4. By natural passages to pleura (tuberculous pleurisy)
5. Transbronchial spread into adjacent lung segments
6. Tuberculous salpingitis into peritoneal cavity
7. Infected sputum into larynx
8. Swallowing of infected sputum
9. Renal lesions.

Primary Tuberculosis

It is the infection of an individual who has not been previously infected or immunised. It is also called 'Ghon's complex or childhood tuberculosis'.

Primary complex or Ghon's complex: It is the lesion produced at the portal of entry with foci in the draining lymphatic vessels and lymph nodes. It has 3 components:

Ghon's focus (Fig. 3.28a): Lesion in the lung is the primary focus or Ghon's focus. It is 1–2 cm, solitary, located peripherally near the fissure, in any part of the lung but more often in the subpleural focus in the upper part of lower lobe or lower part of upper lobe. Microscopically, the lung lesion consists of tuberculous granulomas with caseation necrosis.

Lymphatic vessels: The lymphatics draining the lung lesion may develop tuberculous lymphangitis.

Lymph nodes: Hilar and tracheobronchial lymph nodes in the area drained are enlarged. The affected lymph nodes are matted and show caseation necrosis.

Fate of Primary Tuberculosis

1. Healing by fibrosis and further may undergo calcification and even ossification.
2. Progressive primary tuberculosis where infection is disseminated through bronchi to other parts of the same lung or to the other lung.
3. Primary miliary tuberculosis where bacilli enter circulation and spread to various tissues and organs.
4. Progressive secondary tuberculosis where healed lesions get reactivated. This is seen with lowered host resistance.

Secondary Tuberculosis

It is the infection of an individual who has been previously infected or sensitised. It is also called 'secondary or post-primary or reinfection tuberculosis'.

The infection may be acquired from
- *Endogenous source:* Reactivation of dormant primary complex
- *Exogenous source:* Fresh dose of reinfection by tubercle bacilli.

Fate of Secondary Pulmonary Tuberculosis

The lesions may heal with fibrous scarring and calcification. The lesions may extend to progressive secondary pulmonary tuberculosis with the following pulmonary and extrapulmonary organ or tissue involvement.

1. *Fibrocaseous tuberculosis:* Grossly, tuberculous cavity is spherical with thick fibrous wall, lined by yellowish, caseous, necrotic material and the lumen may be traversed by thrombosed blood vessels. The overlying pleura may also be thickened and

shows adhesions. Microscopically, widespread coalesced tuberculous granulomas composed of epitheloid cells, Langhans' giant cells and peripheral mantle of lymphocytes and having central caseation necrosis are seen. The outer wall of cavity shows fibrosis.

2. Fibrocaseous cavitary tuberculosis (Fig. 3.28b).
3. *Miliary tuberculosis:* There is lymphohaematogenous spread of tuberculous infection. The spread may occur to systemic organs or isolated organ. The spread through pulmonary vein produces disseminated or isolated organ lesion in different extrapulmonary sites (e.g. liver, spleen, kidney, brain and bone marrow). Spread into the pulmonary artery restricts the development of miliary lesions within the lung. The miliary lesions are millet seed-sized (1 mm diameter), yellowish, firm areas (Fig. 3.28c). Microscopically, the lesions show the structure of tubercles with minute areas of caseation necrosis (Fig. 3.28d).
4. *Tuberculous pneumonia:* Individuals with high degree of hypersensitivity, tuberculosis may spread to the rest of the lung producing caseous pneumonia. Microscopically, the lesions show exudative reaction with oedema, fibrin, polymorphs and monocytes but numerous tubercle bacilli can be demonstrated in the exudate.

OBSTRUCTIVE PULMONARY DISEASES

These are associated with airflow obstruction. They are listed below:
1. Chronic obstructive lung/pulmonary disease (COPD)
   i. Chronic bronchitis
   ii. Emphysema
2. Bronchial asthma
3. Bronchiectasis
4. Small airways disease
5. Cystic fibrosis.

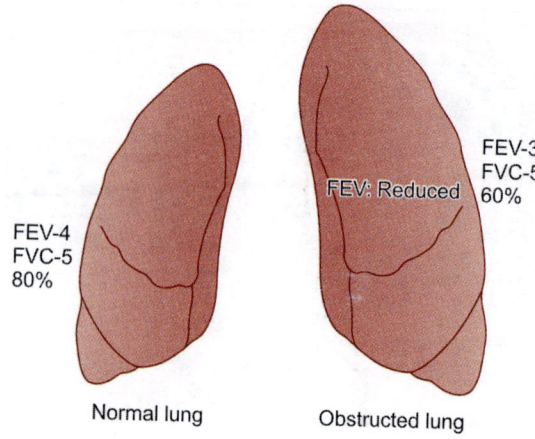

Fig. 3.29: Lung functions in obstructive lung diseases (comparison to normal)

In obstructive lung diseases forced expiratory volume in 1st second (FEV1) is less, forced vital capacity (FVC) is reduced and FEV1/FVC is less than 0.7 (Fig. 3.29).

CHRONIC BRONCHITIS

The diagnosis on clinical grounds should include persistent productive cough for at least three months, in at least two consecutive years in absence of any identifiable cause.

Pathogenesis: Cigarette smoking, other air pollutants such as SO_2, NO_2 may contribute. These irritate leading to hypertrophy and hyperplasia of mucus glands of surface epithelium of smaller bronchi and bronchioles. The irritants cause inflammation with infiltration of CD8+ T cells, macrophages and neutrophils. No eosinophils are present.

Pathology: In large airways, the mucosa is hyperaemic and oedematous. It is covered by mucopurulent secretion. Small bronchi and bronchioles also contain similar secretion. Normally, the Reid index is 0.4. Reid index is ratio of the thickness of the submucous glands to the thickness between the epithelium and the cartilage. In chronic bronchitis, there is hyperplasia and hypertrophy of submucosal glands with Reid index more than 0.4. The small airways (small bronchi and bronchioles) show increase in goblet cells and mucous plugging with inflammation and fibrosis. The

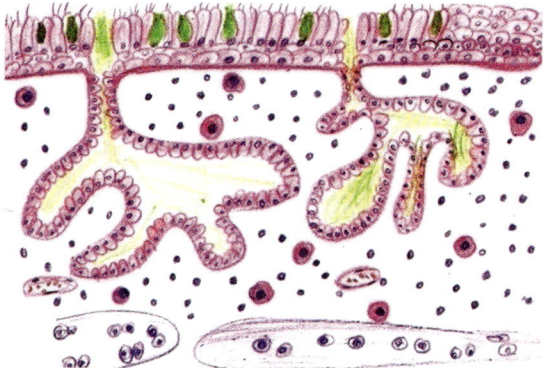

Fig. 3.30: Schematic diagram of changes in chronic bronchitis

bronchial epithelium may show increase in goblet cells, squamous metaplasia, basal cell hyperplasia, mucus plugging, inflammation and fibrosis. There is narrowing of lumen and airway obstruction.

In severe form, complete obstruction of the lumen due to fibrosis can occur. Peribrochiolar fibrosis and luminal narrowing result in airway obstruction.

Clinical features: Patients have cough with copious purulent sputum without ventilatory dysfunction. Some develop outflow obstruction with hypercapnoia, hypoxaemia, cyanosis (blue bloaters), peripheral oedema and polycythemia. In pink puffers chronic bronchitis leads to pulmonary hypertension and cardiac failure (Fig. 3.30).

EMPHYSEMA (Figs 3.31a to c)

Emphysema is defined as permanent dilatation of air spaces distal to the terminal bronchioles with destruction of the walls, without obvious fibrosis.

Emphysema can be classified, according to its anatomic distribution within the lobule into five types:
1. Centriacinar
2. Panacinar (panlobular)
3. Paraseptal (distal acinar)
4. Irregular (para-cicatricial)
5. Mixed (unclassified).

A number of other conditions to which the term 'emphysema' is loosely applied to overinflation, which is given as follows:
- Compensatory overinflation (compensatory emphysema)
- Senile hyperinflation (ageing lung, senile emphysema)

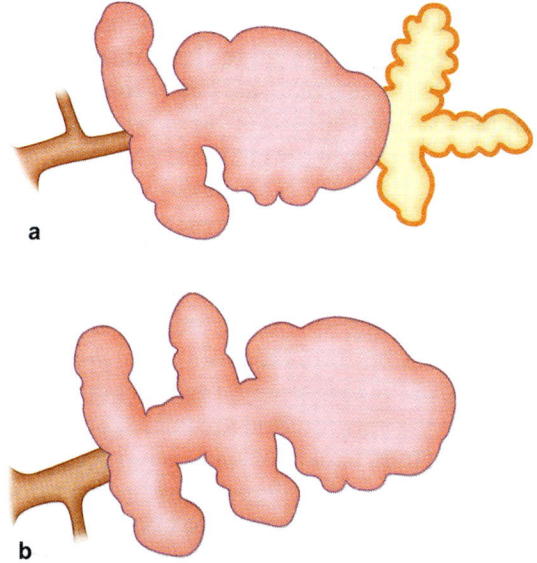

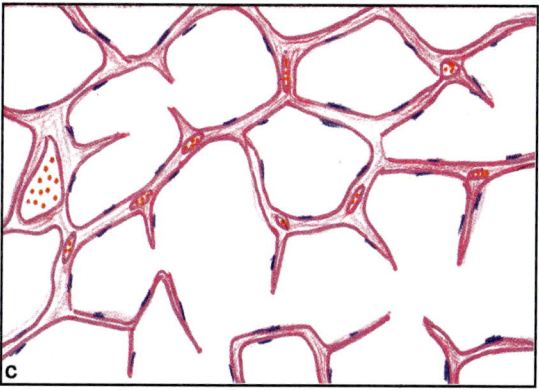

Figs 3.31a to c: Diagrammatic representation of emphysema: (a) Centriacinar, (b) panacinar, (c) schematic diagram of microscopy emphysema lung

- Obstructive overinflation (infantile lobar emphysema)
- Unilateral translucent lung (unilateral emphysema)
- Interstitial emphysema (surgical emphysema).

Etiopathogenesis

The important etiologic factors are tobacco smoke and air pollutants. Other less significant contributory factors are occupational exposure, infection and somewhat poorly understood familial and genetic influences.

However, the pathogenesis of the most significant event in emphysema, the destruction of alveolar walls, is closely related to the deficiency of serum α_1-antitrypsin commonly termed protease-antiprotease theory/hypothesis.

Protease-antiprotease Theory

Alpha-1-antitrypsin (α_1-AT) is a glycoprotein that is normally synthesised in the liver and is distributed in the circulating blood, tissues, body fluids and inflammatory cells. The normal function of α_1-AT is to inhibit proteases and hence its name α_1-protease inhibitor.

In lung, the proteases are derived from neutrophils. Neutrophil elastase has the capability of digesting lung parenchyma but is inhibited from doing so by anti-elastase effect of α_1-AT.

There are several known alleles of α_1-AT which have an autosomal codominant inheritance pattern and are classified as normal, deficient, null type having no detectable level, and dysfunctional type having about half the normal level.

The normal α_1-AT phenotype called PiMM is present in 90% of the population. The most abnormal phenotype homozygous state PiZZ has α_1-AT deficiency and emphysema occurs in early age and has greater severity in smokers.

The mechanism of alveolar wall destruction in emphysema by elastolytic action is based on the imbalance between proteases and antiproteases:
- By decreased anti-elastase activity, i.e. deficiency of α_1-AT.
- By increased activity of elastase, i.e. increased neutrophilic infiltration in the lungs causing excessive elaboration of neutrophil elastase.

Smoking promotes emphysema. Oxidants in cigarette smoke have inhibitory influence on α_1-AT, thus lowering the level of anti-elastase activity. Smokers have up to ten times more phagocytes and neutrophils in their lungs than non-smokers. Thus, they have very high elastase activity.

Pathologic changes: Emphysema can be diagnosed with certainty only by gross and histologic examination of sections of whole lung. The lungs should be perfused with formalin under pressure in inflated state to grade the severity of emphysema with naked eye.

Grossly, the lungs are voluminous, pale with little blood. The edges of the lungs are rounded. Mild cases show dilatation of the air spaces visible with hand lens. Advanced cases show subpleural bullae and blebs bulging outwards from the surface of the lungs with rib marking between them. The bullae are air-filled, cyst-like structures, larger than 1 cm in diameter. The rupture of bullae directly into the subpleural interstitial tissue is the common cause of spontaneous pneumothorax.

Microscopy reveals destruction of alveolar walls, leading to enlarged air spaces. In addition to alveolar loss, the number of alveolar capillaries are diminished. Terminal and respiratory bronchioles may be deformed because of the loss of septa. With loss of elastic tissue in the surrounding alveolar septa, radial traction on the small airways is reduced. As a result, they tend to collapse during expiration, this is an important cause of chronic airflow obstruction in severe emphysema. Bronchiolar inflammation and submucosal fibrosis are consistently present in advanced disease.

Clinical features
- There is a long history of slowly increasing severe exertion dyspnoea.
- Patient is quite distressed with obvious use of accessory muscles of respiration.
- Chest is barrel-shaped and hyper-resonant.
- Cough occurs after dyspnoea starts and is associated with scanty mucoid sputum.
- Recurrent respiratory infections.
- Patients are called 'pink puffers' as they remain well-oxygenated but have tachypnoea.
- Weight loss.
- Features of right heart failure and hypercapnoeic respiratory failure are the usual terminal events.
- Chest X-ray shows small heart with hyperinflated lungs.

Centriacinar (Centrilobular) Emphysema (Fig. 3.29a)

In this type of emphysema, the central or proximal parts of the acini are affected while the distal parts are spared. Grossly, lesions are more common and more severe in the upper lobes of the lungs. Large amount of black pigment is often present in the walls of emphysematous spaces. In more severe cases, distal parts of acini are also involved and the appearance may closely resemble panacinar emphysema. This type of emphysema is common in chronic smokers.

Microscopically, there is distension and destruction of the respiratory bronchiole in the centre of the lobules, surrounded peripherally by normal uninvolved alveoli. The terminal bronchioles supplying the acini show chronic inflammation and are narrowed.

Panacinar (Panlobular) Emphysema (Pan meaning entire acinus) (Fig. 3.29b)

This type of emphysema is seen in α_1-AT deficiency.

Grossly, this condition involves the lower zone of lungs more frequently and more severely than the upper zone. The involvement may be confined to a few lobules or may be more widespread affecting a lobe or part of lobe of the lung. The lungs are enlarged and overinflated.

Microscopically, all the alveoli within a lobule are affected to the same degree. All portions of acini are distended. The respiratory bronchioles, alveolar ducts and alveoli are all dilated and their walls stretched and thin. Ruptured alveolar walls and spurs of broken septa are seen between the adjacent alveoli. The capillaries are stretched and thinned. Special stains show loss of elastic tissue. Inflammatory changes are usually absent.

Paraseptal (Distal Acinar) Emphysema

This type involves the distal part of acinus while the proximal part is normal. It is localised along the pleura and along the perilobular septa. Adjacent to areas of fibrosis, scarring or atelectasis are severe in the upper half of the lungs. Grossly, the subpleural portion of the lung shows air-filled cysts, 0.5 to 2 cm in diameter. Rupture of these bullae can cause pneumothorax in young adults.

Irregular (Paracicatrical) Emphysema

This type is seen surrounding scars from any cause. The involvement is irregular as regards to the portion of the acinus involved as well as within the lung as a whole.

Mixed (Unclassified) Emphysema

Lung may show more than one type of emphysema. There is clear-cut distinction between one type of emphysema and the other.

ASTHMA

Asthma is a chronic inflammatory disorder of airways which causes repeated episode of wheezing, breathlessness, chest tightness and cough. There is hyper-responsiveness to various stimuli leading to bronchospasm and mucus hypersecretion. This may be with:
1. Intermittent and reversible airway obstruction.
2. Chronic bronchiolar inflammation with eosinophils.

3. Bronchial smooth muscle cell hypertrophy and hyperactivity.

Asthma may be classically divided into:
1. Extrinsic (atopic)
2. Intrinsic (non-atopic).

Extrinsic/atopy/allergic asthma: About 70% of the cases, the a etiological agent is extrinsic or atopic due to IgE and T helper 2 mediated immune response. The bronchospasm is induced by inhaled antigens, can occur at any age, but usually begins in childhood with family history of allergic diseases.

Risk factors and triggers: Environmental antigens such as dust, pollen, animal dander, foods or any antigen may be implicated.

Intrinsic/non-atopic asthma: In other 30% of patients it is intrinsic (non-atopic) triggered by non-immune causes. No family history is available in these patients. These can be:
- Infectious asthma
- Exercise induced asthma
- Occupational asthma
- Drug induced asthma
- Air pollution
- Emotional factors
- Obesity
- Diet
- Allergens.

Pathogenesis

The aetiological factors cause type I IgE mediated hypersensitivity (atopy), acute on chronic airway inflammation and bronchial hyper-responsiveness to stimuli to T-helper 2 to release cytokines (IL-4, IL-5, IL-13). IL-4 stimulates IgE production. IL-5 activates eosinophils and IL-13 responsible for mucus production. Epithelial cells are activated to produce chemokines which promote T-helper 2 cells and eosinophils accumulate.

In sensitized person, type I IgE mediated hypersensitivity occurs with acute and late phase response. IgE coated mast cells when exposed to same antigen, there occurs cross-linking of IgE and release of cytokines and cause accumulation of neutrophils, mononuclear cells, mast cells and eosinophils. These release chemical mediators (Table 3.19). Eosinophils are important in late phase reaction. Major basic protein and eosinophil cationic protein of eosinophils cause injury to airway epithelial cells.

The mechanism of bronchial inflammation and hyper-responsiveness is less clear for intrinsic (non-atopic) asthma. These patients have normal serum concentrations of IgE and some negative for skin tests. The disease is usually is adult onset.

Pathology

The changes are seen in prolonged and severe attack (status asthamaticus).

Gross: Lungs are over distended due to over-inflation. Small areas of atelectasis, occlusion of the bronchi and bronchioles by viscid mucus plugs are present.

Microscopy: Lumen has mucus plugs having normal or degenerated respiratory epithelium forming twisted strips called Curschmann's spirals and Charcot-Leyden crystals (crystals

Table 3.19: Action of chemical mediators in asthma

Leukotrienes (LC4, D4, E4)	Vasoconstriction, increased VP, increased mucus secretion
Thromboxane A2	Platelet activation and vasoconstriction
Acetylcholine from motor nerves	Smooth muscle contraction
Histamine	Bronchospasm, increased VP
Bradykinin	Increased vascular permeability, vasodilatation and smooth muscle contraction
Prostaglandin D2	Bronchoconstriction, vasodailation
Platelet activating Factor (PAF)	Aggregation of platelets and release of histamine

of eosinophilic proteins). The bronchial wall shows thickened basement membrane of the bronchial epithelium, submucosal oedema and inflammatory infiltrate consisting of mast cells, eosinophils and other inflammatory cells. There is hypertrophy of submucosal glands as well as of the bronchial smooth muscle.

Clinical features: Characteristic symptoms of asthma are:
1. Wheezing
2. Dyspnoea
3. Coughing

Symptoms are worse at night and patients awake in the morning hours. Some patients may have increased sputum production which is tenacious and difficult to expectorate.

BRONCHIECTASIS (Figs 3.32a and b)

It is defined as permanent dilatation of the bronchi and bronchioles, developing secondary to inflammation with weakening of the bronchial walls. The most characteristic manifestation of bronchiectasis is persistent cough with expectoration of copious amounts of foul smelling and purulent sputum.

Etiopathogenesis

The origin of inflammatory destructive process of bronchial walls is nearly always a result of two basic mechanisms:
1. Obstructive cause
2. Non-obstructive cause: Infection or defects in the defence mechanism.

Obstructive causes: The obstructive causes generally localised to a segment of the lung distal to the site of mechanical obstruction.

The causes of endobronchial obstruction include:
- Foreign bodies.
- Endobronchial tumours.
- Compression by enlarged hilar lymph nodes and postinflammatory scarring (e.g. in healed tuberculosis) all of which favour the development of postobstructive bronchiectasis.
- Mucus plugs as in asthma.

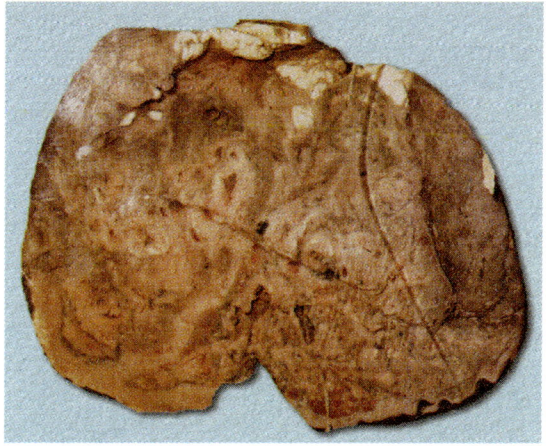

Fig. 3.32a: Gross picture of bronchiectasis, note dilated and prominent bronchioles

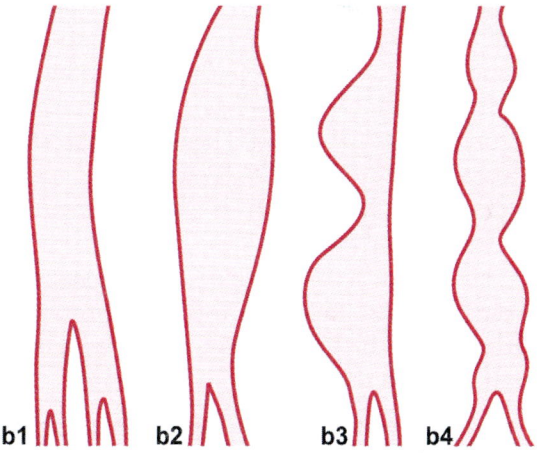

Fig. 3.32b: Schematic diagram of cylindrical (b1), fusiform (b2), secular (b3) vericose types and (b4) of air passages in bronchiectasis

Acquired Disorders Causing Obstruction

- Neurotopic diseases that impair consciousness, swallowing, cough
- Incompetence of the lower oesophageal sphincter
- Nasogastric intubation
- Chronic bronchitis.

Non-obstructive causes

As a secondary complication: Necrotising pneumonias such as in staphylococcal suppurative pneumonia and tuberculosis may develop bronchiectasis as a complication.

Hereditary and congenital factors: Several hereditary and congenital factors may result in diffuse bronchiectasis. These include:
1. *Congenital bronchiectasis:* Caused by developmental defects of the bronchial system.
2. *Cystic fibrosis:* It is a generalised defect of exocrine gland secretions, resulting in obstruction, infection and bronchiectasis.
3. *Hereditary immune deficiency diseases:* They are often associated with high incidence of bronchiectasis.
4. *Immotile cilia syndrome:* It includes Kartagener's syndrome (bronchiectasis, situs inversus and sinusitis) which is characterised by ultrastructural changes in the microtubules causing immotility of cilia of the respiratory tract epithelium, sperms and other cells. Males in this syndrome are often infertile.
5. *Atopic bronchial asthma:* These patients often have positive family history of allergic diseases and may rarely develop diffuse bronchiectasis.

The causes for non-obstructive localised bronchiectasis include childhood bronchopulmonary infections such as measles, pertussis and other bacterial infections.

Pathologic changes: The disease characteristically affects distal bronchi and bronchioles beyond the segmental bronchi.

Grossly, the lungs may be involved diffusely or segmentally. Bilateral involvement of lower lobes occurs most frequently. More vertical air passages of left lower lobe are more often involved than the right. The pleura is usually fibrotic and thickened with adhesions to the chest wall. The dilated airways, depending upon their gross or bronchographic appearance, have been subclassified into the following different types:
- *Cylindrical (Fig. 3.32b1):* The most common type characterised by uniform and moderate tube-like bronchial dilatation.
- *Fusiform (Fig. 3.32b2):* Having spindle-shaped bronchial dilatation.
- *Saccular (Fig. 3.32b3):* Having rounded sac-like bronchial distension, affects the proximal 3rd to 4th branches of the bronchi. The bronchi are severely dilated and end blindly in dilated sacs with collapse and fibrosis of the distal lung parenchyma.
- *Varicose (Fig. 3.32b4):* Having irregular bronchial enlargements.

Cut surface of the affected lobes, generally the lower zones, shows characteristic honey-combed appearance. The bronchi are extensively dilated nearly to the pleura, their walls are thickened and the lumina are filled with mucus or mucopus. The intervening lung parenchyma is reduced and fibrotic.

Microscopically, the bronchial epithelium may be normal, ulcerated or may show squamous metaplasia.

The bronchial wall shows infiltration by acute and chronic inflammatory cells and destruction of normal muscle and elastic tissue with replacement by fibrosis. The intervening lung parenchyma shows fibrosis, while the surrounding lung tissue shows changes of interstitial pneumonia.

Clinical features
- Chronic cough with foul-smelling sputum
- Haemoptysis
- Recurrent pneumonia
- Sinusitis in diffuse bronchiectasis
- Clubbing of fingers
- Amyloidosis
- Cor pulmonale.

RESTRICTIVE LUNG DISEASES

These are also called diffuse interstitial or infiltrative lung diseases. These are heterogeneous group of disorders predominantly involving pulmonary interstitium and also have intra-alveolar components. It is of diffuse and chronic nature. In these diseases the lungs are restricted from fully expanding. The lungs are not able to expand and fill with air. There is decreased total lung capacity (Fig. 3.33).

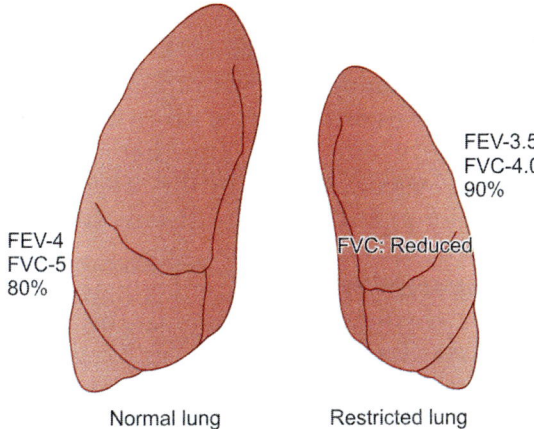

Fig. 3.33: Lung size and functions in restrictive lung diseases (comparision to normal)

In restrictive lung diseases FEV1 is reduced and FVC is much more reduced and FEV1/FVC more than 0.8. These are classified as given in Table 3.20:

Table 3.20: Restrictive lung diseases
Fibrosing
Interstitial pneumonia
Nonspecific interstitial pneumonia
Cryptogenic organising pneumonia
Collagen vascular disease associated
Pneumoconiosis
Therapy related
Granulomatous
Sarcoidosis and other causes
Hypersensitivity pneumonitis
Pulmonary eosinophilia
Smoking related
Desquamative interstitial pneumonia
Respiratory bronchiolitis
Neuromuscular diseases, e.g. amyotrophic lateral sclerosis

Pathogenesis

The initial common manifestation is alveolitis. The septae and alveoli show inflammatory cells.

Injury is usually mild, self-limited and resolution occurs. With the persistence of injurious agent, there is parenchymal injury, and progressive fibrosis. The activated macrophages secrete IL-8 and LB4 which recruit and activate neutrophils. The oxidants and proteases released by these inflammatory cells injure alveolar epithelium and degrade connective tissue. Fibrogenic growth factors like FGR, TFG beta and PDGF attract fibroblasts with proliferation of connective tissue.

Lung Carcinoma

It is the most common primary tumour of the lung. Most common in men and people from industrialised nations are affected.

Etiology

- Smoking
- Atmospheric pollution
- Occupational causes include workers exposed to asbestos, nickel, beryllium, arsenic and metallic iron
- Dietary factors : Vitamin A deficiency
- Genetic factors
- Chronic scarring.

Smoking: More than 90% of the lung cancer is associated with smoking. Two packs of cigarettes/day increases the risk by 6–7 fold while cessation of smoking reduces the risk. Passive smoking and radon gas produced from radioactive decay of uranium found in soil and rocks increases the risk twofold. Polycyclic hydrocarbons and 3, 4 benzo-pyrines present in the tobacco smoke has the highest risk of malignancy. Squamous cell carcinoma is common with smoking while adenocarcinoma can be encountered in non-smokers.

Exposure to industrial pollutants: This has been associated with lung cancer.

Genetic factors: Mutations of K-ras, enzyme aryl hydrocarbon hydroxylase (metabolises benzopyrines and hydrocarbons), P53 and RB genes, Myc gene over-expression (small cell carcinoma), 3p deletions, Bcl-2 over-expression (inhibits apoptosis) can be associated in lung cancer. Classification of lung tumours is given in Table 3.21.

Table 3.21: Classification of lung tumours[8]

Epithelial tumours
Benign—Papilloma, adenoma
Pre-invasive: Adenocarcinoma *in situ*, squamous carcinoma *in situ*
Adenocarcinoma: Lepidic, acinar, papillary, micropapillary, solid, mucinous, non-mucinous
Squamous cell carcinoma: Keratinising, non-keratinising, basaloid
Adenosquamous carcinoma
Neuroendocrine: Small cell carcinoma, combined small cell carcinoma, large cell carcinoma, combined large cell neuroendocrine carcinoma, carcinoid
Sarcomatoid carcinoma
Lymphoepithelioma like carcinoma
NUT carcinoma
Salivary gland type carcinoma
Mesenchymal: Hamartoma, PEComa, pleuropulmonary blastoma, inflammatory myofibroblastic tumour
Lymphohistiocytic tumours: Lymphomas and other related tumours
Tumours of ectopic origin: Germ cell tumour, intrapulmonary thymoma, melanoma and others
Pleural tumours: Benign mesothelioma, malignant mesothelioma
Metastatic tumours

Note: Modified from 2015 WHO classification of lung, pleura, thymus and heart

Pathologic Changes

Gross (Fig. 3.34a)
Squamous cell carcinoma: Most commonly, the lung cancer arises in the main bronchus or one of its segmental branches in the hilar parts of the lung, more often on the right side. The tumour begins as a small roughened area on the bronchial mucosa at the bifurcation. As the tumour enlarges, it thickens, the bronchial mucosa has nodular or ulcerated surface. As the nodules coalesce, the carcinoma grows in to a friable mass, 1 to 5 cm in diameter, narrowing and occluding the lumen.

The cut surface of the tumour is yellowish-white with foci of necrosis and haemorrhage which may produce cavitary lesions. It is common to find secondary changes in bronchogenic carcinoma of lung such as bronchopneumonia, abscess formation and bronchiectasis as a result of obstruction and intercurrent infections. The tumour soon spreads within the lungs by direct extension or by lymphatics, and to distant sites by lymphatic or haematogenous routes.

Adenocarcinoma: A small proportion of lung cancers chiefly adenocarcinomas, originate from a small peripheral bronchioles (Fig. 3.34b). The tumour may be a single nodule or multiple nodules in the periphery of the lung

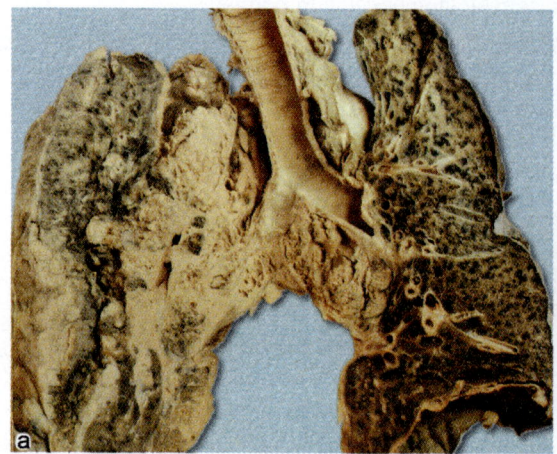

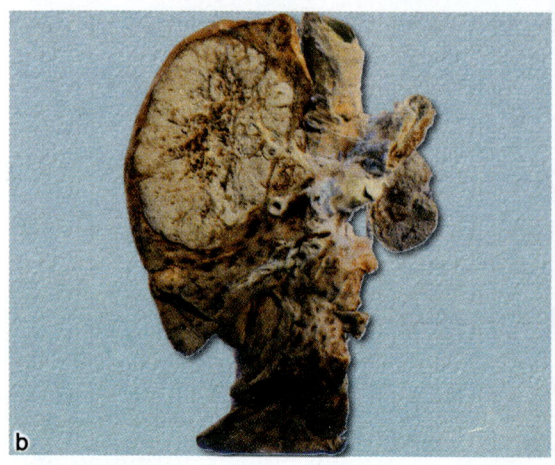

Figs 3.34a and b: Gross picture of carcinoma lung: (a) Squamous cell carcinoma, (b) adenocarcinoma

producing pneumonia-like consolidation of a large part of the lung. The cut surface of the tumour is grayish and mucoid.

Microscopy

Squamous cell carcinoma: It is the most common type of lung carcinoma. They arise in a large bronchus and are prone to massive necrosis and cavitation. It is diagnosed microscopically by intercellular bridges, keratinisation and can be well-differentiated, moderately differentiated or poorly differentiated. Frequently, the edge of the growth and the adjoining uninvolved bronchi show squamous metaplasia, epithelial dysplasia and carcinoma *in situ* changes.

Adenocarcinoma: The predominant patterns include:

1. *Acinar type:* This type has predominance of closely packed glandular or tubular structures separated by fibrous stroma.
2. *Lepidic pattern:* There is recognisable alveolar septa and alveolar architecture and malignant cells line the inner surface..
3. *Papillary adenocarcinoma:* It has pronounced papillary configuration with fibrovascular core lined by columnar to cuboidal cells.
4. *Micropapillary adenocarcinoma:* Papillae lack fibrovascular core.
5. *Solid variant:* Poorly differentiated adenocarcinoma lacking acini, tubules or papillae but having mucus-containing vacuoles in many tumour cells.

Adenosquamous Carcinoma

There is clear evidence of both keratinisation and glandular differentiation.

Small Cell Carcinoma

The cells of small cell carcinoma of lung are derived from neuroendocrine cells and express variety of neuroendocrine markers. It is also accompanied by many paraneoplastic syndromes. The lesion appears as pale gray centrally located mass with early involvement of hilar and mediastinal nodes. These are most aggressive tumours with poor prognosis. These have strong association with smoking. Mutation of P53 and RB gene are common. The cells may express Chromogranin A, synaptophysin, CD56, TTF1, CD117, etc. Ki67 is a proliferative marker. Non-small cell lung tumours (squamous cell carcinoma and adenocarcinoma) have better prognosis than this tumour.

Grossly, the tumour is tan, homogenous, soft, and rubbery and has necrosis. Microscopy shows round, oval or fusiform-shaped, scant cytoplasm, nuclei two to three times of small lymphocyte, nuclear molding present, inconspicuous nucleoli, nuclear chromatin appear salt and pepper pattern. Cells are fragile and show fragmentation and crush artifacts. Mitoses are high. There is basophilic staining of the vascular wall due to deposition of nuclear debri from necrotic tumour cells.

PNEUMOCONIOSES

It is the term used for lung diseases caused by inhalation of dust, mostly at work, also called 'dust diseases' or 'occupational diseases'.

The type of lung disease varies according to the nature of dust inhaled. Some of the dusts are inert and cause no reaction and no damage, while others cause immunologic damage and predispose to tuberculosis or neoplasia (Table 3.22).

The factors which determine the extent of damage caused by inhaled dust are:
- Size and shape of the particles
- Their solubility and physicochemical composition
- The amount of dust retained in the lungs
- The additional effects of other irritants such as tobacco smoke
- Host factors such as efficiency of clearance mechanism and immune status of the host.

In general, most of the inhaled dust particles larger than 5 μ reach the terminal airways where they are ingested by alveolar macrophages. Most of these too are eliminated

Table 3.22: A comprehensive list of various types of occupational lung diseases caused by inorganic (mineral) dusts and organic dusts

Agent	Diseases
Inorganic (mineral) dusts	
Coal dust	Simple coal workers' pneumoconiosis, progressive massive fibrosis, Caplan's syndrome
Silica	Silicosis, Caplan's syndrome
Asbestos	Asbestosis, pleural diseases, tumours
Beryllium	Acute berylliosis, chronic berylliosis
Iron oxide	Pulmonary siderosis
Organic (biologic) dust	
Mouldy hay	Farmer's lungs
Bagasse	Bagassosis
Cotton, flax, hemp dust	Byssinosis
Bird droppings	Bird breeder's lung
Mushroom compost dust	Mushroom workers' lung
Mouldy barley, malt dust	Malt workers' lung
Mouldy maple bark	Maple bark disease
Silage fermentation	Silo filler's disease

by expectoration but the particles 1–5 μ accumulate in alveolar tissue. Of particular interest are the particles smaller than 1 μ which are deposited in the alveoli most efficiently.

Most of the dust-laden macrophages accumulated in the alveoli die, leaving the dust, around which fibrous tissue is formed. Some macrophages enter the lymphatics and reach regional lymph nodes. The tissue response to inhaled dust may be one of the following 3 types:
1. *Fibrous nodules,* e.g. coal workers' pneumoconiosis and silicosis.
2. *Interstitial fibrosis,* e.g. asbestosis.
3. *Hypersensitivity,* e.g. berylliosis.

Coal Workers' Pneumoconiosis

This is the commonest form of pneumoconiosis and is defined as the lung disease resulting from inhalation of coal dust particles especially in coal miners engaged in handling soft bituminous coal for a number of years often 20 to 30 years.

It exists in 2 forms
1. Simple coal workers' pneumoconiosis—a milder form.
2. Progressive massive fibrosis—an advanced form.

Anthracosis on the other hand is not a lung disease in true sense. There is accumulation of carbon dust in the lungs of most urban dwellers due to atmospheric pollution and cigarette smoke.

Anthracotic pigment is deposited in the macrophages, in the alveoli and around the respiratory bronchioles and into the draining lymph nodes but does not produce any respiratory difficulty or radiologic changes.

Pathogenesis

It appears that anthracosis, simple coal-workers pneumoconiosis and progressive massive fibrosis are different stages in the evolution of fully-developed coal workers' pneumoconiosis. However, progressive massive fibrosis develops in a small proportion of cases of simple coal workers' pneumoconiosis. A number of predisposing factors have been implicated in this transformation. These are:
- Older age of the miners
- Coal dust burden
- Duration of exposure (20–30 years)

- Concomitant tuberculosis
- Additional role of silica dust.

Activation of alveolar macrophages plays the most significant role in the pathogenesis of progressive massive fibrosis by release of various mediators:
- Free radicals
- Chemotactic factors like leukotrienes, TNF, IL-8 and IL-6
- Fibrogenic cytokines such as IL-1, TNF and platelet derived growth factors.

Pathologic changes

The pathologic changes in lung in coal workers' pneumoconiosis is graded by radiologic appearance according to the size and extent of opacities.

Simple Coal Workers' Pneumoconiosis

Gross: The lung parenchyma shows small, black focal lesions, measuring less than 5 mm in diameter and evenly distributed throughout the lung but have a tendency to be more numerous in the upper lobes. These are termed coal macules and if palpable, are called nodules. The air spaces around coal macules are dilated with destruction of alveolar walls. Similar blackish pigmented lesions are found on the pleural surface and in the regional lymph nodes.

Microscopy
1. Coal macules are composed of aggregates of dust-laden macrophages. These are present in the alveoli and bronchiolar walls.
2. There is some increase in the network of reticulin and collagen in the coal macules.
3. Respiratory bronchioles and alveoli surrounding the macules are distended without significant destruction of the alveolar walls.

Progressive Massive Fibrosis

Gross: Besides the coal macules and nodules of simple pneumoconiosis, there are larger, hard, black scattered areas measuring more than 2 cm in diameter and sometimes massive. They are usually bilateral and located more often in the upper parts of the lungs posteriorly. Sometimes, these masses breakdown centrally due to ischaemic necrosis or due to tuberculosis forming cavities filled with black semifluid resembling India ink. The pleura and the regional lymph nodes are also blackened and fibrotic.

Microscopy
- The fibrous lesions are composed almost entirely of dense collagen and carbon pigment.
- The wall of respiratory bronchioles and pulmonary vessels included in the massive scars are thickened and their lumina obliterated.
- There is scanty inflammatory infiltrate of lymphocytes and plasma cells around the areas of massive scars.
- The alveoli surrounding the scars are markedly dilated.

Rheumatoid Pneumoconiosis (Caplan's syndrome)

The development or rheumatoid arthritis in a few cases of coal workers' pneumoconiosis, silicosis or asbestosis is termed rheumatoid pneumoconiosis or Caplan's syndrome.

Gross: The lungs have rounded, firm nodules with central necrosis, cavitation or calcification.

Microscopy: The lung lesions are modified rheumatoid nodules with central zone of dust-laden fibrinoid necrosis enclosed by palisading of fibroblasts and mononuclear cells.

Silicosis

Silicosis is caused by the prolonged inhalation of silicon dioxide commonly called silica.

Silica constitutes about one-fourth of the earth's crust. Therefore, a number of people engaged working with siliceous rocks or sand and products manufactured from them are at increased risk. These include miners (e.g. granite, sandstone, slate, coal, gold, tin and copper), quarry workers involved in the manufacture of abrasives containing silica.

Pathogenesis

Silicosis appears after prolonged exposure to silica dust, often after a few decades. Besides it depends upon a number of other factors such as total dose, duration of exposure, the type of silica inhaled and individual host factors.

Mechanism

1. Silica particles of 0.5 to 5 μ size on reaching the alveoli are taken by the macrophages which undergo necrosis. New macrophages engulf the debris and thus a repetitive cycle of phagocytosis is and necrosis is set in.
2. Some silica-laden macrophages are carried to the respiratory bronchioles, alveoli and in the interstitial tissue. Some of the silica dust is transported to the subpleural and interlobar lymphatics and into the regional lymph nodes. The cellular aggregates containing silica are associated with lymphocytes, plasma cells, mast cells and fibroblasts.
3. Silica dust is fibrogenic. Crystalline form, particularly quartz is more fibrogenic than non-crystalline form of silica.
4. Silica is cytotoxic and kills the macrophages which engulf it. The released silica dust activates viable macrophages leading to secretion of macrophage-derived growth factors such as interleukin-1 that favours fibroblast proliferation and collagen synthesis.
5. Simultaneously, there is activation of T and B lymphocytes. This results in increased serum levels of immunoglobulins (IgG and IgM), antinuclear antibodies, rheumatoid factor and circulating immune complexes as well as proliferation of T cells.

Pathologic changes

Gross: The chronic silicotic lung is studded with well-circumscribed, hard, fibrotic nodules of 1–5 mm in diameter.

They are scattered throughout the lung parenchyma but are initially more often located in the upper zones of the lungs.

These nodular lesions frequently have simultaneous deposition of coal dust and may develop calcification.

The pleura is grossly thickened and adherent to the chest wall. There may be similar fibrotic nodules on the pleura and within the regional lymph nodes.

The nodular lesions are detectable as egg-shell shadows in chest X-ray. The lesions may undergo ischaemic necrosis and develop cavitation, or may be complicated by tuberculosis and rheumatoid pneumoconiosis.

Microscopy: The silicotic nodules are located in the region of respiratory bronchioles, adjacent alveoli, pulmonary arteries, in the pleura and the regional lymph nodes.

The silicotic nodules consist of central hyalinised material with scanty cellularity and some amount of dust. The hyalinised centre is surrounded by concentric laminations of collagen which is further enclosed by more cellular connective tissue, dust-filled macrophages and a few lymphocytes and plasma cells. Some of these nodules may have calcium deposits.

The collagenous nodules have cleft-like spaces between the lamellae of collagen which when examined by polarised microscopy may demonstrate numerous birefringent particles of silica.

The severe and progressive form of the disease may result in coalescence of adjacent nodules and cause complicated silicosis similar to progressive massive fibrosis of coal workers' pneumoconiosis.

The intervening lung parenchyma may show hyperinflation or emphysema.

Cavitation when present may be due to ischaemic necrosis in the nodules or may reveal changes of tuberculosis or rheumatoid pneumoconiosis (Caplan's syndrome).

Asbestosis

Asbestos is a Greek word meaning *'unquenchable'*. In general, if coal is with lot of dust and little fibrosis, asbestos is with little dust and lot of fibrosis.

Prolonged exposure for a number of years to asbestos dust produces three types of severe diseases:
1. Asbestosis of lungs
2. Pleural disease
3. Tumours.

In nature, asbestos exists as long thin fibrils which are fire-resistant and can be spun into yarns and fabrics suitable for thermal and electrical insulation and has many applications in industries.

Particularly at risk are workers engaged in mining, fabrication and manufacture of a number of products from asbestos such as asbestos pipes, tiles, roofs, textiles, insulating boards, sewer and water conduit systems, brake lining, clutch castings, etc.

There are two major forms of asbestos:
1. Serpentine consisting of curly and flexible fibres, it includes the most common chemical form chrysotile (white asbestos) comprising more than 90% of commercially used asbestos.
2. Amphibole consists of straight, stiff and rigid fibres, it includes the less common chemical forms crocidolite, amosite, tremolite, anthophyllite and actinolyte. However, the group of amphibole, though less common, is more important since it is associated with induction of malignant pleural tumours, particularly in association with crocidolite.

Pathogenesis
Over exposure to asbestos for more than a decade may produce asbestosis of the lung, pleural lesions and certain tumours.

Mechanism
The inhaled asbestos fibres are phagocytosed by alveolar macrophages from where they reach the interstitium. Some of the engulfed dust is transported via lymphatics to the pleura and regional lymph nodes.

The asbestos-laden macrophages release chemo-attractants for neutrophils and for more macrophages, thus inciting cellular reaction around them.

Asbestos fibres are coated with glycoprotein and endogenous haemosiderin to produce characteristic beaded or dumb-bell-shaped asbestos bodies.

All types of asbestos are fibrogenic and result in interstitial fibrosis. Fibroblastic proliferation may occur via macrophage-derived growth factor such as interleukin-1. Alternatively, fibrosis may occur as a reparative response to tissue injury by lysosomal enzymes released from macrophages and neutrophils or by toxic free radicals.

A few immunological abnormalities such as antinuclear antibodies and rheumatoid factor have been found in cases of asbestosis.

Asbestos fibres are carcinogenic, the most carcinogenic being crocidolite. There is high incidence of bronchogenic carcinoma in asbestosis which is explained on the basis of the role of asbestos fibres as tumour promoters or by causing cell death of the airways so that it is exposed to the carcinogenic effects of cigarette smoke. The development of pleural mesothelioma in these cases is probably by carrying of asbestos fibres via lymphatics to the pleura.

Pathologic changes
Gross: The affected lungs are small and firm with cartilage-like thickening of the pleura. The sectioned surface shows variable degree of pulmonary fibrosis, especially in the subpleural areas of lungs. The advanced cases may show cystic changes.

Microscopy: There is non-specific interstitial fibrosis. There is presence of characteristic asbestos bodies in the involved areas. These are asbestos fibres coated with glycoprotein and haemosiderin and appear beaded or dumb-bell-shaped and these are positive for Prussian blue stain.

There may be changes of emphysema in the pulmonary parenchyma between the areas of interstitial fibrosis.

Pleural Diseases

Pleural effusion: It develops in about 5% of asbestos workers.

Visceral pleural fibrosis: Quite often, asbestosis is associated with dense fibrous thickening of the visceral pleura encasing the lung.

Pleural plaques: Fibrocalcific pleural plaques are the most common lesions associated asbestosis exposure.

Gross: The lesions appear as circumscribed, flat, small (up to 1 cm in diameter), firm or hard, bilateral nodules. They are seen often on the posterolateral part of parietal pleura and on the pleural surface of the diaphragm.

Microscopy: They consist of hyalinised collagenous tissue which may be calcified and are visible on chest X-ray.

Tumours

Asbestos exposure predisposes to a number of cancers, most importantly bronchogenic carcinoma and malignant mesothelioma. A few others are: carcinomas of oesophagus, stomach, colon, kidneys and larynx and various lymphoid malignancies.

Bronchogenic carcinoma: It is the most common malignancy in asbestos workers. Its incidence is 5 times higher in non-smoker asbestos workers than the non-smoker general population and 10 times higher in asbestos workers who smoke than the other smokers.

Malignant mesothelioma: It is an uncommon tumour but association with asbestos exposure is present in 30–80% of cases with mesothelioma.

Exercise

45

Salivary Gland Tumours

The salivary glands give rise to a diversity of tumours. About 80% of tumours occur within the parotid gland. Rest occur in other major salivary glands and minor salivary glands. Males and females are affected about equally. They occur usually in the sixth or seventh decade of life.

They can be classified as given in Table 3.23.

Pleomorphic Adenoma (Mixed tumour of salivary glands)

Because of their histologic diversity, these neoplasms have also been called mixed tumours.

Table 3.23: Classification of salivary gland neoplasms[9]

Benign epithelial tumours	Malignant epithelial tumours	Soft tissue tumours
Pleomorphic adenoma	Acinic cell carcinoma	Haemangioma
Myoepithelioma	Secretory carcinoma	Haematolymphoid tumours
Basal cell adenoma	Mucoepidermoid carcinoma	Hodgkin's lymphoma
Warthin tumour	Adenoid cystic carcinoma	Diffuse large B-cell lymphoma
Oncocytoma	Polymorphous low-grade adenocarcinoma	Extranodal marginal zone
Canalicular adenoma	Epithelial-myoepithelial carcinoma	B-cell lymphoma
Sebaceous adenoma	Clear cell carcinoma, not otherwise specified	
Lymphadenoma	Hyalinising clear cell carcinoma	
Sebaceous	Basal cell adenocarcinoma	
Non-sebaceous	Sebaceous carcinoma	
Ductal papillomas	Cribriform carcinoma	
Inverted ductal papilloma	Intraductal carcinoma	
Intraductal papilloma	Sebaceous lymphadenocarcinoma	
Sialadenoma papilliferum	Cystadenocarcinoma	
Cystadenoma	Low-grade cribriform cystadenocarcinoma	
Sclerosing polycystic adenosis	Mucinous adenocarcinoma	
Intercalated duct hyperplasia	Oncocytic carcinoma	
	Salivary duct carcinoma	
	Adenocarcinoma, not otherwise specified	
	Myoepithelial carcinoma	
	Carcinoma ex pleomorphic adenoma	
	Carcinosarcoma	
	Metastasising pleomorphic adenoma	
	Squamous cell carcinoma	
	Small cell carcinoma	
	Large cell carcinoma	
	Lymphoepithelial carcinoma	
	Sialoblastoma	

It accounts for 90% of the benign tumours of the salivary gland.

This tumour occurs at any age and has female predilection. The parotid gland is frequently affected. The other major and minor salivary glands also can be affected. It is slow growing, causes painless swelling at the angle of jaw and readily palpable as discrete mass. Facial nerve needs to be taken care off while resecting the tumour. Recurrence is known and 2% of these tumours may undergo malignancy. A carcinoma arising in a pleomorphic adenoma is referred to variously as carcinoma ex-pleomorphic adenoma or as malignant mixed tumour.

Gross: The tumour is capsulated, lobulated and usually measures about 5 to 6 cm in diameter. Cut section is grey white with variegated areas (Figs 3.35a and b).

Microscopy: The epithelial cells will be in the form of ducts, irregular tubules or acini. Some of these cells show squamous metaplasia. The myoepithelial cells would be arranged in sheets and show myxoid and chondroid areas. Rarely bone formation may be present (Fig. 3.35c).

Warthin's Tumour (Papillary cystadenoma lymphomatosum)

This is a benign neoplasm and second most common salivary gland neoplasm. It arises almost exclusively in the parotid gland (the only tumour virtually restricted to the parotid) and occurs more commonly in males than in females, usually in the fifth to seventh decades of life. It is more common in smokers and bilateral.

Gross: Warthin tumours are round to oval, encapsulated masses, 2 to 5 cm in diameter, usually arising in the superficial parotid gland, where they are readily palpable. Cut section reveals a pale grey surface punctuated by narrow cystic or cleft-like spaces filled with a mucinous or serous secretion.

Microscopy: The cystic spaces are lined by a double layer of neoplastic epithelial cells

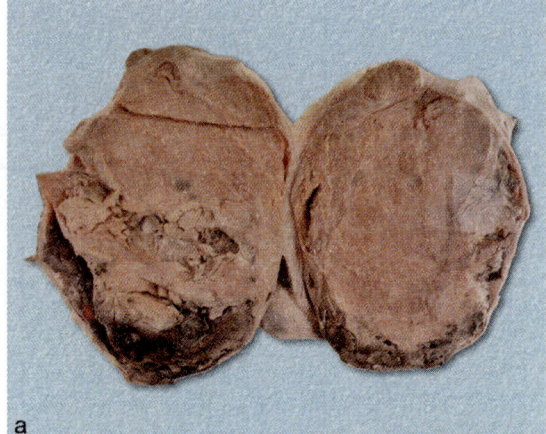
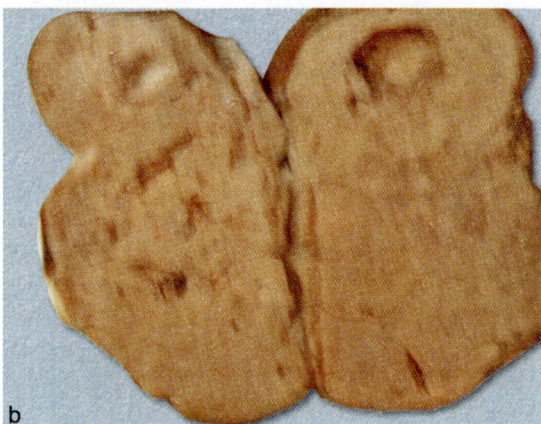

Figs 3.35a and b: Gross picture of pleomorphic adenoma

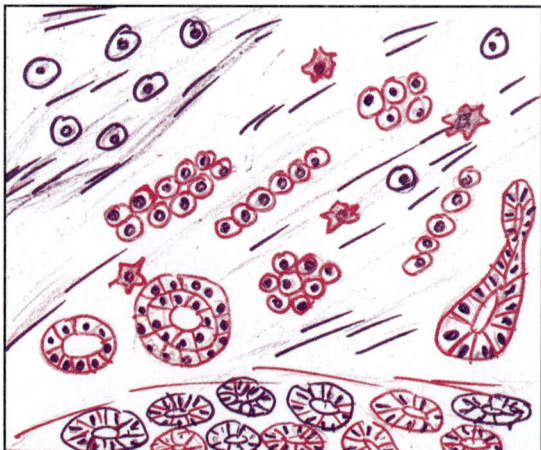

Fig. 3.35c: Schematic diagram of microscopy of pleomorphic adenoma

resting on a dense lymphoid stroma sometimes bearing germinal centres. The double layer of lining cells is distinctive; it consists of columnar cells having an abundant, finely granular, eosinophilic cytoplasm, that imparts an oncocytic appearance, which rests on a layer of cuboidal to polygonal cells. These cells form papillary structures projecting into cystic lumina.

Mucoepidermoid Carcinoma

These are composed of variable mixtures of neoplastic squamous cells, mucus secreting cells, and intermediate cells. They represent about 15% of all salivary gland tumours, and they occur mainly (60 to 70%) in the parotid gland.

Gross: Mucoepidermoid carcinomas can grow as large as 8 cm in diameter and although they are apparently circumscribed, they lack well-defined capsule and are often infiltrative at the margins. Pale and grey-white on cut section, they frequently contain small, mucin-containing cysts.

Microscopy: The basic histologic pattern is that of cords, sheets, or cystic configurations of squamous, mucous, or intermediate cells. Mucoepidermoid carcinomas are subclassified into low, intermediate, or high grade. The low grade tumours are usually well-circumscribed. The mucinous cells predominate and these have clear cytoplasm and eccentrically placed nuclei. These are admixed with epidermoid cells which are squamous-like but lack keratinisation and intercellular bridges. The third type of cells seen are intermediate cells which are smaller than epidermoid cells.

High grade tumours are solid and have infiltrative nature. Marked atypia and frequent mitosis are not the features and when such features are present poorly differentiated adenocarcinoma or adenosquamous carcinoma are to be considered.

Adenoid Cystic Carcinomas

These are common in minor salivary glands and are known for recurrence.

Grossly are solid with infiltrative margins. Microscopy has typical cribriform pattern (sieve-like). The nests and columns of cells are arranged around a space (pseudocyst) and true glands which are filled with PAS positive material.

Acinic Cell Tumours

These are relatively uncommon, representing only 2 to 3% of salivary gland tumours. Most arise in the parotids; these have male preponderance and peak in 3rd decade of life.

Grossly, encapsulated, solid, friable, grey-white and usually are less than 3 cm. Occasionally they present with marked cystic degeneration.

Microscopy has cells with abundant cytoplasm filled with basophilic zymogen granules.

They may be arranged in solid, microcystic, papillary and follicular patterns.

Exercise 46

Lesions of Gastrointestinal Tract

CARCINOMA OF ORAL CAVITY

Squamous cell carcinoma is the commonest malignant tumour of the oral cavity.

Aetiology

- Tobacco consumption (smoking, pipe smoking, betel quid consumption)
- HPV infection
- Genetic predisposition
- Chronic irritation (ill-fitting dentures, Jagged teeth, etc.)
- Actinic radiation
- Premalignant conditions: Leukoplakia, erythroplakia.

Squamous cell carcinoma can arise anywhere in oral cavity but most commonly involved sites are:

- Ventral surface of tongue
- Floor of mouth
- Lower lip
- Soft palate
- Gingiva

Grossly, they may present as verrucous plaques, ulcers, protruding masses with irregular and indurated borders.

Microscopically, similar to squamous cell carcinoma occurring elsewhere. However, degree of differentiation does not correlate with behaviour.

Common sites of metastasis include cervical lymph nodes, mediastinal lymph nodes, lungs, liver and bones.

GASTRIC ULCER / DUODENAL ULCER/PEPTIC ULCER

Peptic ulcers are ulcers defined histologically by breach in the mucosa that extend through the muscularis mucosa into the submucosa or deeper due to action of acid peptic juices. Often solitary and can occur in any portion of gastrointestinal tract which is exposed to action of acid/peptic juices (Fig. 3.36a and b).

Common locations in order of frequency are:

- First part of duodenum
- Lesser curvature and antrum of stomach
- Gastro-oesophageal junction
- Margins of gastrojejunostomy (stomal ulcer)
- Stomach and or jejunum of patients with Zollinger-Ellison syndrome
- Meckel's diverticulum containing ectopic gastric mucosa.

Aetiology: Following are the possible causes for peptic ulcer:

- *H. pylori*
- Chronic use of NSAIDs
- Cigarette smoking
- Alcohol
- Corticosteroid use
- Personality and psychological stress
- Heredity
- *Associated diseases:* Alcoholic cirrhosis, chronic obstructive pulmonary disease (COPD), chronic renal failure, hyperparathyroidism especially in case of duodenal ulcer.

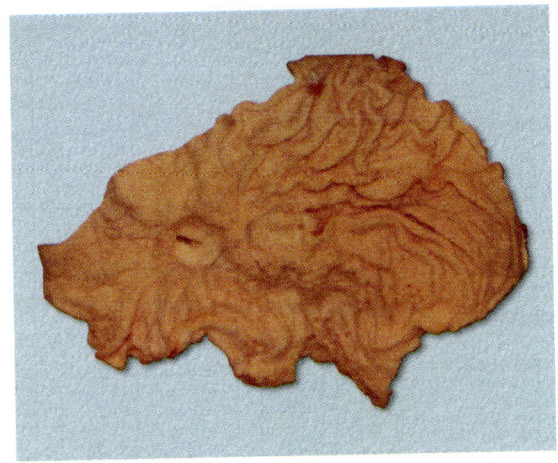

Fig. 3.36a: Gross picture of peptic ulcer

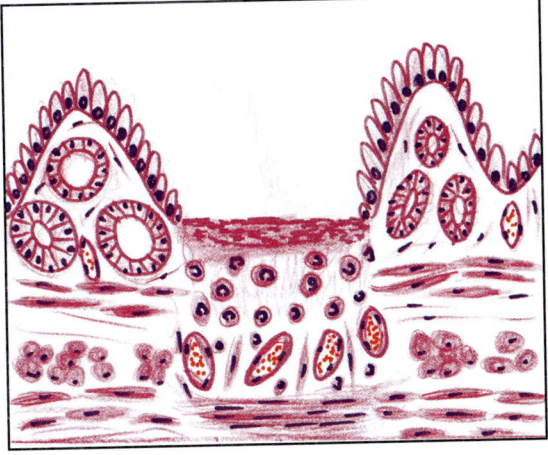

Fig. 3.36b: Schematic diagram of microscopy of peptic ulcer

GASTRIC ULCER

Gastric ulcers (GU) primarily result from altered/defective mucosal defenses. Most patients of gastric ulcer secrete less acid than duodenal ulcer and even sometimes lesser than normal individuals.

Factors implicated include:
- Back diffusion of acid (H ions) into mucosa
- Role of NSAIDS
- *H. pylori* infection
- Decreased parietal cell mass and abnormalities of parietal cells.

Back diffusion of H ions into mucosa: The damaging factors, especially *H. pylori* and NSAIDs, weaken of intercellular junctions, and cause foveolar damage which allows H ions and pepsin to diffuse into lamina propria. The other damaging factors include alcohol and spicy food.

Role of NSAIDs: Prostaglandins which play a major role in maintaining mucosal integrity are inhibited by the NSAIDs and further predispose to mucosal damage. NSAIDs also reduce mucin and bicarbonate production. The antral ulcers usually develop along lesser curvature.

H. pylori infection: *H. pylori* is a major factor in pathogenesis of peptic ulcers/gastric ulcer. The reason for this may be:

1. It induces an intense inflammatory and immune response. There is production of pro-inflammatory cytokines such as interleukins (IL-1, IL-6, IL-8) tumour necrosis factor (TNF). These recruit and activates neutrophils.
2. It secretes urease that breaks down urea to form toxic compounds such as ammonium chloride and monochloramine. They also elaborate phospholipases, proteases that damage surface epithelial cells.
3. Enhances gastric acid secretion and impairs duodenal bicarbonate production.
4. Evokes immunogenic response by activation of B and T-lymphocytes.
5. The bacterial platelet activating factor promote thrombotic occlusion of surface capillaries.

Decreased number and abnormalities of Parietal cells: This suggests that hypersecretion of acid is not the cause of GU.

Sites of gastric ulcer: Lesser curvature and antrum (common), anterior and posterior wall and greater curvature (less common).

DUODENAL ULCER

Duodenal ulcers (DU) are due to increased acid production or due to the effect of acid as evidenced by the following.

1. The gastric acid secreted depends upon the parietal cell mass. Patients of duodenal ulcer may have double of parietal cell mass

and maximum acid secretion compared to controls.
2. Gastric acid secretion stimulated by food is increased in magnitude and duration in patients with duodenal ulcer.
3. Some patients of duodenal ulcer can have increased G cell response to meals and can have increased number of antral G cells.
4. Acid secretion in people with duodenal ulcer may be more sensitive to secretogogues like gastrin than the normal individuals. This is possibly due to increased vagal tone or increased affinity of parietal cells to gastrin.
5. Accelerated or rapid gastric emptying is noted in patients with duodenal ulcers. Thus acidic food enters duodenum.
6. There is hyperacidification of duodenal bulb.
7. There is decreased bicarbonate secretion.
8. Decreased retrograde motility impairs neutralization by pancreatic alkaline secretions.

Morphology

1. Most commonly located in first part of duodenum (anterior wall more often affected) and stomach (more commonly on lesser curvature) usually at antral and corpus junction.
2. Majority are solitary.
3. These are usually less than 2 cm. They may penetrate the muscle tissue.
4. Round to oval, sharply punched out, with straight walls, margins are usually levelled or slightly elevated.
5. Base is smooth and clean.
6. Converging mucosal folds.
7. The blood vessels at the margins may be thrombosed.

Histology Gastric/ Duodenal Ulcer

In active ulcers, shows four different zones (Askanazy zones) from lumen outwards. They are:
1. *Zone of necrotic debri:* Superficial zone has debri.
2. *Zone of inflammation:* This zone shows dead cells and acute inflammatory cells.
3. *Zone of granulation tissue:* Composed of capillaries, fibroblasts, macrophages, lymphocytes and plasma cells.
4. *Zone of fibrosis or collagenous scar:* Beneath granulation tissue collagenous tissue is present. The ulcer may erode muscle and the layers, causing perforation and if blood vessels are eroded bleeding and haemorrhage.

Complications
- Bleeding/haemorrhage
- Perforation
- Obstruction from oedema
- *Scarring:* Can produce pyloric stenosis (Duodenal ulcers) and hourglass deformity (Gastric ulcers)
- Pancreatitis
- Rarely malignant transformation.

Clinical features: Epigastric burning or aching pain is a common feature. Few may have iron deficiency anaemia, haematemesis and perforation. With gastric ulcer, pain worsens after eating as gastric acid production is increased as food enters stomach whereas in duodenal ulcer pain is relieved by meal and manifests 2–3 hours after meal when stomach releases digested food along with acid into duodenum. Nausea, vomiting, bloating, abdominal fullness, water brush, belching are the other features.

GASTRIC CARCINOMA

It is the second most common tumour in the world and the most common malignant tumours of the stomach.

Higher incidence is seen in Japan, Chile, Costa Rica, Columbia, China, Portugal, Russia and Bulgaria. Incidence is lesser in United States, United Kingdom, Canada, Australia, New Zealand, France and Sweden. It is more common in lower socioeconomic groups. Male to female ratio is 2 : 1.

Classification

There are different classifications. Lauren's classification has 2 subtypes (intestinal and diffuse type) and WHO classifies into various cell types.

Lauren's classification for gastric carcinoma[10]

Intestinal type: Bulky tumours with malignant cells in diffuse sheets and glandular pattern
- Usually develops from a precursor lesion
- Older age group (mean age 55 years)
- M : F ratio is 2 : 1

Difffuse type: Malignant cells in diffuse sheets
- No identifiable precursor lesions
- Affects slightly younger (mean age 48 years)
- M : F ratio is 1 : 1

WHO classification for gastric carcinoma[11]

Epithelial tumours
- Intraepithelial neoplasia: Adenoma
- Adenocarcinoma:
  - Papillary adenocarcinoma
  - Tubular adenocarcinoma
  - Mucinous adenocarcinoma
  - Signet ring carcinoma
  - Undifferentiated carcinoma
  - Adenosquamous carcinoma
  - Small cell carcinoma
  - Carcinoid tumour

Non-epithelial tumours
- Leiomyoma
- Schwannoma
- Granular cell tumour
- Leiomyosarcoma
- Gastrointestinal stromal tumour
- Kaposi's sarcoma
- Others
  - Malignant lymphoma

Etiological factors

Environmental factors
- Infection by *H. pylori*
- Diet: Nitrites derived from nitrates (found in water and preserved food)
- Smoked and salted foods, pickled vegetables, excessive spicy food
- Lack of fresh fruits and vegetables
- Low socioeconomic status
- Cigarette smoking.

Host factors
- Chronic gastritis
- Partial gastrectomy
- Gastric adenomas
- Barrette's oesophagus.

Genetic factors
- Blood group 'A' individuals
- Family history
- Hereditary nonpolyposis colon carcinoma syndrome
- Familial gastric carcinoma syndrome (E-cadherin mutation).

Genetic mechanisms: Loss of alleles in various chromosomal loci, microsatellite instability of several genes.

Morphology

Location: Pylorus and antrum (60–65%), cardia (25–30%), and remainder in fundus and body.

Lesser curvature (40%) more involved than greater curvature (15%).

Most common on the lesser curvature of antropyloric region.

Macroscopic growth patterns
- Exophytic
- Flat or depressed
- Excavated
- Linitis plastica (leather bottle appearance).

Depth of invasion

Early gastric carcinomas: Confined to mucosa and submucosa regardless of involvement of perigastric lymph nodes (not same as carcinoma *in situ* where it is confined to the surface epithelial layer).

Advanced gastric carcinomas: Extending below the submucosa, and may infiltrate muscular wall.

Histological subtypes

Intestinal and diffuse types (refer to Lauren's classification).

Gross: Gastric carcinoma can be early gastric cancer or advanced gastric cancer. In early gastrtic cancer, the neoplasm is limited to the

mucosa and submucosa. Grossly, early gastric carcinoma can be of:
a. Exophytic
b. Flat or depressed
c. Excavated types.

Advanced gastric carcinoma can be of:
a. Exophytic (polypoid/fungating)
b. Linitis plastica
c. Excavated types.

Microscopy: In any of these types, the microscopy shows adenocarcinoma (Fig. 3.37) with varying degrees of differentiation. They can be of different subtypes such as papillary, tubular, mucinous, signet ring cell and undifferentiated adenocarcinoma (WHO classification). In diffusely infiltrative pattern, the neoplasm may be associated with desmoplasia.

Spread: Left supraclavicular lymph node (Virchow's node, sentinel node) may be seen in even occult malignancy.

Sister Mary Joseph nodule: Periumbilical metastatic nodule.

Local invasion: To duodenum, pancreas, retroperitoneum.

Metastasis to one or both the ovaries: This is called Krukenberg's tumour.

Clinical features
- Insidious disease, generally asymptomatic until late in the course

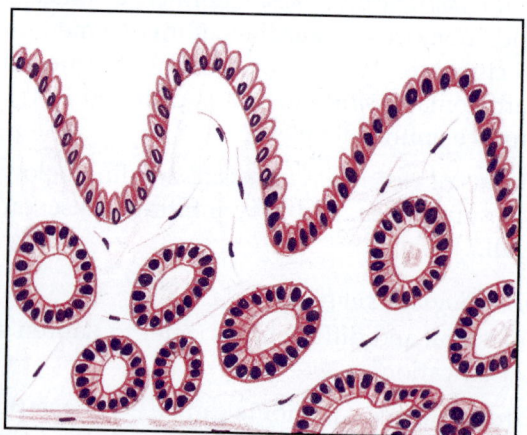

Fig. 3.37: Schematic diagram of microscopy of adenocarcinoma stomach

- Weight loss, anorexia, abdominal pain, vomiting, altered bowel habits, anaemia.

TYPHOID ULCER[12,13]

Grossly (Fig. 3.38a)
1. Characteristic pathology is prominent in the ileum associated with Payer's patches.
2. The intestine shows raised nodules representing hyperplastic Payer's patches.
3. Ulceration, linear ulcers full thickness ulceration of surface epithelium overlying Payer's patches ensues as the disease progresses.
4. Suppurative mesenteric lymphadenitis, perforation and toxic megacolon may complicate typhoid fever.

Microscopically
1. Following hyperplasia of Payer's patches, acute inflammation overlying epithelium develops.
2. Eventually macrophages mixed with lymphocytes, plasma cells, macrophages with erythrophagocytosis are seen. Neutrophils are not usually present.
3. Necrosis of overlying epithelium begins and spreads to neighbouring mucosa.
4. The ulcers are deep, with base at the level of muscularis propria.

TUBERCULOUS ULCER[12,13]

It may be primary or secondary tuberculosis. Primary is common with *Tuberculosis bovis* organisms, but the incidence is reduced with pasteurisation of milk.

Grossly (Fig. 3.38b)
1. Ileocaecal and jejuno-ileal areas are most commonly involved areas followed by appendix and ascending colon.
2. Strictures and ulcers are most common findings along with thickened mucosal folds.
3. Ulcerative, hypertrophic, and ulcerohypertrophic are three morphological types.

The ulcerative type commonly affects the ileum and jejunum. The hypertrophic and

ulcerohypertrophic types commonly affect the ileocaecum and cause obstruction or present as a mass.
4. The ulcers are often circumferential and transverse. Multiple and segmental lesions with skip areas are common.
5. Healing of ulcers leads to stricture formation and may perforate, bleed, or form fistulas.
   Obstruction, perforation, and haemorrhage are common complications.
6. Regional lymph nodes also affected.

Microscopically, shows classical granulomas with caseation necrosis surrounded by epithelioid cells, Langhans' type of giant cells and mantle of lymphocytes with surrounding fibrosis suggestive of tuberculosis as seen in other organs.

These granulomas are seen mainly in the submucosal and serosal layers.

Table 3.24 shows the differences between typhoid and tuberculosis ulcer intestine.

Differential diagnosis for tuberculosis
1. Yersiniosis—granulomas are non-caseating.
2. Crohn's—difficult to differentiate from tuberculosis, grossly linear ulcers are present rather than circumferential ulcers, cobble stoning is typical which is not a feature in tuberculosis.
3. Fungal diseases.

Inflammatory Bowel Diseases

Causes of colitis
- Ulcerative colitis
- Crohn's disease

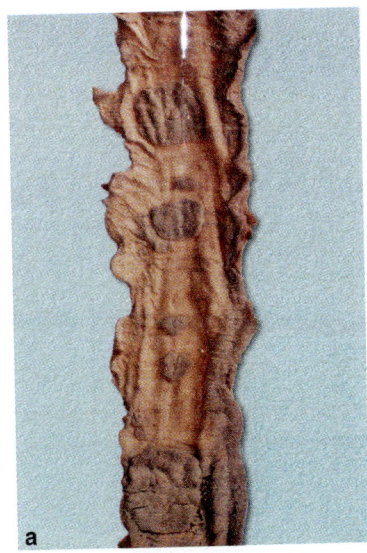
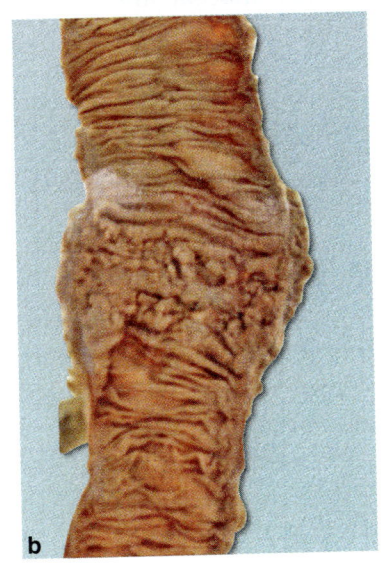

Figs 3.38a and b: (a) Gross picture of typhoid ulcer (b) tuberculous ulcer intestine

	Table 3.24: Differences between typhoid ulcer and tuberculous ulcer intestine	
	Tuberculous ulcer intestine	*Typhoid ulcer*
Site	Anywhere in the intestine, commonly ileocaecal junction	Ileum
Ulcers	Circumferentially placed	Longitudinally placed along the Payer's patches
Gross features	Transverse and circumferential ulcers	Vertical ulcers along the Payer's patches
Microscopy	Granulomas	Erythrophagocytosis
Complications	Stricture, obstruction, adhesions	Perforation, peritonitis
Blood changes	Lymphocytosis, ESR increased	Neutropenia, Widal positive

- Collagenous colitis
- Lymphocytic colitis
- Ischaemic colitis
- Radiation colitis
- Diverticular disease associated colitis
- Allergic proctocolitis.

ULCERATIVE COLITIS

It is a chronic idiopathic inflammatory bowel disease with episodes of bloody diarrhoea and histologically has crypt destruction, colitis with continuous involvement from rectum extending proximally.

Incidence: Uncommon, 4–20/1,00,000 population

Epidemiology
M : F—equal
  Whites higher incidence than other ethnic group.
  Jews higher incidence than other religious group.
  Rare in 1st decade.
Peak: 15–25 years of age major peak
  60–70 years of age minor peak
  25% have family history

Clinical features: Present with recurrent episodes of bloody diarrhoea.

Gross and endoscopic findings
- Unremarkable serosa
- Bowel wall thickness normal
- Continuous involvement from rectum proximally
- May involve entire colon and ileum
- *Active phase:* Mucosa erythematous, bloody, friable, granular with polyps
- *Quiescent phase:* Mucosa granular with punctuate erythema with polyps
- In both phases normal submucosal vascular network is lost.

Microscopy (Fig. 3.39a)
- Crypt architecture distortion
- Mucosal chronic inflammation
- *In active phase:* Cryptitis, crypt abscesses
- Eosinophils may predominate

- Lymphoid aggregate at mucosal and submucosal interphase
- Regenerating epithelium is immature and mucin depleted
- Inflammation superficial
- Transmural inflammation is not present unless it is deep seated ulceration
- Submucosa—oedema and congestion, lacks fibrosis.

Prognosis: It has risk of dysplasia and adenocarcinoma.

Crohn's Disease (Regional enteritis, granulomatous enterocolitis, terminal ileitis)

It is a chronic multifocal, relapsing and remitting progressive inflammatory disease of unknown cause that can affect any portion of GIT. It is characterised by foci of glandular destruction, aphthous (mucosal) ulcerations, serpiginous ulcers, transmural inflammation, fibrosis and granulomas in the small and large intestine.

Incidence: 2–20/1,00,000 population

Epidemiology
M : F—equal
  Whites have higher incidence than other ethnic group.
  Ashkenazi Jews have higher incidence than other religious group.
Peak: 20–30 years of age major peak
  60–70 years of age minor peak
  10% have family history

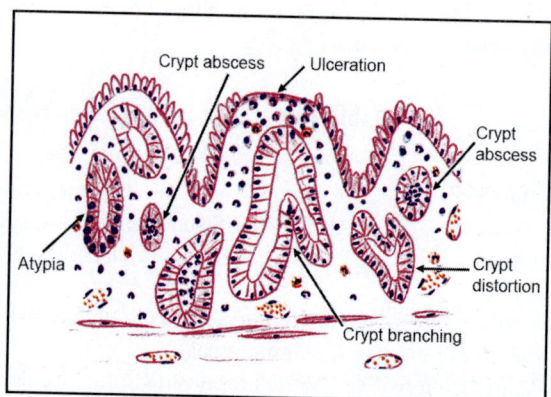

Fig. 3.39a: Schematic diagram of ulcerative colitis

Clinical features
- Cramping pain, non-bloody diarrhoea, fever, malaise and anorexia
- Haemorrhage and bleeding uncommon
- *Upper intestinal involvement:* Dyspepsia, weight loss, hypoalbuminaemia and iron deficiency anaemia
- Fistula and stenosis
- Anal and perianal fistulas and fissures
- Inflammatory changes can be seen in joints, eyes and skin.

Gross and endoscopy findings
- Aphthous ulceration
- Longitudinal ulcers (train tract and rake ulcers) and adjacent normal mucosa
- Cobble stone appearance
- Strictures
- Fissures and fistulas
- Involvement of terminal ileum
- Loss of submucosal vascular network
- Often rectal sparing
- Creeping fat—subserosal fat covers and contracted over involved area
- Firm, thick, pipe-like bowel, wall thickened
- Interloop adhesions
- Inflammatory polyps
- Multifocal
- Occasional confluent involvement.

Microscopic findings (Fig. 3.39b)
- Ulcers separated by normal mucosa
- Mucosal erosions with underlying lymphoid aggregate
- Variable inflammation in single biopsy
- Transmural inflammation
- Epithelioid granuloma
- Duplication of muscularis mucosae
- Hyperplasia of nerve bundle
- Mucin slightly reduced
- Ulceration, fissures and fistulas
- Submucosal fibrosis.

Prognosis: It has risk of malignancy

Differences between Crohn's and ulcerative colitis is given in Table 3.25.

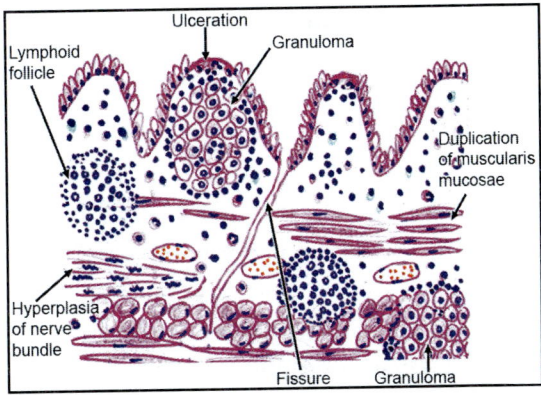

Fig. 3.39b: Schematic diagram of Crohn's disease

		Crohn's	Ulcerative colitis
	Table 3.25: Differences between Crohn's and ulcerative colitis		
Macroscopy	Bowel region	Colon, ileum	Colon
	Distribution	Skip lesions	Diffuse
	Strictures	+	Late/rare
	Wall	Thickened	Normal
	Dilatation	+	+
	Inflammation	Transmural	Mucosal
Microscopy	Inflammation	Transmural	Mucosal
	Ulcers	Deep/linear	Superficial
	Submucosa	Normal/inflammed	Normal
	Crypt abscesses	Uncommon/few	Common
	Oedema	Marked	Minimum
	Hyperaemia	Seldom prominent	Prominent
	Lymphoid reaction	Marked	Mild

Contd.

Table 3.25: Differences between Crohn's and ulcerative colitis *(contd.)*

	Crohn's	Ulcerative colitis
Lymphoid aggregate	+	–
Serositis	Marked/variable	Absent/mild
Mucin producing cells	Slighltly reduced	Depleted
Granuloma	common (50%)	No
Fistula and sinuses	+	–
Neurotic hyperplasia	Common	–
Lymph node	Granuloma +	–
Inflammatory Pseudopolyps	Less common	Common

INTESTINAL POLYPS

The term polyp of the intestine refers to a protruding epithelial lesion into the lumen, from the intestinal mucosa. Polyps are usually asymptomatic but may ulcerate and bleed, cause tenesmus, if in the rectum and when very large, produce intestinal obstruction. Polyps can be:

- Neoplastic
- Hamartomatous—juvenile polyps, Peutz-Jeghers polyps:
- Non-neoplastic.

Adenomas (adenomatous polyps): About two-thirds of all colonic polyps are adenomas. These adenomas have dysplastic foci and thus have malignant potential (Figs 3.40a and b).

Tubular adenomas: Tubular adenomas account for more than 80% of colonic adenomas. They are characterised by a network of branching adenomatous epithelium. To be classified as tubular, the adenoma should have a tubular component of at least 75%.

Villous adenomas: Villous adenomas account for 5 to 15% of adenomas. They are characterised by glands that are long and extend straight down from the surface to the centre of the polyp. To be classified as villous, the adenoma should have a villous component of at least 75%.

Tubulovillous adenomas: These have 26 to 75% villous component. Polyp base is sessile—base is attached to the colon wall, Pedunculated if a mucosal stalk is interposed between the polyp and the wall.

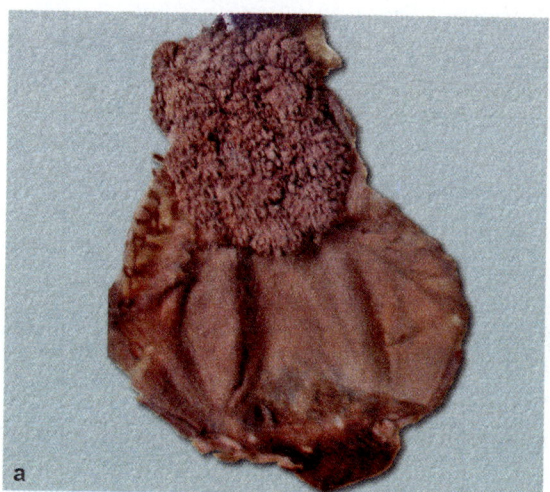

a

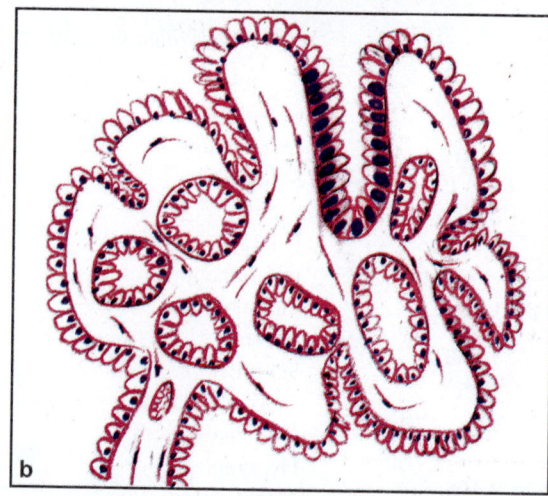

b

Figs 3.40a and b: Gross and schematic diagram of adenoma

Risk Factors for Malignant Potential of Adenomatous Polyps

- Adenomatous polyps >1 cm in diameter
- Adenomatous polyps with high-grade dysplasia
- Adenomatous polyps with >25% villous histology
- Adenomatous polyps with invasive cancer.

Familial juvenile polyposis (FJP): FJP is associated with an increased risk for the development of colorectal cancer, and in some families, gastric cancer, especially where there are both upper and lower gastrointestinal polyps.

Inflammatory pseudopolyps: : Inflammatory pseudopolyps are irregularly shaped islands of residual intact colonic mucosa that are the result of the mucosal ulceration and regeneration that occurs in inflammatory bowel disease (IBD).

Juvenile polyps: Juvenile polyps are hamartomatous lesions that consist of a lamina propria and dilated cystic glands rather than increased numbers of epithelial cells. (Fig. 3.40c).

Peutz-Jeghers polyps: The Peutz-Jeghers polyp is a hamartomatous lesion of glandular epithelium supported by smooth muscle cells that is contiguous with the muscularis mucosa. Patients with PJS are at increased risk of both gastrointestinal (gastric, small bowel, colon, pancreas) and non-gastrointestinal cancers with a cumulative cancer risk of about 50% by age of 60 years. (Fig. 3.40d).

CARCINOMA COLON

Carcinoma colon, in 90% of the cases generally affects patients >50 years.

Hereditary: Family history, younger age of onset, specific gene defects, e.g. familial adenomatous polyposis (FAP), hereditary non-polyposis colorectal cancer (HNPCC or Lynch syndrome).

Sporadic: Absence of family history, older population, isolated lesion.

Familial: Patients having relatives with identified genetic predisposition (e.g. FAP, HNPCC, Peutz-Jeghers syndrome) have risk, patients with colon cancer of <50 years in the family, colon cancer in 1st degree relatives has 2–3 fold increased risk, 1st degree relatives with colon cancer with <50 years 3–4 fold increased risk, 2nd degree relatives 3–4 fold increased risk (1st degree relatives—parents, siblings and children, 2nd degree relatives—grandparents, uncles and aunts).

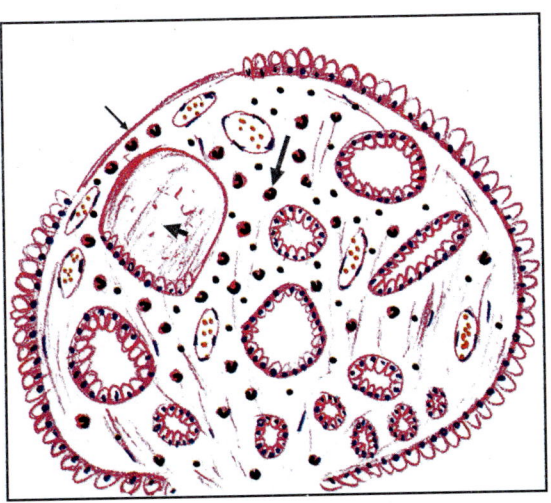

Fig. 3.40c: Schematic diagram of Juvenile polyp. Thin arrow—ulceration, thick arrow—oedema and inflammation, short arrow—mucin in the glands

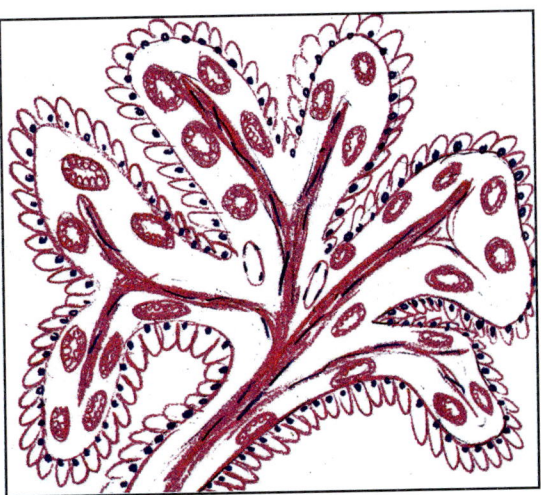

Fig. 3.40d: Schematic diagram of Peutz-Jeghers polyp

Risk factors: Past history of colorectal cancer, pre-existing adenoma, ulcerative colitis, radiation.

Diet—carcinogenic foods

Familial adenomatous polyposis
- FAP account for <1% of all colorectal cancers
- Due to mutation of the adenomatosis *polyposis coli* (APC) gene
- Numerous adenomas appear as early as childhood and virtually 100% have colorectal cancer by age 50 if untreated.

Hereditary non-polyposis colorectal cancer/ Lynch syndrome
- More common than FAP and account for ~1–5% of all colonic adenocarcinomas
- Due to a mutation in one of the mismatch repair genes
- Earlier age of onset of colorectal cancer and predominantly involve the right colon
- HNPCC also increases the risk of:
  - Endometrial, ovarian, breast carcinomas
  - Stomach, small bowel, hepatobiliary carcinomas

Renal pelvis or ureter carcinoma.

Morphology: Most of the colorectal carcinomas occur in caecum or ascending colon, rectum and distal sigmoid, descending colon and proximal sigmoid; the remainder are scattered elsewhere. Most often carcinomas occur singly (Figs 3.41a and b).

Differences between right and left sided colonic cancers are given in Table 3.26

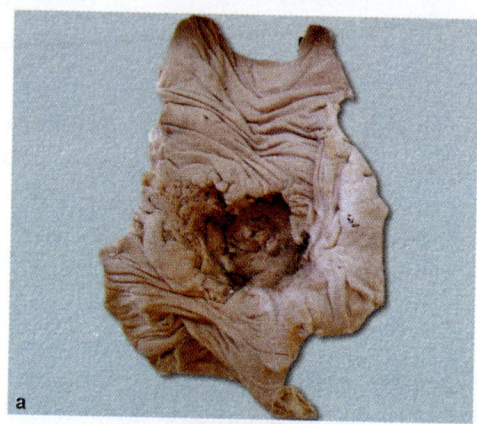

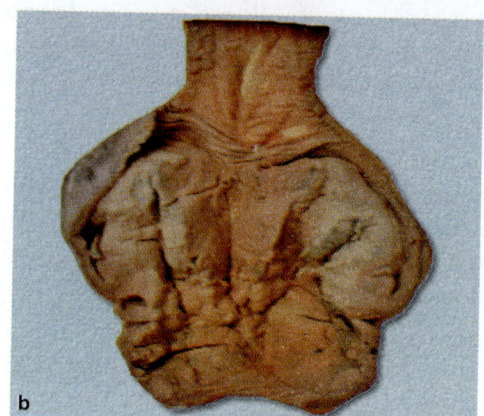

Figs 3.41a and b: Gross pictures of carcinoma colon

Table 3.26: Differences between right and left sided colonic cancers
Colorectal carcinomas begin as *in situ* lesions, they evolve into different morphologic patterns
Carcinoma of proximal colon (right-sided cancer colon): 1. Tend to grow as bulky, exophytic, polypoid mass 2. Occur typically in caecum and ascending colon 3. Rarely result in obstruction 4. Become quite large before clinical presentation
Carcinoma of distal colon (left-sided cancer colon): 1. Tend to be annular, encircling lesions that produce so-called napkin-ring constriction with narrowing of the lumen 2. The margins are heaped up 3. Produce ulcero-nodular lesions with invasion of the wall and desmoplastic stroma 4. Associated with obstruction and proximal dilatation of colon with attenuation and flattening of mucosal folds
Both forms of neoplasms directly penetrate the bowel wall

Microscopically, colorectal cancers are adenocarcinomas which may be well-differentiated to undifferentiated and anaplastic. Many produce mucin and these secretions spread through the gut wall and facilitate cancer extention and worsen the prognosis. Cancers of the anal canal and anorectal junction can be adenosquamous or squamous cell carcinomas.

Diagnosis
- Faecal occult blood
- Colonoscopy
- Anorectal ultrasound
- CT and MRI—staging prior to treatment
- Blood tests for:
  - Anaemia
  - Tumour marker CEA—useful for monitoring progress but not specific for diagnosis.

Exercise 47

Common Lesions of Liver

JAUNDICE

Jaundice is the yellowish discolouration of the skin and sclera resulting due to increased serum bilirubin, a common manifestation of liver disorders causing bile retention. Normal serum bilirubin range is 0.1 to 1.2 mg/dl. Bilirubin levels more than 1.2 mg/dl or for classic definition, bilirubin more than 2.5 mg/dl along with yellowish discolouration of the skin and sclera defines jaundice.

Pathophysiology of Jaundice

Jaundice occurs whenever there is an imbalance between the bilirubin production and its metabolism and clearance. There are four major mechanisms by which jaundice can occur:

1. Increased production of bilirubin [prehepatic].
2. Decreased hepatic uptake of bilirubin [prehepatic].
3. Impaired conjugation of unconjugated bilirubin [hepatic].
4. Decreased hepatocellular excretion [hepatic].
5. Impaired bile flow-intra/extrahepatic [posthepatic].

Increased production of bilirubin: This can occur due to excessive red cell destruction which could be intra- or extra-vascular or due to ineffective erythropoiesis. The liver is unable to conjugate the large amount of bilirubin formed, hence leading to unconjugated hyperbilirubinaemia.

Causes
i. Haemolytic anaemias—thalassaemia, sickle cell anaemia, neonatal jaundice, etc.
ii. Excessive internal haemorrhages—alimentary tract or large haemotomas
iii. Ineffective haemopoiesis.

This is a predominantly unconjugated hyperbilirubinaemia but when associated with parenchymal liver disorders, may have both unconjugated and conjugated bilirubin.

Decreased hepatic uptake: Any defect in the binding of bilirubin with albumin, its transportation to the liver and its binding with the receptor and cytoplasmic protein can cause jaundice which is again predominantly unconjugated. Causes include:
i. Drugs—rifampicin, probenicid
ii. Hepatitis—viral, alcoholic
iii. Sepsis.

Impaired conjugation: The underlying cause can be hereditary like Gilbert's syndrome and Crigler-Najjar syndrome or it could be acquired as in drugs, cirrhosis or hepatitis. Impaired conjugation is also seen in neonatal jaundice. This occurs due to deficiency or defect of the enzyme glucuronyl transferase enzyme.

Decreased hepatocellular excretion of bilirubin: This is also called intrahepatic cholestasis and results in predominantly conjugated hyperbilirubinaemia due to regurgitation of bilirubin in the blood. The underlying pathology may be due to damage to the canalicular plasma membrane, alterations in the contractile properties of the canaliculus or alterations in the permeability of the canalicular membrane. Causes could be hereditary such as Dubin-Johnson syndrome and Rotor syndrome, drugs like oral contraceptives and cyclosporine and diffuse hepatocellular damage due to viral etiology, drug induced or alcoholic hepatitis or cirrhosis.

Impaired bile flow-intrahepatic/extrahepatic: Intrahepatic obstruction to bile could be due to inflammatory damage to of intrahepatic bile ducts as seen in primary biliary cirrhosis, and liver transplantation.

Extrahepatic cholestasis which results in obstruction to the larger bile ducts could be due to gallstones, primary sclerosing cholangitis, tumours, both benign and malignant of the bile duct, head of pancreas and sometimes the duodenum.

Laboratory Workup

To differentiate between various types of Jaundice.

There are various tests to assess the liver function in jaundice which also help us to detect whether the underlying cause of jaundice is prehepatic, hepatic or posthepatic.

Urine bile salts and pigments: These are usually not seen in the urine in prehepatic/haemolytic and some forms of congenital causes of jaundice. In case of hepatic and post-hepatic causes, they are strongly present in the urine.

Serum bilirubin: According to van den Bergh/diazo reaction, bilirubin can be indirect [i.e. uncojugated], direct [i.e. conjugated] and total. Total bilirubin is increased in all types of jaundice to varying degrees depending on the severity of the underlying cause. The type of bilirubin seen in prehepatic jaundice is predominantly indirect whereas it is direct in hepatic and posthepatic/obstructive jaundice.

Liver enzymes: There are four major enzymes involved in the metabolism of liver which can be raised in varying degrees in different types of jaundice.
1. Serum glutamate pyruvate transaminase [SGPT/ALT]
2. Serum glutamate oxaloacetate transaminase [SGOT/AST]
3. Alkaline phosphatase [ALP]
4. Serum gamma-glutamyl transferase [SGGT/GGT].

SGPT and SGOT are increased in jaundice due to hepatic injury—especially viral hepatitis. SGPT levels when more than ten times the normal level indicates acute hepatocellular injury. The levels of these enzymes are not very high in intrahepatic cholestasis or posthepatic biliary obstruction. SGOT might also be increased in myocardial infarction and muscle injury, therefore SGPT is a more specific for liver injury.

Alkaline phosphatase is normal in uncomplicated haemolytic jaundice, moderately increased in hepatic jaundice and markedly in increased in post-hepatic/obstructive jaundice. This is because, ALP is excreted through the biliary system in the same manner as bilirubin.

GGT/SGGT levels are raised in all forms of hepatobiliary disease and especially in intrahepatic obstructive disorders.

Some other relevant liver function tests include serum total proteins, albumin, globulin, A/G ratio and prothrombin time.

It is necessary to differentiate intrahepatic cholestasis from extrahepatic cholestasis. Other than radiological scans, we can differentiate between the two by doing a prothrombin time which is prolonged in extrahepatic obstructive jaundice due to malabsorption of vitamin A, D, E and K and also prolonged in intrahepatic obstructive jaundice due to hepatocellular disease. Administration of vitamin K improves the prothrombin time in obstructive extrahepatic jaundice but not in diffuse hepatocellular disease.

HEPATITIS

Hepatitis is caused by hepatotrophic viruses.
1. Hepatitis A virus (HAV), Hepatitis B virus (HBV), Hepatitis C virus (HCV), Hepatitis D virus (HDV) and Hepatitis E virus (HEV).
2. There can be other viruses causing hepatitis, e.g. Virus causing yellow fever, cytomegalovirus and Epstein-Barr virus.
   Yellow fever is endemic in tropical areas of Africa, Central and South America.

HEPATITIS A VIRUS

Hepatitis A virus (HAV) infection runs a self-limited course. It has an incubation period of 15 to 50 days (average 28 days). HAV does not cause chronic hepatitis, no carrier state and rarely causes fulminant hepatitis. Fatality is less common (0.1%).

Epidemiology

HAV occurs all over the world, endemic in countries with poor hygiene and sanitation. The disease tends to be mild or asymptomatic especially in children. In adults has higher morbidity.

Mode of Spread

Following are important findings as regards to how HAV spreads.
1. HAV spreads through faeco-oral route, directly from person to person or ingestion of contaminated water and foods.
2. Virions are shed in the stool 2–3 weeks before and 1 week after the onset of jaundice.
3. HAV is not shed in the body fluids like saliva, urine and semen.
4. Close contact with infected person during the period of shedding, ingestion of raw vegetables and feco-oral contamination accounts to most of the cases and common with children in schools, play homes and nursery.
5. Viremia is transient, blood borne infection occurs rarely. Hence HAV is not a screening test for donated blood for blood transfusion.

HAV Virion Description

It is small, non-enveloped, single stranded RNA, 27 nm in diameter, belongs to picorna virus group. The virions, through gut reach

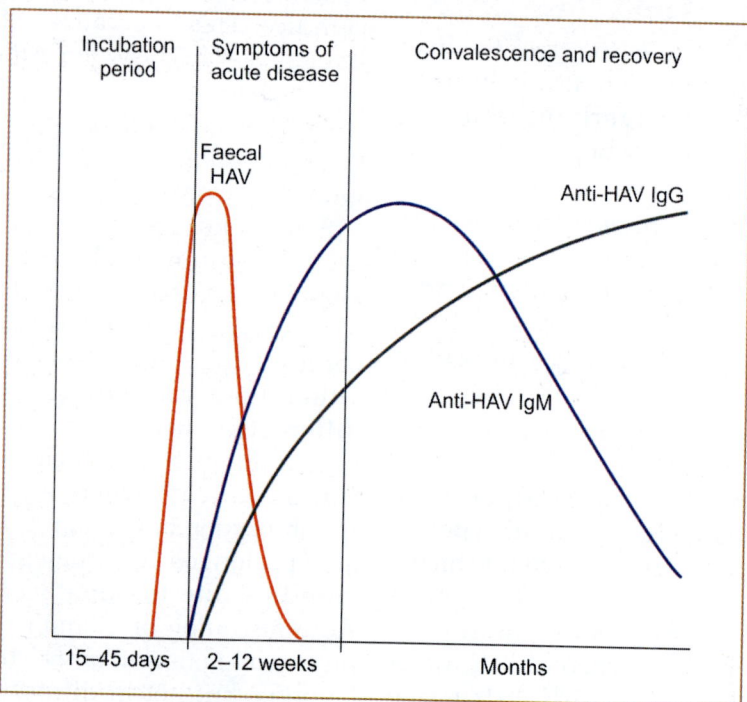

Fig. 3.42a: Diagnostic markers in HAV infection

hepatocytes, multiply and are shed in bile and faeces. There is damage to hepatocytes by T cells.

Diagnosis (Fig. 3.42a)

1. HAV shed in stool and bile.
2. IgM antibodies against HAV (anti-HAV IgM) appear at onset of symptoms and persist for several months. This is diagnostic of current infection with HAV.
3. Anti-HAV-IgG denote past infection, persists during convalescence period and beyond. And protects against re-infection.

Histopathology: HAV produces acute hepatitis, periportal inflammation and necrosis. Plasma cells are prominent. Perivenular cholestasis is seen. There can be fulminant hepatitis with panlobular necrosis with fatty change of surviving cells.

Clinical course: Clinical course is characteristically mild in young individuals.

HEPATITIS B VIRUS

Hepatitis B virus (HBV) can produce:
1. Acute Hepatitis with recovery
2. Non-progressive chronic hepatitis
3. Progressive chronic hepatitis with cirrhosis
4. Fulminant hepatitis.

HBV Structure

HBV belongs to hepadnaviridae group and is a double stranded DNA virus. The virus also called Dane particle. It is 42 nm consists of core containing DNA and a DNA polymerase enzyme. The core is surrounded by double shelled layers.

1. Inner nucleocapsid layer having HBc Ags.
2. Outer surface lipid envelope proteins composed of HBs Ag.

The HBV has following features:
1. Core protein HBcAg retained in hepatocytes, HBeAg-secreted into blood.
2. Envelope glycoprotein hepatitis B surface antigen (HBsAg) secreted in blood.
3. A DNA polymerase with reverse transcriptase activity is present inside the core.
4. HBV X, a transcriptional transactivator plays a role in hepatocellular carcinoma.

Transmission

HBV is a blood borne disease can spread by:
1. Parenteral route—particularly through blood and blood products, dialysis, and IV drug users.
2. It can spread through needle pricks and healthcare workers are at risk of infection.
3. Contact with semen, saliva, sweat, tears, breast milk, and sexual transmission can also spread the disease.

Incubation period: 45–180 days (6 weeks to 6 months). It is present in all body fluids except stool. It can withstand extremes of temperature and humidity.

Acute phase: Follows incubation period, lasts for weeks to months.

Serum markers in acute phase (Fig. 3.42b):
1. HBsAg: Appears before the onset of symptoms, peaks during active phase declines to undetectable levels in 3–6 months.
2. Anti-HBsAb: Does not appear until acute phase is over. Does not appear sometimes several months after disappearance of HBsAg. Anti-HBsAb persists for life, conferring protection.
3. HBeAg, HBV DNA and DNA polymerase appear in serum soon after HBsAg, these represents active viral replication. It is a indicator of viral replication, infectivity and probable progression to chronic hepatitis.
4. Anti-HBeAb: Appear when acute phase is subsiding.
5. IgM anti HBc appear shortly after onset of symptoms correlate with elevated serum amino transferase which is indicative of cell destruction.
6. With decline of IgM anti-HBc, IgM anti-HBc Ab is replaced by IgG anti-HBcAb.

HBV infection can be prevented by vaccination and screening of donors of blood, organs, and tissues.

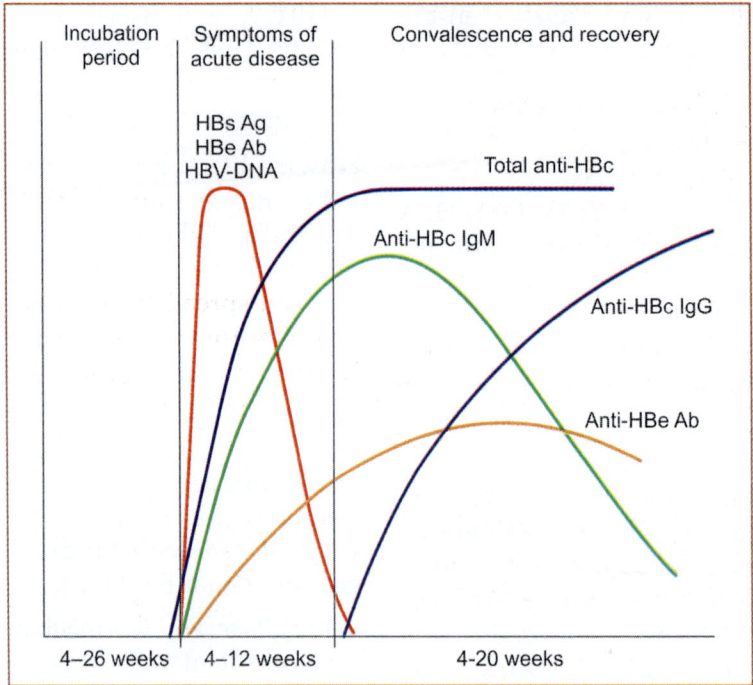

Fig. 3.42b: Diagnostic markers in HBV infection

Histopathology: Histologically, the most distinctive feature of HBV infection is ground glass hepatocytes. The cytoplasm of these cells has finely granular inclusions consisting of proliferated endoplasmic reticulum containing HBsAg. These push the nucleus aside and also create halo separating the nucleus from the cell membrane.

Clinical features: About 65% of the people are asymptomatic. Remaining may have flue like symptoms, nausea, vomiting and jaundice. About 5% of the affected people get chronic hepatitis.

ALCOHOLIC LIVER DISEASE

Alcoholic liver diseases include:
1. Alcoholic steatosis
2. Alcoholic hepatitis
3. Alcoholic cirrhosis.

Alcoholic steatosis is the initial stage which progresses to alcoholic hepatitis followed by alcoholic cirrhosis.

Pathogenesis

Alcohol induced liver damage is a multifactorial process. Primary mechanism is oxidative stress.

1. Alcohol is metabolised to acetate by two enzymes. Alcohol dehydrogenase and Aldehyde dehydrogenase produce acetate and result in steatosis.
2. Microsomal ethanol oxidising system: Hepatocellular damage is due to:
   a. The direct toxic effect of acetaldehyde.
   b. Oxidative stress and free radical injury: Results in mitochondrial damage.
   c. Direct effect on microtubule organization: Causing mallory hyaline/mallory dense bodies
   d. Depletion of reduced glutathione (antioxidant) leading to toxicity of free radicals.
   e. Lipid peroxidation.
   f. Activation of cytochrome p450 leads to transformation of some drugs to toxic metabolites.

g. Steatosis develops due to reduced catabolism, increased lipid biosynthesis, impaired secretion of lipoproteins and increase peripheral mobilization of fat.
h. Abnormal cytokine regulation: Reactive oxygen species and endotoxins derived from gut bacteria release: TNF, IL-6, IL-8 and IL-18 are released.

ALCOHOLIC STEATOSIS

This is the mildest form of alcoholic liver disease. Excessive drinking for 15–20 years produces alcoholic steatosis followed by alcoholic hepatitis.

Hepatic steatosis gives rise to hepatomegaly with mild increase of serum bilirubin and alkaline phosphatase. Complete resolution is possible with cessation of alcohol.

Clinical features of alcoholic hepatitis develop acutely with a bout of heavy drinking. Malaise, anorexia, weight loss, upper abdominal discomfort, tender hepatomegaly and fever are the usual symptoms.

Gross findings: Liver is enlarged, yellow, soft and greasy.

Microscopic findings: Hepatocytes contain fat vacuoles. The accumulation is more in zone 3 area, however it may be panlobular. No inflammation or fibrosis is present.

Note: Refer to topic on fatty liver.

ALCOHOLIC HEPATITIS

Alcoholic hepatitis is the beginning stage of cirrhosis (Fig. 3.43). Alcoholic hepatitis has four characteristic features:

Hepatocyte swelling and necrosis: Hepatocytes undergo ballooning degeneration and necrosis. There is fat and water accumulation in the cells.

Mallory bodies: Tangled intermediate filaments accumulate along with other proteins visible as eosinophilic inclusion in the cytoplasm, perinuclear location in hepatocytes undergoing ballooning degeneration. These are present in:
- Alcoholic liver diseases
- Biliary cirrhosis
- Wilson's disease
- Cholestatic syndromes
- Hepatocellular tumours

Neutrophil infiltration: Neutrophils accumulate around degenerating hepatocytes particularly those containing Mallory bodies. Lymphocytes and macrophages also enter into the portal tract and spill into the parenchyma.

Fibrosis: There is sinusoidal and pericellular fibrosis which surrounds centrilobular hepatocytes. This is referred to as "Chicken Wire Fibrosis'. Periportal fibrosis may predominate with heavy alcohol intake.

There may be cholestasis and deposition of hemosiderin in hepatocytes and Kupffer cells.

Grossly: Liver has bile stained areas. Liver is either normal in size or enlarged. It may contain visible nodules.

ALCOHOLIC CIRRHOSIS

This is an irreversible stage. The disease evolves slowly and insidiously. It has following features:
1. Cirrhotic liver is tan yellow, fatty, enlarged and weighs over 2 kg. Over the years it becomes brown, shrunken, and may weigh less than 1 kg.

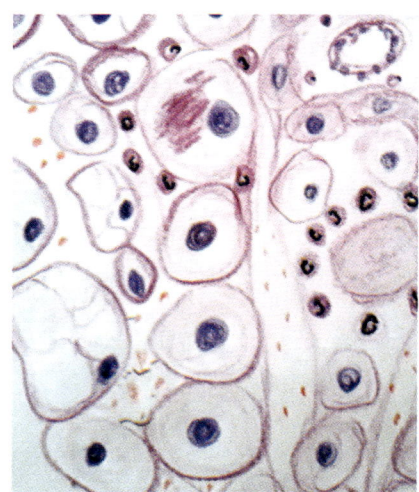

Fig. 3.43: Microscopy in alcoholic hepatitis. Note hydropic degeneration, Mallory hyaline, neutrophils and chicken wire fibrosis

2. Initially, the fibrous septae are delicate and extend through sinusoids from central vein to portal tract and from portal tract to portal tract.
3. Regenerative activity traps parenchymal hepatocytes with uniform sized nodules. These are less than 0.3 cm in diameter. This is termed micronodular cirrhosis.
4. The nodules become more prominent and eventually become macronodules. Thus in a later stage a mixed nodular pattern develops.
5. Bile stasis develops.
6. Microscopic features of cirrhosis are present. Fatty change and Mallory bodies are present.
7. Mallory bodies and fat diminish in late stages and the size shrinks progressively.

Laboratory Findings
- Bilirubin increased
- Alkaline phosphatase increased
- Neutrophilic leukocytosis
- Alanine aminotranferase elevated
- Aspartate aminotranferase elevated.

CIRRHOSIS (Figs 3.44a to c)

Cirrhosis is characterised by the following:
1. It is diffuse and irreversible.
2. There is loss of normal lobular architecture.
3. There is damage to the hepatocytes with replacement of liver tissue by fibrosis (scar tissue). The viable hepatocytes divide and form regenerative nodules.

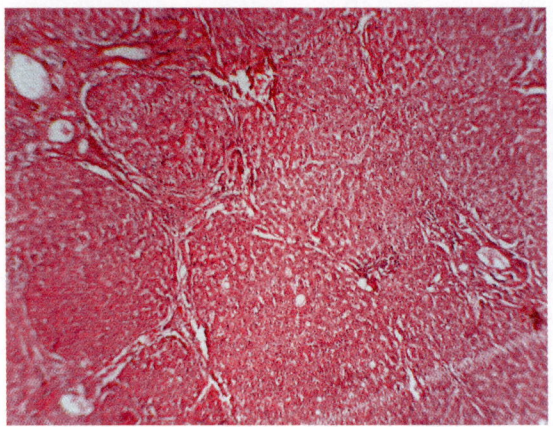

Fig. 3.44b: Photomicrograph of cirrhosis

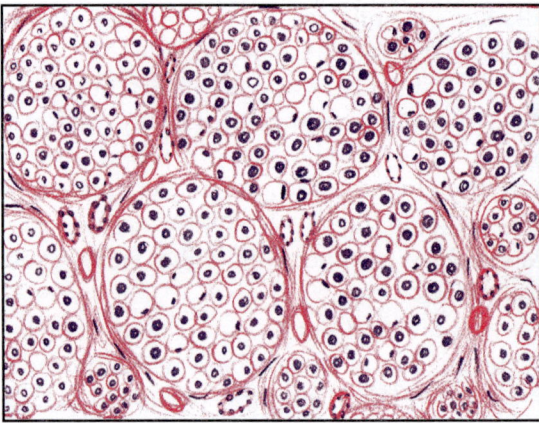

Fig. 3.44c: Schematic diagram of microscopy of cirrhosis

4. There is re-organisation of the vascular channels.
5. These changes lead to loss of liver function.

Clinical features: May be asymptomatic or may present with nonspecific clinical manifestations like anaemia, weight loss and weakness. Advanced cases may present with signs of hepatic failure like GI bleeding, hepatic encephalopathy, hepatorenal syndrome. Death in these patients is due to liver failure, complications related to portal hypertention, and development of hepatocellular carcinoma.

Classification of cirrhosis is given in Tables 3.27 and 3.28.

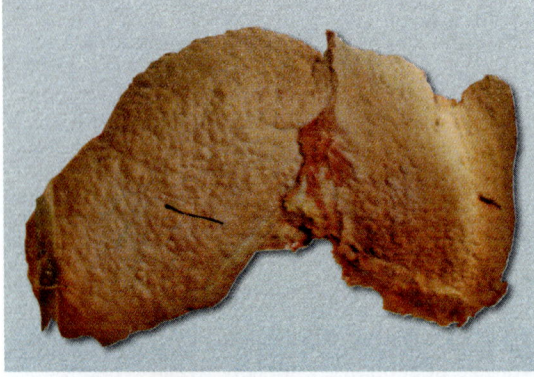

Fig. 3.44a: Gross picture of cirrhosis

Table 3.27: Etiological classification of cirrhosis

Alcoholic liver disease	Metabolic diseases

Chronic hepatitis
  B and C viruses
  Autoimmune hepatitis
  Drugs
Non-alcoholic fatty liver disease (NASH)
Biliary diseases
  Primary biliary cirrhosis
  Extrahepatic biliary obstruction
  Sclerosing cholangitis
Haemochromatosis
Autoimmune hepatitis
Cystic fibrosis
Hepatic venous outflow obstruction
	Wilson's disease
	α_1-antitrypsin deficiency
	Tyrosinemia
	Glycogen storage disease
	Hereditory fructose intolerance
	Indian childhood cirrhosis
	Cryptogenic cirrhosis

Table 3.28: Morphological classification of cirrhosis

Micronodular cirrhosis: Uniform, small nodules up to 3 mm in diameter, thin fibrous septae. Previously this was known as Laennec's cirrhosis.
Often caused by alcohol damage, haemochromatosis, Wilson's disease, primary biliary disease, Indian childhood disease, hepatic venous outflow obstruction
Macronodular cirrhosis: Large irregular nodules, coarse and thick bands of connective tissue, nodules >3 mm. Often seen following hepatitis B infection, toxins and poisoning.
Mixed micro and macronodular cirrhosis: The causes of micronodular cirrhosis can progress to this morphological type.

Investigations

Liver tests—usually elevation of serum aminotransferases, alkaline phosphatase and gammaglutamyl transpeptidase, increase in bilirubin levels.

Tests for synthetic function—serum albumin and prothrombin (reduced).

Endoscopy, ultrasound, CT.

HEPATOCELLULAR CARCINOMA

Hepatocellular carcinoma (HCC) represents 90% of the primary tumours of liver. This accounts for 5% of all the tumors, and third most common cause of death globally. Aetiology of HCC is given in Table 3.29. The highest incidence is seen in geographical areas with higher incidence of hepatitis B

Table 3.29: Aetiology of hepatocellular carcinoma (HCC)

Hepatotrophic viruses—HBV, HCV Pre-existing cirrhosis Alcohol Chemical carcinogens—exposure to thorostat as radiological contrast medium Hemochromatosis Wilson's disease α_1-antitrypsin deficiency Tyrosenemia	Drugs—anabolic steroids contraceptive pills Aflatoxins—metabolic product of *Aspergillus flavus* Schistosomiasis

(most infected are Africa, Asia and pacific islands) and C virus (most infected are Mediterranean and European regions) infections. Males are at higher risk than females.

Signs and symptoms
- Nonspecific symptoms
- Abdominal pain, fullness or with mass
- Fever with chills
- Anorexia and weight loss
- Jaundice
- Cachexia
- GI or oesophageal variceal bleeding
- Liver failure and hepatic coma
- Invasion of hepatic vein and spread to inferior vena cava: Presents with right heart failure.

On examination
- Liver is enlarged
- Splenomegaly
- Ascites.

Macroscopy: Three types
1. Unifocal—single large mass
2. Multifocal—many nodules of varying sizes (Fig. 3.45a)
3. Diffusely infiltrating/spreading type—involves entire liver blending with underlying cirrhosis (Fig. 3.45b).

The tumour tissue is paler than normal surrounding tissue. The tumour tissue sometimes has greenish hue. Tumour emboli in portal vein is a common finding.

Microscopy (Fig. 3.45c): There are four architectural and cytological types (patterns) of hepatocellular carcinoma:
1. Pseudoglandular (adenoid)
2. Pleomorphic (giant cell)
3. Clear cell
4. Fibrolamellar variant.

In well-differentiated forms, tumour cells resemble hepatocytes, form trabeculae, cords and nests, and may contain bile pigment in cytoplasm. The cords and trabeculae are 3–4 cell layer thick and are separated by sinusoids.

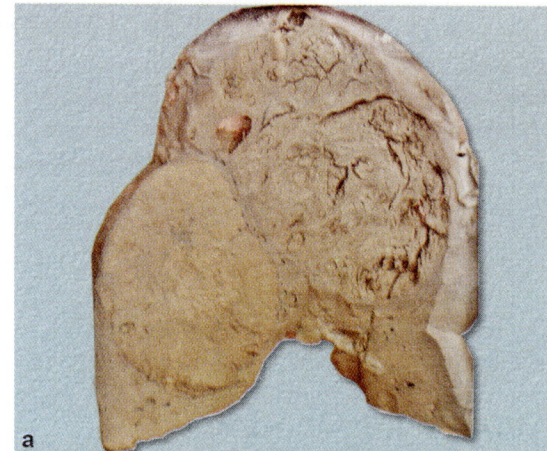

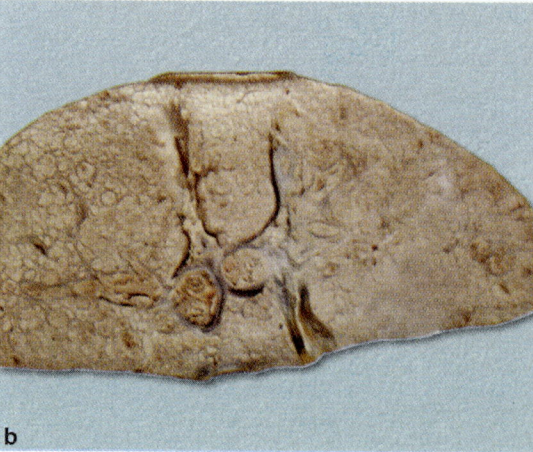

Figs 3.45a and b: Gross pictures of HCC, (a) multifocal, (b) diffusely infiltrative

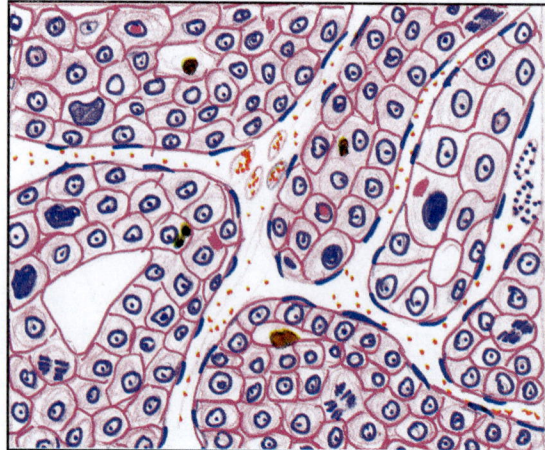

Fig. 3.45c: Schematic diagram of microscopy of HCC

In poorly differentiated forms, malignant epithelial cells show varying degree of differentiation. The tumour cells are discohesive, pleomorphic, anaplastic with tumour giant cells. Abnormal mitosis are frequent. Nucleoli are prominent. Cytoplasm is scanty and basophilic. The tumour cells may exhibit intranuclear pseudoinclusions.

The tumour has a scant stroma and central necrosis because of the poor vascularisation.

The tumour cells have tendency to invade along the hepatic vein.

Important features that guide treatment include:
- Size
- Spread
- Involvement of liver vessels
- Presence of a tumour capsule
- Presence of extrahepatic metastases
- Presence of daughter nodules
- Vascularity of the tumour.

Investigations
- Increased levels of bilirubin
- Alpha fetoproteins (AFP) produced by 70% of HCC and it is >400 ng/ml (cut off 20 ng/ml)
- CT and MRI—localizes the mass
- Biopsy to confirm the diagnosis
- These patients may have hyperglycaemia, hypercalcaemia, polycythemia, hypercholesterolaemia.

FIBROLAMELLAR VARIANT OF HCC

This distinctive variant of hepatocellular carcinoma clinically and pathologically, occurs in young individuals between the age groups of 20 and 40 years of age. This has following features:
1. This has no risk factors.
2. Not associated with chronic hepatitis or cirrhosis.
3. The tumour is well-circumscribed with central scar, microscopy has laminated fibrous layers with tumour cells scattered in between. The tumour cells have low nuclear cytoplasmic ratio with abundant granular eosinophilic (oncocytic) cytoplasm.
4. AFP levels normal or modestly elevated.
5. Prognosis: Has indolent course and 60% are surgically resectable.

Cholangiocarcinoma

Cholangiocarcinoma is a relatively rare primary neoplasm of liver arising from the bile ducts classified under adenocarcinoma (Table 3.30).

Table 3.30: Risk factors for cholangiocarcinoma	
Primary sclerosing cholangitis	Smoking
Ulcerative colitis	Pancreatitis (inflammation of the pancreas)
Parasitic liver diseases—liver fluke	Infection with HIV
Viral hepatitis	Exposure to asbestos
Alcoholic liver disease	Exposure to radon or other radioactive chemicals
Cirrhosis	Exposure to dioxin, nitrosamines, or polychlorinated
Congenital liver diseases	biphenyls (PCBs)

Exercise 48

Neoplasms of Breast

FIBROADENOMA

This benign tumour is common in reproductive age.

Gross: These are sharply circumscribed, freely mobile masses and measure about 1 to 2 cm in diameter (Fig. 3.46a).

Microscopy: There is proliferation of glandular and stromal tissue. The ducts are round to tubular, lined by single or multi-layered epithelium (pericanalicular pattern) or compressed into slit-like spaces having active proliferation of stroma (intracanalicular pattern) (Figs 3.46b and c).

PHYLLODES TUMOUR

The term phyllodes tumour was previously called cystosarcoma phyllodes. Phyllodes tumour generally occurs in older age groups than fibroadenoma.

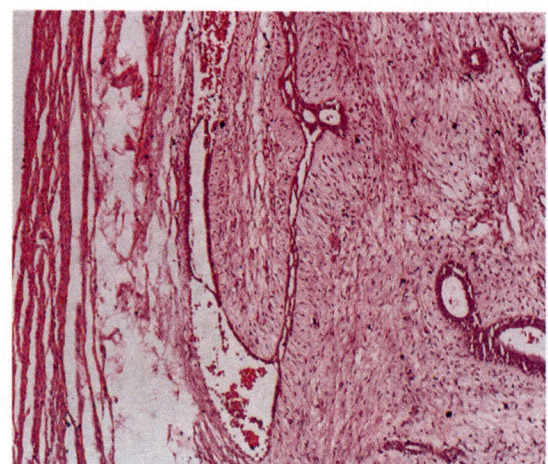

Fig. 3.46b: Photomicrograph of fibroadenoma, note stromal and glandular proliferation

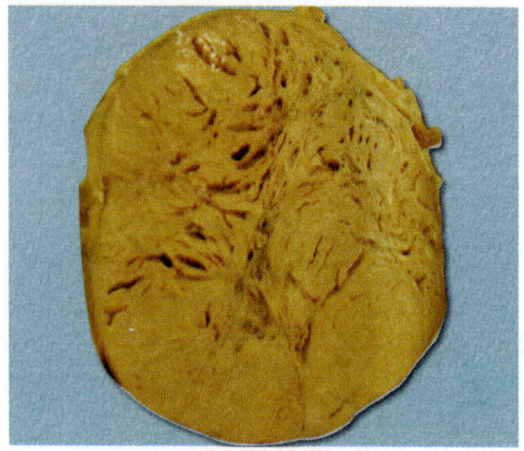

Fig. 3.46a: Gross picture of fibroadenoma

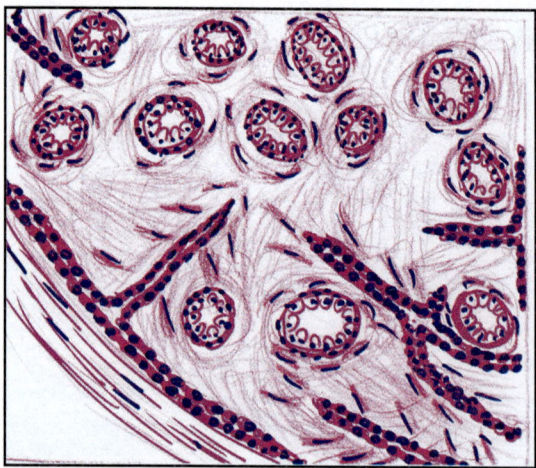

Fig. 3.46c: Schematic diagram of microscopy of fibroadenoma

Gross: These attain large sizes than fibroadenomas. These are fast growing tumours. Cut section, the glands exhibit leaf like clefts and slits, hence the name phyllodes (in Greek *phyllodes* means leaf like).

Microscopy: Phyllodes tumour has features similar to fibroadenoma, but has predominant stromal hypercellularity. Thus, the tissue is composed of epithelial and stromal component. There is predominant proliferation of periductal stroma than the glandular element.

These can be benign, borderline or malignant depending upon histological features, including stromal cellularity, nuclear features and mitoses. Most of the times mitosis less than 5/10 HPF and between 5 and 10/HPF suggests benign and borderline phyllodes respectively. The features suggestive of malignancy are:
- Mitotic activity > 10/10 HPF
- Atypia of stroma
- Stromal overgrowth
- Infiltrating margins
- Haemorrhage and necrosis.

Metaplasia in stroma is more frequent than fibroadenomas. Stromal metaplasia to fatty tissue, bone, cartilage and skeletal muscle are known. Epithelium can show hyperplasia and squamous metaplasia. Apocrine metaplasia is less frequent than fibroadenoma.

Most of the benign phyllodes tumours remain localised and can be cured by wide excision (Figs 3.47a and b). About 15% of the malignant tumours may metastasise to distant sites. Recurrences are known in benign, borderline and malignant tumours.

FIBROCYSTIC DISEASE

Fibrocystic disease (FCD) is an important lesion as it may simulate the clinical, radiographical, and gross appearance of carcinoma and also its possible association with carcinoma. Alternative terms like fibrocystic change, mammary dysplasia, etc. have been used. FCD usually has the following morphological changes:
- Epithelial hyperplasia with or without atypia
- Apocrine change
- Cyst formation
- Chronic inflammation
- Fibrosis
- Fibroadenomatoid change
- Calcification.

Epithelial Hyperplasia with or Without Atypia

The lobules, ducts and ductules may be filled with proliferated cuboidal epithelium. Sometimes papillary excrescences project into the lumen which is termed ductal papillomatosis. Epithelial hyperplasia can be with or without atypia. The degree of hyperplasia can be mild, moderate or severe. The epithelium may show atypical changes in

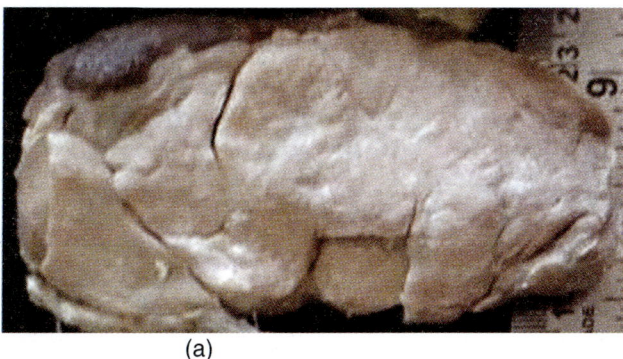
(a)

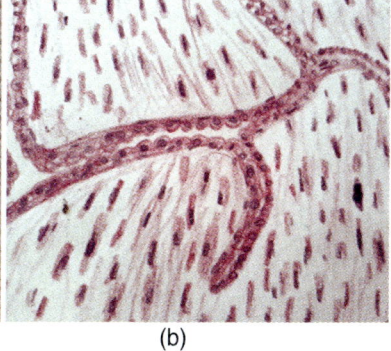
(b)

Figs 3.47a and b: (a) Gross picture of phyllodes tumour, note extensive stromal proliferation with slits or leaf-like clefts (*Courtesy:* HOD and staff of Pathology, SDM College, Dharwad), (b) Microscopy of phyllodes tumour

the lobular or ductular hyperplasia, the recognition of which is very important. These are associated with fivefold increase in risk of developing carcinoma. When associated with family history, the risk increases by tenfold.

Apocrine change: This is very common change and is observed in dilated and cystic structures.

Cyst formation: These can be microscopic or grossly visible cysts. They usually contain cloudy yellow or clear fluid. The cysts may rupture and elicit an inflammatory response in the stroma with abundant foamy macrophages and cholesterol clefts. The cysts may have flattened epithelium or may only have a fibrous wall with or without the epithelium.

Chronic inflammation: This is common but secondary feature in FCD. This is related to rupture of the cysts and release of secretions in the stroma. Lymphocytes, plasma cells and foamy histiocytes are the predominant cells.

Fibrosis: This change is often present, but varies in degree. This is probably due to secondary reaction to rupture of the cysts.

Fibroadenomatoid change: This has microscopic picture reminiscent of fibroadenoma, but lacking the sharp circumscription and is less common change in FCD.

Calcification: This is less common.

NONINVASIVE BREAST CARCINOMAS

Duct carcinoma in situ (DCIS): This has different are achitectural patterns like solid, comedo, cribriform, papillary, micropapillary and clinging types. Necrosis may be present. The nuclear features may be of low grade to high grade (Fig. 3.48).

Comedo type of DCIS: This has high grade nuclear features with central extensive necrosis. The resected tissue sample when pressed, the necrotic material protrudes like toothpaste or worm. Calcification is frequently seen. The progrosis of DCIS is excellent after simple mastectomy.

Lobular carcinoma in Situ (LCIS): This has uniform monomorphic cells with bland, round

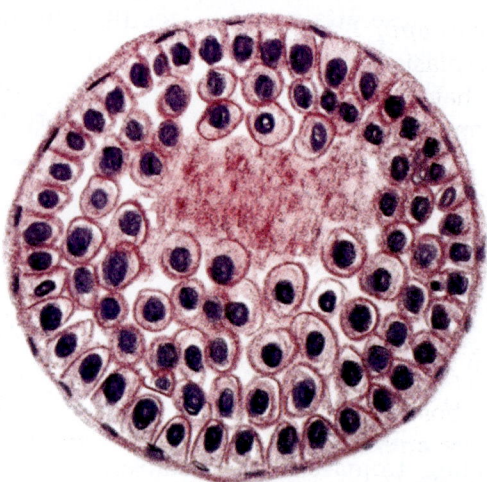

Fig. 3.48: Microscopy in duct carcinoma *in situ* (DCIS), note intact basement membrane and necrosis

nuclei and occur in loosely cohesive clusters inside the lobules. Signet ring cells are common. No calcification in present. LCIS will eventually develop into lobular carcinoma.

GYNAECOMASTIA

Gynaecomastia is the enlargement of male breast resulting from hypertrophy and hyperplasia of both glandular and stromal components.

Causes:
- Increased estrogen activity—exogenous or endogenous
- Decreased androgen activity
  Before the age of 25 years, it is usually related to hormonal pubertal changes.
  Later ages it may be because of following causes:
  1. Hormonally active tumours: Leydig cell tumours of testis, HCG secreting germ cell tumours, carcinoma lung or others
  2. Cirrhosis
  3. Medication: Digitalis, phenytoin.

Clinical features: The mass lies below the nipple. It may be unilateral or bilateral.

Pathology

Gross: It is an oval mass and has elastic consistency with well-circumscribed borders.

Microscopy: There is ductal and stromal hyperplasia surrounded by myxoid stroma with halo effect containing large amounts of mucopolysaccharides (hyaluronic acid).

BREAST CARCINOMA

It is familial and has about 1.5 to 2 times higher risk in women who are having first degree relatives with breast carcinoma. Mutations of p53 gene are present. Estrogen is known to play a role. Women who are on oral contraceptives, those with increased length of reproductive life and also nulliparous women have increased risk of breast carcinoma. 17q21 (BRCA1) is the breast carcinoma susceptibility gene and there is amplification of erbB/neu gene in these patients.

INFILTRATING (INVASIVE) CARCINOMA

The most common histological type of invasive breast carcinoma is invasive ductal carcinoma (Table 3.31). The salient features of these are described below.

Infiltrating duct carcinoma: Not otherwise specified (IDS-NOS)/No special type (IDS NST— majority of invasive duct carcinomas fall in this type (Fig. 3.49a). This is also called schirrhous carcinoma.

Gross: The gross appearance of this is typical with irregular and stellate outline. They are delimited, firm or hard, about 1 to 2 cms masses and they infiltrate into the surrounding tissue with fixation to the chest wall. Cut section of the tumour is retracted below the cut surface and it is gritty to cut (Fig 3.49b).

Table 3.31: Histological typing of breast carcinoma WHO (2012)[14]

Benign epithelial tumours: Sclerosing adenosis, apocrine adenosis, adenomas
Intraductal proliferation: Ductal hyperplasia, atypical ductal hyperplasia
Precursor lesions: Duct carcinoma *in situ*, lobular carcinoma *in situ*, atypical lobular hyperplasia
Papillary lesions: Intraductal papilloma, intraductal papillary carcinoma, solid papillary carcinoma
Epithelial myoepithelial: Pleomorphic adenoma, adenoid cystic carcinoma
Epithelial tumours
    Invasive carcinoma—No special type /not otherwise specified
    Invasive lobular carcinoma—Classic, solid, alveolar, pleomorphic
    Tubular carcinoma
    Mucinous carcinoma
    Cribriform carcinoma
    Medullary pattern: Medullary carcinoma, atypical medullary carcinoma, invasive carcinoma
              No special type with medullary feat
    Carcinoma with apocrine differentiation
    Carcinoma with signet ring differentiation
    Secretary carcinoma
    Invasive papillary
    Salivary gland tumours
Neuroendocrine tumours
Metaplastic carcinoma with mesenchymal differentiation
    Adenosarcoma
    Squamous cell carcinoma
    Spindle cell carcinoma
    With mesenchymal differentiation
Mesenchymal tumours
Fibroepithelial tumours
Malignant lymphomas
Metastatic tumours

Microscopy: The malignant cells are in cords, solid cell nests, tubules and glandular pattern. Depending upon the nuclear atypia, tubule formation and mitosis, they are categorized into well, moderately or poorly differentiated varieties (Fig. 3.49c).

Some of the Invasive Breast Carcinomas with Favourable Prognosis

- Tubular carcinoma
- Mucinous carcinoma
- Cribriform carcinoma
- Medullary carcinoma
- Secretary carcinoma.

Other Breast Carcinomas

- Metaplastic carcinoma
- Inflammatory carcinoma.

Tubular carcinoma: The average age of the patients for tubular carcinoma is around 50 years. These are well-differentiated tumours and have favourable prognosis. Grossly, these do not differ much from IDC-NOS. They are less than 2 cm, hard consistency and poorly circumscribed margins.

Microscopically, the glands are well-differentiated, there is absence of necrosis, no mitoses, and scanty pleomorphism. There are irregularly arranged tubules lined by single layer of epithelium with low mitoses and little pleomorphism. The cytoplasmic apical snouts are frequently seen. The glandular lumina is open and have angulated outlines. The intervening stroma is fibroblastic. The tubular carcinoma should be called only when tubular component is more than 90%.

Mucinous carcinoma: This is also called mucoid, colloid and gelatinous carcinoma. This usually occurs in postmenopausal women. Grossly, well-circumscribed, soft, crepitant on palpation and contains jelly like material or gelatinous mass. Foci of haemorrhage are frequent. This variant has favourable prognosis.

Microscopically, has small cluster of malignant tumour cells showing little pleomorphism and low mitoses; and these cells are floating in a sea or pool of mucin which is

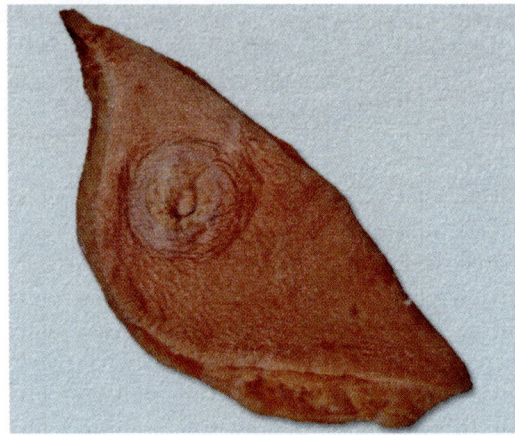

Fig. 3.49a: Gross picture of infiltrating duct carcinoma breast, note retracted nipple

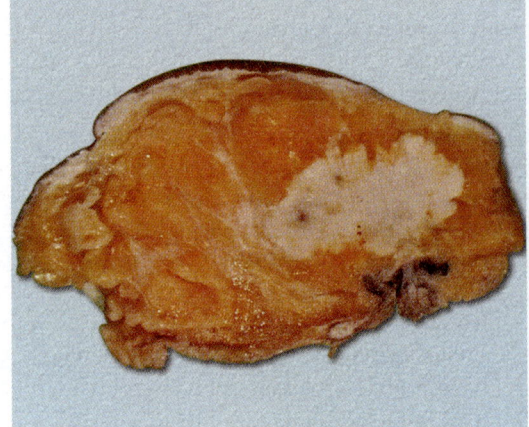

Fig. 3.49b: Gross picture (C/S) of infiltrating duct carcinoma breast

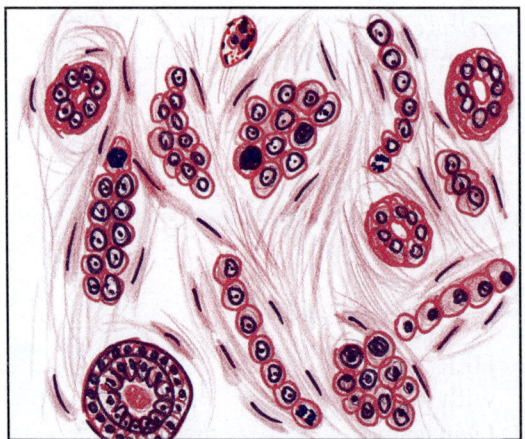

Fig. 3.49c: Schematic diagram of microscopy of infiltrating duct carcinoma breast

surrounded by bands of fibrous connective tissue. Intracellular mucin may be seen.

Medullary carcinoma: This occurs usually in patients of less than 50 years of age. It is well-circumscribed, soft in consistency and often large with fleshy tumour mass. Cut section is solid, homogenous, and gray with small foci of necrosis. These have favourable prognosis. Microscopically, has syncytial growth pattern, with cells in sheets and and anastomosing bands. Stroma is sparse. This pattern should be more than 75% of the tumour to call as medullary carcinoma. There is lymphocytic and plasma cell infiltration in the stroma and necrosis is frequent. The malignant cells are large, with marked nuclear pleomorphism, prominent nucleoli, and frequent mitoses. Tumour giant cells may be present. Sometimes squamous metaplasia may be observed. The plasma-lymphocytic infiltrate and syncytial growth pattern of cells are important to designate the tumour as medullary carcinoma.

Prognostic Factors

1. *Age of the patient:* Age of the patient of lesser than 50 years has better prognosis.
2. *Histologic types:* Special types of invasive carcinomas (tubular, mucinous, papillary and secretary) have long survival.
3. *Tumour grade:* With Bloom Richardson grading, well-differentiated grade 1 tumours- have long survival (Table 3.32).
4. *Estrogen and progesterone receptors:* Tumours with hormone receptors positive cancer have better prognosis. 80% tumours with estrogen and progesterone receptors respond to hormone manipulation. Tumours with estrogen/progesterone receptors negativity less likely respond to hormone manipulation.
5. *During pregnancy and lactation:* Aggressive behaviour.
6. HER 2/neu over expression is associated with poor prognosis.
7. *Lympho-vascular invasion:* Poor prognosis.
8. *Tumours with high proliferation rate (S phase fraction, Ki 67):* Have a worse prognosis.

Table 3.32: Modified Bloom Richardson grading

Tubule formation, nuclear features and mitosis	score
Tubule formation	
More than 75%	1
10–75%	2
Less than 10%	3
Nuclear pleomorphism	
Small, regular, uniform	1
Moderately increased, variable size	2
Marked variation	3
Mitotic count	
0–9	1
10–19	2
More than 20	3

Leitz or Ortholux 25x objective or field diameter of 0.59 mm

Grade

3–5 points	Grade I	Well-differentiated
6–7 points	Grade II	Moderately differentiated
8–9 points	Grade III	Poorly differentiated

9. *DNA content:* Aneuploid tumours abnormal DNA indices have a slightly worse prognosis.
10. BRCA1 and BRCA2 mutations are associated with worse overall survival.
11. Early diagnosis with small tumours and devoid of lymph node metastasis has lesser stage and favourable survival.
12. Size of breast carcinoma less than 1 cm and associated with negative lymph nodes have better prognosis.
13. Tumours with pushing margins have better prognosis.
14. Tumour necrosis, increased lymph node metastasis and high grade tumours have decreased survival.
15. Increased micro-vessel density around the tumour has aggressive course.

MOLECULAR CLASSIFICATION

Luminal A: The breast carcinoma of this type is ER/PR positive, luminal CK positive, HER2 negative (50%) and responds to hormone therapy, response to chemotherapy variable, and includes tubular, cribriform, low grade infiltrating duct carcinoma-NOS and classic lobular carcinoma. This type of breast carcinoma has good prognosis.

Luminal B: Luminal B type of breast carcinoma is ER/PR variable, luminal CK positive, HER2 variable. This type has higher proliferative activity than luminal A, higher histological grade, includes high grade infiltrating duct carcinoma-NOS and micropapillary carcinoma, responds to hormone therapy not as good as luminal A, response to chemotherapy is variable and prognosis is not good when compared to luminal A type of breast carcinoma.

HER2 positive: HER2 postive breast carcinoma are p53 positive, high grade, responds to herceptin and anthracyclin based chemotherapy. This includes high grade infiltrating duct carcinoma-NOS.

Basal like: In this type, basal epithelial genes positive (cytokeratin 5/6 and others, EGFR) and ER/PR negative, HER2 negative, p53 positive, BRCA1 mutations positive, most are triple negative, includes high grade infiltrating duct carcinoma-NOS, metaplastic carcinoma and medullary carcinoma. This type of tumour does not respond to herceptin (Transtuzumab). This occurs in young women. It is sensitive to platinum-based chemotherapy, relapse is rapid and has poor prognosis.

Note: Even though medullary carcinoma is included in this type, it may have better prognosis.

Following is the ER/PR and HER2 status with relation age of occurrence, survival, recurrence, etc.

1. *ER positive, HER2 negative:* These have low proliferation rate, occur in older females, detected by mammography, bone metastasis is 70%, viscera 25% and brain less than 10%, associated with long survival and relapse later than 10 years.
2. *ER positive/negative and HER2 positive:* Occurs in young females, associated with p53 mutations, relapse is short and has survival less than 10 years.
3. *Triple negative (ER negative, PR negative, HER2 negative):* These occur in younger females, associated with BRCA1 mutations and have short survival.

Exercise 49

Kidney Lesions

GLOMERULAR DISEASES

Classification of Glomerular Diseases

1. *Primary glomerular diseases:* The disease begins in glomerulus and causes direct damage only to the glomerulus. Primary glomerular diseases include the following:
   - Acute proliferative glomerulonephritis
     - Post-streptococcal
     - Non-streptococcal causes
   - IgA nephropathy
   - Hereditary nephritis: Alports, Fabry's and thin basement membrane lesion
   - C3 glomerulopathy/dense deposit disease
   - Rapidly progressive glomerulonephritis/ Crescentic glomerulonephritis:
     - Due to anti-GBM antibodies: Goodpasture's syndrome
     Due to immune complex deposition
     - ANCA-associated glomerulonephritis:
   - Both anti-GBM disease and ANCAs-associated glomerulonephritis
   - Minimal change disease
   - Membranous glomerulopathy
   - Focal and segmental glomerulosclerosis
   - Membranoproliferative glomerulonephritis
   - Chronic glomerulonephritis.
2. *Secondary glomerular diseases:* Glomerular diseases that occur secondary to certain systemic diseases.
   - Lupus nephritis
   - Diabetic nephropathy
   - Amyloidosis
   - Cast nephropathy
   - Goodpasture's syndrome
   - Microscopic polyangitis
   - Wegener's granulomatosis
   - Henoch-Schönlein purpura
   - Bacterial endocarditis
   - Microscopic polyarteritis/polyangitis
   - GN due to extrarenal infection
   - Thrombotic microangiopathy

PATHOGENESIS OF GLOMERULAR DISEASES

The important mechanisms established are:
1. Antibody-mediated injury
   i. *In situ* immune complex deposition
      - Antibodies directed against glomerular cell components
      - Antibodies against planted antigens
      - Heymann nephritis.
   ii. Circulating immune complex deposition: Injury resulting from deposition of soluble circulating antigen-antibody immune complexes in the glomerulus
2. Complement system-mediated injury
3. Cell-mediated immune response.

Antibody-Mediated Injury

In situ immune complex deposition mediated glomerular injury: This can be with following mechanisms:

Anti-GBM antibodies directed against normal components of the glomerular basement membrane: The Anti-GBM antibodies bind to intrinsic antigens in the GBM, results in linear pattern of staining by immunofluorescence technique. The Anti-GBM antibodies cross react with basement membrane component of other tissues especially of the lung alveoli causing simultaneous lung and kidney lesions. This is termed Goodpasture's syndrome. The antibodies are to the GBM component which is non-collagenous domain NC1 of the alpha 3 chain of type IV collagen (Fig. 3.50).

Antibodies against planted antigens: In this type nephritis, the antibodies react with planted antigens in the glomerulus which are normally not present. The planted antigens include cationic molecules which bind to anionic components of the glomerulus. These are DNA, nucleosome, and other nuclear proteins. Viruses, bacteria and parasitic products and drugs may also get planted. Antibodies to these planted antigens induce a discrete pattern of immunoglobulin deposition which is granular by immunofluorescence and indistinguishable from intrinsic antigens (Fig. 3.51).

The Heymann nephritis: Human counterpart of membranous nephropathy which is well-explained by Heymann nephritis model in the rats is mediated by Th2 response, which is observed by increase in percentage of IL-4 and IL-10 in the peripheral blood T-cells. This correlates well with the amount of proteinuria. Once the disease sets in antibodies against megalin (gp 330) gets deposited at the subepithelial space of glomerulus and trigger podocytes injury.

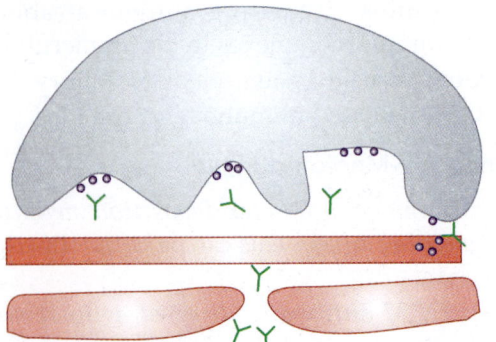

Fig. 3.50: Anti-GBM antibodies directed against normal components of the glomerular basement membrane

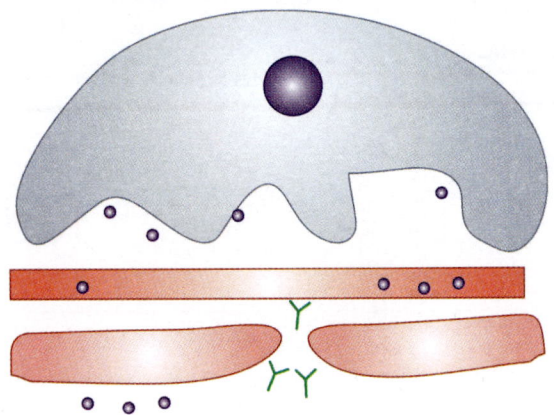

Fig. 3.51: Schematic diagram, antibodies to the planted antigens in glomerulus

Circulating immune complex deposition: Injury resulting from deposition of soluble circulating antigen–antibody immune complexes in the glomerulus. Here the antigen is endogenous origin as in SLE or exogenous as in streptococcal infection, Hepatitis B viral infection, parasitic as in *Plasmodium falciparum* malaria and spirochete infection (*Trepanema pallidum*). The antigen-antibody complexes are formed *in situ* or in the circulation and then they are trapped in the glomerulus (Fig. 3.52). Here they produce injury, activate complement and recruit leukocytes.

Thus, there is leukocytic infiltration, proliferation glomerular cells like endothelial, mesangeal, and parietal epithelial cells. Electron microscopy reveals these immune complexes as electron dense deposits or lumps/clumps which may lie at any of the three locations like:

1. Mesangium
2. Subendothelial location (between the endothelial cells and the GBM).
3. Subepithelial location (between the GBM and podocytes).

The immunoglobulins and complement in these deposits can be demonstrated by immunofluorescence microscopy.

Mesangial deposits are usually observed in IgA nephropathy and class I and II of lupus nephritis. These deposits lead to activation of

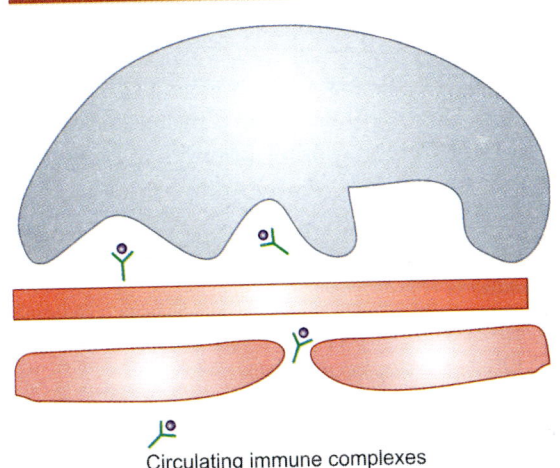

Fig. 3.52: Schematic diagram, deposition of soluble circulating antigen–antibody immune complexes in the glomerulus

mesangial cells which initiate activation of the complement, coagulation and release of cytokines and growth factors. The C5b-9 mediated mechanism has been implicated in the pathogenesis of mesangial deposits and proliferation of mesangial cells leading to glomerular hypercellularity.

Subendothelial deposits in type 1 MPGN and class III and IV of lupus nephritis, these immune complexes recruit circulating inflammatory cells like neutrophils, lymphocytes, macrophages and platelets activate effector cells and cause injury. C5a and IL-8 recruit neutrophils at the site of injury, phagocytose immune complex aggregates get activated and generate reactive oxygen species following respiratory burst.

Subepithelial deposition are characteristic as in AGN (humps) and MGN with formation of spike like deposits.

Complement-Mediated Injury

The major pathway for antibody initiated injury is complement leukocyte-mediated. There is generation of complement components which are chemotactic mainly C5a. There is recruiting of neutrophils and monocytes. The neutrophils release proteases which damage and degrade the GBM. Oxygen derived free radicals cause cell damage. In some cases the C5-C9 membrane attack complex cause damage to epithelial cells and detachment. Components of complement stimulate mesangeal and epithelial cells to secrete various mediators of cell injury. There is increased TGF beta which stimulates synthesis of extracellular matrix and altered GBM composition and thickening.

In complement-mediated injury, there is persistent activation of alternate complement pathway by following mechanisms.

Autoantibodies

- *C3 nephritic factor (C3Nef):* This is an autoantibody to the alternate complement pathway's C3 convertase.
- *Autoantibodies to the complement alternative pathway regulatory proteins:* Complement factor H (CFH) and factor B.

Genetic abnormalities of complement component genes:
- C3 mutation
- Factor H mutation
- Allelic variants of complement factor I (CFI), CFH, C3.

Various renal diseases exhibit deposition of complement in the glomeruli like dense deposit disease, C3 glomerulopathy and C1q nephropathy. Certain renal diseases also show presence of immunoglobulins along with complement deposition like post-infectious glomerulonephritis, membranous nephropathy, IgA nephropathy and lupus nephritis.

Cell-Mediated Immune Response

The sensitised T cells formed during cell-mediated immune reaction can cause glomerular injury.

The cell-mediated immune responses are implicated in pathogenesis of minimal change disease, focal and segmental glomerulosclerosis (FSGS), pauci-immune crescentic glomerulonephritis and class IV lupus nephritis. The lymphocytes and macrophages recruited usually release tissue factors and TGF-β that initiate fibrin deposition as well as extracellular matrix deposition. The crescentic GN is predominantly thought to be of Th1-mediated response. Macrophages release ROS and inflammatory cytokines causing Bowman capsule injury, mediating formation of crescents and influx of inflammatory cells.

Many glomerulonephritis are result of an autoimmune process. Loss of self-tolerance and exposure to a aetiological agents lead to immune complex formation, mostly by the mechanism of molecular mimicry and epitope spreading. Some antigens that are implicated are listed below:

Non-collagenous domain of the alpha-III chain of type IV collage	Goodpasture's syndrome
DNA-nucleosome complex	Lupus nephrits (non-renal self antigens)
HCV antigen- containing cryoglobulins	HCV associated MPGN

NEPHRITIC SYNDROME

Nephritic syndrome is characterised by:
- Haematuria
- Urine sediment: Manifested by dysmorphic RBCs and RBC casts and often white blood cells
- Reduced glomerular filtration rate (GFR),
- High serum creatinine and blood urea nitrogen levels
- Variable degrees of hypertension
- Oliguria
- Oedema.

The primary glomerular diseases which fall under nephritic syndrome are:
- Acute postinfectious glomerulonephritis
- IgA nephropathy (Berger's disease)
- Hereditary nephritis
- C3 glomerulonephritis and dense deposit disease.

NEPHROTIC SYNDROME

The primary and secondary to glomerular diseases which fall under nephrotic syndrome are:

Primary Glomerular Diseases
- Minimal change disease
- Focal segmental glomerulosclerosis
- Membranous glomerulonephritis
- Membranoproliferative glomerulonephritis
- IgA nephropathy.

Secondary Glomerular Diseases
- Lupus nephritis
- Diabetic nephropathy
- Amyloidosis
- Cast nephropathy
- Goodpasture's syndrome
- Microscopic polyangitis
- Wegener's granulomatosis
- Henoch-Schönlein purpura
- Bacterial endocarditis
- Microscopic polyarteritis/polyangitis
- GN due to extrarenal infection
- Thrombotic microangiopathy.

The classical features are:
- Heavy, albumin-dominant proteinuria (>3000 mg/day or spot urine protein/protein to creatinine ratio of >3000 mg of protein/gram of creatinine)
- Hypoalbuminemia
- Oedema
- Hyperlipidemia
- Lipiduria.

Acute Glomerulonephritis (AGN)

Post-streptococcal Acute Glomerulonephritis

- It is seen 1 to 4 weeks after a streptococcal infection of the pharynx or skin (impetigo)
- Caused by group A β-haemolytic streptococci are nephritogenic, types 12, 4, and 1
- Affects children 6 to 10 years of age
- It is immunologically mediated disease
- It is characterised by diffuse proliferation of glomerular cells
- The exogenous antigen-induced disease pattern is postinfectious glomerulonephritis
- The endogenous antigen-induced disease is the nephritis of SLE.

General Pathology and Systemic Pathology

Pathogenesis
- Principal antigenic determinants are streptococcal pyogenic exotoxin B (SpeB) and its zymogen precursor (zSpeB)
- Activation of the complement system and consumption of complement components leads to low serum complement levels.
- Granular immune deposits in the glomeruli.

Clinical course
- In children, malaise, fever, nausea, oliguria
- Periorbital oedema
- Mild to moderate hypertension
- Haematuria (smoky or cola-coloured urine) 1 to 2 weeks after recovery from a sore throat
- In adults—sudden hypertension or edema, with elevation of BUN.

Investigations
- Urine-red cell casts in the urine, mild proteinuria (usually less than 1 g/day)
- Elevations of antistreptococcal antibody titers
- Decline in the serum concentration of C3 and other components of the complement cascade.

Complications: Can progress to rapidly progressive glomerulonephritis or chronic glomerulonephritis.

Morphology (Fig. 3.53a)
- The classic diagnostic picture is one of enlarged, hypercellular glomeruli
- The hypercellularity is caused by leukocytic infiltration, proliferation of endothelial and mesangial cells; and crescent formation
- Interstitial oedema and inflammation
- Tubules contains red cell casts.

Immunofluorescence microscopy granular deposits of IgG, IgM, and C3 in the mesangium and along the glomerular basement membrane (GBM).

Electron microscopic findings are discrete, amorphous, electron-dense deposits on the epithelial side of the membrane, often having the appearance of "humps" representing the antigen-antibody complexes at the epithelial cell surface.

Subendothelial and intramembranous deposits and mesangial deposits may be present.

Non-streptococcal Acute Glomerulonephritis
Occurs sporadically in association with other infections, including:
- Bacterial (e.g. staphylococcal endocarditis, pneumococcal pneumonia, and meningococcemia)
- Viral (e.g. hepatitis B, hepatitis C, mumps, human immunodeficiency virus [HIV] infection, varicella, and infectious mononucleosis)
- Parasitic (malaria, toxoplasmosis)
- Granular immunofluorescent deposits and subepithelial humps characteristic of immune complex nephritis are present.

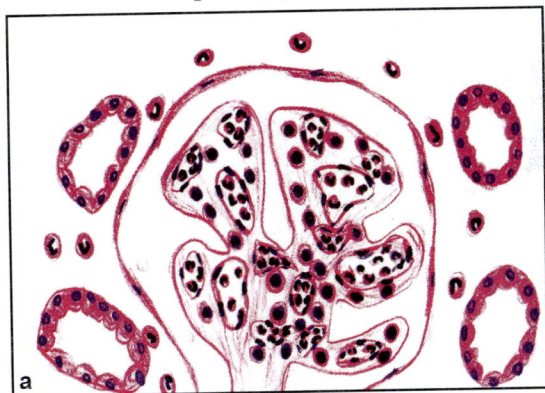

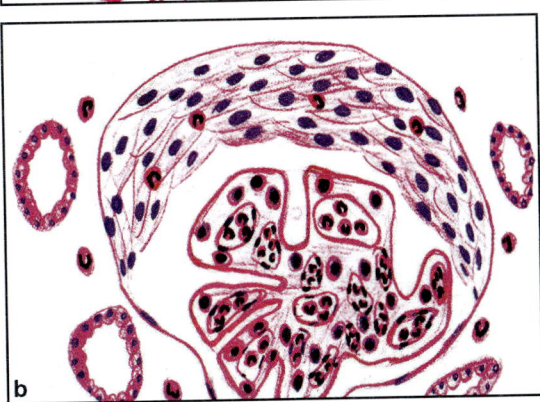

Figs 3.53a and b: (a) Schematic diagrams, microscopy AGN, (b) RPGN

Rapidly Progressive (Crescentic) Glomerulonephritis (Fig. 3.53b)

It is a syndrome characterised clinically by rapid and progressive loss of renal function associated with severe oliguria and signs of nephritic syndrome. Most common histologic picture is the presence of crescents.

Classification and pathogenesis: Rapidly progressive glomerulonephritis (RPGN) is categorised into three groups on the basis of immunological findings.

Type I (anti-GBM antibody) crescentic GN is characterised by linear deposits of IgG and in many cases C3 on the GBM. In some individuals the anti-GBM antibodies cross-react with pulmonary alveolar basement membranes causing pulmonary haemorrhage associate causing with renal failure. This is termed Goodpasture's syndrome.

Type II (immune complex) crescentic GN can be a complication of any of the immune complex nephritides, including postinfectious glomerulonephritis, lupus nephritis, IgA nephropathy, and Henoch-Schönlein purpura.

There is severe injury to the glomeruli with segmental necrosis. GBM breaks with resultant crescent formation with diffuse cellular proliferation, and leukocyte exudation within the glomerular tuft.

Immunofluorescence shows granular (lumpy bumpy) pattern of immune complex deposition.

Type III (pauci-immune) is defined by the lack of anti-GBM antibodies or immune complexes by immunofluorescence and electron microscopy.

Most of the individuals have circulating antineutrophil cytoplasmic antibodies (ANCAs) that produce cytoplasmic (c) or perinuclear (p) staining patterns.

It is a component of a systemic vasculitis such as Wegener granulomatosis or microscopic polyangiitis.

Clinical course
- Haematuria with red blood cell casts in the urine
- Moderate proteinuria
- Hypertension and oedema
- In Goodpasture's syndrome—recurrent hemoptysis or even life-threatening pulmonary haemorrhage.

Gross: The kidneys are enlarged and pale, often with petechial haemorrhages on the cortical surfaces.

Microscopy
1. Glomeruli—focal necrosis, diffuse or focal endothelial proliferation, and mesangial proliferation.
2. Crescents are formed by proliferation of parietal cells and by migration of monocytes and macrophages into the urinary space.
3. Fibrin strands are frequently prominent between the cellular layers in the crescents.

Immunofluorescent microscopy
- Immune complex—mediated cases show granular immune deposits
- Goodpasture's syndrome—linear GBM fluorescence for IgG and complement
- Pauci-immune—little or no deposition of immune reactants.

Electron microscopy shows immune complex deposition (type II).

Serum analyses for anti-GBM antibodies, antinuclear antibodies, and ANCAs.

Treatment
- Goodpasture's syndrome—plasmapheresis with steroids and cytotoxic agents in other forms of RPGN respond well to steroids and cytotoxic agents.
- Chronic dialysis or transplantation. Figures 3.43c and d show the gross specimen and microscopy of chronic glomerulonephritis.

Chronic Pyelonephritis (PN) and Reflux Nephropathy (Figs 3.53c to f)

Chronic pyelonephritis is a disorder in which chronic tubulointerstitial inflammation and

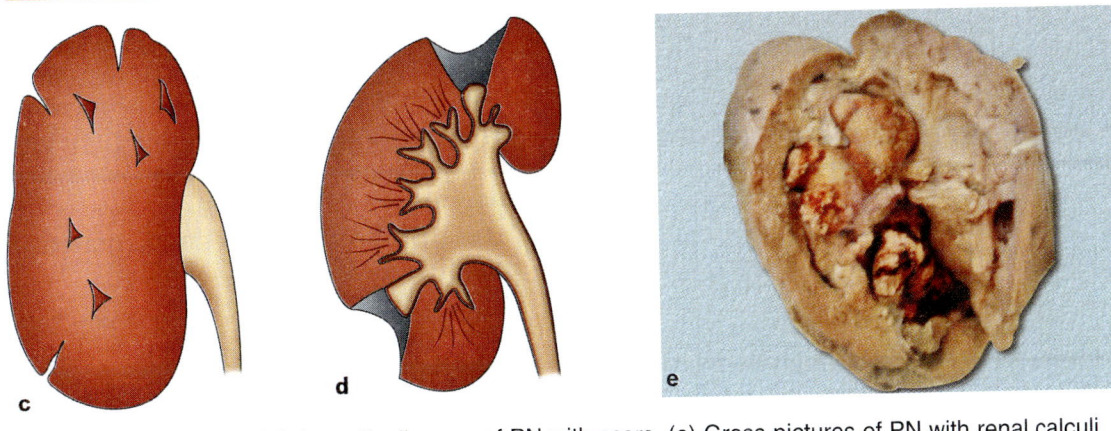

Figs 3.53c to e: (c, d) Schematic diagram of PN with scars, (e) Gross pictures of PN with renal calculi

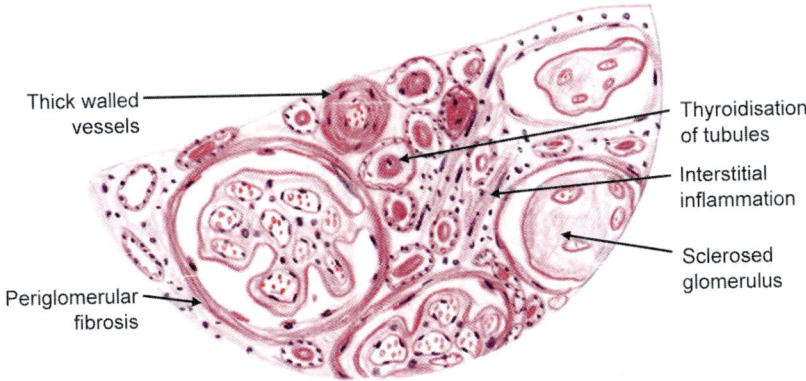

Figs 3.53f: Microscopy in PN

renal scarring are associated with pathologic involvement of the calyces and pelvis. Chronic pyelonephritis is an important cause of end-stage kidney disease.

Chronic pyelonephritis can be divided into two forms:
1. Chronic reflux-associated
2. Chronic obstructive PN.

Reflux nephropathy
- Occurs early in childhood
- There is superimposition of a urinary infection on congenital vesicoureteral reflux and intrarenal reflux
- It may cause scarring and atrophy of one kidney or involve both, leading to chronic renal insufficiency.

Chronic obstructive PN
- Obstruction predisposes the kidney to infection
- Recurrent infections superimposed on diffuse or localised obstructive lesions lead to recurrent bouts of renal inflammation and scarring
- Parenchymal atrophy.

Clinical features
- Insidious in onset or presents with back pain, fever, frequent pyuria, and bacteriuria
- Polyuria and nocturia (because kidney looses its ability to concentrate urine).

Morphology
Gross
- Kidneys are irregularly and asymmetrically scarred.

- Calyces are dilated, blunted, or deformed and flattening of the papillae.

Microscopy
- Involve predominantly tubules and interstitium
- The tubules are atrophied
- Dilated tubules with flattened epithelium may be filled with colloid casts (thyroidisation)
- Chronic interstitial inflammation and fibrosis of cortex and medulla
- Arcuate and interlobular vessels show obliterative intimal sclerosis
- Glomeruli have periglomerular fibrosis

X-ray findings
- Asymmetrically contracted kidneys with coarse scars and blunting and deformity of the calyceal system
- Significant bacteriuria may be present, but it is absent in the late stages
- Proteinuria is mild.

Complication
Secondary focal segmental glomerulosclerosis with significant proteinuria.

The appearance of proteinuria and focal segmental glomerulosclerosis is a poor prognostic sign.

HYDRONEPHROSIS

Hydronephrosis (HN) is dilatation of renal pelvis and calyces with atrophy of renal parenchyma.

This may be due to obstruction to outflow of urine. Obstruction may be sudden or insidious.

Obstruction can be at any level from urethra to renal pelvis. Causes include the following:
1. **Congenital causes:** Atresia of urethra, posterior urethral valves, pyeloureteral junction stenosis and ureteral valves, aberrant renal artery compressing ureter (aberrant renal artery to the inferior pole cross anteriorly to the ureter) and kinking of ureter.
2. **Acquired causes:**
   Foreign bodies: Calculi and necrotic papillae
   Tumours: Nodular hyperplasia of prostate, prostatic carcinoma, bladder tumours, retro-peritoneal tumours, carcinoma cervix and uterus.
   Infections: Prostatitis, urethritis, ureteritis, retroperitoneal fibrosis.
   Neurogenic: Spinal cord damage with neurogenic bladder.
   Pregnancy

Pathogenesis
With obstruction, there is back pressure on pelvicalyceal system with dilatation and gradually causing pressure atrophy of renal parenchyma. The high pressure also compresses vasculature causing arterial insufficiency and venous stasis. The tubules loose concentrating capacity and later stages eventually glomerular filtration is reduced.

Pathology
- It can be unilateral or bilateral
- Bilateral obstruction occurs when obstruction is below the ureters
- Unilateral obstruction occurs with obstruction to ureter.

Gross: One or both kidneys massively enlarged depending on level and nature of obstruction (Fig. 3.53g).

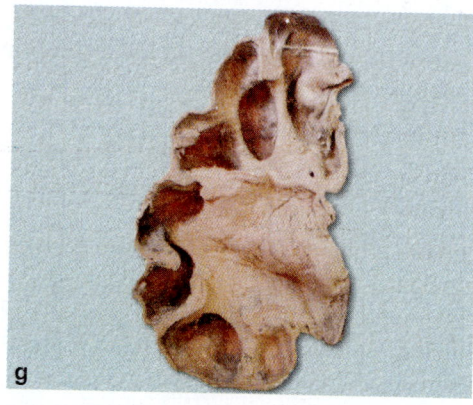

Fig. 3.53g: Gross picture of hydronephrosis

Pelvicalyceal system is dilated. Renal parenchyma is compressed and atrophied with obliteration of papillae and flattening of pyramids.

Microscopy: Tubules dilated. Atrophy and fibrosis replace tubules with relatives paring of glomeruli. In severe cases glomeruli show atrophy and disappear with loss of reduced kidney paranchyma and renal papillae may show necrosis. Obstruction may cause infection causing pyelonephritis.

Clinical features:

- Anuria
- With incomplete obstruction—polyuria and defects in glomerular filtration
- Unilateral may remain silent.

VASCULAR DISEASES OF KIDNEY

Benign Nephrosclerosis (NS)

Benign nephrosclerosis associated with sclerosis of renal arterioles and small arteries resulting in ischaemia of parenchyma.

Pathogenesis

Two processes participate in the arterial lesions:

1. Medial and intimal thickening, as a response to haemodynamic changes, ageing or genetic defects.
2. Hyaline deposition in arterioles.

Three groups of hypertensive patients with benign nephrosclerosis are at increased risk of developing renal failure:

1. People of African descent.
2. People with more severe blood pressure elevations.
3. Persons with a second underlying disease, especially diabetes.

Clinical features

- Uremia
- Mild proteinuria.

Morphology of Kidney in Benign Nephrosclerosis

Gross

- The kidneys are either normal or moderately reduced in size, with average weight between 110 and 130 g.
- The cortical surfaces have fine and even granularity.
- The loss of mass is due to mainly cortical scarring and shrinking (Fig. 3.53h).

Microscopy

- There is narrowing of the lumens of arterioles and small arteries, caused by thickening and hyalinisation of the walls (hyaline arteriolosclerosis).
- Fine surface granulations are microscopic subcapsular scars with sclerotic glomeruli and tubular dropout (Fig. 3.53i).

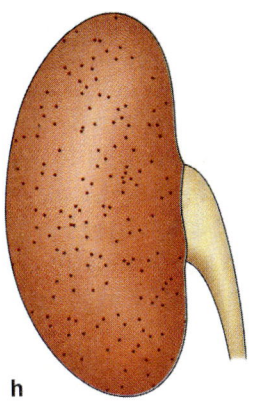

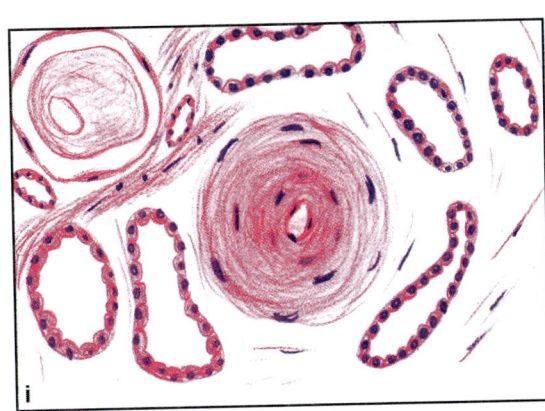

Figs 3.53h and i: (h) Granular contracted kidney in NS, (i) Schematic diagram in NS

- The interlobular and arcuate arteries show medial hypertrophy, reduplication of the elastic lamina, and increased myofibroblastic tissue in the intima, which narrow the lumen. This change, is called fibroelastic hyperplasia.
- There is patchy ischaemic atrophy which consists of:
  a. Foci of tubular atrophy and interstitial fibrosis
  b. A variety of glomerular alterations—collapse of the GBM, deposition of collagen within the Bowman's space, periglomerular fibrosis, and total sclerosis of glomeruli.

MALIGNANT NEPHROSCLEROSIS

Malignant hypertension is less common than benign hypertension and accounts for only 5% of the individuals with raised blood pressure. The blood pressure is usually more than 180/120 mm Hg. It may occur *de novo* without pre-existing hypertension or may appear suddenly in a person who had mild hypertension.

The pathogenesis is not clear, but there is long-standing benign hypertension with vascular wall damage especially of the kidneys.

Gross: The kidneys are normal or slightly reduced in size and surface shows pinpoint haemorrhagic lesions giving the flea bitten appearance.

Microscopy: The vessels show necrotizing arteriolitis, fibrinoid necrosis, there is proliferation of intimal smooth muscle cells with onion skin concentric lamellated thickening of the arterioles with progressive narrowing. This is called hyperplastic arteriolosclerosis.

Prognosis: There is rapid progression of kidneys to end organ damage with renal failure, hypertensive encephalopathy, left ventricular failure, retinal haemorrhages, exudates and papillaoedema. Death is mostly due to uremia and in small percentage of individuals due to cerebral haemorrhage and cardiac failure.

Kidney Stones

Stones may be formed at any level in the urinary tract, but most commonly they arise in the kidney itself.

M : F ratio is 4 : 1. Predominant age of onset is 3–5 decade.

Clinical features
- Pain and haematuria
- Pain is severe and abrupt.

Causes and pathogenesis

The common stones are:
1. Calcium containing (Fig. 3.53j) stones (70%)—calcium oxalate, calcium phosphate or mixture of these two.
2. Triple phosphate stones (15%)—comprised of magnesium, ammonium, phosphate and calcium carbonate.
3. Uric acid stones (5–10%).
4. Cystine stones (1–2%).

There are many causes for initiation and propogation of stone formation, most important is an increased urinary concentration of stone constituents that exceeds their solubility in urine, i.e. supersaturation.

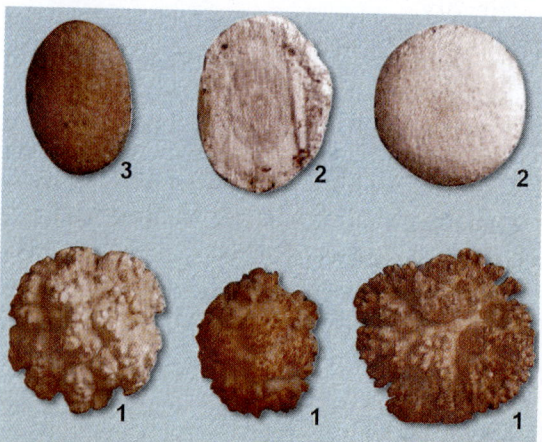

Fig. 3.53j: Gross pictures of renal stones, (1) note calcium oxalate stones with spikes, (2) smooth surfaced calcium phosphate stones, and (3) yellowish brown cystine stone

A low urine volume also may favour supersaturation.

Calcium Phosphate Stones

- These are formed in alkaline urine
- In conditions like renal tubular acidosis and hyperparathyroidism
- These may be large in size
- These have smooth surface

Calcium Oxalate Stones

- These are formed in acidic urine
- They are associated with hypercalcaemia and hypercalciuria
- They are also associated with increased uric acid secretion
- These have spiky surface
- These cause acute pain and haematuria.

Triple Phosphate Stones

1. These are associated with infections of urea splitting oraganisms (proteus and some staphylococci) which convert urea to ammonia. The resultant alkaline urine causes precipitation of magnesium, ammonium phosphate salts.
2. Stag horn calculi (Fig. 3.60g) belongs to this category.
3. These are big in size and can damage the kidney.

Uric Acid Stones

1. These are formed in acidic urine.
2. These are found in patients with hyperuricaemia such as gout and diseases with rapid turnover like leukaemias.
3. Uric acid stones are radiolucent.

Cystine Stones

1. These are formed in acidic urine.
2. These are caused by genetic defects in renal re-absorption of amino acids along with cystine leading to cystinuria.
3. The cystine crystals are flat hexagons in urine.

Complications

These can cause parenchymal changes like infection and obstruction leading to:
1. Pyelonephritis
2. Hydronephrosis (Fig. 3.60i)
3. Renal failure.

TUMOURS OF KIDNEY

Renal Cell Carcinoma

Renal cell carcinoma (RCC), also called hypernephroma is the most common type of renal carcinoma in adults. It accounts for approximately 3% of adult malignancies and 90–95% of neoplasms arising from the kidney.

Renal cell carcinoma is more common in people of Northern European ancestry and North Americans than in those of Asian or African descent. In United States, its incidence is slightly higher among black persons than among white individuals. Incidence is slightly higher in men than in women (M : F ratio—1.6 : 1). Usually age of occurrence is in 5th–6th decades of life, but may occur at earlier age.

Aetiology

A number of environmental and genetic factors have been studied as possible causes for renal cell carcinoma (RCC) such as the following:

1. Cigarette smoking doubles the risk of renal cell carcinoma and contributes to as many as one-third of all cases.
2. Obesity is another risk factor, particularly in women.
3. Hypertension may be associated with an increased incidence of renal cell carcinoma.
4. In patients undergoing long-term renal dialysis, there is an increased incidence of acquired cystic disease of the kidney, which predisposes to renal cell cancer.
5. Tuberous sclerosis appears to be associated with renal cell carcinoma, although the exact nature of this is unclear.
6. In renal transplant recipients, acquired renal cystic disease of the native kidney also predisposes to renal cell cancer.

7. von Hippel-Lindau disease is an inherited disease associated with renal cell carcinoma.

Pathogenesis
RCC originates from the proximal convoluted tubular epithelium. It occurs in a sporadic (non-hereditary) and a hereditary form, and both forms are associated with structural alterations of the short arm of chromosome 3(3p). Mutations of tumour suppressor genes (VHL, TSC) or oncogenes (MET) are also noticed in families with high-risk of renal cancer.

At least 4 hereditary syndromes associated with renal cell carcinoma are recognised
- von Hippel-Lindau (VHL) syndrome
- Hereditary papillary renal carcinoma (HPRC)
- Familial renal oncocytoma (FRO) associated with Birt-Hogg-Dube syndrome (BHDS)
- Hereditary renal carcinoma (HRC).

von Hippel-Lindau Syndrome
von Hippel-Lindau disease is an autosomal dominant syndrome that confers predisposition to a variety of neoplasms, including the following:
- Renal cell carcinoma with clear cell histologic features
- Pheochromocytoma
- Pancreatic cysts and islet cell tumours
- Retinal angiomas
- Central nervous system (CNS) hemangioblastomas
- Epididymal cystadenomas.

Renal cell carcinoma develops in nearly 40% of patients with von Hippel-Lindau disease and is a major cause of death among these patients.

Deletions of 3p occur commonly in renal cell carcinoma associated with von Hippel-Lindau disease. The VHL gene is mutated in a high percentage of tumours and cell lines from patients with sporadic (non-hereditary) clear cell renal carcinoma.

Mutations of the VHL gene result in accumulation of hypoxia inducible factors (HIFs) that stimulate angiogenesis through vascular endothelial growth factor (VEGF) and its receptor (VEGFR). VEGF and VEGFR are important new therapeutic targets.

Hereditary Papillary Renal Carcinoma
Hereditary papillary renal carcinoma is an inherited disorder with an autosomal dominant inheritance pattern; affected individuals develop bilateral, multifocal papillary renal carcinoma. Germline mutations in the tyrosine kinase domain of the MET gene have been identified.

Familial Renal Oncocytoma and Birt-Hogg-Dube Syndrome
Individuals affected with familial renal oncocytoma can develop bilateral, multifocal oncocytoma or oncocytic neoplasms in the kidney. Patients with Birt-Hogg-Dube syndrome have a dominantly inherited predisposition to develop benign tumours of the hair follicle (i.e. fibrofolliculomas), predominantly on the face, neck, and upper trunk, and these individuals are at risk of developing renal tumours, colonic polyps or tumours, and pulmonary cysts.

Hereditary Renal Carcinoma
Affected individuals with this inherited condition have an increased tendency to develop oncocytomas, benign renal tumours that have a low malignant potential.

Clinical features
The most common presentations include haematuria (40%), flank pain (40%), and a palpable mass in the flank or abdomen (25%). Other signs and symptoms include weight loss (33%), fever (20%), hypertension (20%), hypercalcaemia (5%), night sweats, malaise and varicocoele usually left-sided due to obstruction of the testicular vein (2% of males).

Renal cell carcinoma is a unique and challenging tumour because of the frequent occurrence of paraneoplastic syndromes, including hypercalcaemia, erythrocytosis, and non-metastatic hepatic dysfunction (Stauffer syndrome). Polyneuromyopathy, amyloidosis, anaemia, fever, cachexia, weight loss, dermatomyositis, increased erythrocyte sedimentation rate (ESR), and hypertension are also associated with renal cell carcinoma.

Pathology

Gross: Clear renal cell carcinoma is typically a solitary tumour. Tumour size usually ranges from 0.3 to 30 cm in maximal diameter, with a mean of 6–7 cm. The tumour may be multifocal and bilateral in some cases.

The tumour is bosselated, well-circumscribed mass with a capsule or pseudocapsule and a pushing margins. On cut section, it is typically yellow to golden coloured because of accumulation of lipid in the malignant cells, while areas of haemorrhage (brown), fibrosis (gray), necrosis, and cystic degeneration often give a variegated appearance (Fig. 3.54a).

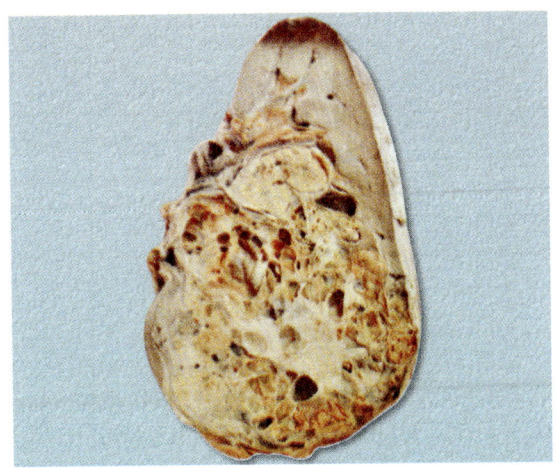

Fig. 3.54a: Gross picture of renal cell carcinoma

Microscopy (Fig. 3.54b)

Typical clear renal cell carcinoma is characterised by epithelial cells with clear cytoplasm and a well-defined cell membrane, interspersed within a highly vascularised stroma. The transparency of the cytoplasm results from accumulated droplets of glycogen, phospholipids, and neutral lipids—in particular, cholesterol ester. Glycogen can be demonstrated by periodic-acid Schiff (PAS) stain, whereas neutral lipids can be identified using the oil red O-stain on unfixed tissue but are dissolved by histological processing.

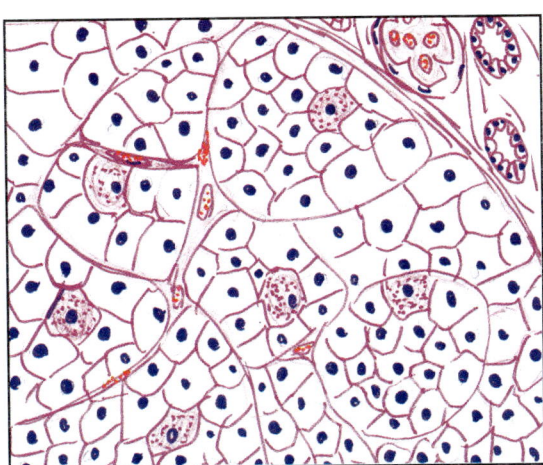

Fig. 3.54b: Schematic diagram of microscopy of renal cell carcinoma

Various architectural patterns like compact—alveolar (nested), tubular (acinar), microcystic, papillary or pseudopapillary patterns may seen histologically.

Clear cell variety may contain a variable proportion of cells with granular eosinophilic cytoplasm. Rarely, these granular cells are the predominant or even the only cell type.

Prognosis

The five-year survival rate is around 90–95% for tumours less than 4 cm. For larger tumours confined to the kidney without venous invasion, survival is still relatively good. For tumours that extend through the renal capsule and out of the local fascial investments, the survivability reduces to near 60%. If it has metastasised to the lymph nodes, the 5-year survival is around 5 to 15%. If it has spread metastatically to other organs, the 5-year survival rate is less than 5%.

Wilms' Tumour

Wilms' tumour (also known as nephroblastoma) is a rare malignant tumour of the kidney that primarily affects children. It is the most common tumour of the kidney in children and accounts for 6% of all paediatric tumours. Wilms' tumour most often, affects children at peak ages 2–5 years, 90% are less than 10 years old.

Wilms' tumour most commonly affects one kidney and is bilateral in 5% of the cases. A minority of these are associated with syndromes or congenital anomalies.

Aetiopathogenesis: Genetic mutations of nephrogenic rests (benign foci of embryonal kidney cells that persist abnormally into postnatal life) and frequently associated with deletions or mutations of WT1.

Beckwith-Wiedeman Syndrome

- Hemihypertrophy
- Organomegaly
- High birth weight
- Omphalocele
- Neonatal hypoglycaemia
- Wilms' tumour, hepatoblastoma (5%)
- 11p15 loss of imprinting IGF2/H19 genes.

WAGR Syndrome

- Wilms' tumour
- Aniridia
- Genitourinary malformations
- Hypospadias
- Undescended testes
- Mental retardation
- 30% chance of Wilms'
- 11p13 deletions
- Germline mutations of WT1.

Denys-Drash Syndrome

- Gonadal dysgenesis (male pseudohermaphroditism)
- Nephropathy—renal failure
- Germline anomalies of WT1 (renal and gonadal development)
- Gonadoblastoma.

Pathology

Most Wilms' tumours are unilateral, being bilateral in less than 5% of the cases, although patients with Denys-Drash syndrome mostly have bilateral or multiple tumours. They tend to be encapsulated and vascularised tumours that do not cross the midline of the abdomen.

Gross: Solitary/multiple cystic mass, soft, bulging, gray-white with focal haemorrhage and necrosis (Fig. 3.55).

Microscopy: Wilms' tumour with classic triphasic combination has three elements namely, blastemal, epithelial and stromal derivatives (Fig. 3.55).

- Blastemal components are in the form of sheets of small blue cells without differentiation.
- Characteristic is the presence of abortive tubules and glomeruli (epithelial components) surrounded by a spindled cell stroma.
- The stromal or the mesenchymal components may include striated muscle, cartilage, bone, fat tissue and fibrous tissue.

The tumour usually compresses the normal kidney parenchyma.

The mesenchymal component may include cells showing rhabdomyoid differentiation.

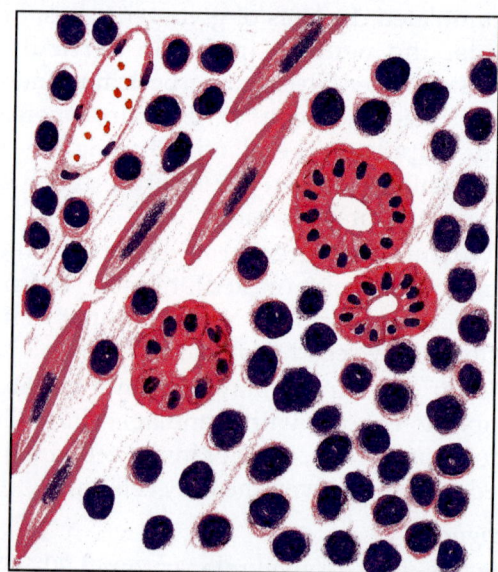

Fig. 3.55: Schematic diagram of microscopy of Wilms' tumour. Note triphasic pattern

The rhabdomyoid component may itself show features of malignancy (rhabdomyosarcomatous Wilms') (Fig. 3.55).

Clinical manifestations
- In an isolated case may present with asymptomatic/palpable abdominal mass, hypertension (25%), haematuria (25%), fever (25%), pain and intestinal obstruction.
- It may present with any of the syndromes mentioned with a renal mass.

Prognosis: It is a tumour with very good prognosis. It is highly responsive to treatment, (nephrectomy + chemotherapy). 5-year survival rate is 90%.

Neoplasms Arising from Stratified Squamous Epithelium

SQUAMOUS CELL PAPILLOMA

This benign tumour arises from the epithelial surface. The epithelium proliferates and is thrown into papillary folds which become increasingly complex. The proliferation is accompanied by a corresponding growth of supportive connective tissue.

Aetiology

Chronic irritation and infection with human papillomavirus (HPV) are two proposed aetiologies. HPV 6 and HPV 11 have been implicated for squamous cell papilloma in different sites.

Gross: It is a warty growth with finger-like projections (Fig. 3.56a).

Microscopy: This benign neoplasm shows a papillomatous lesion lined by hyperplastic and hyperkeratotic stratified squamous epithelium. The thin core of the papillae has lymphatics and blood vessels, e.g. Wart (Fig. 3.56b).

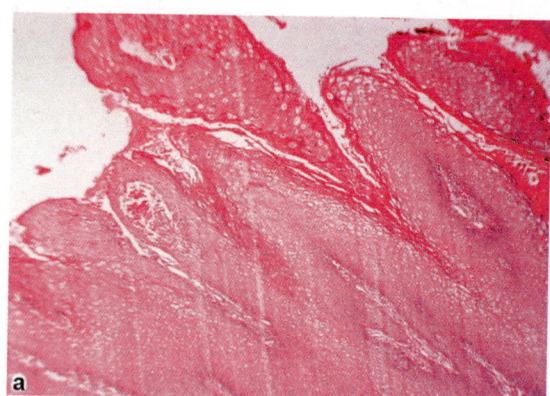

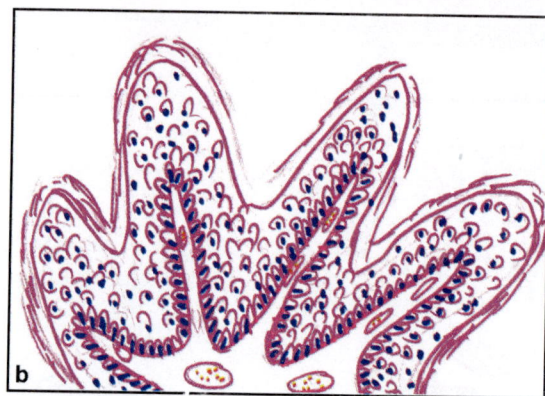

Figs 3.56a and b: Photomicrograph of squamous cell papilloma, note papillae lined by stratified squamous epithelium; (a) shows hyperkeratosis, (b) schematic diagram of microscopy of squamous cell papilloma

SQUAMOUS CELL CARCINOMA

Predisposing factors for this malignant tumour are as follows: Exposure to UV light, chemicals (tars and oils), chronic ulcers such as Marjolin's ulcer, burn scars, osteomyelitis, radiation, tobacco and betel nut chewing, xeroderma pigmentosa and so on.

HPV 16 and 18 are associated with squamous cell carcinoma of skin as well as squamous cell carcinoma of genital system.

Gross: The tumour presents as a nodular cauliflower-like growth. It is prone to bleed and ulcerate (Fig. 3.57a).

Microscopy (Figs 3.57b and c): The epithelium shows atypical squamous cells. There is a

General Pathology and Systemic Pathology

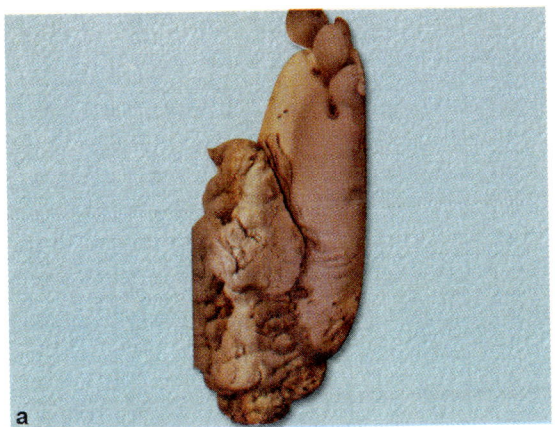

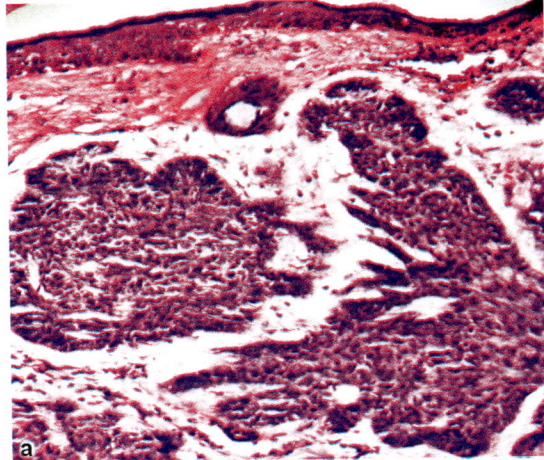

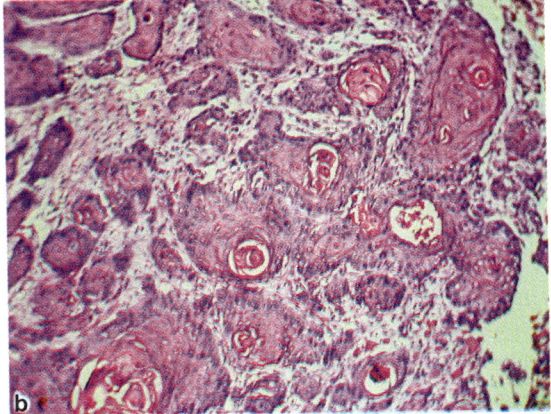

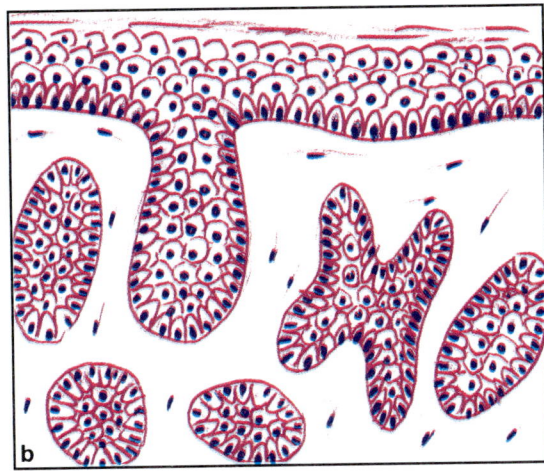

Figs 3.58a and b: Photomicrograph of basal cell carcinoma, (a) note islands of cells and peripheral cells showing palisaded nuclei, (b) schematic diagram

morphic nuclei, arranged in sheets and exhibit good amount of keratinisation (well-differentiated keratinising) to highly anaplastic cells with single cell keratinisation (poorly differentiated/non-keratinising).

BASAL CELL CARCINOMA (BCC)

It is a slow growing, locally malignant tumour which rarely metastasises (Figs 3.58a and b).

Predisposing factors include: Light pigmented people (whites), immunosuppression and other predisposing factors similar to squamous cell carcinoma.

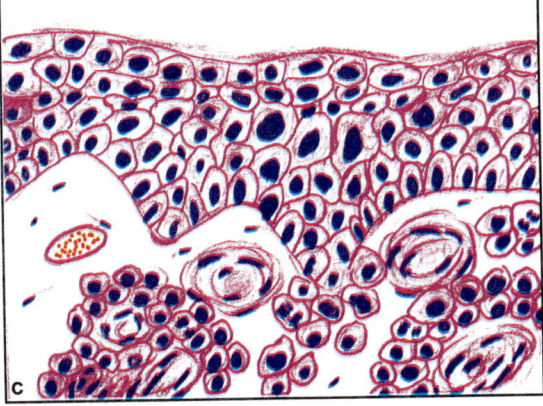

Figs 3.57a to c: (a) Gross, (b) photomicrograph of squamous cell carcinoma, (c) schematic diagram of malignant squamous cells with epithelial cells

breach in the basement membrane and the neoplastic cells invade the subepithelial tissue. The cells are polygonal with atypical pleo-

It occurs in elderly people. It arises from the basal epithelium or from the follicular epithelium.

Clinically there are three types
a. *Nodular BCC:* It is pearly white, firm nodule with ulceration and adjacent telangiectasia.
b. *Superficial BCC:* This presents as erythematous flat lesion having distinct pearly white raised border with adjacent telangiectasia.
c. *Morpheic BCC:* It shows depressed white plaque with erythematous border.

Microscopy: The cells grow from basal epithelium downwards into the dermis as cords or islands. The neoplastic cells are basophilic with slight nuclear enlargement and hyperchromatic nuclei. The nuclei of the peripheral cells are arranged in palisading pattern.

Exercise 51

Tumours of Melanocytes

NAEVUS

Mole or melanocytic naevus is generally used to designate localised benign lesion of melanocytes.

These are acquired or congenital.

Majority are located in the skin and mucous membranes (Figs 3.59a and b).

These naevi can be categorised as:
- Junctional naevus
- Intradermal naevus
- Compound naevus

Junctional Naevus

The melanocyte proliferation is restricted to the basal portion of the epithelium (junctional area).

Naevi of palms and soles are of this type.

Grossly, flat or slightly elevated, non-hairy, fawn coloured.

Microscopically, nests of melanocytes are seen on epithelial side of the dermoepidermal junction.

Malignant melanoma can arise from these lesions.

Intradermal Naevus

The proliferated melanocytes are in the dermis. It may be flat, pedunculated or papillomatous.

Compound Naevus

Juctional and dermal components, melanin production is abundant.

MALIGNANT MELANOMA

Majority of the melanomas arise from
- Skin especially of head and neck area and lower extremities
- The other sites are:
  – Oral and anogenital mucous membranes
  – Palms and soles
  – Subungual region
  – Oesophagus
  – Meninges
  – Eye—uvea, choroid, ciliary body, conjunctiva and eyelid.

Aetiology and predisposing factors
- Sunlight plays an important role
- People who develop freckles after sun exposure are susceptible
- Lightly pigmented individuals (whites/fair skinned) are more prone than the deeply pigmented individuals
- Occurs in pre-existing dysplastic naevus
- Mutations of B-raf oncogene, CMM1 gene on chromosome 1p36 and tumour suppressor gene mapped on 9p21 are found in some family members.

Clinical features

Malignant melanomas are usually asymptomatic.

Itching or pain may be early sign.

Change in colour with shades of black, brown, red dark blue, and grey is striking feature in malignant melanoma unlike benign naevi. The borders are not smooth.

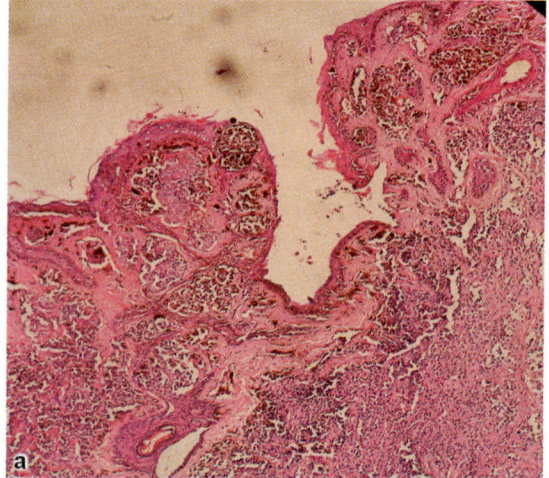

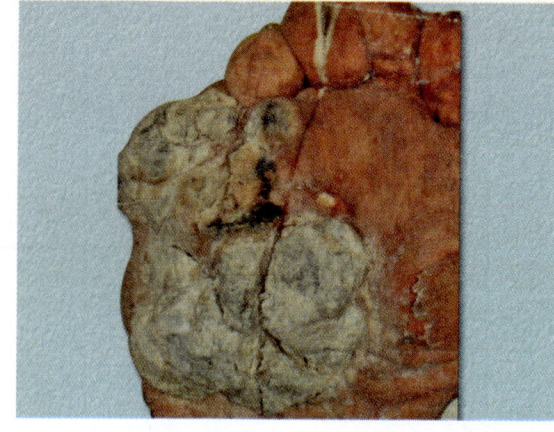

Fig. 3.60a: Gross picture of malignant melanoma

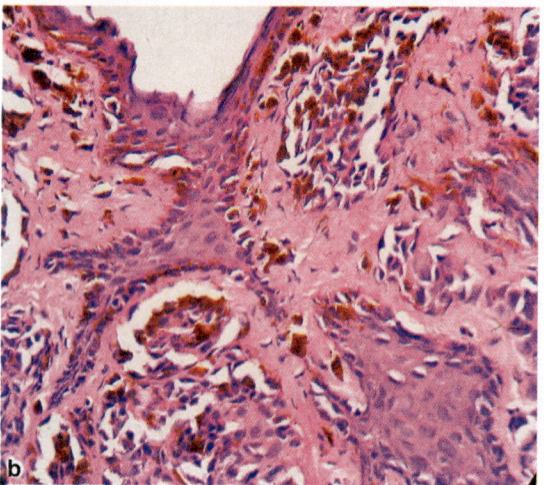

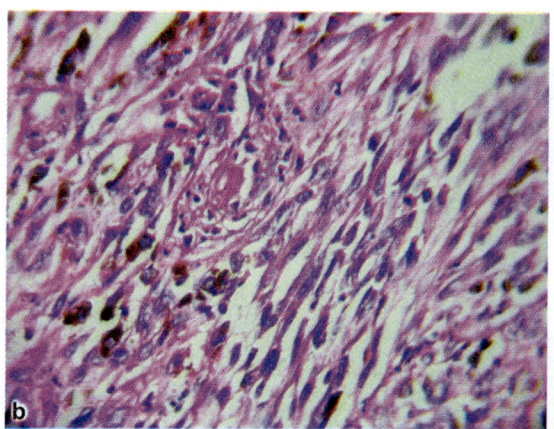

Figs 3.59a and b: Photomicrograph of naevus (compound naevus)

The warning signs of malignant melanoma (ABCD rule) are:
- Asymmetry of shape
- Border irregularity
- Colour variation
- Diameter more than 6 mm.

Morphological Features in General, in Malignant Melanoma (Fig. 3.60a)

Gross: Malignant melanoma usually presents as ulceronodular friable mass. It is grey to black in colour. The naevus with malignant change shows irregular enlarging borders; it has itching and shows change of colours.

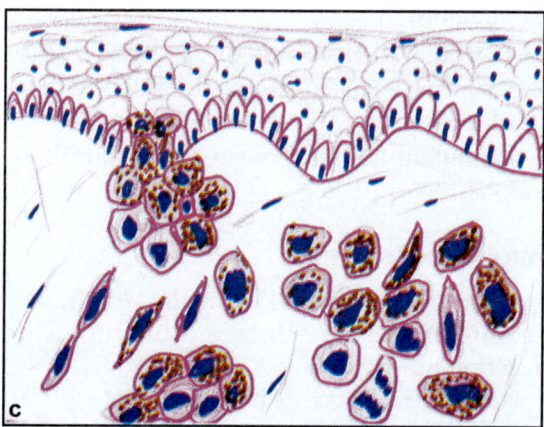

Figs 3.60b and c: Photomicrograph of malignant melanoma and schematic diagram

Microscopy (Figs 3.60b and c): There is junctional activity of melanocytes. The neoplastic cells may be epithelioid or spindle-shaped. The cells may be extremely bizarre. The cytoplasm can be eosinophilic, basophilic, foamy or clear. Melanin pigment in the cytoplasm of these cells may be abundant, scant or absent. The nuclei are markedly atypical. The cells have vertical growth phase and radial growth phase.

Malignant melanoma cells are positive for vimentin, S-100, HMB-45, Melan-A (Mart-1), and tyrosinase. However, desmoplastic variety is positive for S-100; HMB-45 and Melan-A are negative.

The different types of malignant melanomas are:
- Superficial spreading melanoma
- Nodular melanoma
- Acral (lentigenous) melanoma
- Lentigo maligna (Hutchinson's freckle) melanoma.

Superficial Spreading Melanoma

1. This is the most common form. It has variegated appearance, has different shades of colours from blue admixed with tan, brown or black.
2. The surface is slightly elevated, margins are barely palpable.
3. May have white areas.
4. The borders are irregular and notched.
5. With deep invasion, there is appearance of elevated nodule on the surface.
6. Microscopically, has transepidermal proliferation of atypical melanocytes with nest formation and pagetoid appearance.

Nodular Melanoma

1. It is an uncommon form, appears in short duration, in younger people.
2. Presents as circumscribed elevated, spheroidal smooth nodule covered with normal epithelium, as an elevated blue black plaque, or as polypoid ulcerated mass.
3. It has vertical growth.
4. Lateral flat component is not seen grossly or microscopically.

Acral (Lentigenous) Melanoma

1. Has intraepidermal radial and vertical growth.
2. Atypical melanocytes are present in dermo-epidermal junction with focal upward growth. In vertical growth phase atypical melanocytes fill and expand the papillary dermis.

Lentigo Maligna (Hutchinson's Freckle) Melanoma

- Typically seen in elderly
- Sun exposed areas
- Fair skinned people or whites
- Flat slowly growing lesion
- Colour varying from tan to black
- Microscopically, proliferation of atypical melanocytes at the basal layer distributed individually and in nests
- Spindle cell type with low degree of aggressiveness.

Most of the malignant melanomas produce melanin pigment; however, some may not and in such instances demonstration of presence of an enzyme thyrosinase by DOPA reaction can diagnose amelanotic melanomas.

DOPA Reaction

Melanin is produced from thyrosine by the action of an enzyme thyrosinase (DOPA oxidase). To know the presence of an enzyme, DOPA reaction test is done. If the enzyme is present in the tissue (as in amelanotic melanoma) acts on dihydroxyphenylalanine (DOPA) and demonstrates the presence of an enzyme DOPA oxidase which converts DOPA into melanin-like pigment.

This can be done on paraffin sections or frozen sections.

Note: False positive results may be seen with mast cells.

Mast cells can be confirmed by metachromatic stains.

IHC for Mart-1, Melan-A, S-100 HMB-45 are usual for diagnosing amelanotic melanoma.

The Clark level refers to how deep the tumour has penetrated into layers of the skin. This system was originally developed by WH Clark, in 1966. Clark levels are defined in Table 3.33.

Breslow thickness[15]: First reported by Alexander Breslow in 1970, the Breslow thickness is defined as the total vertical height of the melanoma, from the granular layer of the overlying epidermis or from the ulcer base to the area of deepest penetration in the skin (Table 3.33a).

Table 3.34 defines the staging system for cutaneous melanoma of the American Joint Commitee on Cancer.

Table 3.33: Depth of invasion according to Clark levels

- *Level I:* Confined to the epidermis (intraepidermal/ *in situ* melanoma)
- *Level II:* Invasion of the papillary (upper) dermis
- *Level III:* Filling of the papillary dermis, but no extension into the reticular (lower) dermis
- *Level IV:* Invasion of the reticular dermis
- *Level V:* Invasion of the deep subcutaneous tissue

Table 3.33a: Depth of invasion according to Breslow thickness

Risk	Depth of invasion
Low risk	Up to 0.76 mm
Intermediate risk	0.76 to 1.5 mm
High risk	More than 1.5 mm

An instrument ocular micrometer is used to measure the thickness of the excised tumour. Depending upon the depth, melanoma are categorised as given in Table 3.34

Table 3.34: Staging system for cutaneous melanoma of the American Joint Committee on Cancer[16]

Stage	Description
0	Melanoma *in situ*, Clark level I (pTisN0M0)
IA	Localised melanoma ≤ 0.75 mm thick or Clark level II (pT1N0M0)
IB	Localised melanoma 0.76–1.50 mm thick or Clark level III (pT2N0M0)
IIA	Localised melanoma 1.51–4.00 mm thick or Clark level IV (pT3N0M0)
IIB	Localised melanoma > 4.00 mm thick or Clark level V (pT4N0M0)
IIIA	Regional lymph node(s) metastasis ≤ 3 cm in greatest dimension (any pT, N1M0)
IIIB	Regional lymph node(s) metastasis > 3 cm in greatest dimension and/or in-transit metastasis (any pT, N2M0)
IV	Distant metastasis (any pT, any N, M1)

pT: primary tumour; N0: lymph node; M0: no distant metastasis; M1: distant metastasis

Exercise 52

Endometrium and Uterus, Trophoblastic Diseases and Cervix the Normal Endometrium

Normal Endometrium

The endometrium has two components:
1. *Stratum basalis:* This does not respond to hormones.
2. *Stratum functionalis:* This is superficial layer which responds to hormonal changes of the normal ovulatory cycle.

Gonadotropin releasing hormone (GnRH) from hypothalamus stimulates production of follicle stimulating hormone (FSH) and later Luteinising hormone (LH) from the anterior pituitary gland. Both these hormones stimulate growth of follicles in the ovary with oestrogen production in proliferative phase, i.e. before ovulation. After ovulation, in secretory phase LH converts granulosa and theca cells to secrete more progesterone and reduces oestrogen secretion. Hormone inhibin secreted by the corpus luteum, inhibits secretion of FSH and LH. Two days before menstruation, corpus luteum involutes with reduced secretion of oestrogen, progesterone and inhibin, removes negative feedback and stimulates secretion of FSH and later LH from anterior pituitary and thus the cycle continues.

Proliferative Phase (Follicular phase)

The first 14 days of a 28 days menstrual cycle, prior to ovulation is proliferative phase. In response to pituitary FSH and LH, oestrogen is secreted by the granulosa and theca cells of the developing follicle. During the early period of this phase, glands are straight and tubular and stroma is immature. Later from 10 to 14th day glands become more tortuous due to epithelial proliferation.

Early proliferative (days 4–7): Thin surface epithelium, straight short glands, compact stroma, minimal mitotic activity and large nuclei.

Mid proliferative (days 8–10): Columnar surface epithelium; longer curving glands, variable stromal oedema and numerous mitotic figures.

Late proliferative (days 11–14): Has tortuous glands with prominent mitotic activity and pseudostratification. The stroma is dense.

Secretory Phase

Secretory phase is assumed to start after ovulation, i.e. starts from day 14th in a 28 days cycle, but may vary.

Progesterone secretion inhibits endometrial proliferative activity and induces secretory activity.

Early secretory phase is for first 4 days after ovulation. In this phase there is appearance of subnuclear vacuolations. On 3rd and 4th postovulatory day, the subnuclear vacuolations are seen in most of the glands.

Mid secretory phase (5 to 9th postovulatory day): Secretions reach peak on 7th postovulatory day. The glands are tortuous, lumen is distended and stroma is oedematous. Spiral atrerioles are inconspicuous.

Late secretory phase (10th to 14th postovulatory day), there is exhaustion of glandular secretions, glands become serrated, and tortuous, stromal oedema reduces. Predecidual change develops in the stromal cells around the spiral arterioles. The spiral arterioles are prominent and are well-muscularised.

Endometrial Hyperplasia

An excess of estrogen relative to progesterone, if sufficiently prolonged or marked, will induce exaggerated endometrial proliferation/hyperplasia. There is increased proliferation of the endometrial glands relative to the stroma. This results in increased gland to stromal ratio (glands are more compared to stroma).

It is one of the important causes for abnormal uterine bleeding. It can occur at any age during reproductive period, but common age is around 4th to 5th decade, predominantly at two extremes of reproductive life (peri- and postmenopausal period and in teenage around menarche).

Hyperestrinism with prolonged estrogenic stimulation of the endometrium results in continued proliferation and hyperplasia of the glands.

Causes for excessive estrogen are:
- Failure of ovulation, such as is seen around the menopause
- Obesity (peripheral conversion of androgens to estrogens)
- Tumors of the ovary producing estrogen, viz. granulosa cell tumour, thecoma.
- Polycystic ovarian syndrome (including Stein-Leventhal syndrome), follicular cysts of ovary, ovarian cortical stromal hyperplasia.
- Prolonged administration of estrogen (iatrogenic estrogen replacement therapy) during menopause.
- Excessive adrenocortical function.

There are different classifications. Following is one of the recommended classifications. In this, the severity of hyperplasia is classified based on architectural crowding and cytologic atypia into:

- Simple hyperplasia
- Complex hyperplasia
- Atypical hyperplasia.

The latter two can be also classified as:
- Complex hyperplasia without atypia
- Complex hyperplasia with atypia.

WHO 2014[17] *classifies endometrial hyperplasia as below:*
1. Hyperplasia without atypia
2. Hyperplasia with atypia.

Hyperplasia was thought to represent a continuum of morphological changes due to estrogen excess. The risk of developing carcinoma is dependent on the severity of the hyperplasic changes and associated cellular atypia. When atypical hyperplasia is discovered, it must be carefully evaluated for the presence of cancer and must be monitored by repeated endometrial biopsy. However, some studies suggest that:
1. Endometrial hyperplasia and neoplasia are two biologically different diseases.
2. Important feature is presence or absence of cellular atypia.

Simple hyperplasia carries a negligible risk, while a female with atypical hyperplasia with cellular atypia has a 28% risk of developing endometrial carcinoma.[18]

Simple hyperplasia is a true hyperplasia with increase in endometrial bulk, it is a diffuse process involving basal and functional zones. The glands show proliferative endometrium. The glands vary in size. Some are small, some large and some are cystically dilated. The stroma is cellular; however gland to stroma ratio is normal.

Complex hyperplasia is focal, mainly involves glandular component. The glands are variable in size, larger, more numerous, closely packed or crowded, irregular in contour with reduction in the intervening stroma. The glands show out-pouchings or budding. The glandular epithelium is tall columnar or cuboidal with basal or central nuclei, multi-layering, no loss of nuclear polarity, mitoses are numerous and are of normal form.

Atypical hyperplasia is focal and involves glandular component. The glands are closely packed or crowded with reduction in the intervening stroma. The glands show back to back arrangement and similar to complex hyperplasia are irregular in shape, show outpouchings or budding and intraluminal tufting. The glandular epithelium is tall columnar or cuboidal with basal or central nuclei, multilayering (stratification) is marked with loss of nuclear polarity, mitoses are numerous and are normal. There is nuclear atypia and N : C ratio is increased.

ENDOMETRIOSIS AND ADENOMYOSIS

Endometriosis

It is characterised by endometrial glands and stroma, in a location outside the endometrium and myometrium.

It occurs in as many as 10% of women in their reproductive years and in nearly half of women with infertility.

It is a common cause of dysmenorrhoea, and pelvic pain, and may present as a pelvic mass filled with degenerating blood (chocolate cyst).

It is frequently multifocal and may involve tissue in the pelvis (ovaries, pouch of Douglas, uterine ligaments, tubes, and rectovaginal septum), surgical scars particularly of caesarian section, less frequently in more remote sites of the peritoneal cavity and about the umbilicus and uncommonly lymph nodes, lungs, and even heart, skeletal muscle, or bone.

Three Possibilities/Theories

- The regurgitation theory, proposes menstrual backflow through the fallopian tubes with subsequent implantation. Indeed, menstrual endometrium is viable and survives when injected into the anterior abdominal wall; however, this theory cannot explain lesions in the lymph nodes, skeletal muscle, or lungs.
- The metaplastic theory proposes endometrial differentiation of coelomic epithelium, which is the origin of the endometrium itself. This theory, too, cannot explain endometriotic lesions in the lungs or lymph nodes.
- The vascular or lymphatic dissemination theory can explain extrapelvic or intranodal implants.

Grossly, endometriosis appears as bluish cystic nodules often surrounded by fibrosis. Sometimes may appear polypoid simulating neoplastic process.

Microscopically, has endometrial glands and stroma, often embedded in fibrous stroma. May have fresh or old haemorrhage with haemosiderin laden macrophages.

Adenomyosis

Adenomyosis refers to presence of glands and stroma deep within the myometrium.

Grossly, the uterus is enlarged and globular because of myometrial hypertrophy. The enlargement is asymmetrical, cut section has depressed cystic spaces embedded in bulged myometrial tissue and may contain haemorrhagic foci.

Microscopically, glands and stroma are seen in the myometrium at a distance of at least one low power field from the endometrial and myometrial junction. The endometrial glands are in proliferative phase.

LEIOMYOMA

This is a common tumour in women referred to as fibroids, arises from smooth muscles of uterus. Overall incidence is 4–11%. The tumours are found in at least 25% of the women in active reproductive age and are more common in blacks. These are oestrogen responsive. They regress or even calcify after menopause.

The size may rapidly increase in pregnancy, and may cause complications like spontaneous abortion, foetal malpresentations, uterine inertia and postpartum haemorrhage. Malignant transformation is extremely rare.

These tumours can occur subserosally beneath the serosa, intramurally within the myometrium and submucosally beneath the endometrium and produce symptoms depending upon their size and location.

Submucosal leiomyomas usually produce metrorrhagia (abnormal bleeding), intramucosal leiomyomas menorrhagia, and subserosal may remain asymptomatic or may produce pain. The large once may block the uterus, produce urinary frequency, because of compression of urinary bladder and may interfere with pregnancy. Red degeneration may also produce pain.

Grossly (Fig. 3.61a), they are sharply circumscribed, round, firm, grey white, can be easily enucleated, has whirled appearance. They vary from small to enormous size and location varies. They may show degenerative changes like hyaline change, mucoid change, hydropic change, etc.

Microscopically (Figs 3.61b and c), the tumour is composed by whirled, interlacing bundles of smooth muscle cells separated by vascularised connective tissue. The muscle cells are uniform in size and shape, have oval nucleus and long slender bipolar cytoplasmic processes. Mitoses are sparse.

The histological variants are:
- Cellular leiomyoma
- Atypical, bizarre, symplastic or pleomorphic leiomyoma
- Mitotically active leiomyoma
- Leiomyolipoma
- Palisaded leiomyoma
- Epithelioid (clear cell) leiomyoma
- Parasitic leiomyoma
- Angio leiomyoma.

ENDOMETRIAL CARCINOMA

A primary malignant epithelial tumour, usually with glandular differentiation, arising in the endometrium has the potential to invade into the myometrium and spread to distant sites.

Epidemiology and Pathogenesis

While the disease affects mainly postmenopausal women frequently between the ages of

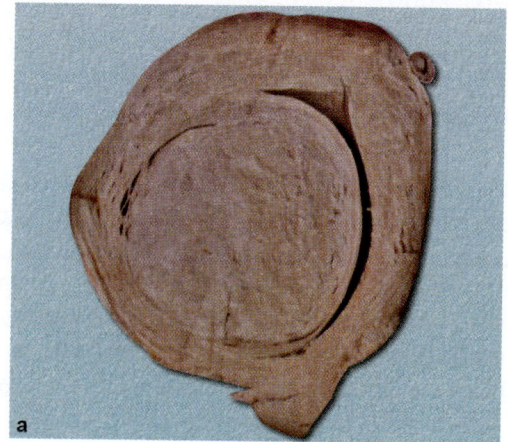

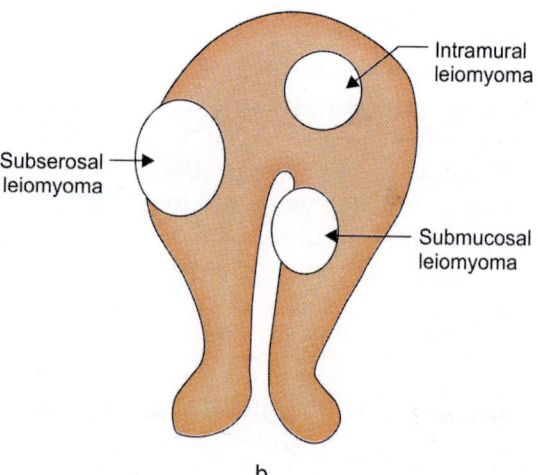

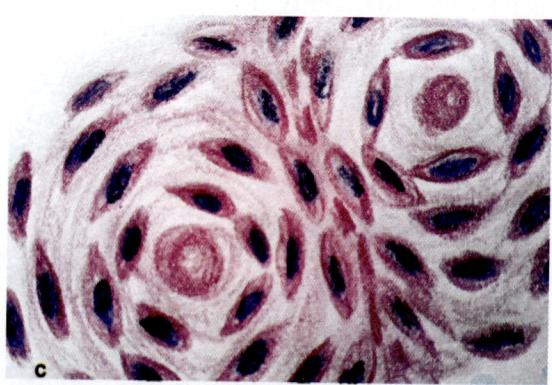

Figs 3.61a, b, c: (a) Gross picture of Leiomyoma uterus, (b) Schematic diagram of Leiomyoma uterus to show submucosal, subserosal and intramural leiomyoma (c) microscopy of leiomyoma

55–65, approximately 20% of the cases occur in premenopausal women. It is a most common malignant tumour of female genital tract. It occurs commonly in:
- Developed countries
- Obese, Diabetic, nulliparous, hypertensive.

80–85%—Estrogen dependent tumours, are the low grade, well/moderately differentiated predominantly endometrioid type.

10–15%—Non-estrogen dependent tumours are the higher grade-serous/clear cell carcinoma in older postmenopausal women.

Risk Factors for Endometrial Cancer

- Early menarche (<age 12)
- Late menopause (>age 52)
- Infertility or nulliparous
- Obesity, diabetes, caucasian women, diet high in animal fat
- Treatment with tamoxifen for breast cancer
- Estrogen replacement therapy (ERT) after menopause
- Age greater than 40 years
- Family history of endometrial cancer or hereditary non polyposis colon cancer (HNPCC)
- Personal and family history of breast or ovarian cancer
- Prior radiation therapy for pelvic cancer.

Symptoms of Endometrial Cancer

- Heavy bleeding postmenopausal bleeding or discharge
- Dysuria
- Pain and/or mass in pelvic area
- Weight loss
- Back pain.

Pathology

Endometrial cancer includes:
1. Those arising in the endometrial lining (endometrial carcinoma)—these make up about 95% of all uterine cancers.
2. Those arising in the uterine stroma or myometrial cells (uterine sarcomas).

Gross: Endometrial cancer is seen as raised, rough, polypoid lesion which protrudes into the cavity and also infiltrates the wall. With extensive infiltration, there can be uterine enlargement. The infiltration of the tumour appear as firm grey white tissue with linear extensions from the base of the tumour. Myometrial invasion may be visible to the naked eye. The invasion of myometrial wall whether less than half or more than half has to be documented which helps in staging of the endometrial carcinoma (Fig. 3.62). The size of the uterus may remain normal too. It often arises in the fundal region of the uterus. Mass may arise from body, isthmus and cornual part of uterus.

Microscopy: Endometrial carcinomas (80%) are adenocarcinomas characterised by glandular pattern resembling normal endometrial epithelium. The glandular/villoglandular structures are lined by simple to pseudostratified columnar cells with their long-axis perpendicular to basement membrane with elongated nuclei polarised in the same direction. Grade of endometrioid carcinoma is based on architectural pattern, nuclear features or both.

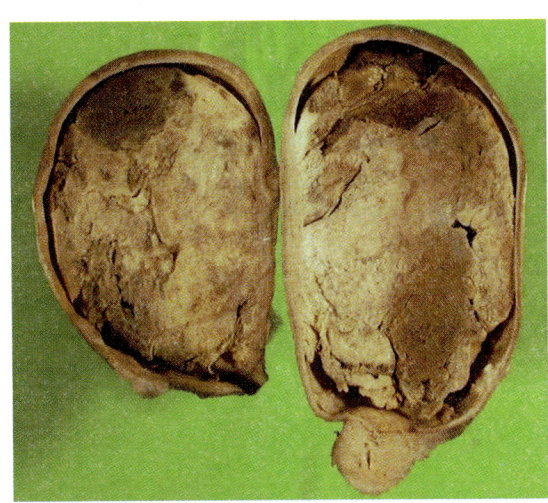

Fig. 3.62: Gross specimen, cut section of endometrial carcinoma filling the endometrial cavity

Histological Sub-types of Endometrial Cancer

- Endometrioid adenocarcinoma
- Adenosquamous
- Serous papillary
- Sarcomas/leomyosarcomas
- Carcinosarcomas
- Clear cell.

The other variants include:
- Adenoacanthoma
- Glassy cell carcinoma
- Secretary carcinoma
- Ciliated carcinoma
- Mucinous carcinoma
- Undifferentiated carcinoma
- Small cell (neuroendocrine) carcinoma
- Squamous cell carcinoma
- Endometrial carcinoma with trophoblastic differentiation.

The most frequent histological type is endometrioid carcinoma or conventional adenocarcinoma. The histological (microscopic) grading is done based on the architectural pattern and nuclear features or both. The histological grading of the tumour tissue is given below:

Grade 1: Tumour has 5% or less non-squamous solid growth, nuclei are oval, mildly enlarged and has evenly dispersed chromatin (well-differentiated).

Grade 2: Tumour tissue has 6–50% non-squamous solid growth, nuclear features are inbetween grade 1 and 3 (moderately differentiated).

Grade 3: Tumour tissue has more than 50% non-squamous solid growth, nuclei markedly enlarged, pleomorphic, coarse chromatin and prominent eosinophilic nuclei (poorly differentiated).

Grades 1 and 2 (well-differentiated and moderately differentiated) cancers have a better prognosis than Grade 3 cancers. Mitosis less than 5/HPF has good outcome. More than 10/HPF has worse prognosis.

Endometrioid Carcinoma with Squamous Differentiation

Squamous elements should constitute 10% of a tumour qualify as an adenocarcinoma with squamous differentiation.

1. Adenoacanthoma—adenocarcinoma with benign appearing squamous elements has good prognosis.
2. Adenosquamous carcinoma—adenocarcinoma with malignant appearing squamous epithelium has worse prognosis.

GESTATIONAL TROPHOBLASTIC DISEASES

Gestational trophoblastic disease is a spectrum of disorders with abnormal proliferation and maturation of villous or trophoblastic tissue, as well as neoplasms derived from trophoblast that originate in the placenta.

Classification:
1. Hydatidiform mole
   - Complete and
   - Partial mole } Noninvasive mole
2. Placental site trophoblastic tumours
3. Invasive moles
4. Choriocarcinomas.

HYDATIDIFORM MOLE (VESICULAR MOLE)

Hydatidiform mole is a noninvasive abnormal placental neoplasm characterised by voluminous mass of swollen enlarged, oedematous and avascular chorionic villi accompanied by variable amounts of proliferated trophoblastic epithelium. Moles are common before the age of 20 or after the age of 40.

The incidence is 1 to 1.5 in 2000 pregnancies. Higher incidence is seen in Asian countries.

Two categories:
- Complete hydatidiform mole
- Partial hydatidiform mole.

Complete Hydatidiform Mole

1. Characterised by hydropic swelling of all the villi and a variable degree of trophoblastic proliferation.

2. Does not permit embryogenesis. Fetal tissue is not usually present.

Cytogenetics: Complete mole results from fertilisation of an empty ovum that lacks functional maternal DNA. Most commonly, a haploid (23X) set of paternal chromosomes introduced by monospermy duplicates to 46XX, but dispermic 46XX and 46XY moles also occur. Because the embryo dies at a very early stage before placental circulation has developed, few chorionic villi develop blood vessels, and fetal parts are absent (Figs 3.63a to c).

Clinical features
- Usually discovered between 12 and 14 weeks of gestational age.
- Vaginal bleeding with passage of vesicles after a period of amenorrhea.
- Uterus is abnormally enlarged and soft.
- Hyperemesis gravidarum and PIH may be associated.
- USG abdomen shows "snowstorm appearance".
- Serum HCG levels are elevated.

Pathological features

Gross: Oedematous villi forming characteristic grape-like transparent vesicles.

Lack of embryonic tissue is characteristic.

Microscopy
- Diffuse hydropic swelling of majority of villi with central acellular cistern formation.
- The villi are avascular.
- Diffuse, irregular, circumferential, exuberant, proliferation of trophoblasts.
- Absent fetal parts.

Diagnosis

Elevated serum HCG levels and absence of fetal parts or absence of fetal heart sounds are diagnostic.

Sequelae: 2–3% of these cases go for choriocarcinoma

Partial Hydatidiform Mole

Occur between 9 and 34 weeks of gestation. Uterine size is generally small for gestational age. Abnormal uterine bleeding is common feature. Missed or spontaneous abortion is common in cases of incomplete molar pregnancy. Serum HCG levels are in the normal or low range for gestational age.

Pre-eclampsia occurs in some cases.

Cytogenetics: Partial hydatidiform mole is a distinct form of mole that almost never evolves into choriocarcinoma. These moles have 69 chromosomes (triploidy), of which one haploid set is maternal and two are paternal in origin. This abnormal chromosomal complement results from fertilisation of a normal ovum (23X) by two normal spermatozoa, each carrying 23 chromosomes, or a single spermatozoon that has not undergone meiotic reduction and bears 46 chromosomes. This results from fertilisation of a haploid ovum and duplication of the paternal haploid chromosomes or from dispermy (single ovum and two sperms 23x or 23y) thus in partial mole karyotype is triploid. 69XXY is most common karyotype (70–80%) followed by 69XXX (20–25%) and rarely 69XYY may also be encountered. The foetus associated with a partial mole usually dies after 10 weeks gestation, and the mole is aborted shortly thereafter. In contrast to a complete mole, fetal parts may be present.

Gross: Villi may be evident as vesicles. Foetus or foetal parts are always present.

Microscopy
1. Normal villi and villi with hydropic changes
2. Inconspicous/no central cistern formation
3. Trophoblastic hyperplasia is focally present
4. Foetal parts present.

Complications: May rarely develop into choriocarcinoma.

Comparative features of complete and partial hydatidiform mole are given in Table 3.35.

Table 3.35: Comparative features of complete and partial hydatidiform mole

Features	Complete mole	Partial mole
Karyotype	46XX and rarely 46XY	Triploid 69XXY or 69XXX, rarely 69XYY
Parental origin of haploid genome sets	Both paternal	1 maternal, 2 paternal
Preoperative diagnosis	Mole	Missed abortion
Marked vaginal bleeding	Marked	Mild
Uterus size	Large for gestational age	Small for gestational age
Serum hCG	Markedly elevated	Less elevated than complete mole
hCG in tissue	3+	1+
Hydropic villi	All	Some
Trophoblastic proliferation	Diffuse	Focal
Atypia	Minimal	Minimal or Absent
Embryo	No	Fetal parts may be present
Blood vessels	Absent	Present
Nucleated erythrocytes	No	Sometimes seen
Choriocarcinoma	2% after mole	No choriocarcinoma

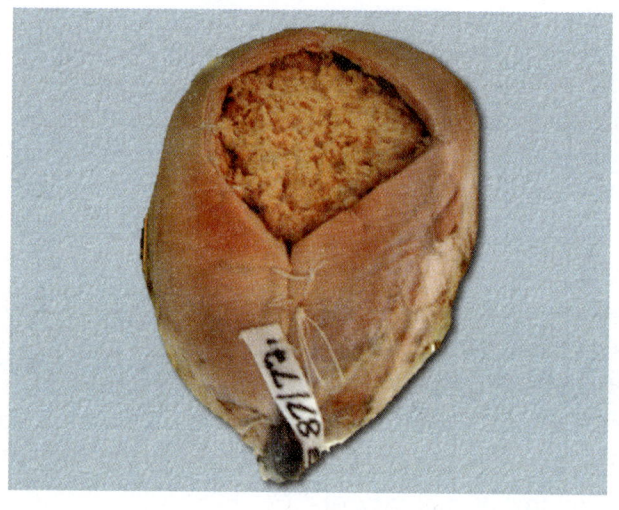

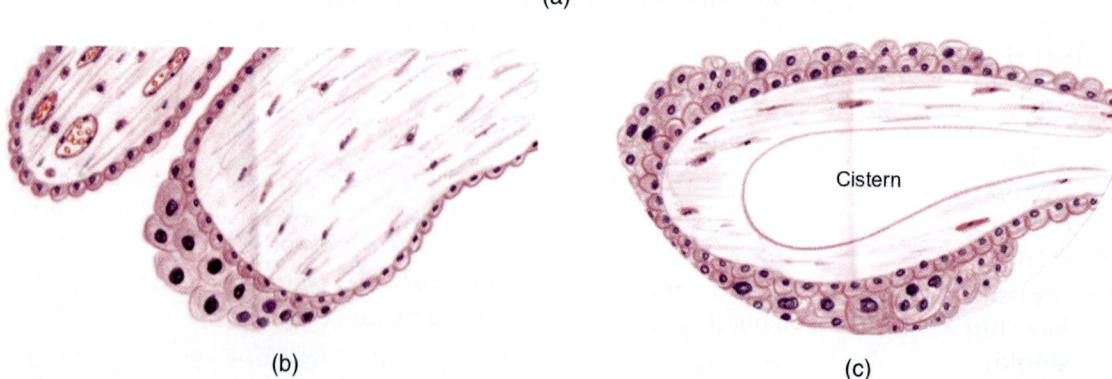

Figs 3.63a to c: (a) Gross picture of vesicular mole, schematic diagrams, microscopy of vesicular mole partial (b), and complete (c). Note the changes in partial and complete mole

CARCINOMA CERVIX

It is a malignant tumour of cervix. Squamous cell carcinoma is the commonest malignant tumour occurring in 80–90% of the cases. Remaining 20% are adenocarcinoma and adenosquamous carcinoma (Fig. 3.64a).

Peak age: 40–45 years.

Precursor lesion: Cervical intraepithelial neoplasm (CIN).

Etiology and Pathogenesis

1. About 99.7% of the cancers and premalignant lesions are associated with oncogenic HPV subtypes. More than 90% of cervical carcinoma contains DNA sequences of specific HPV types, especially HPV 16 and HPV 18. The distribution of HPV types in invasive cervical cancers shows only minor geographic variations. Globally, HPV 16 is most frequently detected in invasive cervical cancer, followed by HPV 18. HPV types 31, 33, 35, 45, 52, and 58 are the next most common types found in cervical cancers.

   A cervical cancer vaccine has recently been approved and recommended for females between the ages of 9 and 26, which in clinical trials has decreased the risk of cervical cancer. Vaccinated women developed neither HPV-associated pre-cancer nor invasive cervical cancer.

2. The other sexually transmitted diseases like herpes simplex virus 2 may play concurrent role.

Other risk factors

- Lower education attainment, older age, obesity, smoking, poverty (socioeconomical status), parity, use of oral contraceptives, sexual activity and lowered immunity (immune-suppression) are independently related to high rates of cancer.
- *Cigarette smoking:* Both passive and active have higher risk. HPV infection along with smoking has two-to-threefold increased risk.
- Alcohol.
- Drug abuse.
- *Parity:* Increased parity has more risk. Nulliparous females have reduced risk.
- *Oral contraceptives (OC) and progesterone use:* Long term use of combination OC or progesterone use has increased risk. HPV with OC association increases risk four fold.
- *Sexual activity:* HPV infection is related to number of sexual partners. Early age of first intercourse (at the age of 20–21years) increases the risk of HPV infection and carcinoma cervix.
- *Immunity:* Immunocompromised women have more risk of cervical cancer.

Mechanism of Cancer Development

The molecular mechanisms involved in carcinogenesis are complex and not fully understood. Increasing evidence suggests that HPV oncoproteins are the critical components of cancer cell proliferation. The high-risk HPV oncoproteins get integrated into the host DNA. The early viral replication proteins E1 and E2 makes the virus to replicate within the cervical cells. The E6 oncoproteins degrades the p53 gene and inhibits apoptosis while E7 oncoprotein binds to RB gene and degrades it. Thus, both of these are involved in proliferation and survival of the transformed cells. Markers of actively of dividing cells like

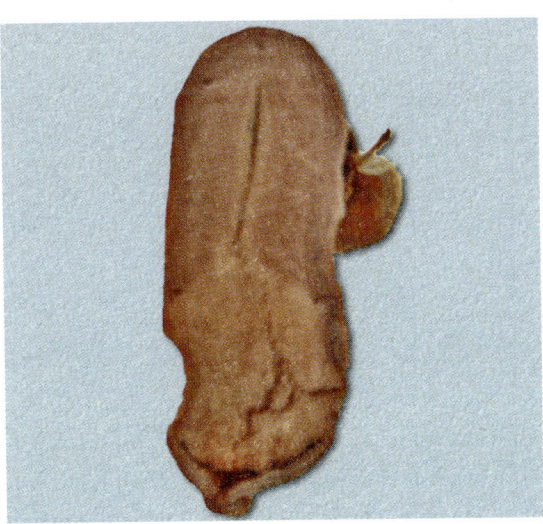

Fig. 3.64a: Gross picture of squamous cell carcinoma cervix

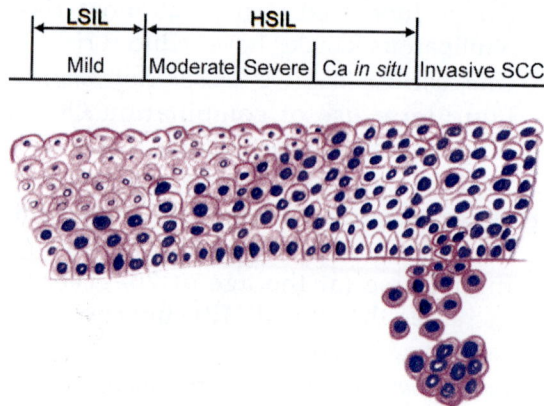

Fig. 3.64b: Schematic diagram of dysplasia, carcinoma *in situ* and malignant transformation (invasive squamous cell carcinoma)

Ki-67, P-16, a cyclin dependent kinase inhibitor are over expressed in upper layers of the epithelium. Ki-67 and P-16 staining is highly correlated with high grade HPV infection. In addition, E6 upregulates the expression of telomerase, which leads to immortalisation of the cells.

Pathology

Squamous cell carcinoma is the most common histologic subtype accounting for 70–80% of invasive carcinomas. Adenocarcinoma and adenosquamous carcinoma comprise 10–15% of all cases, and all other variants account for another 10–15% of the cervical cancer cases.

Morphology

Grossly has fungating, ulcerating and infiltrative lesions.

Microscopically, can have large cell keratinising type, large cell nonkeratinising type and small cell nonkeratinising types (Fig. 3.64b).

In large cell keratinizing type the cells are polyhedral and present in sheets or individually. Increased and abnormal mitosis are present. The cells vary in size and shape have irregular hyperchromatic nuclei. Individual cell keratinisation and epithelial pearl formation are present.

Large cell non-keratinising is composed of histologically recognisable squamous cells, which are large and polygonal with eosinophilic cytoplasm and indistinct cell borders, lack keratin pearl formation or nests of squamous cells with keratinisation, there is greater degree of nuclear pleomorphism and infiltrative border with associated inflammation is often seen.

Exercise 53

Common Ovarian Tumours

Histogenesis

Most of the surface epithelial tumours are derived from ovarian surface epithelium. Serous Tubal Intraepithelial Carcinoma (STIC) is gaining importance as a precursor lesion for serous high grade tumours.

Aetiology

Several hypotheses are proposed for development of ovarian cancer. These are the following:
1. *Incessant ovulation hypothesis:* During ovulation, the surface epithelium of the ovary is damaged with repair which increases the opportunity for developing mutations that promote carcinogenesis.
2. *Gonadotropin overstimulation hypothesis:* Overstimulation of the ovarian surface epithelial cells by gonadotropins (follicle stimulating hormone and luteinizing hormone) increases cell division and mutations that promote carcinogenesis.
3. *Hormonal stimulation:* High concentrations of androgens promote carcinogenesis and progestins decrease the risk.
4. *Inflammatory response:* Ovulation is accompanied by release of inflammatory mediators which promote malignant transformation.
5. *Genetic and familial predisposition:* BRCA1 (located in the long arm of chromosome 13) or BRCA2 (located in the long arm of chromosome 17) mutations produces high-grade carcinomas, with a poor prognosis.
6. Risk factors associated with ovarian carcinoma:
   a. Low parity, delayed childbearing, early age at menarche and late age at menopause are associated with increased number of ovulations.
   b. Oral contraceptives, breastfeeding and multiparity are the factors with reduced ovulation and decreased risk of cancer.
   c. Infertile women treated with clomiphene, age, family history and obesity have increased risk.
   d. Hormone replacement therapy (HRT) and endometrisis have increased risk.
   e. Smoking has increased risk of ovarian tumours.

Epidemiology

Benign tumours are common in the age range of 20–40 years and over 70% of ovarian cancer occurs after the age of 50 years. Ovarian cancer ranks third, next to breast and cervix cancers.

Clinical Features

Epithelial ovarian cancer presents with a wide variety of nonspecific symptoms. These are:
1. Abdominal pain, pelvic pain, abdominal bloating, increased abdominal size, difficulty in eating and feeling full quickly after eating.
2. Torsion or rupture of the tumour can result in acute abdominal symptoms.
3. Ovarian cancer is bilateral in 25% of cases.
4. Presence of ascites is mostly suggestive of carcinoma.

5. Patients with functional sex cord stromal tumours may be with features related excess estrogen or androgens.
6. Granulosa cell tumours occurring in a young girl may have precocious puberty

Ovarian mass, in a female over the age of 45 years should raise the suspicion of ovarian cancer and should be evaluated. The identification of solid or complex mass by ultrasonography is worrisome.

Histological classification of tumours (WHO, 2014) is given in Table 3.36.

Table 3.36: WHO histological classification of tumours of the ovary (WHO, 2014)[19]

Surface epithelial-stromal tumours
Serous tumours:
Benign: Cystadenoma, adenofibroma, cystadenofibroma
Borderline tumour: Serous borderline tumour, micropapillary variant
Malignant: Low grade and high grade Adenocarcinoma
Mucinous tumours:
Benign: Cystadenoma, adenofibroma, cystadenofibroma
Borderline tumour
Malignant: Adenocarcinoma
Mucinous cystic tumour with pseudomyxoma peritonei
Endometrioid tumours including variants with squamous differentiation
Clear cell tumours
Transitional cell tumours
 a. *Malignant:* Transitional cell carcinoma (non-Brenner type), malignant Brenner tumours
 b. Borderline
 c. Benign: Brenner tumours
Seromucinous tumours
  Benign: cystadenoma, adenofibroma
  Borderline: Borderline seromucinous tumour
  Malignant: Seromucinous carcinoma
Squamous cell *tumours*
Mixed epithelial tumours (specify components)
Undifferentiated and unclassified tumours
Sex-cord stromal tumours
Granulosa-stromal cell tumours
Thecoma-fibroma group
Sertoli-stromal cell tumours
Steroid cell tumours

Contd.

Germ cell tumours
1. Dysgerminoma
2. Yolk sac tumour
3. Embryonal carcinoma
4. Polyembryoma
5. Non gestational choriocarcinoma
6. Mixed germ cell tumour (specify components)
7. Immature teratoma
8. Mature teratoma–solid, cystic (dermoid cyst)
9. Monodermal teratoma and highly specialised types
    Thyroid tumour group—struma ovarii, benign and malignant
    Carcinoid group
    Neuroectodermal tumour group
    Carcinomas (SCC and adenocarcinoma)
    Sebaceous carcinoma
10. Others

Sex cord-stromal tumours
  Pure sex cord tumors: GCT
  Sertoli cell tumour
  Sex cord tumour with annular tubules
  Pure stromal
  Fibroma/sarcoma
  Thecoma
  Sclerosing stromal tumour
  Leydig cell tumour
  Steroid cell tumour
  Gonadoblastoma
  Mixed germ cell-sex cord-stromal tumour
Tumours of the rete ovarii
Miscellaneous tumours
Tumour-like conditions
Lymphoid and haematopoetic tumours
Secondary tumours
(WHO 2014 classification with slight modification)

Serous Cystadenoma Ovary

Gross: The surface is smooth and occasionally papillary excrescences are observed over the surface. These tumours contain thin watery fluid. The inner surface of the cyst wall is smooth and may display papillary structures (Fig. 3.65a).

Microscopy: This tumour shows single layer of ciliated or nonciliated columnar epithelium lining the cyst wall and the papillae (Fig. 3.65b).

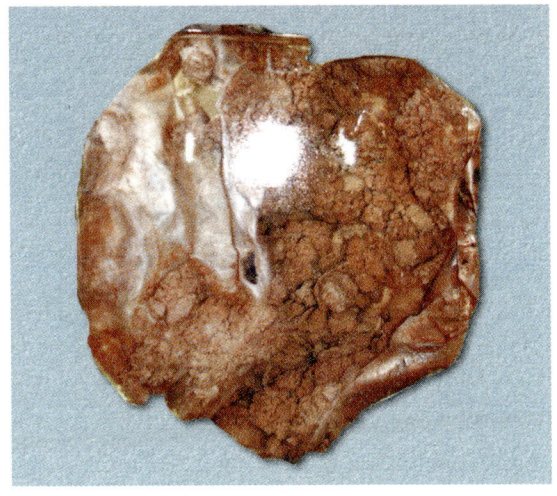

Fig. 3.65a: Gross picture, papillary serous cyst adenoma

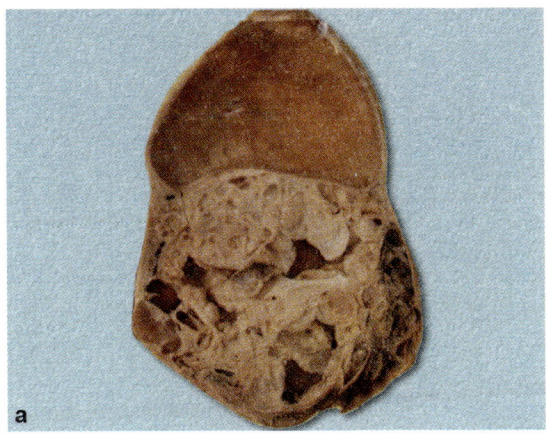

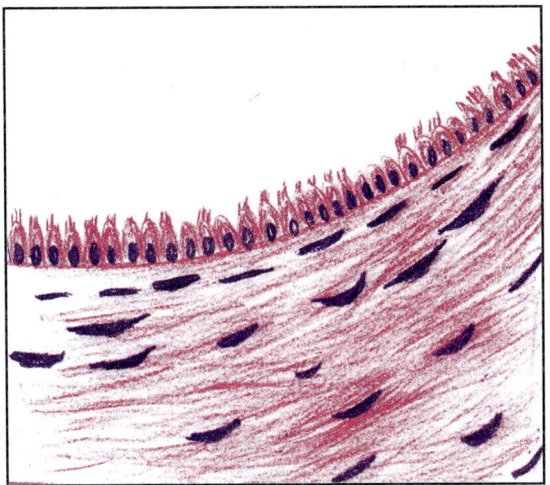

Fig. 3.65b: Photomicrograph of serous cyst adenoma, note—tall columnar ciliated epithelial cells

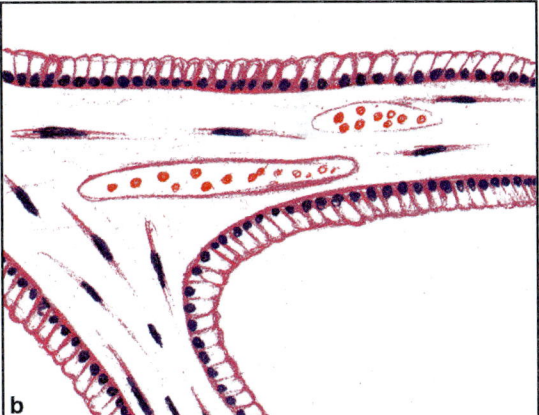

Figs 3.66a and b: (a) Gross and (b) schematic diagram of mucinous cystadenoma, note—tall columnar mucin secreting epithelium with basal nuclei

Mucinous Cystadenoma Ovary

Gross: These are round, ovoid or irregularly lobulated masses. They have smooth outer surface with a whitish or bluish colour. The content of the cyst is a viscid fluid, sometimes very thick or thin. These tumours are frequently multiloculated (Fig. 3.66a).

Microscopy: The tumour microscopy shows single layer of nonciliated tall columnar epithelium with pale stained cytoplasm. The nuclei are placed at the base (Fig. 3.66b). Paneth cells, goblet cells and endocrine cells may be noticed in these tumours.

Mature Cystic Teratoma Ovary

Gross: This tumour has a thick capsule, usually unilocular and contains a pale yellow greasy material composed of frequently keratin, sebum and hair. There is often a solid portion at one pole of the cyst, which contains the bulk of the cellular elements. Teeth are found in many of the cases (Fig. 3.67a).

Microscopy: The mature elements derived from mesoderm, endoderm and ectoderm are observed. Skin and its appendages are frequently present followed by neural tissue, cartilage, respiratory epithelium and gastrointestinal epithelium (Fig. 3.67b).

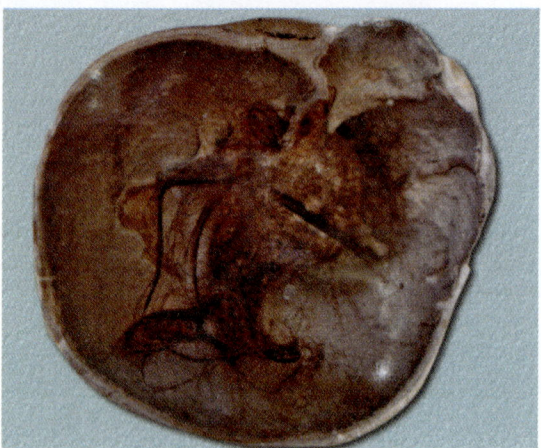

Fig. 3.67a: Gross picture of mature teratoma (dermoid cyst)

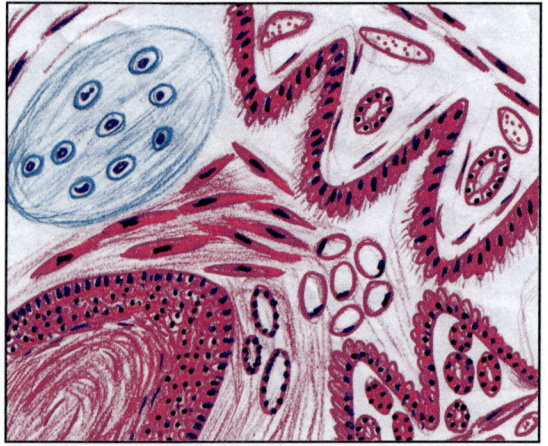

Fig. 3.67b: Schematic diagram of mature teratoma, note—skin with its appendages and other mature elements

FUNCTIONAL/HORMONE SECRETING OVARIAN TUMOUR

Sex-cord Stromal Tumour

Nearly 90% of hormone producing ovarian tumours are sex-cord stromal tumour. These can be:
1. Pure stromal tumour
   Thecoma (estrogens)
   Leydig cell tumour (androgens)
   Steroid cell tumour.
2. Pure sex cord tumour
   Granulosa cell tumour (estrogens, rarely androgens)
   Sertoli cell tumour (androgens, rarely estrogens).
3. Mixed sex-cord stromal tumour.
   Sertoli Leydig cell tumour also called gynandroblastoma or arrhenoblastoma
   Sex cord stromal tumours (not otherwise classified).

The other hormone secreting ovarian tumours are:

Carcinoid tumours of ovary: These can be primary or metastatic (mainly from GIT). These secrete variety of neuro-humoral substances including serotonin, histamine, brachykinin, bradykinin, prostaglandins etc.

Struma ovary: Rare monodermal teratoma with predominant presence of thyroid tissue.

Choriocarcinoma of ovary: Aggressive tumour of trophoblastic cells and secrete beta HCG.

Exercise 54

Common Testicular Lesions

CRYPTORCHIDISM

This represents testicular non-descent into the scrotum. Normally, testes develop in relation to lumbar region, they reach the iliac fossa during 3rd month and deep inguinal ring by 7th month of intrauterine life. By the end of 8th month, they reach the scrotal sac.

Cryptorchidism is present in 1% of the male population. About 10% of these are bilateral. Hormonal abnormalities, testicular abnormalities, mechanical problems like obstruction of the inguinal canal may interfere with testicular descent. It is also seen with Prader-Willi syndrome.

The cause is not known in many of the cases. Unilateral or bilateral cryptorchidism causes sterility and atrophy. Unilateral cryptorchidism may be associated with atrophy of other side testis which is descended and also contributes to infertility.

Unilateral or bilateral cryptorchidism is associated with fivefold increase risk of malignancy.

Pathology: The affected cryptorchid testis is normal in size in early life or may be reduced at the time of puberty. There is tubular atrophy by 5–6 years of age and hyalinisation by puberty. Following are the important features:
- Loss of tubules
- Thickened basement membrane
- Hyperplasia of Leydig cells
- Foci of intratubular germ cell neoplasia may be observed in cryptorchid testes.

Atrophic changes similar to cryptorchid testes may be seen in chronic ischaemia, trauma, radiation, chemotherapy or with increased levels of estrogen as seen in cirrhosis. This may not develop intratubular neoplasia.

TESTICULAR TUMOURS

Many types of testicular tumours originating from germ cells or sex cord stromal tumours are known.

Aetiology

1. *Undescended testis (cryptorchidism):* 10% of testicular tumours are associated with cryptorchidism.
2. *Environmental factors:* Pesticides and non-steroidal estrogen (Di-ethylstilbesterol or DES) exposure *in utero* is known with testicular dysgenesis syndromes (cryptorchidism, hypospadiasis and poor germ quality).
3. *Genetics:* Familial association is known in testicular tumours.

Pathogenesis

Most tumours arise from precursor lesion called intratubular germ cell neoplasia. The exception to this is paediatric tumours (yolk sac tumours, mature teratoma) and spermatocytic seminoma. The term carcinoma *in situ* was used earlier to this lesion. Following is the classification of testicular tumours (Table 3.37).

Table 3.37: Classification of testicular tumours[20]

Germ cell tumours derived from germ cell neoplasia *in situ*
    Noninvasive germ cell neoplasia
        Germ cell neoplasia *in situ*
        Specific forms of intratubular germ cell neoplasia
    Tumours of single histological type
        Seminomatous germ cell tumours
            Seminoma
        Nonseminomatous germ cell tumours
            Spermatocytic seminoma
            Embryonal carcinoma
            Yolk sac tumour
            Trophoblastic tumours
                Choriocarcinoma
                Non-choricarcinomatous trophoblastic tumours
                Placental site trophoblastic tumour
                Epithelioid trophoblastic tumour
            Teratoma postpubertal type
        Germ cell tumours of more than one histological type
            Mixed germ cell tumours
Sex cord stromal tumours
    Pure tumours
        Leydig cell tumours
        Sertoli cell tumour
        Granulosa cell tumour
        Fibroma thecoma
        Mixed
        Gonadoblastoma
        Unclassified
Miscellaneous tumours
Haematolymphoid tumours
(WHO 2016 classification with modification)

GERM CELL NEOPLASIA *IN SITU*

This was earlier termed intratubular germ cell neoplasia or testicular intraepithelial neoplasia. Now has been known as germ cell neoplasia *in situ* (GCNIS). Many germ cell tumours of testis arise from this precursor lesion. But tumours like spermatocytic seminoma, yolk sac tumour and teratoma do not originate from this lesion. This can be classified as below.

1. Differentiated seminomatous GCNIS
2. Differentiated non-seminomatous GCNIS
3. Undifferentiated GCNIS.

Microscopy: In seminomatous GCNIS, the affected tubules are filled with large polygonal cells with prominent nuclei and clear cytoplasm. These are usually sertoli cells and normal germ cells. The morphology is spermatogenesis is absent. Placental alkaline phosphatase and OCT3/4 are positive. In nonseminomatous GCNIS, intratubular embryonal carcinoma, intratubular yolk sac tumour, intratubular teratoma, etc., can occur.

Seminoma Testis

This is the most common testicular tumour. Typical (classical) seminoma accounts for 85–90% of the cases and occurs in the age range of 35–45 years. It is rare in old age as well as in young age. It is associated with cryptorchidism. The testis is enlarged with or without pain. The serum levels of HCG and PLAP may be increased. About 75% of the seminomas are confined to the testis at the time of presentation in contrast to about 50–70% of the nonseminomatous germ cell tumours which could have had metastasis by the time they are diagnosed.

Gross: The tumour is well-demarcated, homogenous, firm, grey white and lobulated (Fig. 3.68a).

Microscopy: There is a diffuse proliferation of large uniform tumour cells. The tumour cells are separated into lobules by supporting stroma which contains variable number of lymphocytes. They have distinct cell membrane. The nuclei are centrally placed; they are large and round with sharp nuclear membrane and they have prominent nucleoli (Fig. 3.68b). The cytoplasm is abundant and usually clear/eosinophilic/amphophilic. Mitoses are common. The stroma may show scattered syncytiotrophoblastic giant cells. The PAS stain demonstrates glycogen in the cytoplasm of these tumour cells.

Teratoma Testis

Teratoma refers to various cellular or organoid components derived from more than one germ layer. These tumours may occur at any age

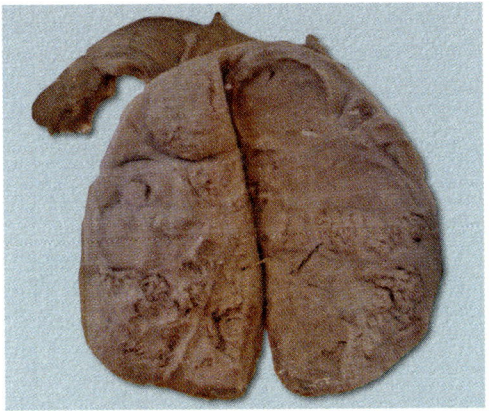

Fig. 3.68a: Gross picture of seminoma testis

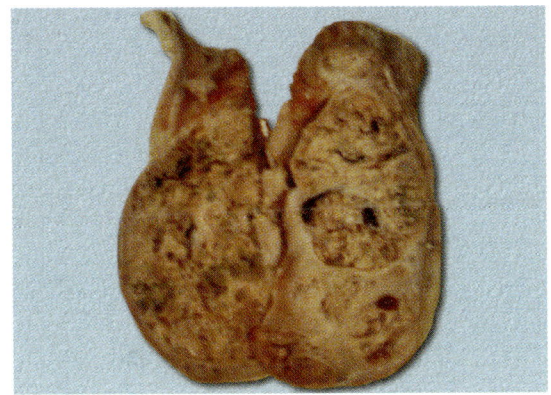

Fig. 3.69a: Gross picture of teratoma testis

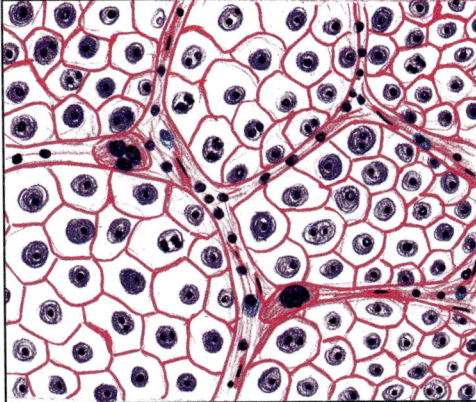

Fig. 3.68b: Schematic diagram of seminoma

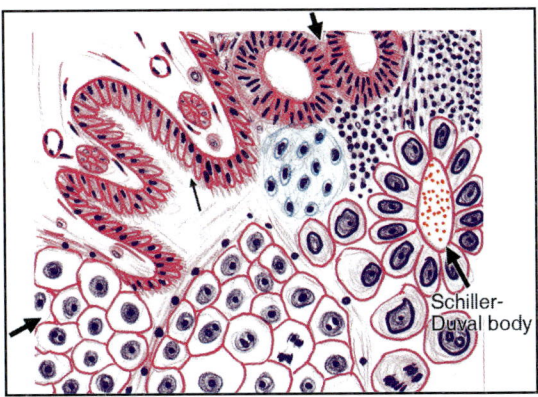

Fig. 3.69b: Schematic diagram of teratoma testis. *Note:* Mixed germ cell tumour components—seminoma component (thick arrow), immature (short arrow) and mature teratoma (thin arrow) components and yolk sac tumour component with Schiller-Duval body

from infancy to adult life, pure forms are common in infants and children and these are second in frequency to yolk sac tumours. In adults pure forms are rare. Teratoma in combination with other germ cell tumours is common.

Gross: Teratoma testis is a large tumour measuring about 5 to 10 cm in diameter. The cut section is heterogenous with solid to cystic and cartilaginous areas. Haemorrhage and necrosis are common features (Fig. 3.69a).

Microscopy: Teratomas comprise different tissues like neural tissue, muscle, islands of cartilage, squamous epithelium, thyroid tissue, respiratory epithelium, intestinal epithelium and so on. These elements may be mature or immature. Malignant transformation of any of these elements can be present. There can be combination of other germ cell tumours too (Fig. 3.69b).

Tumour markers in germ cell tumours: The following markers are helpful in detection of the germ cell tumours:
  i. Alpha-fetoproteins for yolk sac tumour
  ii. HCG for choriocarcinoma
  iii. HCG, placental alkaline phosphatase and placental lactogen for seminoma.
  iv. Lactate dehydrogenase for tumour burden.

The tumour markers are helpful in
  i. Histological typing of the tumour.
  ii. For staging of the testicular germ cell tumours.
  iii. Assessing tumour burden.
  iv. In monitoring response to therapy.

Exercise 55

Lesions of Prostate

Nodular Hyperplasia of Prostate

Usually called benign prostatic hypertrophy, recently it is termed nodular hyperplasia by Moore as it is the disease presents with nodular enlargement of the gland caused by hyperplasia of glandular and stromal components.

About 20% of men at the age of 40 years have nodular hyperplasia of prostate which increases to 70% by the age of 60 years and to 90% by the age of 70 years. The proliferation is related to dihydrotestosterone (DHT) which is synthesised from testosterone by the action of an enzyme 5α-reductase type 2. DHT binds to nuclear androgen receptors and stimulates the growth of prostate.

Gross: Prostate is enlarged, weighs up to 200 g. Cut section is nodular with milky white ooze. When predominantly fibromuscular, it is firm, pale grey and has less fluid.

Microscopy: There is glandular and fibromuscular proliferation. The glandular element shows cystically dilated glands lined by two layers—inner columnar and outer cuboidal to flattened epithelium. The epithelium is thrown into papillae (Fig. 3.70). The lumen shows corpora amylacea and foci of squamous metaplasia. The stroma may show chronic inflammation, abscesses or infarction.

Prostatic Intraepithelial Neoplasia (PIN)

It is a precursor lesion of prostate cancer. It has rearrangement involving ETS genes which are also found in invasive prostate cancer.

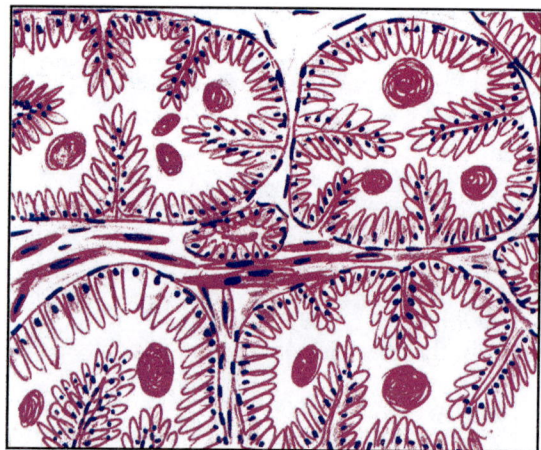

Fig. 3.70: Photomicrograph of nodular hyperplasia of prostate to show proliferation of glands and stroma

Both PIN and invasive cancer typically predominate in the peripheral zone. Prostates containing cancer have a higher frequency and greater extent of PIN and often seen in proximity to cancer.

Morphology

Consists of prostatic acini or ducts lined by cytologically atypical cells with enlarged nuclei, having prominent nucleoli and show marked crowding. PIN glands are surrounded by a patchy layer of basal cells and an intact basement membrane.

Prostatic intraepithelial neoplasia was originally graded from 1 to 3, currently divided into two grades depending upon degree of atypia, i.e. the nuclear features regardless of architecture:

1. Low grade
2. High grade

Grade 1 is considered as low grade PIN, whereas grades 2 and 3 are currently considered together as high grade PIN.

Low grade PIN has more architectural complexity than hyperplasia, occasional enlarged and hyperchromatic nuclei, rare nucleoli.

High grade of PIN is associated with cytologically atypical cells with enlarged nuclei, having prominent nucleoli and progressive disruption of the basal cell layer. Architecturally four main patterns of high-grade PIN have been described; they are tufting, micropapillary, cribriform, and flat. High-grade is always associated with adenocarcinoma.

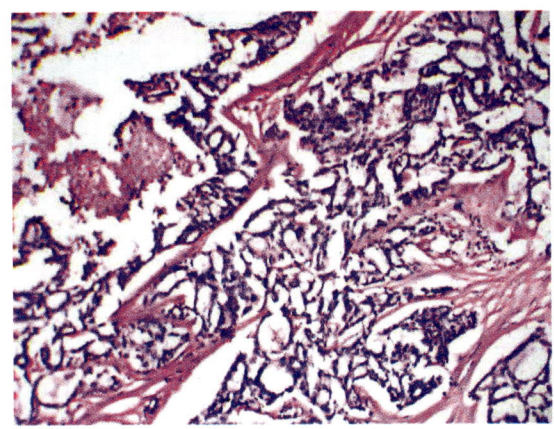

Fig. 3.71a: Photomicrograph of prostatic carcinoma

Prostatic Carcinoma (Figs 3.71a and b)

In about 70% of the cases, carcinoma prostate arise in the peripheral zone of the gland, classically in a posterior location. On cut section, the mass is gritty and firm.

Microscopy: Prostatic carcinoma is an adenocarcinoma with glands lined by single layer of uniform cuboidal to columnar cells. The glands are crowded and the cytoplasm is pale to clear or amphophilic. The nuclei lining these glands are large with some variation in size and shape having one or more nucleoli. Microscopic findings can be graded according to Gleason's grading of prostatic carcinoma (Table 3.38).

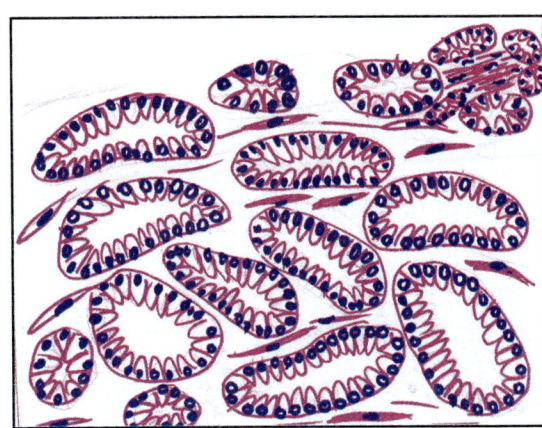

Fig. 3.71b: Schematic diagram of microscopy of prostatic carcinoma

Table 3.38: Gleason's microscopic grading of prostatic carcinoma	
Grade	Description
1	Single, separate, uniform glands in closely packed masses with a definite, usually rounded edge limiting the tumour
2	Single, separate, slightly less uniform glands, loosely packed with less sharp edge
3a	Single, separate, much more variable glands, may be closely packed but irregularly separated, ragged poorly defined edge
3b	Like 3a, but very small glands or tiny cell clusters
3c	Sharply or smoothly circumscribed rounded masses of papillary or cribriform tumour
4a	Raggedly outlined, raggedly infiltrating, fused glandular tumour
4b	Like 4a, with large pale cells (hypernephroid)
5a	Sharply circumscribed, rounded masses of almost solid cribriform tumour, with central necrosis (comedocarcinoma)
5b	Ragged masses of anaplastic carcinoma with only enough gland formation, or vacuoles to identify as adenocarcinoma

Exercise

56

Common Bone Lesions

Osteomyelitis (OM)

Osteomyelitis denotes inflammation of bone and marrow. It may be complication of a systemic infection or occur as a isolated focus. It may be acute (pyogenic), subacute or chronic process.

Bacterial or Pyogenic Osteomyelitis

Spread
Haematogenous dissemination
Direct inoculation: Compound fractures, surgeries.
Contiguous spread: Infection in adjacent bone and soft tissue.

Organisms
Coagulase positive *Staphylococcus aureus* (70–90% cases), *Salmonella* in sickle cell anaemia patients, *Klebsiella*, *E. coli*, *Pseudomonas* in genitourinary tract patients and intravenous drug abusers.
Others organisms—*Haemophilus influenzae*, Group B *Streptococcus*.

Sites involved
Neonates—epiphysis and metaphysis
Children—metaphysis
Adults—epiphysis, metaphysis or diaphysis.

Morphology
Depends on
a. Stage: Acute, subacute or chronic
b. Location of infection
c. Age involved
d. Virulence of the organisms
e. Resistance of the host.

The bacteria proliferate, induce inflammation. Within 48 hours the entrapped bone undergoes necrosis. The infection reaches the periosteum through Haversian system.

In children, the periosteum is loosely attached to the cortex. Subperiosteal abscesses formed. Lifting periosteum further impairs blood supply and both ischaemic injury and suppurative cause segmental bone necrosis and the dead piece of bone is known as sequestrum (Fig. 3.72a).

In infants, the infection spreads to adjoining joint to produce suppurative arthritis,

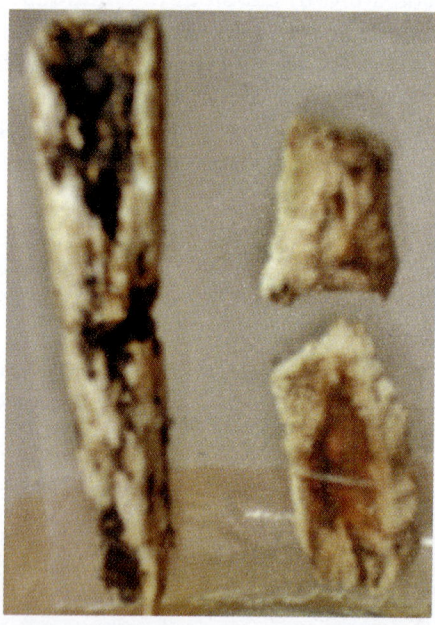

Fig. 3.72a: Gross picture of OM, note—dead bone sequestrum

sometimes with extensive destruction of articular cartilage and permanent disability.

Rupture of periosteum leads to a soft tissue abscess and formation of a draining sinus.

After first week, chronic inflammatory cells become more numerous, release cytokines, stimulates osteoclastic bone resorption, ingrowth of fibrous tissue, deposition of reactive bone in the periphery.

Newly deposited bone forms a sleeve of living tissue around devitalised infected bone, it is known as involucrum.

Microscopically, admixer of inflammatory cells including neutrophils, lymphocytes, plasma cells, fibrosis, bone necrosis (necrotic bony spicules) and new bone formation are evident (Fig. 3.72b).

Clinical features: Malaise, fever, chills, leukocytosis, throbbing pain.

Complications

Chronic osteomyelitis remains as long as infected dead bone remains.

There may be sinus tracts lined by granulation tissue and stratified squamous epithelium, in long-standing cases, the lining epithelium may develop squamous cell carcinoma.

Following are the variations in OM
1. Brodie abscess—small intraosseous abscess frequently involving cortex and is walled off by reactive bone.
2. Sclerosing osteomyelitis of Garre—develops in jaw bones and is associated with extensive new bone formation that obscures much of the underlying osseous structure.

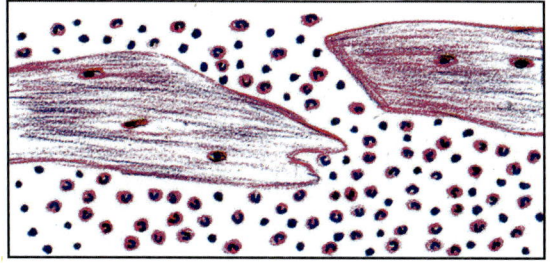

Fig. 3.72b: Schematic diagram, microscopy of OM

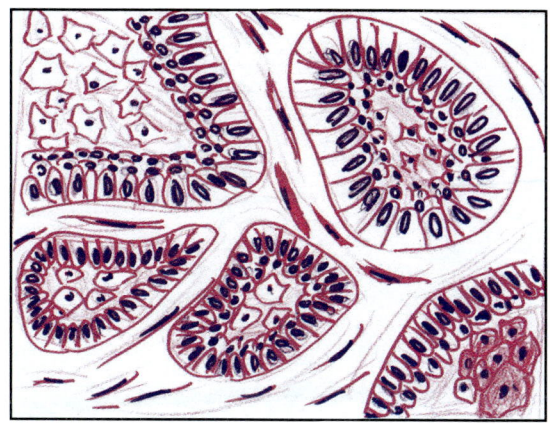

Fig. 3.73: Schematic diagram of microscopy of ameloblastoma

Ameloblastoma

Gross: The tumour is grey white with solid to cystic areas expanding the affected bone.

Microscopy: There are different histological patterns such as follicular, plexiform, acanthomatous and granular cell pattern. The follicular pattern is more common. There is central area of stellate cells resembling stellate reticulum and peripheral layer of cuboidal to columnar epithelium with polarisation of the nuclei away from the basement membrane (Fig. 3.73).

Osteosarcoma

Osteosarcoma is a malignant mesenchymal tumour. It occurs frequently before the age of 20 years. It may also occur in elderly patients with Paget's disease, bone infarcts and in patients with prior irradiation. The tumour arises in the metaphyseal region of the long bones; most commonly around the knee, upper end of the femur, humerus and jaw bones.

Gross: These tumours are bulky masses, grey white in colour and have areas of haemorrhage and cystic degeneration. They can destroy the cortex and produce soft tissue masses (Fig. 3.74a).

Microscopy: The tumour cells are pleomorphic with hyperchromatic nuclei. There

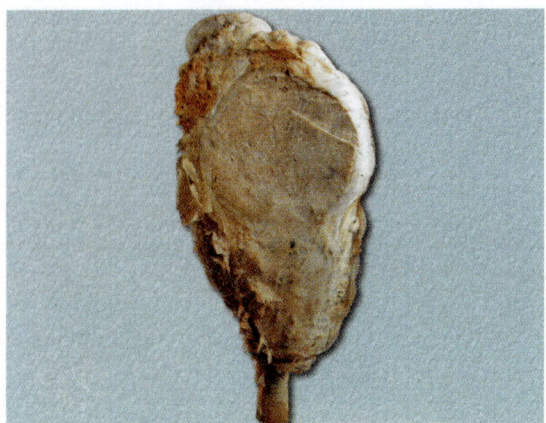

Fig. 3.74a: Gross picture of osteosarcoma

are good number of bizarre tumour giant cells. There is a formation of osteoid by the tumour cells (Fig. 3.74b). There may be chondroblastic and fibroblastic differentiation. Vascular invasion is common.

Histological variants of osteosarcoma: There are different histological variants of osteosarcoma such as conventional osteosarcoma, fibroblastic, chondroblastic, telangiectatic, small cell, fibrohistiocytic, anaplastic and well-differentiated intramedullary osteosarcomas.

Osteoclastoma

This is a locally aggressive tumour and is believed to arise from monocyte-macrophage lineage. It occurs in the age range of 20 to 40 years and involves the epiphysis and metaphysis. It occurs most commonly around the knee and lower end of the radius; but any bone may be involved. It is associated with pathological fracture. X-ray shows lytic lesion with soap bubble appearance.

Gross: Osteoclastoma is a large tumour with club-shaped deformity. The cut section shows red-brown solid areas and cystic areas containing haemorrhage (Fig. 3.75a).

Microscopy: These tumours have oval mononuclear stromal cells which may exhibit atypical features. The background has numerous osteoclastic giant cells (Fig. 3.75b). Necrosis, haemorrhage and haemosiderin deposition are common features (Fig. 3.75c).

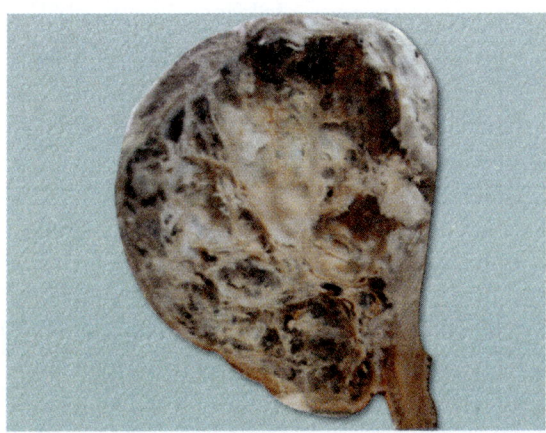

Fig. 3.75a: Gross picture of osteoclastoma

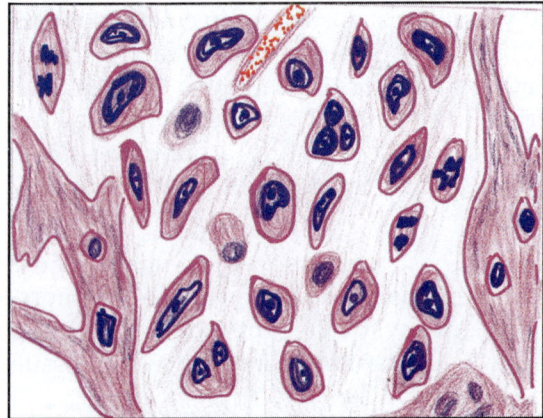

Fig. 3.74b: Schematic diagram, microscopy of osteosarcoma

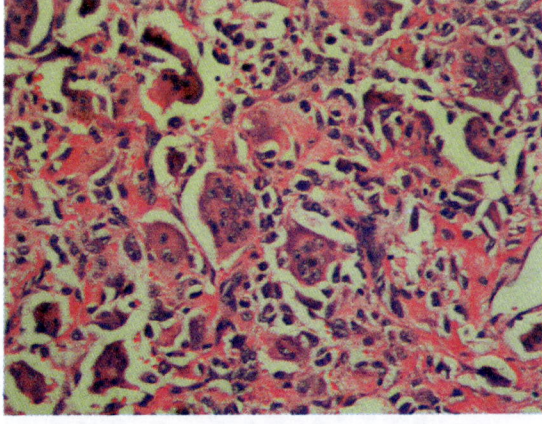

Fig. 3.75b: Photomicrograph of osteoclastoma, note—numerous osteoclastic giant cells

Ewing's Sarcoma[22]

Ewing's sarcoma accounts for 5–10% of primary bone tumours and is the second most common tumour in childhood next to osteosarcoma in children. It occurs predominantly in children and young adults and shows a slight predilection for males.

It is characterised by recurrent chromosomal translocations [t(11;22) EWSR1-FLI1 or t(21;22) EWSR1-ERG] and membranous MIC2/CD99 overexpression.

Ewing's sarcoma usually arises from diaphysis or metadiaphyseal region of long bones, pelvic bones and ribs. The rare locations are the skull bones, vertebra, scapula, and the small bones of hands and feet. Any soft tissue site can be affected. Ewing's sarcoma shows a permeative pattern with periosteal reaction.

The radiological findings are essential for histopathological diagnosis.

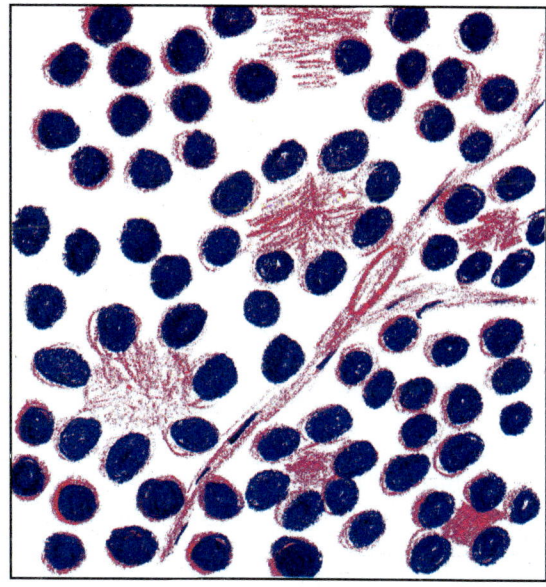

Fig. 3.76: Schematic diagram, microscopy of Ewing's sarcoma, note—rosettes

X-ray Findings

1. Destructive, lytic tumour with reactive periosteal bone resembling 'onion skin'.
2. Widening of medullary canal

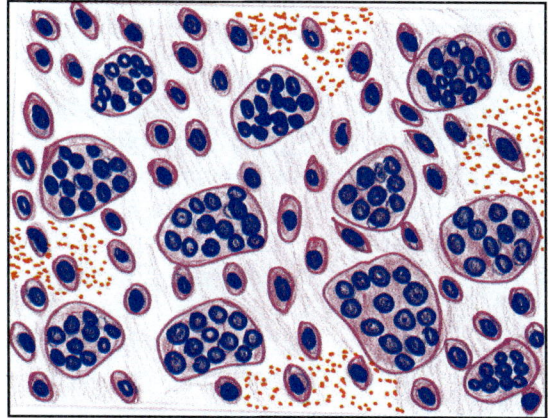

Fig. 3.75c: Schematic diagram of microscopy of osteoclastoma

Gross: This tumour arises in medullary cavity, invades cortex and periosteum producing soft tissue mass. The tumour is tan white in colour and has areas of haemorrhage and necrosis.

Microscopy: Ewing's sarcoma is a highly malignant small round blue cell tumour, histologically, composed of sheets of small cells with high nuclear to cytoplasmic ratio. The cytoplasm is scant, eosinophilic, and usually contains glycogen, which is detected by periodic acid-Schiff stain and is diastase degradable.

The nuclei are round, with finely dispersed chromatin, and one or more tiny nucleoli. Rosette formation is also seen. This tumour frequently undergoes necrosis and shows a "peritheliomatous" or a perivascular distribution. Homer-Wright rosettes, cells arranged in a circle around a central fibrillary structure is indicative of a neural differentiation (Fig. 3.76).

Exercise 57

Lesions of Thyroid

Thyroid gland has two lateral lobes connected by isthmus. It is located below and anterior to larynx. Weight of normal thyroid gland is 15 to 25 g. In response to thyrotropin releasing hormone (TRH) from hypothalamus, TSH is released from the anterior pituitary and this raises the T_3 and T_4. Elevated levels in turn suppress TRH and TSH.

Thyroglobulin secreted by the follicular cells is rich in tyrosine. Iodinisation of tyrosine later gets converted into T_3 and T_4 and following steps are involved.

Iodide circulating in blood is taken up and this is called iodine trapping.

This undergoes oxidation from iodide to iodine.

$$\text{Iodide} \xrightarrow{\text{Peroxidase enzyme and hydrogen peroxide}} \text{Iodine}$$

Iodine binds to thyroglobin → Organification

Tyrosine is iodised to monoiodotyrosine and then to diiodotyrosine.

Two molecules of diiodotyrosine forms T_4.

One molecule of monoiodotyrosine and one molecule of diiodotyrosine forms T_3

T_3 has 10 times more affinity than T_4 for thyroid hormone receptors.

Following are the causes of hypothyroidism
Primary
- Iodine deficiency—endemic/food faddism
- Drugs—lithium
- Congenital biosynthetic defect
- Postablative
- Hashimoto thyroiditis.

Secondary
Pituitary.

COLLOID GOITRE (Figs 3.77a and b)

The colloid goitre has hyperplastic phase and involution phase. In hyperplastic phase, the thyroid gland is diffusely and symmetrically enlarged. The follicles vary in size; some are large and some are small. These are lined by cuboidal to columnar epithelium which pile up at places. In the involution phase, the cut section shows brownish translucent material. The follicles are large and are lined by cuboidal epithelium. The lumen contains abundant colloid.

The episodes of hyperplasia and involution produces multinodular goitre. At this stage grossly, the thyroid gland is multilobulated, asymmetrical and at some instances, the nodules may be prominent. Variable amount of colloid, areas of fibrosis, haemorrhage, calcification and cystic degeneration are present. Microscopy shows colloid rich follicles lined by flattened epithelium and areas of follicular epithelial hyperplasia.

PAPILLARY CARCINOMA THYROID

Commonly found in 20–50 years of age group.
Gross
1. Non-encapsulated, infiltrative masses.
2. Occasionally capsulated.
3. Firm and white due to fibrous tissue.

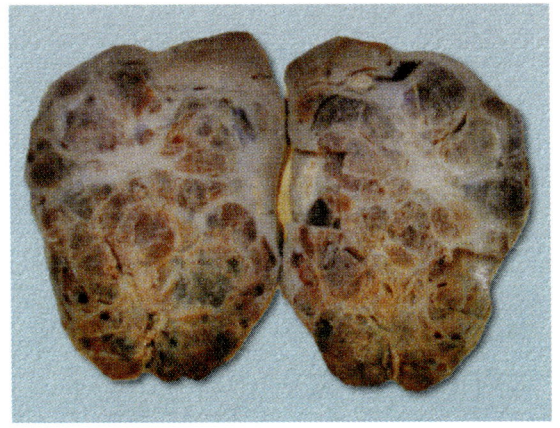

Fig. 3.77a: Gross picture of multinodular goitre

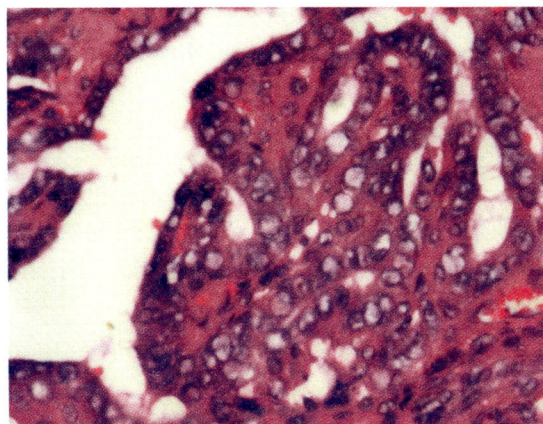

Fig. 3.78a: Microscopy of papillary carcinoma thyroid

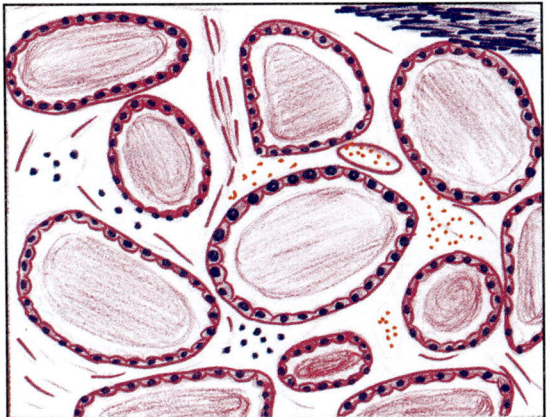

Fig. 3.77b: Schematic diagram, microscopy of multinodular goitre, note—haemorrhage and calcification

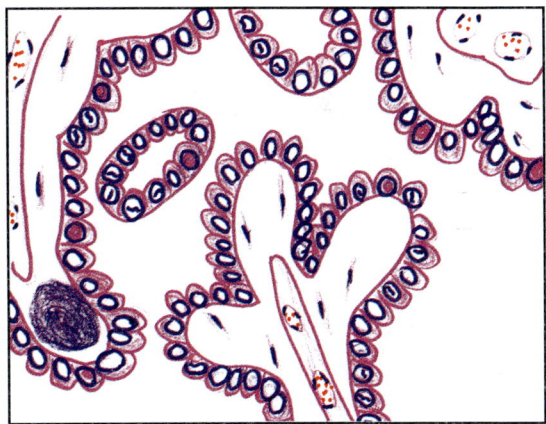

Fig. 3.78b: Schematic diagram, microscopy of papillary carcinoma thyroid, note, psammoma body, nuclei with peripheral clumping of chromatin, nuclear overlapping, nuclear grooves and intranuclear eosinophilic cytoplasmic inclusions

Microscopy (Figs 3.78a and b)
- Papillae with fibrovascular core
- Single or stratified lining of cuboidal or columnar cells
- Nuclei large with groundglass or peripheral clumping of chromatin (Orphan Annie eye nuclei)
- Eosinophilic inclusions in the nuclei (cytoplasmic invaginations)
- Nuclear grooves and nuclear overlapping
- Psammoma bodies in the stroma.

These tumours metastasise via lymphatics.

FOLLICULAR ADENOMA

These present as solitary nodules, rarely may synthesise excess T_3 or T_4 and appear as hot nodules on isotope scan and sometimes cause thyrotoxicosis.

Gross

1. Follicular adenomas are well-circumscribed masses.
2. Solid, encapsulated capsule is complete, compress surrounding normal thyroid tissue.

Microscopy (Fig. 3.79)
- Compact micro- or macrofollicles with little colloid.
- Intact capsule
- No capsular or vascular invasion.

FOLLICULAR CARCINOMA

These tumours account for 15–30% of the thyroid tumours.

Common above the age of 40 years.

F : M = 3 : 1

Common in endemic areas with iodine deficiency.

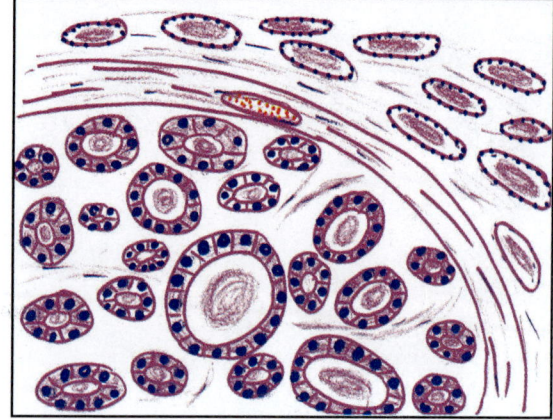

Fig. 3.79: Schematic diagram, microscopy of follicular adenoma

Gross
- Vary in size
- Yellow tan coloured
- Thick fibrous capsule with invasion
- Haemorrhage, necrosis and cystic degeneration present
- These can be minimally or widely invasive, depending upon capsular invasion.

Microscopy
- Microfollicles and macrofollicles
- Haemorrhage and necrosis present
- Mitoses common
- No papillae are seen
- Neoplasm extends through the capsule, shows vascular invasion. Also extends into the surrounding soft tissue.

Exercise 58

Lesions of Lymph Node

HODGKIN'S DISEASE (HODGKIN'S LYMPHOMA)

Hodgkin's lymphoma (HL) is a malignant neoplasm of the lymphoid system with the potential to spread to many sites and produce of large tumourous masses containing dysplastic cells (RS cells).

Classification of Hodgkin's Lymphoma (WHO)

1. Classical Hodgkin's lymphoma
   Nodular sclerosis
   Lymphocyte-rich
   Mixed cellularity
   Lymphocyte depleted
2. Nodular lymphocyte predominant Hodgkin's lymphoma

In general, in Hodgkin's disease

Gross: The lymph nodes are enlarged, grey white, and are of rubbery consistency.

Microscopy: Depending upon the type of Hodgkin's disease (Figs 3.80a and c).

In mixed cellularity, there is diffuse effacement of the lymph node architecture with polymorphic cellular infiltrate which includes small lymphocytes, eosinophils, plasma cells and macrophages admixed with plenty of Reed-Sternberg (RS) cells (classical and mononuclear varieties).

The nodular sclerosis Hodgkin's disease may show abundant fibrosis; the classical RS cells are less frequent and show lacunar variety of RS cells.

Lymphocyte-rich Hodgkin's disease shows lymphocyte predominance with mononuclear and classical RS cells. In lymphocyte

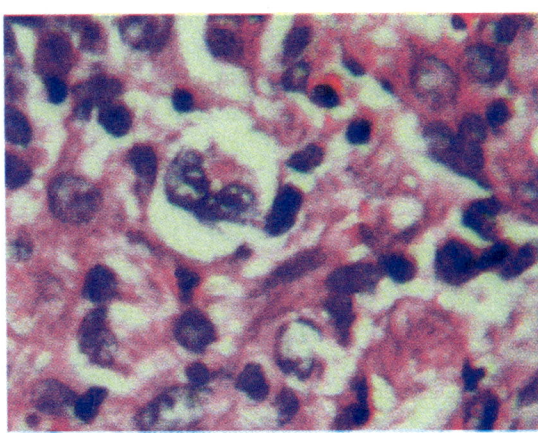

Fig. 3.80a: Photomicrograph of Hodgkin's disease, note, RS cell

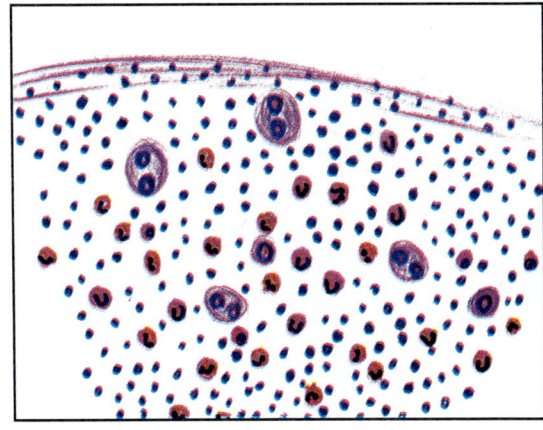

Fig. 3.80b: Schematic diagram, microscopy of Hodgkin's disease (mixed cellularity)

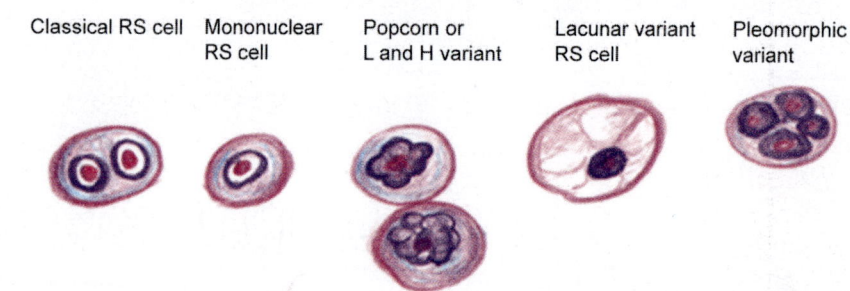

Fig. 3.80c: Types of RS cells

depletion, large number of classical RS cells, RS cells with bizarre configuration and atypical mononuclear variants are present.

In lymphocyte predominance, there is a nodal effacement which shows nodular infiltrate of small lymphocytes admixed with histiocytes. In this histological type, the classical RS cells are difficult to find and however, they have L and H variants (popcorn cells).

The details are given regarding other features HL share the following characteristics:

1. Usually arise in the lymph nodes preferably cervical lymph node.
2. Majority of them manifest clinically in young adults.
3. It is characterised by a heterogeneous cellularity comprising a minority of specific neoplastic cells, the Hodgkin's cells and the Reed-Sternberg cells and a majority of reactive non-neoplastic cells.
4. The tumour cells are usually ringed by T lymphocytes in a rosette like manner.

The important finding in Hodgkin's lymphoma is the Reed-Sternberg (RS) cell. This is a large cell (15–45 µm in diameter) with mirror image nuclei, exceptionally prominent nucleoli, distinct nuclear membrane and abundant, usually slightly eosinophilic, cytoplasm. The nucleus has inclusion-like acidophilic nucleolus surrounded by a distinctive clear zone; together they impart an owl-eye appearance.

Classical Hodgkin's Lymphoma

Classical Hodgkin's lymphoma (CHL) is characterised by clonal proliferation of typical mononuclear Hodgkin's cells and multinucleated Reed-Sternberg cells. Expression of the lymphocytic activation antigen CD30 unites the different types of CHL. A variable inflammatory background of lymphocytes, eosinophils, macrophages, neutrophils, plasma cells, fibroblasts, and collagenous tissue determines the morphologic appearance.

Four different types of CHL are defined: lymphocyte-rich, nodular-sclerosis, mixed-cellularity, and lymphocyte-depleted variants.

Nodular Sclerosis Hodgkin's Lymphoma (NSHL)

Most common form of HL.

Accounts for 70% of CHL.

Affects adolescent girls and young women in the age range of 15 to 35 years.

Manifest as lower cervical, supraclavicular and mediastinal adenopathy (stage II). Symptoms occur in up to 40% of patients.

Microscopy: NSHL features nodular architecture in which lymphoid tissue is surrounded by fibrosis. There is presence of a particular variant of the RS cell, the lacunar cell. This cell is large and has a single multilobate nucleus with multiple small nucleoli and an abundant, pale-staining cytoplasm. In formalin-fixed tissue, the cytoplasm often retracts, giving rise to the appearance of cells lying in empty spaces, or lacunae. The fibrosis may be scant or abundant, and the cellular infiltrate may show varying proportions of lymphocytes, eosinophils, histiocytes, and lacunar cells. Classic RS cells are infrequent.

IHC: The lacunar variants express CD15 and CD30 and usually do not express B and T cell-specific antigens.

The prognosis is good, with a cure rate of 80 to 85%. Untreated, NSHL is fatal, with a 10-year survival rate of only 1%. With irradiation and chemotherapy, a 70% cure rate can be achieved.

Mixed Cellularity Hodgkin's Lymphoma

1. Most common form of Hodgkin's lymphoma in older patients (> 50 years)
2. Most frequent HL subtype in HIV-1-infected patients and shows the highest association with EBV.
3. Accounts for 25% of cases.
4. Male predominance.
5. Most common site is cervical lymph nodes. However, after staging, most patients are found to have stage II or III disease. A minority have visceral involvement (stage IV).
6. Mediastinal involvement is uncommon.

Microscopy: Histology is like that of the nodular sclerosis variety, but collagen bands are missing. Classic RS cells are plentiful within a distinctive heterogeneous cellular infiltrate, which includes small lymphocytes, eosinophils, plasma cells, and histiocytes.

Compared with the other common subtypes, more patients with mixed cellularity have disseminated disease and systemic manifestations.

The prognosis is intermediate, with a cure rate of 75%.

Lymphocyte Rich Hodgkin's Lymphoma (LRHL)

It is characterised by classical RS cells in an abundant background of small lymphocytes. Mixed inflammatory cells and collagen bands are missing.

Lymphocyte Depleted Hodgkin's Lymphoma (LDHL)

1. Least common type of CHL.
2. Most clinically aggressive type.
3. Frequently associated with HIV infection and most are positive for EBV.
4. Advanced stage and symptoms are seen in more than 70% of patients.
5. Affects middle-aged to elderly men.
6. Advanced clinical stage (III and IV) and signs and symptoms are present in two-thirds of patients.
7. Those with the diffuse fibrosis subtype of LDHL commonly present with fever of undetermined origin, pancytopenia, and wasting.
8. There is usually no peripheral or mediastinal adenopathy. However, retroperitoneal adenopathy is frequently prominent and involvement of the spleen, liver, and bone marrow is common.
9. *Microscopy:* Shows marked absence of background lymphocytes.
10. The overall cure rate in both types of LDHL is 40–50%.
11. Without treatment, this type of HL has the worst prognosis profound immunodeficiency develops and death commonly results from secondary infections.

Nodular Lymphocyte Predominant Hodgkin's Lymphoma

1. Accounts for 5% of HL cases.
2. Present with isolated cervical or axillary lymphadenopathy.
3. *Microscopy:* It is characterised by a large number of small resting lymphocytes admixed with a variable number of histiocytes, often within large, poorly defined nodules. Other types of reactive cells, such as eosinophils, neutrophils, and plasma cells are scanty or absent, and classic RS cells are extremely difficult to find. Scattered among the reactive cells are lymphohistiocytic (L & H) variant RS cells that have a delicate multilobed, nucleus that

has been likened in appearance to popcorn ("popcorn cell").
4. *IHC:* The L & H variants express B cell markers (e.g. CD20).
5. L & H variants have rearranged and somatically hypermutated IgH genes, strongly supporting a follicular B cell origin.
6. Excellent prognosis.

NON-HODGKIN'S LYMPHOMA

Non-Hodgkin's lymphoma (NHL) or malignant lymphomas (ML) are neoplastic disorders which originate from the lymphoid tissue similar to Hodgkin's disease but do have the RS cells. NHL are common in men than women. It is common malignancy occurring in developed countries accounting for 4.3% of all malignancies in USA.

Risk Factors and Aetiology

The risk factors for development of lymphoma are not fully understood. However following factors are implicated and association is seen in the causation of the disease.
1. Environmental association with pesticides, chemicals, hair dyes, radiation and chemotherapy are known.
2. Viruses: HIV infection, EBV in Burkitt lymphoma, Human T cell leukaemia Virus-1(HTLV-1) in T cell lymphomas and leukaemias
3. Immune-suppression with inherited disorders like severe combined immunodeficiency disease, Wiskott-Aldrich syndrome.
4. Infection with *H. pylori* with ongoing antigenic stimulation is known to cause NHLs and especially MALT lymphomas.
5. Patients with chronic diseases.
6. Patients with autoimmune diseases: Hashimoto's thyroiditis is known to cause primary NHL in thyroid gland.
7. Chromosomal translocations play an important in the causation NHLs. Chromosomal traslocations like t(14:18) in follicular lymphoma, t(11:14) in mantal cell lymphoma, etc. are known in Non-Hodgkin's lymphomas (Table 3.39).

Table 3.39: 2016 WHO classification of mature lymphoid, histiocytic and dendritic neoplasms[23]

Non-Hodgkin's lymphoma
Mature B neoplasms
Chronic lymphocytic leukaemia/small lymphocytic leukaemia (CLL/SLL)
Monoclonal B cell lymphocytosis
B-prolymphocytic leukaemia
Splenic Marginal Zone Lymphoma
Hairy cell leukemia (HCL)
Splenic B cell lymphoma/ leukaemia
Lymphoplasmacytic Lymphoma (Waldenstrom's macroglobulinaemia)
MUGS-IgM/IgG/IgA
Heavy chain diseases (Mue, gamma and alpha)
Plasma cell myeloma
Solitary plasmacytoma of bone
Extraosseous plasmacytoma
MALT lymphoma
Nodal marginal zone lymphoma
Follicular lymphoma
Large B cell lymphoma
Mantle cell lymphoma
Diffuse large B cell lymphoma (DLBCL)
T cell rich large B cell lymphoma
CNS large B cell lymphoma
Thymic /mediastinal large B cell lymphoma
ALK positive large B cell lymphoma
Plasmablastic lymphoma
Burkitt lymphoma
High grade B cell lymphoma

Mature T and NK cell neoplasms
T cell prolymphocytic leukaemia
T cell large cell lymphoma
Aggressive NK cell leukemia
Adult T cell lymphoma/leukaemia
Extranodal T/K cell lymphoma, nasal type
Enteropathy associated T cell lymphoma
Mycosis fungoides
Sezary syndrome
Primary cutaneous CD30 positive T cell lymphoproliferative disease
Peripheral T cell lymphoma
Angio-immunoblastic lymphoma
Anaplastic large cell lymphoma (ALK+ /ALK)
Hodgkin's lymphoma
Post-transplant lymphoproliferative disorders (PTLD)
Histiocytic and dendritic cell neoplasms

In SLL/CLL, lymph nodes are enlarged and the architecture is effaced. There is diffuse proliferation of small round lymphocytes with regular nuclear contours, inconspicuous nucleoli, scanty cytoplasm, mitoses are minimal and scattered larger cells (prolymphocytes and paraimmunoblasts) with vesicular nuclei and prominent nucleoli.

Bone marrow, spleen and liver are also infiltrated with such cells. There is absolute lymphocytosis and these cells are fragile and gets disrupted during preparation of smears. These are called smudge cells. Smear also shows variable number of larger activated lymphocytes.

Immunophenotype, karyotype and molecular features: The cells express pan B cell markers (CD19, CD20, CD23 and surface Ig heavy and light chains). The cells also express CD5 similar to cells of mantle cell lymphoma. These are negative for CD10. ZAP-70 positivity has unfavouable prognosis.

Clinical features: The patients are elderly or middle aged; often have fewer or no symptoms. The symptoms are nonspecific and these include easy fatigability, weight loss and anorexia. Generalised lymphadenopathy and hepatomegaly are present in 50–60% of the cases. The total count is increased and may exceed 2 lakh cells/cmm. Hypogammaglobinaemia is present in 50% of the cases late in the disease process and this is the reason for increased susceptibility to bacterial infections.

Follicular Lymphoma (FL) is relatively common and accounts for 40% of the adult NHLs. They are unusual before 20 years of age.

Pathology: The lymph nodes are enlarged. The architecture is effaced and cortex and medulla show nodular pattern of growth of lymphoid follicles. The cells are larger than resting B cells, angular cleaved nuclei, nuclear chromatin is coarse and condensed and nucleoli are indistinct. These cells are mixed with larger centroblasts having vesicular chromatin, several nucleoli with moderate amount of cytoplasm. Mitoses are infrequent; apoptotic cells are not seen. Uniform follicles and indistinct/fading of lymphoid follicles are common. Condensation of reticulin fibres around the follicles helps to distinguish follicular lymphoma from follicular hyperplasia.

Immunophenotype, karyotype and molecular features: The cells express pan B markers CD19, CD10 and CD20. CD5 and CD43 are negative. t(14:18) (q13;q32) is found in 85% of FL.

Clinical features: Follicular lymphoma predominantly occurs in adults or elderly persons, males and females are equally affected. It presents with painless generalised lymphadenopathy, extranodal involvement is common. Bone marrow is almost always involved at the time of diagnosis. It may progress to diffuse large B cell lymphoma with or without treatment.

Differences between Hodgkin's and non-Hodgkin's lymphomas are given in Table 3.40.

Table 3.40: Differences between Hodgkin's lymphoma and non-Hodgkin's lymphoma

Hodgkin's lymphoma	Non-Hodgkin's lymphoma
More often localised to single group of lymph nodes (either cervical, mediastinal or para-aortic)	Multiple groups of lymph nodes are involved
Spread by contiguity	Noncontiguous spread
Mesenteric lymph nodes and Waldeyer ring rarely involved	Mesenteric lymph nodes and Waldeyer ring commonly involved
Extranodal involvement less common	Extranodal involvement more common
Leukaemic phase absent	Leukaemic phase present
Has association with virus EBV	Has association with virus HIV and immunosuppression
Low grade fever, night sweats and weight loss are common constitutional symptoms	Fewer symptoms
Responsive to treatment	Depends upon type of NHL
Curable with 5 year survival 90%	Prognosis varies with type of NHL and overall survival lesser compared to HD

METASTATIC LYMPH NODE

The primary malignant tumours can metastasise to regional lymph nodes (Fig. 3.81). The common groups of lymph nodes involved are:

1. *Cervical (high jugular, posterior cervical) lymph nodes:* Head and neck malignancies (nasopharynx, tonsils, tongue, floor of mouth, thyroid, extrinsic larynx, facial skin, scalp).
2. *Low cervical group lymph nodes:* Intrathoracic (lungs) and intra-abdominal malignancies.
3. *Supraclavicular (left supraclavicular) lymph nodes:* Gastric malignancy.
4. *Axillary lymph nodes:* Breast and upper extremities malignancies.
5. *Inguinal lymph nodes:* Malignancies of lower extremities, vulva, cervix, endometrium, ovary, penis, prostate, rectum, anus.
6. *Pelvic lymph nodes:* Prostate, testes, female genital tract, lower extremities.

Sometimes lymph node metastasis can be the earliest manifestation as in occult malignancies of head and neck and thyroid papillary carcinoma.

The tumour cells in nests, islands, and cords are seen in the sinusoids of the lymph node with preservation of the integrity of the capsule.

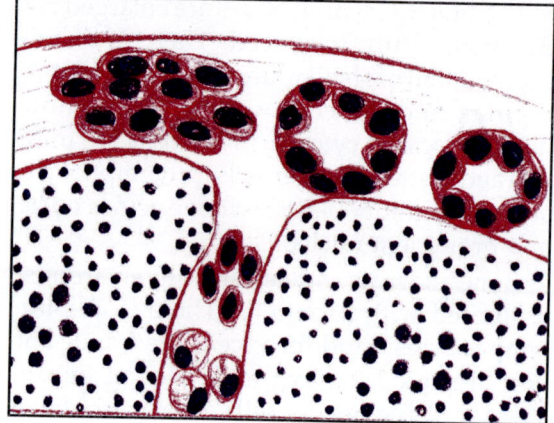

Fig. 3.81: Schematic diagram, microscopy of metastatic adenocarcinoma lymph node

The sites of origin of other metastatic tumours may be indicated by the following:
- Glandular or papillary structures in adenocarcinoma. Papillary structures with occasional psammoma bodies in carcinomas of the thyroid and ovary
- Keratin pearls in squamous cell carcinomas
- Melanin pigment in melanomas
- Neurofibrils in neuroblastomas
- Neurosecretory granules in neuroendocrine tumours
- Argyrophil granules in carcinoid tumours.

Exercise 59

Lesions of Brain

BRAIN TUMOURS: CLASSIFICATION

Central nervous system (CNS) constitutes 2% of all the cancers and in paediatric population it accounts for 20% of all childhood tumours. About 70% of the childhood tumours occur in the posterior fossa whereas most of the adult CNS tumours occur within the cerebral hemispheres. Metastatic tumours are more common than the primary tumours.

The CNS tumours need special attention due to the following reasons:
1. The clinical course of a patient with brain tumour is strongly influenced by patterns of growth and location. Even low grade tumours may have infiltrative margins, clinical deficits and poor outcome.
2. The tumour may not be amenable to surgical resection due to infiltrative margins.
3. Even benign tumours may compress vital organs, if the tumors are adjacent to the vital structures.
4. The tumors may spread through CSF pathway and implants can be present along brain and spinal cord in distant sites away from primary tumour.

Classification of CNS Tumours

In the year 2007 WHO has classified the brain tumours on the basis of phenotype into grade I to IV, however in the year 2016 WHO revised the classification of the CNS tumours based on molecular changes, i.e. genotypic and phenotypic classification which is target therapy based. The detailed classification is beyond the scope of this book.

Depending upon the cell of origin, the CNS tumours are named as below:
Glioma: Arising from the glial cells
Astrocytes: Astrocytoma
Oligodendrocytes: Oligodendroglioma
Ependymal cells: Ependymoma
Choroid plexus: Choroid plexus papilloma
Meningeal cells: Meningioma
Ganglion cells and neural cells: Ganglioneuroma

The simplified WHO 2016 classification of CNS tumours is presented in Table 3.41.

Table 3.41: Classification of CNS tumours

Astrocytic and oligodendroglial tumours	Mixed glial and neuronal
Astrocytoma	Ganglioneuroma
Diffuse astrocytoma IDH mutant	**Embryonal tumours**
Diffuse astrocytoma NOS	Medulloblastoma
Gemistocytic astrocytoma	– WNT activated
Anaplastic astrocytoma IDH mutant	– SHH activated and TP53 mutant
Glioblastoma IDH mutant and IDH wild type	– Non-WNT and NON-SHH activated
Glioblastoma NOS	– Classical

Contd.

Table 3.41: Classification of CNS tumours[24] (Contd.)

Oligodendroglioma NOS Oligodendroglioma IDH mutant and 1p/19q codeleted Oligoastrocytoma NOS Anaplastic oligodendroglioma IDH mutant nd 1p/19q codeleted **Other astrocytic tumours** Pilocytic astrocytoma Subependymal giant cell astrocytoma Pleomorphic xanthoastrocytoma Anaplastic pleomorphic xanthoastrocytoma **Ependymal** Subependymoma Ependymoma RELA fusion positive Myxopapillary ependymoma Papillary ependymoma Clear cell ependymoma Anaplastic ependymoma **Choroid plexus** Choroid plexus papilloma Atypical choroid plexus papilloma Choroid plexus carcinoma **Tumours of neural origin** Ganglioneuroma Neuroblastoma	– Desmoplastic – Anaplastic – NOS Pineloblastoma Neuroblastoma Atypical teratoid rhobdoid tumour **Nerve sheath tumours** Neurofibroma Schwannoma Malignant Peripheral Nerve Sheath Tumour (MPNST) **Meningiomas** Meningioma Atypical meningioma Anaplastic meningioma **Tumours of sellar origin** Pituitary adenoma Craniophyringioma **Miscellaneous** CNS lymphoma Germ cell tumour Hamangioblastoma Malignant melanoma **Metastatic tumours**

ASTROCYTOMA

Different types of astrocytic tumours are recognised. These occur in the cerebral hemispheres and may also occur in the cerebellum, brainstem or spinal cord. They commonly occur during 4–6th decades.

Astrocytomas can be:

1. Localised (grade I astrocytoma): Pilocytic astrocytoma and subependymal giant cell astrocytoma.
2. Infiltrating (grade II to grade IV astrocytomas).

Clinical features in general to gliomas

The most common presenting signs and symptoms are seizures, headache, and focal neurologic deficits related to the anatomic site of involvement.

Infiltrating astrocytomas can be:

1. Diffuse astrocytomas.
2. Anaplastic astrocytoma.
3. Glioblastoma.

Diffuse Astrocytoma

This is WHO grade II and has following different histological types:

1. Pleomorphic xanthoastrocytoma
2. Gemistocytic astrocytoma

The protoplasmic astrocytoma and fibrillary astrocytoma have been taken out in WHO 2016 classification.

Site: Supratentorial region commonly frontal lobes

Age: 20–30 years.

Gross: These tumors, as the name suggests, are having highly infiltrative type of growth, they diffusely involve the white matter of the brain. It extends to different parts of the brain and the borders cannot be determined. Cut section is firm or soft and gelatinous. Cystic degeneration may be seen.

Microscopy: The tumour is cellular and shows fibrillary background. There is variable degree of pleomorphism. Necrosis and mitoses indicates higher grade and aggressive course.

The cells having abundant eosinophilic glassy cytoplasm with eccentric nuclei and prominent nucleoli are called gemistocytic astrocytoma. The background of the tumour has fibrillary network and GFAP and Vimentin are positive.

Anaplastic astrocytoma: This is of WHO grade III and have densely cellular areas and have greater degree of pleomorphism. The cells show increased mitotic activity.

Glioblastoma: This was previously called glioblastoma multiforme (GBM), corresponds to WHO grade IV (Fig. 3.82a).

Age: Above 40 years of age

Types: De novo primary

Secondary: Develops from the pre-existing anaplastic astrocytoma

Sites: This tumour can occur in any part of the brain but more common in the supratentorial region, rare in cerebellum and spinal cord.

Gross: GBM is having infiltrative type of growth; they have variegated appearance solid, cystic and soft areas represent necrosis and haemorrhage.

Microscopy: The tumour cells are highly anaplastic with pleomorphic nuclei. The cells range from spindle to epithelial, bizarre giant cells sometimes round cells seen. Good numbers of mitotic figures are seen. The hallmark and diagnostic point is the presence of necrosis and vascular proliferation. A criterion for vascular endothelial proliferation is vessel having more than two endothelial layers. With marked vascular cell proliferation the tuft forms a ball-like structure, called the glomeruloid body.

PILOCYTIC ASTROCYTOMA

Pilocytic astrocytomas are grade I astrocytomas, occur in children and young adults and these are relatively benign tumours. They are located in the cerebellum but may also appear in the floor and walls of the third ventricle, the optic nerve and occasionally cerebral hemispheres.

Gross: Pilocytic astrocytoma is often cystic and if solid, well-circumscribed. They have localised growth.

Microscopy: The tumour is composed of bipolar cells with long, thin "hairlike" processes that are GFAP-positive and form dense fibrillary meshwork. Cystic areas, Rosenthal fibres and eosinophilic granular bodies are often present. Necrosis and mitoses are absent.

Site: Cerebellum, spinal cord, optic nerve.

Treatment and prognosis: Amenable to excision with good prognosis.

OLIGODENDROGLIOMA

These account for 5–15% of gliomas.

Occur in fourth and fifth decades.

The lesions are found mostly in the cerebral hemispheres, with a predilection for white matter.

Morphology

On gross examination, oligodendrogliomas are gelatinous, gray masses, often with cysts, focal haemorrhage and calcification (Fig. 3.82).

On microscopic examination, the tumors are composed of sheets of regular cells with spherical nuclei containing finely granular chromatin and containing small nucleoli. Perinuclear halo is present giving "fried egg" appearance.

The tumour typically contains a delicate network of anastomosing capillaries ('Chicken wire network'). Calcification is seen in 90% of the cases.

Anaplastic oligodendrogliomas are characterised by increased cellular density, nuclear anaplasia, increased mitotic activity and necrosis.

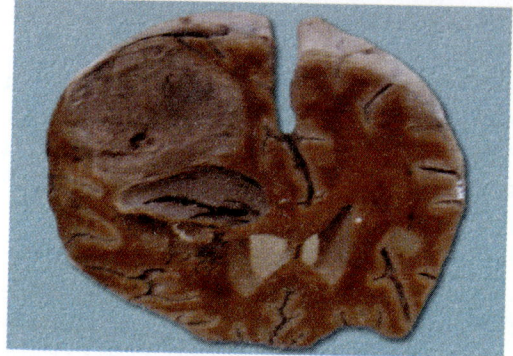

Fig. 3.83: Gross picture of brain tumour (astrocytoma)

MOLECULAR MARKERS IN GLIOMAS

Mutations of isocitrate dehydrogenase (IDH) 1 and 2 mutations and 1p/19q deletion are used as prognostic markers.[25] The gliomas with these mutations and deletions are associated with overall good survival and progression free survival of the patient. IDH mutant forms have good prognosis and progression free survival compared to wild type.[26]

Glioblastoma occur in two forms primary and secondary. Primary glioblastoma are *de novo* occurs without the pre-existing tumours and associated with mutation in PTEN, deletion of chromosome 10 and amplification of EGFR. Secondary glioblastoma arise from the anaplastic astrocytoma are associated with mutation of IDH1 and IDH2, over expression of PDGFRA and p53 mutations (Fig. 3.83).

NOS is applied when (1) genetic testing is not available, (2) genetic testing does not show diagnostic alterations or (3) uncertainity of tumour architecture/cytological features or insufficient tissue.[27]

KIAA 1549 -BRAF15-9 fusion are common with midline pilocytic astrocytoma than within the cerebellum.

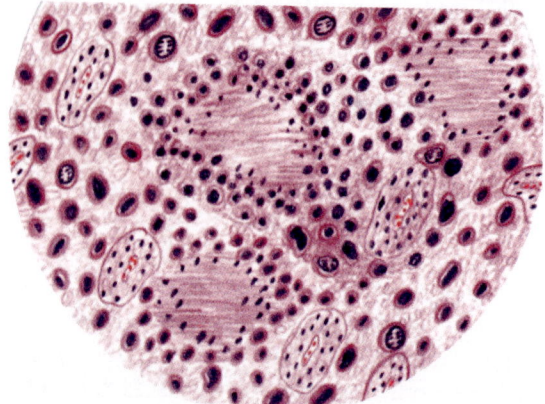

Fig. 3.82a: Schematic diagram, microscopy of astrocytoma (high grade glioblastoma)

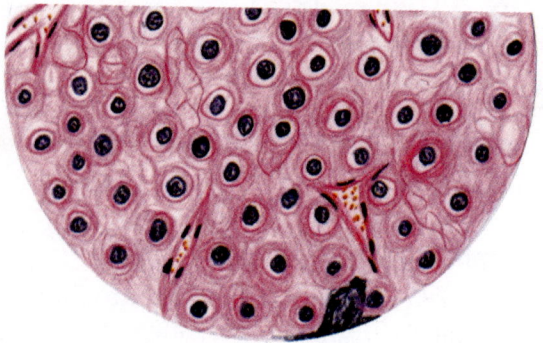

Fig. 3.82b: Oligodendroglioma

Section IV

Histopathology Techniques

Exercise 60. Accessing Procedures in Surgical Pathology
Exercise 61. Fixatives
Exercise 62. Processing
Exercise 63. Haematoxylin and Eosin (H & E) Staining
Exercise 64. Microtomes and Microtomy
Exercise 65. Frozen Section
Exercise 66. Decalcification
Exercise 67. Special Stains
Exercise 68. Theoretical Aspects of Some of the Special Stains

Exercise 60

Accessing Procedures in Surgical Pathology

GENERAL CONSIDERATIONS

- Material to the pathology laboratory is received from the clinicians.
- Name of the patient, middle name, last name, hospital registration number or any other demographic information like age, sex, etc. should be recorded without fail. Failure to do so may invite diagnostic disaster for the physician and the patient.
- Biopsy samples of the same type and of same general description should be handled with maximum care, e.g. gastric biopsies, prostatic needle biopsies, skin biopsies and many other specimens.
- The requisition should be complete in all respects including clinical details, nature of specimen, site and all related particulars.
- Bar codes and other computer driven information should be given strong consideration as compared to the handwritten/ type written labels or both can be used.

RECEIVING OF SPECIMENS TO THE LABORATORY

As soon as any specimen is received with its requisition form, the following should be verified:

1. Name, age, sex, registration number, etc. and tally with the label on the container.
2. Check the content of the container which should tally with the specimen written on the requisition form.

Assign accession number. Record the name, age, sex, referring doctor, accession number, indoor patient number, etc. in the record register.

THE GROSS ROOM

- Delivery of specimens from the operating rooms to the pathology laboratory accessing area and gross room should be undertaken several times in a day.
- Each time meticulous care has to be taken in paper work and labelling to verify, so that no error should be encountered later.
- The pathologist should take responsibility of the gross room.
- The surgical pathologist and all the personnel working in the surgical pathology should have awareness with the proper prosecution of all types of surgical specimens and the technique employed.
- The gross room should be large enough to permit simultaneous work of all the pathologists concerned.
- A cutting board, shelves for specimen container, ready access to water, dissecting area in connection with the sink, dictation equipment actuated by a pedal, computer systems, instruments like scissors, toothed and non-toothed forceps, malleable probes, scalpel blades, disposable blades, long knives, and pins for fixing/attaching specimens to the cork surface should be present while grossing.

- A box with cassettes and labels should be kept ready.
- Formalin, photography facility, X-ray facility, refrigerator, saw, balances and weighing machine should be easily accessible.
- Fixation, processing, H & E staining, facility for imprints, special fixatives, facility for frozen sections, surface marking facility, cytogenetics and EM facility also should be readily accessible.
- For fixation, the volume of fixative should be 10–20 times more than the volume of the specimen. The container should have an opening large enough, so that the tissue could be easily removed after it is fixed. The fixative should surround the specimen and the large specimens should be covered with gauze.
- Fixation should be carried out at room temperature.
- The speed of penetration of fixative is 1 mm/hour and speed can be increased when required by heating the formalin up to 60°C.

General Principles of Grossing

- Proper identification and orientation of specimen is always of primary importance.
- Unlabelled specimens should never be processed.
- If there are difficulties in the orientation of the specimen, then surgeon/clinician should be contacted and their cooperation is sought in identifying position, landmarks and surgical margins.
- The pathologist should be aware of the anatomy and the procedure of operation conducted.
- The specimen should be inspected and a record of the following are made: type of specimen, structures included, dimensions, weight, shape, colour, surgical margins.
- Gross photographs and photographs of the cut sections are to be taken for documentation.
- Description of the cut surface whether solid, cystic or the area of myxoid degeneration, calcification, necrosis, bony areas, cartilage, etc. are noted down.
- If the specimen is large, the abnormality is identified. Sections are given from such abnormal areas. Sometimes, the entire capsule or surgical margins need to be studied for tumour extension. The surgical margins can be coloured or inked for identification.
- If the specimen is small, the whole specimen can be given for study.
- If no abnormality is detected, then random sections are to be given.
- All lymph nodes have to be submitted for processing.
- Specimen radiograph may be taken for evidence of calcification, foreign body (metal chips) and in case of bony lesion to know osteolytic or osteoblastic lesion.
- In pathology of vessels, ducts, urinary tract, etc. radio-opaque dye study with pathological correlation may be undertaken.
- Sections of 2 to 3 mm thickness are given for processing. The size of the tissue has to be 10 to 15 mm in length and breadth.
- Sections of lymph nodes are to be still thinner.
- Metal chips, foreign body, suture material, etc. when present with the tissue are to be removed and then tissue should be submitted for processing.
- Bone and calcified tissue are necessarily submitted for decalcification.
- Tissues with mucosa and skin are embedded perpendicular to the mucosa/epithelium, then the embedding surface has to be marked and put in the capsule facing downwards.

RECORD KEEPING IN SURGICAL PATHOLOGY

- All the tissues should be under the care of the surgical pathologist and not under the clinician or researcher otherwise would cause disaster to the patient and to the pathologist.

- Surgical pathologist serves as maintenance personnel for legal integrity of all the pathologic materials.
- Permanent record should be maintained for research purpose and for legal purpose and in this connection, the following records should be maintained:
  - Histopathology register
  - Requisition file
  - Duplicate report file
  - Dispatch record.
- The histopathology register has to contain the entry of accession number, the name of the patient, patient's age, sex, doctor referred and such relevant details.
- All the request forms with gross and microscopy of the lesion are to be filed in the requisition file. The name of the grossing person, date of grossing, date when the slides are prepared, details of grossing and report also should be entered.
- All the duplicate reports are to be filed.
- Dispatch record has the record of the date when the report is dispatched and to whom.
- Computer disc read only memory computer text entry documents can replace the paper case records.
- To evaluate the promptness and efficiency of the surgical pathology personnel, the record of turn around time (TAT) and also lost tissue record should be maintained.

STORAGE AND FILING OF SLIDES

- All the slides and blocks with accession number on them should be stored properly, if facilities are available.
- If the same patient comes again, the previous records should be searched and those retrieved slides have to be reviewed.
- Slides referred from outside also should be reviewed before therapy and that too very critically.

CODING OF HISTOPATHOLOGY LESIONS

- While writing the diagnosis—the organ, site of biopsy and the type of operation are to be recorded, e.g. Bone-femur-biopsy-osteosarcoma. This helps in coding of the specimens.
- The lesions should be indexed noting the year and accession number for future reference.
- Systemised nomenclature of medicine (SNOMED) coding[28] can be followed. It is a multiaxial classification system. There are 11 axes like T: Topography—anatomic site, M: Morphology—changes found in cells, tissues and organs; L: Living organisms—bacteria and viruses; C: Chemical—drugs, F: Function—signs and symptoms; J: Occupation; D: Diagnosis; P: Procedure followed: A: Devices and agents associated with disease; S: Social relation and G: General.

Exercise 61

Fixatives

Classification of Fixatives

I. Depending on the chemical nature fixatives could be classified as:
- Aldehydes—formaldehyde, glutaraldehyde, acrolein, glyoxal
- Oxidising agents—osmium tetroxide, potassium permanganate, potassium dichromate
- Protein denaturing agents—acetic acid, methyl alcohol, ethyl alcohol
- Other cross linking agents—carbodiimides
- Physical—heat, microwave
- Unknown mechanism—mercuric chloride, picric acid

II. Fixatives can also be classified as
- *Micro-anatomical fixatives:* These are used to preserve the anatomy of the tissue with its correct relationship of the tissue layers and a large aggregates of cells. The fixatives for routine use should be chosen from this group.
  - Formalin based fixatives
  - Buffered glutaraldehyde
  - Formal sublimate
  - Heidenhain's susa
  - Zenker's fluid
  - Zenker's formal
  - Bouin's fluid
  - Gendre's fluid
  - Rossman's fluid.
- *Cytological fixatives*

These are classified as follows:

Nuclear fixatives
- Carnoy's fluid
- Clarke's fluid
- Newcomer's fluid
- Fleming's fluid.

Cytoplasmic fixatives
- Champy's fluid
- Regaud's fluid
- Formal saline and formal calcium
- Zenker's formal
- Schaudinn's fluid
- Ether—alcohol.

Spray fixation: This is achieved by alcohol-based fixatives and they contain wax. Soluble wax acts as a barrier against contamination by dust. For details refer to fixatives in cytology.

- *Histochemical fixatives*
  - Formal saline
  - Cold acetone
  - Absolute alcohol

Postchroming and Secondary Fixation

Postchroming is the treatment of tissues with 3% potassium dichromate following normal fixation. This aids in an improved preservation and in demonstration of mitochondria and myelin.

The postchroming can be carried out both before processing or even after processing. Before processing, the tissue is left in dichromate solution for 6 to 8 days. After processing for 12–24 hours the tissue is immersed in dichromate solution before the staining procedure. In each case, the sections need proper washing in running tap water.

Secondary fixation is sequential application of the two fixatives. This gives more brilliant staining, e.g. fixation in formal saline followed by mercury containing fixatives.

Vapour Fixation

For this kind of fixation, formaldehyde, glutaraldehyde, acrolein, osmium tetroxide, diacetyl, acetic acid, glyoxylic acid, glyoxal and acetaldehyde are used.

These are used to demonstrate glycogen on cryostat cut sections or blocks of frozen dried tissue. Such sections mounted on the slides and may be placed in a closed vessel above the paraformaldehyde and the vessel has to be placed in the oven at 60–70°C for 2 hours. Then the stains are applied.

Microanatomical Fixatives

Formaldehyde (HCHO)

Formaldehyde is a gas that is soluble in water by 40% of its weight. It is known as formaldehyde (40%) or formalin. It contains 10–14% of methanol which is added for its action as stabiliser. The concentrated solution is acidic in nature and becomes still more acidic on storage because of formic acid formation. Neutralisation is done by adding buffers like magnesium or calcium carbonate to the dilute formalin.

Magnesium or calcium carbonates should never be added to concentrated formalin because of formation of CO_2 and also there is a chance of explosion.

The concentrated solution becomes turbid because of formation of paraformaldehyde and this reduces the strength of the solution. It can be filtered and reused.

Formalin pigment is altered blood (acid formaldehyde haematin) by the action of acidic formalin. This is brown granular, extracellular and birefringent. This is avoided by buffering the formalin. Formalin pigment can be removed from the sections by treatment (in a jar) with saturated alcoholic solution of picric acid for 20 minutes. Alcoholic solution of both sodium and potassium hydroxide (e.g. 1% alcoholic solution of 1% sodium hydroxide) will also remove the pigment but these may have deleterious effects on subsequent staining techniques. Treatment with 10% ammonium hydroxide in 70% alcohol for 5–15 minutes will remove this pigment and is less harmful to the tissue sections than the other hydroxides. This pigment needs to be differentiated from the malarial pigment which is intracellular.

Different Formalin-based Fixatives

1. 10% formalin (4% formaldehyde)
40% formaldehyde	100 ml
Distilled/tap water	900 ml

   This is commonly used.

2. Neutral buffered formalin (pH 6.8–7)
40% formaldehyde	100 ml
Distilled/tap water	900 ml
Sodium dihydrogen phosphate monohydrate	4 g
Disodium hydrogen phosphate anhydrous	6.5 g

3. Formal saline
40% formaldehyde	100 ml
Sodium chloride	9 g
Distilled/tap water	900 ml

4. Formal-calcium
40% formaldehyde	100 ml
Distilled/tap water	900 ml
10% calcium chloride	100 ml

Picric Acid Containing Fixatives

Bouin's Fluid

Saturated aqueous picric acid	75 ml
40% formaldehyde	25 ml
Glacial acetic acid	5 ml

This fixative is used in demonstration of glycogen. It penetrates the tissues rapidly and causes little shrinkage. In order to remove picric acid, prolonged washing or treatment with alcohol is needed.

Mercuric Chloride Containing Fixatives

Zenker's Fluid

Distilled water	950 ml
Potassium dichromate	25 g
Mercuric chloride	50 g
Glacial acetic acid	50 g

There are number of variants of this fluid, e.g. Helly's fluid.

This gives a rapid and even penetration; but mercury deposits have to be removed before staining, by using 0.5% iodine solution in 70% ethanol for 5–10 minutes.

Cytological Fixatives

Nuclear fixatives
1. *Carnoy's fluid*

Absolute alcohol	60 ml
Chloroform	30 ml
Glacial acetic acid	10 ml

    This acts as a rapid fixative and is used for preservation of Nissl substance and glycogen; however, it causes shrinkage and destroys cytoplasm. Fixation is complete in 1–2 hours.

2. *Clarke's fluid*

Glacial acetic acid	25 ml
Absolute alcohol	75 ml

    This is also a rapid fixative; it is a good nuclear fixative and preserves cytoplasmic elements.

Cytoplasmic Fixatives

1. *Champy's fluid*

3% potassium dichromate	7 ml
1% chromic acid	7 ml
2% osmium tetroxide	4 ml

    This fluid preserves mitochondria and fat.

2. Formal saline and formal calcium are good cytoplasmic and microanatomical fixatives.
3. Ether—alcohol

70% alcohol	1 part
Diethyl ether	1 part

    This is a rapid cytological fixative but it is highly flammable.
4. Zenker's-formal is a good cytoplasmic and microanatomical fixative.

Histochemical Fixatives

1. Formal saline and absolute alcohol are frequently used fixatives.
2. Cold acetone of 0–4°C is used for enzyme studies particularly phosphatases.

Factors Involved in Fixation

Many factors are involved such as:

1. *Buffers and hydrogen ion concentration*

    Satisfactory fixation occurs at pH between 6 and 8.

    Buffering is achieved by phosphates, veronal acetate, bicarbonates, tris and cacodylate.

    For particular fixative particular buffer is chosen.

2. *Temperature*

    Fixation for paraffin section is carried out at room temperature. For electron microscopy, temperature of 0–4°C is preferred.

3. *Penetration of fixatives*

    The depth (d) penetrated by the fixative is proportional to the square root of time (t) usually expressed as where, k is constant and it is specific for each fixative.

    The values obtained usually are lower because fixed tissue acts as a barrier for inward diffusion of the fixative. It also depends upon the reaction between the tissue components. A slow rate of diffusion reaction gives various zones of tissue which have fixed to different grades.

Coefficients of diffusibility (k) for commonly used fixatives

Fixative	Fixative concentration (%)	k (tissue)
Acetic acid	5	1.2
Chromium trioxide	0.5	0.25
Formaldehyde	4	0.78
Ethanol	100	1.0
Glutaraldehyde	6	0.25
Methanol	100	–
Osmium tetroxide	0.5 to 2	0.29–0.58
Potassium dichromate	3	1.33

4. *Volume changes*

The shrinkage during fixation to embedding of paraffin wax is around 30–40%. The shrinkage is induced by dehydrating agents and hot wax infiltration.

Duration of Fixation

Duration for fixation varies according to the fixative used. With formalin 2 to 6 hours is needed for small tissues and 6 to 12 hours for big tissues. Big tissue specimens have to be cut at definite intervals for proper fixation.

Exercise 62

Processing

Fixation

The tissues are generally fixed for 6 to 12 hours. 10% formalin is the routinely used fixative. For further details, refer to the topic on fixatives.

Dehydration

Dehydration involves removal of water from the tissues. Different solutions can be used to dehydrate and following is the list of dehydrating agents.
- Alcohol
- Spirit (74° OP)
- Methanol
- Propan-2-ol
- Isopropyl alcohol
- Acetone
- Dioxane
- Tetrahydrofuran—dehydrating and clearing agent.

Most commonly, upgraded alcohol solutions are used for effective dehydration. By using upgraded alcohols, water is removed slowly and gradually, in such a way that there is no much shrinkage of the tissue.

In the last jar of alcohol, a layer of anhydrous copper sulphate of about 0.5 to 2.5 cm is usually placed. When the water content of the alcohol increases, the colourless anhydrous copper sulphate absorbs water and becomes bluish in colour. At this stage, alcohol has to be changed.

Clearing

- The term 'clearing' relates to the appearance of the tissues after they have been treated by the fluid chosen to remove dehydrating agent.
- These clearing solutions have refractive index similar to proteins which consequently renders the tissue translucent.
- Clearing agent is necessary because the dehydrating agent is not miscible with paraffin. The clearing agent is miscible with both dehydrating agent as well as paraffin.
- Following is the list of different clearing agents which can be used:
  – Chloroform
  – Xylene
  – Benzene
  – Toluene
  – Carbon tetrachloride
  – Petrol
  – Cedar wood oil
  – Clove oil
  – Citrus fruit oil
  – CNP 30 and inhibisol; of late these are used as clearing agents.

Chloroform and Xylene have been already discussed.

Benzene: This is similar to xylene in its chemical activity but being carcinogenic, it is avoided and therefore not recommended.

Toluene: Though similar to xylene in action it is less damaging. It is flammable and potentially dangerous.

Carbon tetrachloride: This happens to be similar to chloroform, it is toxic and also releases phosgene gas but it is cheaper.

Cedar wood oil: As a clearing agent it is slow in action.

Clove oil: It is similar to cedar wood oil but it is found to be expensive.

Citrus fruit oils: Oil extracted from orange and lemon rinds are commercially available as clearing agents and these are nontoxic.

Impregnation

Paraffin wax with low melting point (MP) of 56 to 58°C is used for impregnation. The following additives are to be added to increase the stickiness of wax so as to produce ribbons of sections.

- Micro-crystalline wax (25% is added to paraffin wax).
- Cerecin
- Rubber
- Beeswax
- Dental wax.

Embedding and Block Making

Wax of slightly higher melting point 58 to 60°C is used for embedding and block making.

The different embedding agents used are
- Paraffin wax of MP of 58 to 60°C
- Water soluble wax
- Ester wax
- Polyester wax
- Microcrystalline wax
- Resins-Acrylic
  Epoxy
  Urea-formaldehyde
- Agar
- Gelatin
- Celloidin.

Block making needs moulds and such required moulds are prepared using Leuckhart's L pieces and metal plates. By adjusting the L pieces, the size and shape of the mould can be decided. At first, the moulds are filled with molten wax after which the tissue is placed at the bottom and pressed with a rod. When the wax gets solidified, the block can be easily separated from L pieces and metal plates and then the block is labelled.

Processing steps used in automatic tissue processor (Histokinette, Riechart Jung Ltd.).

Exercise 63

Haematoxylin and Eosin (H & E) Staining

Method: Regressive staining is usually employed for H&E staining of tissues. Haematoxylin, in this stain is a nuclear stain and eosin is a cytoplasmic stain.

Following are the steps of H&E staining
- Deparaffinisation with xylene—5 minutes
- Deparaffinisation with xylene—5 minutes
- Absolute alcohol—5 minutes
- Wash in water (hydration)
- Stain with haematoxylin—3 to 5 minutes
- Wash in water
- Differentiate in 1% acid alcohol—1 dip
- Wash in water
- Blueing with saturated solution of lithium carbonate—2 to 3 minutes.
- Rinse in water
- Stain with 1% eosin—1 minute
- Wash with tap water
- Dehydrate with absolute alcohol
- Clear with xylene
- Mount with DPX.

Results

Nuclei, calcium	Blue
Muscle, fibrin, keratin	Bright red
Collagen	Pink
RBCs	Red/orange

Composition of Harri's haematoxylin

Haematoxylin	2.5 g
Absolute alcohol	50 ml
Ammonium alum	50 g
Distilled water	500 ml
Mercuric oxide	1.25 g
Glacial acetic acid	20 ml

Preparation of Harri's Haematoxylin

Dissolve haematoxylin in absolute alcohol and alum in hot water separately, after which mix these two and heat to boiling. Then add mercuric oxide, off the fire, cool rapidly by keeping the flask into cold water (when mercuric oxide is added bubbles appear, to avoid this put off the flame and cool immediately). Mix well again, boil for 1–2 minutes and then cool, filter the solution and add glacial acetic acid. For 100 ml of stain, about 2 to 4 ml of glacial acetic acid is to be added.

Other haematoxylins: Two of them are explained below.

1. *Mayer's haematoxylin:* This is used in H & E staining in the progressive method.

   Composition

Haematoxylin	1 g
Distilled water	1000 ml
Ammonium alum/potassium alum	50 g
Sodium iodate	0.2 g
Citric acid	1 g
Chloral hydrate	50 g

   Chlorate hydrate is preservative and citric acid is a acidifier.

2. *Ehrlich's haematoxylin:* This is used in the regressive method of H & E staining.

Composition

Haematoxylin	2 g
Absolute alcohol	100 ml
Distiled water	100 ml
Glycerol	100 ml
Glacial acetic acid	10 ml
Potassium alum in excess	15 g approx

The stain is ripened by natural ripening method or by adding sodium iodate.

Preparation of 1% acid alcohol

Mix 1 ml hydrochloric acid in 99 ml of 70% alcohol.

Preparation of eosin for H&E staining: Eosin is usually called eosin y (eosin yellow, it is water soluble eosin).

1% Eosin stock solution

Dissolve 1 g of eosin in 20 ml of distilled water and add 80 ml of 95% alcohol.

Working eosin solution

Eosin stock solution	1 part
Alcohol 80%	3 parts

Before use, add 0.5 ml of glacial acetic acid to 10 ml of the stain.

Points to Note

- Haematoxylin is obtained from logwood of a tree known as haematoxylon campechianum which was native of Mexico, now mainly cultivated in West Indies. Oxidation of haematoxylin produces a coloured substance called haematin which itself is a poor dye but in the presence of metallic mordant it develops into a powerful stain.
- *Differentiation:* The sections after staining with haematoxylin for 3 to 5 minutes, in regressive staining, are dipped into 1% acid alcohol, then washed in water to be examined under microscope under low power. With differentiation, the excess haematoxylin is removed; the nucleus is clearly visible and the cytoplasm is rendered colourless.
- *Blueing:* When the sections are dipped in 1% acid alcohol, the pH of the sections would become acidic and look pink. By placing the sections in lithium carbonate (alkaline pH) the pH will be neutralised. At this point, the sections appear blue. Hence, this process is called blueing. If already the tap water is alkaline, then there is no need to add lithium carbonate.
- *Mordant:* Mordant is an intermediate substance which binds the tissue and a dye. The dye and the mordant should be simultaneously applied. Salts of aluminium, iron, lead, molybdenum and tungsten are used as mordants.
  Aluminium potassium sulphate (potash alum) and aluminium ammonium sulphate (ammonium alum) are commonly and routinely used as mordants.
- *Ripening:* Ripening is achieved by natural oxidation by exposing the stain to light or air.
  This is, of course, a slow process, sometimes taking up to 3 to 4 months but it retains its staining ability for longer time. Ehrlich's haematoxylin is a good example of natural ripening.
  Ripening by chemical oxidation is achieved by sodium iodate (as in Mayer's haematoxylin) and mercuric oxide (as in Harri's haematoxylin). These convert haematoxylin into haematin instantaneously, so that the resulting solutions are ready for immediate use. But they have a shorter life than the ones which are oxidised by natural ripening.
- Glycerol is added to haematoxylin because it acts as a stabiliser and reduces evaporation and prevents over oxidation.

Exercise

64

Microtomes and Microtomy

Microtomy is the process by means of which the tissue can be sectioned. The basic instrument used for microtomy is microtome.

MICROTOMES

Microtomes are mechanical devices for cutting thin and uniform sections. There are different types of microtomes. These include:

1. Rotary microtome
2. Rocking microtome
3. Base sledge microtome
4. Sliding microtome
5. Freezing microtome

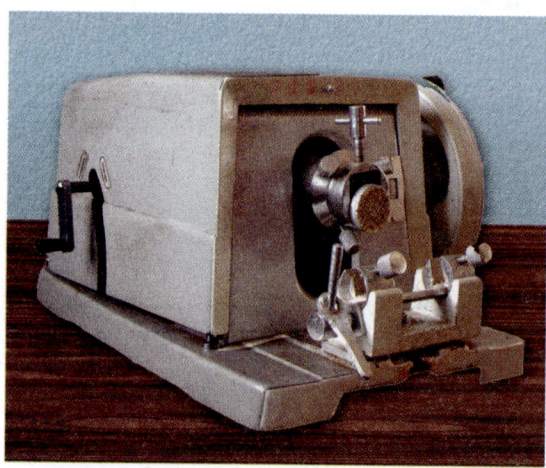

Fig. 4.1: Rotary microtome

Rotary Microtome

This is the most widely used of all the microtomes. The rotary action of the hand wheel helps in cutting. The block holder is mounted on a steel carriage, which moves up and down in grooves and it can be advanced by a micrometer screw (Fig. 4.1).

It is heavy, more stable than the rocking microtome. A large number of blocks can be cut. It is an ideal microtome for serial sections.

Teaching institutions use this microtome because a large number of blocks are to be cut. The cutting angle has to be adjusted. The advantage is that, in this microtome there are less vibrations. The knife is heavier and wedge shaped; however, in recent days disposable knives are available.

Rocking Microtome

In Cambridge rocking microtome, the knife is fixed. The block of tissue moves through an arc and strikes against the knife; between the strokes, the block is moved towards the knife for required thickness of sections. In Great Britain, this was in use for a long time and was called rocking microtome because of its rocking action of the arm; later this was replaced by sledge and rotary microtomes, but still this microtome is in use in some of the laboratories.

Disadvantages

1. Blocks cut with this microtome are less compared to the recent microtomes.
2. Another of its shortcoming is that the arm moves in an arc and hence the sections are cut in a curved plane.

Base Sledge Microtome

This kind of microtome is heavy, stable and as such no vibrations are produced; moreover the knife is long (24 cm) and it is fixed. The block holder slides backwards and forwards against the knife. The whole of the brain sections or any large sections can suitably be taken with this type of microtome.

Sliding Microtome

It is so-called, as in this microtome the knife moves; whereas the block is fixed. This is used for celloidin embedded and paraffin sections.

Freezing Microtome

This kind of microtome is clamped to the edge of a bench and is connected to a cylinder of CO_2. The pressure inside the cylinder is about 1000 lb/in^2 which will keep CO_2 in a liquid state that renders cooling effect.

SECTION CUTTING

While undertaking section cutting, the following things are to be considered:

Clearance angle of 2 to 4° helps to prevent friction between the knife and the block. Clearance angle is formed by the line drawn along the block surface and the lower bevel of the knife.

Rake angle is the angle between the upper bevel of knife and a line drawn at 90° to the block surface. Greater the rake angle, better are the sections for soft tissue and the rake angle is reduced, while cutting hard tissues.

While undertaking section cutting, the following procedure is to be followed:

- Insert the knife in the knife holder and screw it tightly.
- Trim the excess wax on the sides of the cutting surface of the block; or this step may be omitted.
- Fix the block to the block holder.
- Fix the block along with the block holder to the microtome.
- Move the block holder with the block forward and upward till the knife edge touches the block.
- Ensure that the block surface is parallel to the knife and adjust all the screws.
- Trim the block to expose the tissue surface. For this purpose any old knife could be used and the microtome is set at 15 μ. Operate the microtome until the complete sections of the tissue are being cut.
- Reset the thickness gauge at 3 to 4 μ.
- Cut the sections.
- Any teasing needle or any brush is used to lift the sections.
- During the cutting procedure, paraffin wax embedded sections become slightly compressed and creased. To remove the creases, the sections are floated on 50% alcohol and then on water bath at a temperature of which is 10°C lesser than MP of wax (if MP of wax is 56°, water bath temperature is to be around 46°C). Temperature of 5–6°C lesser than MP of wax is also permissible.
- If creases do not disappear with this procedure, gentle pressure is applied with the teasing needle to remove the creases. Apply ice to cool the surface of the block to minimise the creases.
- Take a clean slide and put some egg albumin on the slide.
- Take the sections on the centre of the slide from the water bath. It is preferable to leave about ¾ inch at both the ends of the slide. One end is used for labelling.
- Keep the sections on a hot plate. The temperature of the hot plate has to be 55 to 60°C and keep for 10 to 15 minutes or in the oven at 50°C for 1 hour.

With this, the sections adhere to the slide; as egg albumin coagulates and holds the sections and the sections will not get detached during the staining procedure.

Likely faulty paraffin sectioning and remedial suggestions

Cause/Fault	Remedies

A. Alternative sections thick and thin
  1. Wax too soft
  2. Block or knife loose
  3. Insufficient clearance angle
	1. Cool block surface with ice or re-embed in higher melting point wax
	2. Tighten the screws
	3. Increase slightly the clearance angle

B. Thick and thin zones on a section (chatters)
  1. Knife or block loose
  2. Excessively steep knife angle
  3. Tissue or wax too hard
  4. Calcified area in the tissue
	1. Tighten the screws
	2. Reduce angle but still leave some clearance angle
	3. Use sharp heavy duty knife, use softening agent
	4. Rehydrate and decalcify or do surface decalcification

C. Scoring or splitting of section
  1. Nick in knife
  2. Hard particles in tissue
  3. Hard particles in wax
	1. Sharpen or use different part of knife
	2. If bone, decalcify; if mineral or other material remove them
	3. Re-embed in filtered fresh wax

D. Sections will not form ribbon
  1. Wax too hard
  2. Debris on knife edge
  3. Knife angle too steep or shallow
	1. Cool the block or re-embed in lower melting point wax
	2. Clean with xylene
	3. Adjust optimal angle

E. Sections attached to block on return stroke
  1. Less clearance angle
  2. Wax debris on knife
  3. Debris on block edge
	1. Increase clearance angle
	2. Clean with xylene
	3. Trim with sharp scalpel

F. Sections crumble on cutting
  1. Wax too soft
  2. Wax crystallised due to slow
  3. Bevel of knife too wide or blunt
	1. Apply ice or use high melting point wax
	2. Re-embed in fresh wax cooling
	3. Resharpen to produce narrow bevel

G. Sections expand and disintegrate on water surface
  1. Poor impregnation
  2. Water temperature too high
	1. Repeat impregnation
	2. Cool

Preparation of egg albumin (Mayer's glycerol albumin)

Egg white	50 ml
Glycerol	50 ml
Sodium salicylate	1 ml

Mix the above and filter or equal volume of glycerol, distilled water and egg white can also may be mixed and filtered through a coarse filter paper. The crystals of thymol are added so as to prevent any possible growth of moulds and kept in the refrigerator.

Serial Sections

Ribbons of about 10 to 12 inches in length are cut and every section is taken on the slide.

Cutting of Hard Tissues

The block should be soaked in Mollifex overnight and then cut in the usual manner the next morning.

Fragmentation of Tissue

Inspite of application of ice, some sections tend to break and especially when they contain large amounts of blood. In such cases, apply 1% celloidin and allow it to dry. Of course, care has to be taken while floating; because, the celloidin layer is at the top and the celloidin on the section has to be removed with equal parts of ether and alcohol before removing the wax with xylene.

Adhesives

Different adhesives are used. Some of them include:

Albumin: This is commonly used adhesive; however, it gives dirty background with reticulin stain. One has to be aware that thymol resistant organisms can grow and cause confusion with Gram's stain.

Gelatin: This is used in frozen section.

Chromic gelatin: 0.1% chrome alum in 1% gelatin may be used as adhesive.

Starch paste: This may be used; however, it gives PAS positivity.

Preparation of starch paste: 1 g powdered starch is mixed in 10 ml of cold water; pour this in 20 ml of boiling water; add 2 drops of N/1 hydrochloric acid and boil for 4 to 5 minutes.

Poly-L-lysin: 0.1% solution has to be diluted in distilled water with 1 : 10 ratio.

3-aminopropyl triethoxysilane (APES): The slides are dipped in 2% APES in acetone, drained and then dipped in acetone and finally dipped in distilled water after which they are dried and used. This adhesive is not suitable for cytology.

Points to note

- Generally, glass slides are of 76 × 25 × 1.0–1.2 mm
  Glass slides of larger size are also available.
- Coverslips: These are available in different sizes, commonly used coverslips are of 22 × 22 mm or 22 × 40 mm or 20 × 30 mm.

Embedding Media

The most commonly used embedding medium is paraffin wax. It is the most popular embedding medium for light microscopy as it is cheap, it can be easily handled and the section production provides few difficulties. It has much wider range of melting point and this unique property has the advantage for various climatic regions of the world. Paraffin wax is a mixture of hydrocarbons produced in the cracking of mineral oils. Its melting point (MP) ranges between 40 and 70°C. Higher melting point wax is harder than the one with low melting point. Hence, to promote good ribbons of sections, the wax with suitable hardness at room temperature is chosen, usually of 54°–58°C is satisfactory for routine use.

Paraplast is highly purified paraffin and has a higher degree of elasticity than the normal paraffin wax and yields wrinkle-free sections. It does not require any cooling before cutting, thus the use of ice could be easily avoided.

Beeswax, ceresin, rubber, dental wax and diethylene glycol distearate any of these can be added as additives to paraffin wax.

Recent years, commercial paraffin waxes with added resins of various types are readily available in the market.

Other Embedding Media

There are some cases or occasions for processing, paraffin wax cannot be used or it could be that paraffin wax is not a suitable medium; such as the circumstances occasionally arise are:

1. The processing agent destroys or removes the tissue components that are the main objects of investigation.
2. When thinner sections are required.
3. The use of heat in the processing may adversely affect the tissue.
4. The impregnating medium needs to be harder to support the tissue.

The alternative embedding media to paraffin wax include the following:

Other waxes	Resins	Other media
Water soluble wax, e.g. polyethylene glycol	Acrylic	Agar
Ester wax	Epoxy	Gelatin
Polyester wax	Urea-formaldehyde	Celloidin

Micro-crystalline wax
- With the advent of a wider range of acrylic resins with flexible controllable properties and commercial availability of paraffin waxes with resins; additives and other waxes are not in common use at present.
- Resins have been playing an important role in electron microscopy for thin sectioning and for high resolution.
- *Agar:* Agar gel alone does not provide sufficient support. It is a cohesive agent for small friable pieces. These fragments are embedded in molten agar and then solidified, trimmed and processed for paraffin sectioning.
- Celloidin or low viscosity nitrocellulose are now of limited use.

Mounting Media

Mounting media are syrupy fluids that are used between the section and the coverslip. We should ensure that their refractive index be as near as possible to that of glass (1.518). Two main types of mounting media are available:
1. Resinous media, for preparation of dehydrated and cleared in xylene tissues
2. Aqueous media for mounting sections directly from water, where any treatment with alcohol or xylene would be detrimental to the stain.

Resinous Media

Xylene balsam: About 60% of dried natural resin Canada-balsam is dissolved in xylene in the incubator. However, we should remember that xylene balsam should be kept in dark coloured glass bottles.

DPX: A mixture of distrene (a polystyrene) a plasticiser (tricresyl phosphate) and xylene: thus called DPX was introduced in 1939, and later modified by substitution of a more satisfactory plasticiser that is dibutylphthalate.

Distrene 80	10 g
Dibutylphthalate	5 ml
Xylene	35 ml

This is a commonly used mountant.

Aqueous Media

Kaiser's glycerol jelly

Gelatin	10 g
Distilled water	60 ml
Glycerol	70 ml
Phenol crystals	0.25 g

To prepare this media dissolve gelatin in water in a beaker placed in a water bath before adding glycerol and phenol.

Apathy's mountant

Pure gum arabic (crystals)	50 g
Pure cane sugar	50 g
Distilled water	50 ml
Thymol	0.05 g

Dissolve the ingredients with the aid of gentle heat and store the mountant in tightly stoppered or screw-capped container.

MICROTOME KNIFE

Microtome knives are manufactured by using hard steel with high carbon content or tool steel. They are suitable for paraffin wax embedded tissue cutting. These knives are classified according to their shapes and are described below (Fig. 4.2).

Wedge Knife

Wedge knife is commonly used. It is rigid and used for frozen and paraffin section cutting.

Plano-concave Knife

This is used for cutting nitrocellulose/celloidin embedded tissue; blade is comparatively thinner and vibrates if used to cut harder tissues.

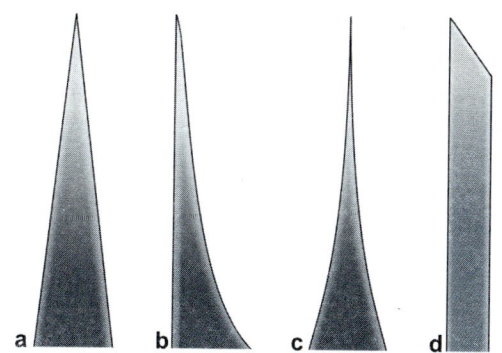

Fig. 4.2: Type of knives: (a) Plane wedge, (b) plano-concave, (c) biconcave, (d) tool edge wedge knife (plane wedge)

Tool Edge or D-profile (Chisel edge)

This is specifically meant for hard tissue cutting. For instance, this is used for cutting hard tissues like bone.

Biconcave Knife

This type of knife is used in rocking microtome (Heiffor knife) and the sledge microtome. Diamond or glass knives are also available.

In recent days, disposable blades are in use.

Production of fine edge of knife depends upon the hardness of the metal used in its manufacture and also on the angles of the facets (18–35°). The hardness is usually 400 to 900 on Vicker's hardness scale, 700 being commonly used. With hardness of more than 900, the knives are brittle and likely to break.

The knife has its own suitable back and can be fitted to a handle. The back is used to produce a suitable angle, so that the sharpening edge touches the surface. During section cutting, the following angles are created:
  i. Rake angle
  ii. Cutting angle (bevel angle)
  iii. Clearance angle.

Points to remember
1. As the rake angle increases, it becomes easier for section cutting and the adjusted angle provides robust edges which are less easily damaged or blunted by hard materials.
2. The clearance angle of 20 to 40° is used to prevent any likely friction between the knife and the block particularly on the return stroke.
3. The cutting angle of 17 to 23° range is preferred for paraffin sectioning.

The knife could be either fixed as in rocking microtome or rotary microtome or it may be kept moving as is in base sledge microtome.

Knives are of different sizes; usually around 8 cm in length, as in freezing and rotary microtomes. A knife of 24 cm in length is used in base sledge microtome.

For descriptive purposes, terms like 'heel' and 'toe' of the knife are used. In this contest, the term 'heel' of the knife is an angle formed by the cutting edge and the end of the knife nearest to the handle. Similarly 'toe' is an angle formed by the cutting edge and that end of the knife farthest from the handle.

MICROTOME KNIFE HONING

Honing is a procedure to sharpen the cutting edge.

Technique of Honing

- The back of the knife and the handle are attached to the knife. Hold the handle of the knife between thumb and forefinger with the cutting edge facing away from the operator and the knife is laid on the nearest end of the hone. The tips of the finger and the thumb of the other hand rest on the other end of the knife, ensuring an even pressure along the whole edge of the knife during honing. The knife is pushed forward diagonally from heel to toe using slight pressure on the knife, turning it over on its back and bringing back diagonally from heel to toe with a figure of 8 movements.
- The knife should be placed in its box to retain the sharpness.
- For honing, different stones are used, e.g. Belgian black vein, Arkansas, Aloxite and carborundum.

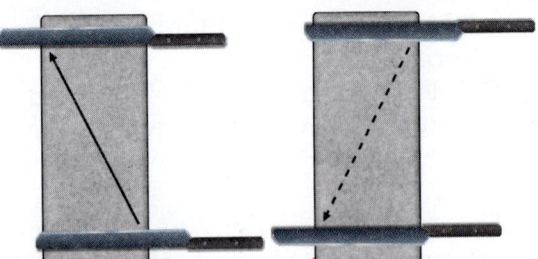

Fig. 4.3: Knife sharpening on a stone

- Glass, copper or bronze plate also could be used. Though copper and bronze plates are expensive, they are superior.
- Suitable abrasives are used while honing, e.g. water, soap water, coconut oil, 3 in 1 oil, aluminium oxide (alumina), iron oxide (jewellers' rouge) and silicon carbide.
- Crystals of 200 to 1000 µ size fine and coarse granules are used in sequence.
- *Uses of back:* While honing the knife with the back, the non-cutting edge is raised above the honing surface, so that the sharpening edge touches the surface and a suitable angle is produced for sharpening (Fig. 4.3).

STROPPING

Stropping is the process of polishing a sharp knife. A blunt knife cannot be sharpened on a strop.

Types of Strops

- The best strops are made from hide from rump of a horse. These can be either flexible (hanging) or rigid.
- The rigid type has a leather strop stretched over a wooden frame of 12 × 2 × 2 inches in size.

Technique of Stropping

The knife is laid on the near end of the strop with the cutting edge towards the operator (opposite of honing). It is held between the forefinger and the thumb to facilitate easy rotation. At the end of each stroke, the knife should be turned on its back to avoid cutting the strop itself.

Exercise 65

Frozen Section

- This method is to produce sections without the use of either the dehydrating agents or clearing agents.
- **Principle:** When the tissue is frozen, the water in it turns into ice, making the tissue firm and the ice itself acts as an embedding medium.
- **The uses of frozen section are**
  1. Demonstration of fats and lipids
  2. Enzyme histochemistry
  3. Early reporting of biopsy specimens particularly during emergency.
- To get frozen sections, following methods or instruments can be employed:
  - Freezing microtome
  - Cryostat
  - Freeze drying
  - Freeze substitution.
- Freezing microtome is attached to a cylinder of liquid CO_2 or a thermomodule unit. The CO_2 is fed to the microtome block stage, so that it maintains the tissue in a frozen state. In thermomodule, the Peltier effect is observed, i.e. heat generated across one surface is lost at the opposite surface, when direct current passes through two dissimilar metals. With thermomodule, –30°C temperature can be obtained.
- Cryostat is a refrigerated cabinet in which rotary microtome is fitted. The temperature can be adjusted between –5°C and –30°C. Usually –16°C is preferred. Freon 22, a gas is used for its cooling effect. An anti-roll plate placed parallel to the knife blade is a glass device coated with perspex. This plate is meant to prevent any possible curling of the tissue.
- Freezing can be also achieved by liquid nitrogen (–190°C), isopentane cooled by liquid nitrogen (–150°C), solid carbon dioxide also called dry ice or cardice (–70°C), carbon dioxide gas under pressure and aerosol sprays (–50°C). The tissue has to be held between two pieces of dry ice.
- Normally, wedge knife is used for taking frozen sections.
- The sections have to be 5–10 µ thick. Thinner sections are difficult to cut. The sections are cut and with the help of a brush, the sections are floated on a water bath and the necessary stains are applied. After staining, again these sections are floated on water bath and collected on albuminised slides and spread properly. A drop of glycerol is put followed by a coverslip; and observed under microscope.

Stains applied routinely are
1. For study of malignant cells—methylene blue H & E stain are employed.
2. For fat demonstration oil red 'O' stain is employed.

Exercise 66

Decalcification

Decalcification is a process of removal of inorganic calcium ions from mineralised bone or organic collagen matrix as well as calcified cartilage.

Decalcification can be achieved by
- Acids
- Chelating agents
- Surface decalcification
- Electrophoresis
- Ion exchange resins.

Criteria for Decalcifying Agent
- Complete removal of calcium
- Minimal damage to the cells and the tissue
- Non-impairment of the subsequent staining
- With reasonable speed.

The choice of the decalcifier depends upon
- The urgency of reporting
- Degree of mineralisation
- The scope of investigation and the subsequent staining technique.

Factors Influencing Decalcifier
i. *Concentration:* Any increase in concentration hastens decalcification, but at the same time, it adversely affects and it may destroy the tissue.

ii. *Temperature:* Any increase in temperature also hastens decalcification but room temperature or 25°C temperature is preferred.

iii. *Agitation:* Continuous agitation is known to hasten decalcification.

iv. *Suspension:* Suspending the tissue in a decalcifier exposes all the surfaces of the tissue for decalcification. Bone samples can be suspended in the fluid with a thread or placed inside some cloth bags tied with a thread. Any perforated platforms deviced to raise the tissue above the container bottom to permit the fluid access to the tissue also are preferred.

v. 1 : 20 ratio of tissue to decalcifying agent is preferred.

Decalcifying Agents

Acids: Strong or weak acids can be used.

Strong acids: Aqueous solution of 5–10% nitric acid or hydrochloric acid is used. This decalcifies at a faster rate. We should remember that the nucleic acids fail to take haematoxylin when these decalcifying agents are employed.

Weak acids: About 5–10% solution of formic acid or acetic acid or picric acid is used. Formic acid is extensively used and decalcification is completed within 1 to 10 days.

These weak acids are preferred for tissues with little calcification; wherein decalcification would be completed in a short-time. These are not suitable for heavily mineralised tissues.

Some of the acid-based decalcifying agents
1. 10% nitric acid
    - Concentrated nitric acid   10 ml
    - Distilled water   90 ml
2. Perenyi's fluid
    - 10% nitric acid   40 ml
    - Absolute alcohol   30 ml
    - 0.5% chromic acid   30 ml

    Mix all the above reagents before use (the solution turns to light blue); when the solution turns to greenish coloured fluid, it should be discarded.
3. Formalin-nitric acid
    - 40% formalin   10 ml
    - Nitric acid   10 ml
    - Distilled water   80 ml
4. Aqueous formic acid
    - 90% stock formic acid   5–10 ml
    - Distilled water to make   100 ml
5. Formic acid-formalin
    - 90% stock formic acid   5–10 ml
    - Formaldehyde 40%   5 ml
    - Distilled water to make   100 ml
6. Buffered formic acid
    - 20% aqueous sodium citrate 65 ml
    - 90% stock formic acid   35 ml

One part of the 20% aqueous sodium citrate and one part of 50% formic acid mixture also can be used.

Nitric acid (as 5–10% aqueous solution) is a rapid decalcifier. But it discolours the tissue to yellow colour and can interfere with the staining process.

However, little damage is caused to the tissue if it is removed from decalcifying agent as soon as decalcification is over. An experienced person can identify completeness of decalcification by just a gentle feel of the tissue.

To change the acidic nature of the tissue to neutral, overnight washing in tap-water or in alkaline solution would be effective.

Sometimes, it is recommended to have two changes of 70% alcohol for 12–18 hours before taking that tissue for dehydration.

The tissue decalcified in acid needs to be kept in haematoxylin for a longer time (for 5 minutes) than the usual section. Eosin staining needs lesser time (30 seconds) and it stains bright pink.

Chelating Agents

Ethylenediamine tetra-acetic acid (EDTA) also called sequestrene or versene is slow in action; this binds to ionic calcium of bone, at the same time, removes first the outer layer and then the inner layer. Up to 14% solution of EDTA could be used.

Other EDTA containing solutions
  i. EDTA solution (Hillemann and Lee)
    - EDTA, disodium salt   5.5 g
    - Distilled water   90 ml
    - Formalin (40%)   10 ml
  ii. Neutral EDTA
    - EDTA, disodium salt   250 g
    - Distilled water   1750 ml

When we want to use EDTA, a wash in formal saline for 12 hours is required.

Surface Decalcification

Sometimes, an area of calcification becomes apparent while sectioning a paraffin wax block. If a small area is involved, then it is possible to decalcify the surface layer by inverting the block in 5% hydrochloric acid for 1 hour or so. However, before cutting the tissue, the block should be rinsed in water to avoid contaminating the knife or the microtome with the acid.

Electrophoretic Decalcification

Though this method is employed for decalcification, it has found little favour and it depends on the theory that calcium ions are attracted to the cathode.

Ion Exchange Resins

Ion exchange resins in decalcifying fluids are used to remove the calcium ions from the tissue at a faster rate.

The resin (commonly an ammonium form of sulphonated polystyrene resin) is layered on the bottom of the container to a depth of approximately 1 cm (it should not be less than 10% of the bulk of the decalcifying agent). The specimen is allowed to rest on it. The volume of fluid employed in this technique needs to be 20–30 times more than the bulk of the specimen.

The use of resin is limited to those decalcifying fluids that do not contain any mineral acids; usually formic acid is recommended. After its use, the resin may be regenerated by washing twice with dilute N/10 hydrochloric acid, followed by three washes in distilled water. This way, the resin could be reused for a longer period without requiring any renewal.

The End Point of Decalcification

To prevent any harmful effects of an acid on the tissue, the tissue should be kept in a decalcifying fluid for a minimum time possible. Some accurate determination of the end point of decalcification, is therefore, necessary.

Any experienced personnel can assess the time needed for decalcification depending upon the size and the structure of the tissue. Small biopsies of cancellous bone should be examined after 24 hours and the other specimens daily or after two or three days. Any experienced personnel could evaluate by the feel of the tissue if decalcification is virtually complete. Probing the tissue with a needle is not recommended; judicious bending or trimming can be of great help in assessing the completeness of decalcification and accurate determination could be obtained by X-ray or chemical tests.

Radiography is the most efficient test for the end point decalcification and several specimens could be exposed on the same X-ray: of course care has to be taken over identification.

A chemical test called calcium oxalate test depends upon the identification of the presence of calcium in the decalcifying solution by precipitation of insoluble calcium hydroxide or calcium oxalate. However, this method cannot be used after EDTA decalcification.

The method employed in this case is to take 5 ml of decalcifying fluid, then neutralise it with N/2 sodium hydroxide or ammonia hydroxide. This may be adjusted using pH paper or pH meter. Thereafter, add 5 ml of saturated ammonium oxalate solution and shake well. Then allow the solution to stand for 30 minutes.

Results would be as follows: A white precipitate (calcium hydroxide) forms after adding ammonia hydroxide/sodium hydroxide which suggests the presence of large amounts of calcium in the decalcifying fluid. There is no need for further steps, as this would be positive enough and at this point, we have to change to fresh decalcifying solution which becomes necessary.

If the fluid remains clear after addition of ammonia hydroxide/sodium hydroxide and the precipitate appears with ammonium oxalate, it means less calcium is present in the solution. If the fluid remains clear after 30 minutes, it is safe to assume that decalcification is completed.

A test known as 'bubble test' is based on the theory that acids react with calcium carbonate in bone to produce carbon dioxide; it is visible as bubble on the bone surface. The bubbles disperse with agitation on shaking but reform. As an end point test, bubble test is subjective and unreliable but could be used as a guide to check the progress of decalcification, i.e. tiny bubbles indicate that the presence of calcium is less in quantity.

Exercise 67

Special Stains

Procedures of some of the special stains commonly used for tissue sections in histopathology are given below.

VERHOEFF STAIN

Procedure

- Deparaffinise
- Bring sections to water
- Stain with Verhoeff's iron haematoxylin for a period of 15–20 minutes that is until sections are jet black
- Differentiate in 2% ferric chloride until elastic fibres are clearly seen. Then rinse in tap water and examine under microscope
- Wash in water, then in 95% alcohol in order to remove iodine colouration
- Wash in water for 5 minutes
- Counterstain with van Gieson stain for a duration of 3 minutes
- Dehydrate, clear and mount.

Reagents for Verhoeff's Iron Haematoxylin

- 5% haematoxylin in absolute alcohol — 20 ml
- 10% ferric chloride — 8 ml
- Verhoeff's iodine — 8 ml

(2 g of iodine + 4 g of potassium iodide + distilled water 100 ml)

The reagents are freshly prepared and mixed in the order as specified above.

Results

Elastic fibres	Black
Collagen	Red
Muscles	Yellow
Nuclei	Black

VAN GIESON STAIN

Procedure

- Deparaffinise
- Bring sections to water
- Stain with Weigert's iron haematoxylin for 15–20 minutes (Weigert's haematoxylin and ferric alum in equal parts)
- Water wash
- Differentiate in 1% hydrochloric acid in 70% alcohol
- Wash well in running tap water
- Counter stain with van Gieson's stain for 2 minutes
- Dehydrate with alcohol to which picric acid has been already added
- Clear and mount.

van Gieson's solution consists of

- Picric acid — 100 ml
- 1% acid fuchsin — 10 ml

Results

Nuclei	Black
Collagen	Red
Other tissues including muscle and RBCs	Yellow

MASSON TRICHROME STAIN

Procedure

- Deparaffinise
- Bring sections to water
- Stain in Weigert's iron haematoxylin for 20–30 minutes (Weigert's haematoxylin and ferric alum in equal parts)
- Differentiate in 1% acid alcohol
- Wash in tap water until sections are blue (called blueing)
- Stain in 1% Panceau '2R' in 1% acetic acid or stain with acid fuchsin solution—5 minutes
- Rinse in distilled water
- Mordant in 2.5% aqueous phosphomolybdic acid for 5 minutes
- Pour 2.5% aniline blue in 2.5% acetic acid or 2% light green in 2% acetic acid—5 minutes
- Differentiate in 1% acetic acid for 1 minute
- Dehydrate, clear and mount.

Acid fuchsin solution is prepared thus:

Acid fuchsin	0.5 g
Glacial acetic acid	0.5 ml
Distilled water	100 ml

Result

Nuclei	Blue black
Cytoplasm, muscle	Red
Collagen	Blue/green

RETICULIN STAIN (GORDON AND SWEET'S METHOD)

Procedure

- Deparaffinise
- Bring sections to water
- Oxidise with acidified potassium permanganate for 3 minutes
- Wash with distilled water
- Bleach with oxalic acid for 1 minute
- Wash well in distilled water
- Mordant with 2.5% ferric alum for 20 minutes
- Wash with distilled water
- Impregnate with Gordon and Sweet's silver solution till sections become transparent but scum appears after 2 minutes
- Wash with distilled water
- Reduce with 10% formalin for 2 minutes, sections become either brown or jet black
- Wash with tap water
- Tone with gold chloride (0.2%) for 3 minutes.
- Wash with tap water
- Fix in sodium thiosulphate (5%) for 3 minutes
- Wash well with tap water
- Counterstain if desired with eosin for 1 minute
- Dehydrate, clear and mount.

Acidified potassium permanganate solution is prepared as below

0.5% aqueous potassium permanganate	95 ml
3.0% sulphuric acid	5 ml

Preparation of Silver Solution

Take 0.5 g of silver nitrate in 5 ml of distilled water. Ensure that there is no turbidity. Add ammonia drop by drop till turbidity appears and disappears. Then, add 5 ml of potassium hydroxide to the above solution. It becomes black. Now, add ammonia drop by drop till the solution becomes just clear. Make it to 50 ml by adding distilled water.

Results

Reticulin fibres—black.

PAS STAIN (PERIODIC ACID-SCHIFF STAIN)

Procedure

- Deparaffinise
- Bring sections to water
- Oxidise with 1% periodic acid for 5 minutes
- Wash with distilled water for 2 minutes and then rinse in several changes of distilled water

- Treat with Schiff's reagent for 20 minutes
- Wash with tap water for 10 minutes till the sections become pink in colour
7. If desired, stain with Harri's or Ehrlich's haematoxylin for 2 minutes. Wash in tap water. Differentiate in 1% HCl in 70% alcohol, wash with tap water (blueing)
8. Dehydrate, clear and mount.

Results

Glycogen and other periodate reactive substances—magenta pink

Nuclei—blue.

The points to be noted are
- In diastase treated sections, glycogen will not stain with PAS
- Mucin containing reactive hexose component is PAS positive (neutral mucins, N-acetyl sialomucins)
- Sulphated mucins—PAS positive
- O-acetyl sialomucins—PAS negative
- Connective tissue mucins (proteoglycans)—PAS negative
- Hyaluronic acid, chondroitin sulphate (uronic acid containing substances)—PAS positive
- Keratan sulphate (lacks uronic acid)—PAS negative
- Sphingomyelin—PAS positive
- Mucoproteins (basement membrane)—PAS positive.

Exercise 68

Theoretical Aspects of some of the Special Stains

PAS STAIN

The PAS reaction is a useful indicator regarding the presence or absence of tissue carbohydrates and particularly for glycogen when the technique incorporates a diastase digestion stage.

The principle behind this reaction is that periodic acid will bring about oxidative cleavage of the carbon to carbon bond in 1,2-glycols or their amino or alkylamino derivatives so as to form di-aldehydes. These aldehydes in turn will react with fuchsin-sulphurous acid that combines with basic pararosaniline to form a magenta coloured compound. The compound formed has shown to be alkyl sulphonate in type.

Periodic acid is the oxidant of choice and it does not progressively over-oxidise the formed aldehydes to form carboxylic acid which would result in weak Schiff reaction.

Periodic acid solution consists of
Periodic acid   1 g
Distilled water   200 ml

Preparation of Schiff's Reagent

Dissolve 1 g basic fuchsin in 200 ml of boiling distilled water in a flask. Then remove the flask from the fire. Cool to 50°C and then add 2 g of potassium metabisulphite. Cool to room temperature, then add 2 ml of concentrated hydrochloric acid and mix well. Add 2 g of activated charcoal and leave overnight in the dark at room temperature. Filter through a No. 1 Whatman paper, by then the solution should be clear or pale yellow. Store in dark container at 4°C.

While preparing the Schiff's reagent, the basic fuchsin solution is sulphurated by adding potassium metabisulphite. There would be rearrangement of chromophoric groups that are present in the basic fuchsin by sulphuration. Any excess sulphur remaining in the solution is removed by treating it with activated charcoal, by which the sulphur particles are adsorbed and thus removed.

RETICULIN STAIN

Reticulin (reticular) fibres can be demonstrated by using metal impregnation methods and dyes. But the dye techniques are not reliable and they do not readily differentiate between collagen and reticulin fibres. The metal impregnation technique provides a clear contrast enabling the finest fibres to be resolved.

Metal impregnation technique mainly employs silver salts in alkaline solution. The silver is in a state that is readily able to precipitate as metallic silver. Reticulin fibres have an affinity for silver salts and require pretreatment with heavy metal salt solutions such as ferric ammonium sulphate; sensitised sites of silver in reduced form are created on reticulin fibres and silver is taken in unreduced form. Upon treatment with the reducing agent, silver in the tissue in unreduced form is converted into metallic silver. The remaining silver if any is removed by sodium thiosulphate. The silver may be partially converted into gold impregnation by treatment with gold chloride and at the same time increases the contrast.

While preparing the silver solution, the solvent has to be distilled water or deionised water to prevent precipitation of insoluble silver salts. Some carbonate or hydroxide is added to a solution of silver nitrate to produce a precipitate. The precipitate is just redissolved by adding ammonia solution. Care has to be taken regarding the cleanliness of glassware. The solutions prepared should be of proper weight and proper volumes accurately measured. Any excess ammonia in the solution may result in great loss of sensitivity.

TRICHROME STAIN

There is some selective demonstration in trichrome stain, regarding the presence of muscle, collagen fibres and erythrocytes.

The size of the dye molecule is significant in these stains. Smaller sized dye molecule will penetrate any of the tissue types. Medium sized ones will penetrate muscle and collagen, whereas, larger sized molecules will penetrate only collagen thus leaving the muscle and the erythrocytes unstained, e.g. van Gieson's stain collagen stains red with acid fuchsin (large molecules) and muscle stains yellow with much smaller dye picric acid.

VERHOEFF STAIN

Elastic fibres will stain quite intensively but not always selectively. The elastic fibres are cross-linked by bisulphide bridges. Following oxidative treatment with iodine as in Verhoeff's haematoxylin, these bisulphide bonds are converted into anionic sulphonic acid derivatives. These derivatives will inhibit the dye uptake by chromatin and stain the coarse fibres more intensively than the fine fibres.

Section V

Cytology Techniques

Exercise 69. Cytological Fixatives
Exercise 70. Lysing Fixatives
Exercise 71. Criteria to Evaluate Screening Tests
Exercise 72. Different Staining Techniques in Cytology
Exercise 73. Cytopreparatory Techniques
Exercise 74. Technique of Fine Needle Aspiration Cytology (FNAC)
Exercise 75. Pleural, Pericardial and Peritoneal Fluids
Exercise 76. Cerebrospinal Fluid (CSF)
Exercise 77. Synovial Fluid
Exercise 78. Sampling, Cytopreparatory Techniques and Cytology of Oral Cavity and Alimentary Tract (Oesophagus, Stomach and Duodenum)
Exercise 79. Sampling, Cytopreparatory Techniques and Cytology of Respiratory Tract
Exercise 80. Sampling, Cytopreparatory Techniques and Cytology of Urinary Tract
Exercise 81. FNAC of Thyroid, Salivary Gland and Breast Lesions
Exercise 82. Cytology of Female Genital System
Exercise 83. Hormone Cytology
Exercise 84. Barr Body

Exercise 69

Cytological Fixatives

There are different types of cytological fixatives. For details refer to the topic on fixation. Spray fixation is described here.

SPRAY FIXATION

Spray fixative contains an alcoholic base and a waxy substance (carbowax) that provides protective coating for the cells. After reaching the laboratory the slide has to undergo two separate rinses of 95% ethanol:
  i. To remove carbowax
  ii. To complete fixation before staining.

Procedure

Immediate fixation is done with wet cell sample. The nozzle of the spray should be held at a distance from the slide. About 6–12 inches is the preferred distance. One should obtain an even spray across the entire slide. Avoid spraying the labelled part.

Composition of Spray Fixative

Polyethylene glycol (carbowax)	50 ml
95% ether alcohol	950 ml

Before staining, keep the slides in two separate changes of 95% ethanol. In the first fresh 95% ethanol keep the slides for 30 minutes and discard after use. In the second fresh 95% ethanol keep the slides for 15 minutes.

Exercise 70

Lysing Fixatives

Lysing fixatives are used for blood cell samples; presence of erythrocytes partially or completely occludes the epithelial cells which have to be observed. To lyse the erythrocytes following fixatives can be used.

i. *Carnoy's fixative:* This contains absolute ethanol, chloroform and glacial acetic acid in 6 : 3 : 1 ratio, always prepare a fresh solution. Modified Carnoy's fixatives with mixture of 95% ethanol, glacial acetic acid and/or chloroform can be used.

ii. *Clarke's fixative:* This contains absolute alcohol and glacial acetic acid in 3 : 1 ratio.

iii. One drop of concentrated hydrochloric acid in 500 ml of 95% ethanol.

iv. 10% glacial acetic acid followed by placing the slide in 95% ethanol.

v. 2M urea solution (120 g powdered urea per litre of distilled water).

Exercise 71: Criteria to Evaluate Screening Tests

Sensitivity: This is the ability of the test to detect the disease when it is present.

Sensitivity = True positive/True positive + False negative × 100%

Specificity: This is the ability of the test to indicate non-disease state when it is not present.

Specificity = True negative/True negative + False positive × 100%

Positive predictive value: This value conveys what proportion of the subjects with positive test results have the disease.

Negative predictive value: This value conveys what proportion of the subjects with negative test results are truly free from the disease.

Exercise 72

Different Staining Techniques in Cytology

The most commonly used staining techniques are given below.

PAPANICOLAOU STAINING

   i. Fix the smears in 95% alcohol for 30 minutes.
  ii. Bring the smears to 80% alcohol—1 minute.
 iii. Bring the smears to 70% alcohol—1 minute.
  iv. Bring the smears to 50% alcohol—1 minute.
   v. Wash the smears in tap water—2 to 3 minutes.
  vi. Stain with Harris haematoxylin—45 seconds.
 vii. Wash in running tap water
viii. Bring the smears to 50% alcohol—1 minute.
  ix. Bring the smears to 70% alcohol—1 minute.
   x. Bring the smears to 80% alcohol—1 minute.
  xi. Bring the smears to 95% alcohol—1 minute.
 xii. Bring the smears to 95% alcohol—1 minute.
xiii. Stain with orange G-6—2½ minutes
 xiv. Bring the smears to 95% alcohol—1 minute
  xv. Bring the smears to 95% alcohol—1 minute.
 xvi. Stain with EA-65—5 minutes
xvii. Bring the smears to 95% alcohol—1 minute.
xviii. Bring the smears to 95% alcohol—1 minute.
 xix. Bring the smears to absolute alcohol—1 minute.
  xx. Bring the smears to absolute alcohol—1 minute.
 xxi. Air dry/warm the smears.
xxii. Clear and mount with DPX.

Results

Nucleus—blue
Cytoplasm—non-keratinising squamous
Cells—blue/green keratinising squamous
Cells—pink/orange
RBCs—orange/pink

Modifications of papanicolaou technique can be done and one should standardise the staining method to achieve reproducible results.

RAPID PAPANICOLAOU METHOD

i.	Prepare smears in usual fashion and air dry	
ii.	Normal saline	30 seconds
iii.	Alcoholic formalin	10 seconds
iv.	Water wash	6 slow dips (1 dip/second)
v.	Richard-Allen haematoxylin	22 slow dips
vi.	Water wash	6 slow dips
vii.	95% ethanol	6 slow dips

viii. Richard-Allen cytostain 4 slow dips
ix. 95% ether alcohol 6 slow dips
x. Absolute alcohol 6 slow dips
xi. Xylene 10 slow dips
xii. Mount with DPX

Richard-Allen haematoxylin and Richard-Allen cytostain are available from Richard-Allen, Richland, MI.

Alcoholic formalin is prepared as below
300 ml of 40% formalin, 2053 ml of 95% ethanol and 647 ml of distilled water (65% ethanol and 4% formaldehyde) are mixed.

Preparation of Papanicolaou (Pap) Stain

1. Harris haematoxylin

Haematoxylin	5 g
Ammonium aluminium sulphate	100 g (mordant)
Ethyl alcohol	50 ml
Distilled water	1000 ml
Mercuric oxide	2.5 g (oxidising agent)

Preparation
- Dissolve haematoxylin in alcohol
- Add ammonium aluminium sulphate to water in a beaker and heat to boiling
- Add haematoxylin solution and bring to boiling once again
- Remove from the flame and add mercuric oxide
- Swirl quickly until a black purple colour appears; the colour appears in a matter of seconds
- Plunge the beaker into cold water rapidly
- When cold, filter into dark bottle. This is stock Harris haematoxylin
- To prepare haematoxylin for staining, add 4 ml of glacial acetic acid per 100 ml of stock Harris haematoxylin.

2. OG-6

Prepare 10% aqueous stock solution of orange G using distilled water.

Working solution of OG-6 is prepared as follows:

95% ethyl alcohol	950 ml
Orange G 10% stock solution	50 ml
Phosphotungstic acid	0.15 g (mordant and differential stain) or
OG-6 powder	2.5 g
Phosphotungstic acid	200 mg

Dissolve both powders in 20 ml of distilled water, then add 200 ml of absolute alcohol. Filter and use the solution.

3. EA-65

EA-65 is prepared as follows

Alcoholic stock solution of light green SF (0.05% solution 95% alcohol)	180 ml
Alcoholic stock solution of Bismarck brown (0.5% solution in 95% alcohol)	40 ml
Alcohol stock solution of eosin yellow (eosin yellow 0.65% solution in 95% alcohol)	180 ml
Phosphotungstic acid (Mordant)	2.4 g

or

Light green SF powder	1 g
Bismarck brown Y	500 mg
Eosin yellow	1 g
Phosphotungstic acid	200 mg

Dissolve all these powders in 20 ml of distilled water, and then add 200 ml of absolute alcohol. Filter and use the solution.

MGG STAINING

Following are required for MGG staining
- May-Grunwald's stain
- Giemsa stain
- Methanol
- Glycerol
- Phosphate buffer (pH 6.8).

Steps of Staining Procedure

i. Air dried smears are fixed in methanol for 10 minutes.
ii. May-Grunwald's stain is diluted with equal part of phosphate buffer or tap water.

iii. Giemsa stain is diluted with 9 parts of phosphate buffer.
iv. Pour May-Grunwald's stain on the smears and wait for 5 minutes.
v. Remove the stain and pour diluted Giemsa stain on the smears and wait for 10 minutes.
vi. Wash with phosphate buffer.
vii. Air dry and mount with DPX.

Preparation of Stains

Preparation of May-Grunwald's stain: 0.3 g of powdered dye is weighed and transferred to a conical flask of 200–250 ml capacity. 100 ml of methanol is added and the mixture is warmed to 50°C. The flask is then allowed to cool to room temperature and shaken several times. Allow it to stand for 24 hours and filter. It is ready for use.

Preparation of Giemsa stain: 1.0 g of Giemsa powder is dissolved in 54 ml of glycerol. Mixed in 84 ml of methanol and filtered.

DIFF-QUICK STAINING

This is a modified Wright's stain and has three solutions. It is fast, practical and provides good cellular details. The stain is comparable to May-Grunwald-Giemsa stain.

- Fixation of smears in methanol containing 1.8 mg/L triaryl methane dye
- Solution I—buffered eosin yellow
- Solution II—buffered solution of thiazide dye methylene blue and azure A (azure A undergoes slow oxidation to azure B).

Procedure

- Fixation
- Solution I—5 dips (5 seconds)
- Water wash
- Solution II—5 dips (5 seconds)
- Rinsed in water and dried
- Clear with xylene
- Mount with DPX.

Exercise 73

Cytopreparatory Techniques

The following are the different cytopreparatory techniques.
a. Toluidine blue stained wet film
b. Permanent smears
   - Wet fixed smear stained with Pap stain
   - Air dried smears stained with MGG/Diff-quick stain
c. Cell block sections
   - Stained with H & E
   - Used for IHC/special stains.

TOLUIDINE BLUE STAINED WET FILM

a. If any clots or fragments of tissue are present, remove them and fix in 10% buffered formalin for 30 minutes and process the fragments as tissues or make cell blocks.
b. Centrifuge the remaining fluid in centrifuge tube for 5 minutes at 2000 RPM.
c. Pour off or pipette off supernatant.
d. Prepare a toluidine blue stained wet film.

Technique

Put a drop of sediment on the centre of the glass slide and put an equal drop of toluidine blue (0.1–0.5%) stain. Mix together with corner of the coverslip and examine immediately.

Permanent Smear

Put 1 to 2 drops of sediment on the centre of a glass slide and spread the material on the slide. Before the smear is dry, immerse the slide in 95% ethanol.

Alternate fixative for 95% ethanol is 95% propanol.

Air dried smears are stained with MGG or Diff-quick stain.

CELL-BLOCK TECHNIQUE

After preparing wet films and smears for Pap stain or MGG stain, prepare a cell-block of the residual sediment. Any of the following procedures can be used to hold the cells together before processing.

i. Add 2 or 3 drops of plasma (outdated plasma from blood bank can be used) to the remaining residual sediment and mix.
ii. Add 3 or 4 drops of thrombin, mix and allow to clot.
iii. Add 10% buffered formalin and fix for 30 minutes. Pour this in a Petri dish containing spontaneously formed clots and process the fragments.
iv. Add few ml of melted agar, mix and refrigerate to solidify.
v. Add 0.5 ml of liquefied Histogel and solidify at room temperature or lesser temperature.

Preparation of thrombin solution: Add 10 ml distilled water to a vial containing 5000 units of powdered thrombin.

Toluidine blue stain: The toluidine blue stain is prepared as below.

Toluidine blue	0.5 g
95% ethanol	20 ml
Distilled water	80 ml

Store the stain in refrigerator to prevent fungal growth.

Uses of wet films

- Wet films reveal diagnostic picture.
- Report can be issued within 10 to 15 minutes after receiving the specimen.
- In case, neoplastic cells are suspected more smears can be prepared; studied with Pap and MGG stains.
- Certain constituents which are not seen in permanent smears such as cholesterol crystals and Charcot-Leyden crystals can be observed. Haemosiderin crystals in the blood effusions, detached ciliary tufts/ciliocytophthoria in peritoneal fluid and psammoma bodies stand out clearly as they are not stained by toluidine blue.

Exercise 74

Technique of Fine Needle Aspiration Cytology (FNAC)

For the fine needle aspirations to be successful, the following criteria are to be fulfilled.
  i. Aspiration of adequate and representative material.
  ii. Interpretation of the lesion and issue of accurate report.

Cytopathologists/clinicians can perform the aspirate or cytopathologists can assist the clinicians in the preparation of the slides. Image-guided aspirations are usually done by a radiologist. In such instances, it is helpful if a cytopathologist also attends, so that the site of aspiration and the exact location can be appreciated prior to the microscopic examination.

Techniques of aspirations of superficial lesions are carried out in an outpatient clinic or laboratory suite which is equipped with necessary instruments for the examination of fine needle aspirations (FNAs).

INSTRUMENTS NECESSARY FOR FNA

  i. Sterile gloves.
  ii. Alcohol swabs for cleaning skin.
  iii. Cameco syringe holder.
  iv. 10 and 20 ml disposable syringes.
  v. 21 to 25 gauge disposable needle.
  vi. Glass slides.
  vii. Watch glass.
  viii. Pencil for labelling slides.
  ix. Reagents for Pap/Diff-quick/MGG staining.
  x. Spray fixative/cytological fixative.
  xi. Rack for air dried smears.
  xii. Empty tubes for cyst fluids.
  xiii. Cell culture medium.
  xiv. Tube with 10% buffered formalin.
  xv. Tube with necessary medium for microbiological investigations, if culture is needed.
  xvi. 1% glutaraldehyde if electron microscopy is required.
  xvii. Gauge swabs.
  xviii. Tissue paper.
  xix. Request forms.
  xx. Biohazard bags.
  xxi. Container for discarding needles and syringes.

Technique (Figs 5.1a to g)

- Aspirations are best performed with the syringe in Cameco syringe holder which has the advantage of freeing one hand to stabilise the lump under aspiration.
- The mass is held between thumb and index finger.
- A 22-gauge needle of 2.5 to 4 cm length is attached to a 10 ml disposable syringe and is introduced into the lesion which is to be aspirated.
- Vacuum is created in the syringe and the lesion is probed several times in different directions.
- Larger masses should be aspirated from the periphery, as centre may be necrotic. The

suction/vacuum is released, the needle along with syringe is withdrawn.
- Release the needle from the syringe. Small quantity of air is drawn up into the syringe and is re-attached to the needle.
- The contents of the needle are blown out onto a labelled glass slide and material is spread.
- The blood specimens can be expelled into a watchglass and selectively sampled or the contents of the needle and syringe can be flushed into an aliquot of normal saline or lysing solution and processed further.
- For the delay in processing or if the slides have to be transported from long distance to the laboratory, the slides should be fixed in 50% ethyl alcohol or spray fixative.
- Fragment of tissue has to be preserved in 10% buffered formalin for paraffin sectioning.
- Cysts, particularly of breast should be completely evacuated and contents should be expelled into a clean dry tube.
- When the aspiration is complete, the patient should be reassured. Puncture site is covered with gauze swab and adhesive tape and gentle pressure is applied to minimise the risk of bleeding.
- Adequacy of material should be checked before the patient departs. If the first attempt is unsatisfactory the procedure can be repeated.

Causes of Failure

- Poor localisation of lesion
- Poor aspiration technique
- Tangential aspiration so that the needle misses the lesion
- Necrosis/cystic change, viable cells are not obtained

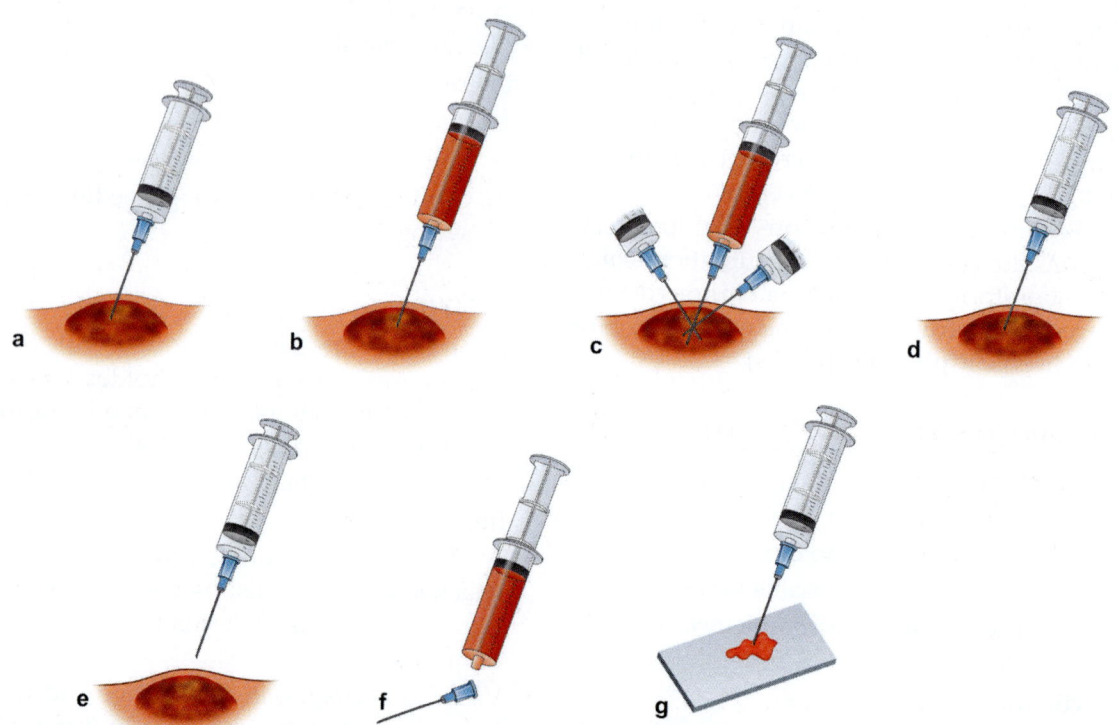

Figs 5.1a to g: Technique of FNA: (a) Insertion of needle into mass, (b) withdrawal of plunger, (c) aspiration with needle in different directions, (d) release of vacuum, (e) withdraw of needle from mass, (f) separation of needle from syringe and air is drawn into syringe, (g) contents of needle are blown out

- Desmoplastic tissue, cells are difficult to aspirate from surrounding fibrous tissue.

Preparation of Smear

- A few drops of grey white/pink blown out material is smeared with the help of another slide and gently pulled apart. The smears are wet fixed (fixed before smear dries) in 95% alcohol. Procedure can be repeated if material is more. The fixed smears are stained with Pap stain. Some smears are air dried and stained with MGG/Diff-quick stain. To check for adequacy, smears can be stained with Diff-quick method for immediate microscopy.
- If fluid is aspirated, sediment or cytocentrifuged preparations are done.
- If the slides are sent from long distance, the specimen is checked against patient details on request form, number of slides and tubes sent are noted. Documentation is made including all these things.
- In case of bloody smears, blood is removed by lysing solution and processed further. Cell blocks and tissue fragments are fixed in buffered formalin and processed for paraffin sections.

Exercise 75

Pleural, Pericardial and Peritoneal Fluids

The body cavities are lined by single layer of flat cells called mesothelium supported by connective tissue, blood vessels and nerves. The parietal and visceral layers are separated by a small volume of lubricating fluid.

Serous body fluids from these body cavities are:

a. Pleural fluid
b. Pericardial fluid
c. Peritoneal fluid.

These body cavities contain a small amount of body fluid that cannot be aspirated. This fluid facilitates the movement of membranes against each other. It is a plasma filtrate containing salts and low molecular weight substances, i.e. glucose and urea. The cellular content is comprised of mesothelial cells with occasional macrophages or lymphocytes. Effusion of these fluids is because of increase of venous pressure, increased capillary permeability or due to interference with lymph flow. The effusions can be transudate or exudate (Table 5.1).

Sampling Techniques of Serous Fluids

- Serous fluids can be sampled by inserting a wide bore needle (under local anaesthesia) through the body wall into fluid containing

Table 5.1: The differences between transudate and exudate

Transudate	Exudate
Accumulates due to non-inflammatory processes such as disturbances with circulation—passive congestion and oedema	Accumulates due to inflammatory processes
Appearance	
Clear	Clear/turbid
Serous	Serous/purulent
Pale yellow	Haemorrhagic
Specific gravity	
Less than 1.015	More than 1.015
Clot	
Absent	Clots spontaneously
Proteins	
Less than 3 g/dl	More than 3 g/dl
Cells	
Mesothelial cells	Neutrophils in acute inflammation
Lymphocytes	Lymphocytes in chronic inflammation and RBCs

cavity. Peritoneal fluid is obtained by abdominal paracentesis, pleural fluid by thoracocentesis and pericardial fluid by pericardiocentesis.

- Washing is obtained by instilling normal saline solution into various recesses of the peritoneal cavity. It is done in patients undergoing abdominal exploration for gynaecological neoplasm to detect peritoneal dissemination.
- Peritoneal dialysate from patients undergoing long-term peritoneal dialysis for renal failure is occasionally submitted for examination.

Collection

- The fluid is collected in a clean, dry container which need not be sterile and sent to the laboratory immediately. If there is a delay in examination, refrigerate the sample at 4°C and do not freeze.
- Anticoagulants are not necessary; however, use of heparin does not interfere with the cytological details.
- Formalin, alcohol or other preservatives are not added and if added, these preservatives will interfere with Pap stain, prevent cells adhering to a slide and coagulate proteins.

Gross Examination of Serous Fluid

Naked eye examination reveals clues about the cause of the effusion and the nature of its cellular contents and hence a note of following is made:

1. Volume, colour, clarity and any unusual features such as malodour, opalescence or high viscosity are noted.
2. A blood-stained serous fluid may be of traumatic cause and carefully looked for cancer cells, especially the ones with orange or deep red colour.
3. Fluids rich in cells and those containing cancer cells sediment spontaneously.
4. Any visible particle in the fluid should be carefully looked for cancer cells.
5. Fluids with chocolate brown colour may have melanoma cells and lighter brown colour may be because of haemosiderophages. Fluids from jaundice patient will have greenish or yellowish tint.
6. Serous fluids in mesothelioma are of high viscosity due to high content of hyaluronic acid.
7. Fluids with cholesterol crystals are yellow and the crystals swirl when agitated.
8. Chylous fluids are creamy due to emulsified lipids.

Microscopic Examination of Serous Fluids

- Cell count is made similar to WBC count.
- *Wet films:* A few drops of sediment or cytocentrifuged cells are placed on a slide and mixed with a drop of toluidine blue stain. A cover slip is placed and observed immediately.
- The smears are prepared with the sediment or cytocentrifuged material and fixed in 95% alcohol for Pap stain and air dried for MGG stain.

The Cells Found in Serous Fluids

Mesothelial cells: These are the only cells specific to serous membranes. When serosa is injured as in inflammation or stimulation, the mesothelial cells undergo proliferation. These are round cells, 9 to 60 µ in diameter; they have abundant delicate pink foamy cytoplasm and often have an indistinct cytoplasmic membrane. The perinuclear halo may be occasionally observed. The nuclei are regular with granular chromatin and they have prominent nucleoli. The cytoplasm of these cells has PAS positive fine granules. Narrow gaps or windows separate these cells from each other. Examination by electron microscopy reveals that the mesothelial cell surface has microvilli. Tissue fragments with mesothelial cells have knobby/smooth contours. The old mesothelial cells may have cytoplasmic vacuoles (Fig. 5.2).

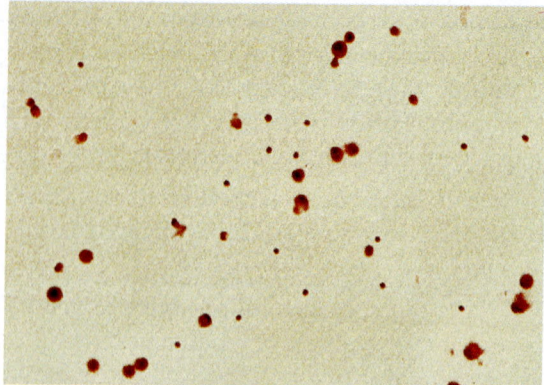

Fig. 5.2: Photomicrograph of mesothelial cells

Reactive and atypical mesothelial cells: The monolayered mesothelial membrane with irritation becomes multilayered. The cells are shed singly or in clusters. They may be arranged in pseudoacini. The cytoplasm is scant to abundant. It is thick and homogenous. The nuclei are placed centrally or eccentrically. The chromatin is clumped and distributed uniformly. The nuclear borders are smooth and sharp, multinucleation may be present. Sometimes, these cells need to be differentiated from malignant cells of adenocarcinoma.

Some of the differentiating points in favour of reactive or atypical mesothelial cells are:
- The cytoplasm and the nucleus are stained with equal intensity
- The cells are in monolayered sheets
- The windows in between the cells are indicative of mesothelial cells
- With PAS stain, the mesothelial cells have fine granules in the cytoplasm.

Some of the points in favour of malignant cells are
- The malignant cells are densely packed and often overlap
- The nuclei are stained densely and are hyperchromatic with increased nuclear cytoplasmic ratio
- The nucleoli are often prominent
- The cells have large droplets of PAS positive material
- In presence of cells in papillae, acini and in three-dimensional clusters, malignancy must be suspected.

The other cells found in serous fluids are:
Macrophages: These cells vary in size. Cytoplasm is vacuolated. The phagocytic activity with engulfed leukocytes, red cells or cellular debris may be noted.

Lymphocytes: The small lymphocytes are commonly found.

Neutrophils: These are numerous in inflammation, infarction and rupture of an organ.

Eosinophils: These cells are found in pleural effusions in allergy, autoimmune diseases, pneumonia, parasitic infection, pulmonary tuberculosis, malignancies, etc.

Plasma cells: These cells may be found in chronic inflammation of the serous cavities.

Mast cells and basophils: These cells are rarely found.

Red cells: A few red cells can be found in serous fluid.

Megakaryocytes: These cells are seldom found in abnormalities of haemopoiesis.

The different conditions for effusions are as follows:
- Non-neoplastic conditions
- Non-specific effusions.

Specific Effusions

Some of the conditions are listed below:
- Rheumatoid disease
- Systemic lupus erythematosus
- Pneumonia
- Tuberculosis
- Cirrhosis
- CCF
- Infarction
- Parasitic, protozoal, fungal and viral infections.

Neoplastic Conditions

- Mesothelioma
- Metastatic carcinoma.

Types of Effusions

Pleural effusion: This may be observed in various conditions such as pneumonia, pulmonary infarct, lung abscess, pleuritis, tuberculosis, heart failure, cirrhosis, malignancy, mesothelioma, pulmonary embolism and viral infection.

Peritoneal effusion: Some of the conditions include pyogenic peritonitis, tuberculosis, rupture of viscera, pancreatitis, CCF, cirrhosis and neoplasms.

Pericardial effusion: The conditions include pericarditis, tuberculosis, uraemia, rheumatic heart disease and myocardial infarction.

Exercise 76

Cerebrospinal Fluid (CSF)

- Cerebrospinal fluid (CSF) is present in the cavity (subarachnoid space) surrounding brain and spinal cord.
- It is produced by ultrafiltration and secretion through choroid plexus, ependymal lining of ventricles and cerebral subarachnoid space.
- CSF drains into venous sinuses enclosed within the dura mater via the arachnoid granulations.
- The functions of CSF are:
  - Collects wastes
  - Circulates nutrients
  - Acts as cushion and lubricates the CNS
- The blood–brain barrier maintains homeostasis in CSF.
- Normal quantity of CSF:
  Adults: 90–150 ml and neonates: 10–60 ml

Normal composition of CSF: The normal composition of CSF is as follows:
  i. Appearance is colourless and clear.
  ii. Pressure is 60 to 180 mm of water in lying position and 200 to 250 mm of water in sitting position.
  iii. pH 7.3–7.4.
  iv. Specific gravity 1.007.
  v. Proteins 15–45 mg/dl.
  vi. Glucose 40–80 mg/dl.
  vii. Chlorides 115–130 mmol/L.
  viii. Cells in CSF are 0–5 lymphocytes/cmm and infrequently occasional monocytes, polymorphs, cells from choroid plexus and ependymal cells may be encountered. Small to medium-sized cuboidal to low columnar cells of choroid plexus may be seen as tissue fragments.

Indications: The indications of CSF aspiration are as follows:
- Diagnostic purpose
  - CSF to study various constituents
  - Measurement of intracranial pressure
  - Testing for spinal block
- Radiological purpose
- Therapeutic purpose
- Anaesthetic purpose

CSF is obtained by the following procedures:
- Lumbar puncture
- Cisternal puncture
- Shunt drainage
- Directly from ventricles (by operation or burr hole) or in infants by transfontanelle puncture holes.

Note: It is important to be aware of the relationship of timing of sampling to previous surgery, invasive or therapeutic procedure such as myelogram. Reactive cells, foreign material and tissue fragments from sinuses may be present in some instances.

Processing of CSF

For CSF analysis these are necessary:
- Fresh specimen is preferred
- Note down pressure

- *Gross examination:* CSF is noted for:
  - Colour—colourless/pink/red
  - Appearance—turbid/clear
  - Clot formation and cobweb formation
- Cells count
- *Wet preparation:* Different methods can be followed for wet preparation.

  Direct smears from the sediment with a drop of toluidine blue stain.

  Cytocentrifuged preparation (1000 RPM × 5 minutes) yields excellent cell recovery.

  Filtration method may be followed.

  Cytocentrifuged preparations are preferred.
- *Biochemical analysis:*
  - Total proteins
  - Glucose
  - Chlorides
- Microbiological examination:
  - Gram's stain
  - Culture
- Pink/red CSF may be seen in haemorrhage, traumatic tap, intracerebral haemorrhage or infarcts.

Differential Diagnosis of Bloody CSF

- Bloody CSF clears between 1st and 3rd tube collected, and suggests traumatic tap
- In haemorrhage, colour remains uniform in all the tubes
- Xanthochromia suggests haemorrhage
- In traumatic and recent haemorrhage intact RBCs are seen. In old haemorrhage erythrophagocytosis and macrophage containing haemosiderin are present.

Xanthochromia: Supernatant of centrifuged CSF has pink/orange/yellow colour due to lysis of RBCs.

Xanthochromia is observed in
- Red cell lysis if CSF is not refrigerated or examination is delayed. The RBCs are lysed within 1 to 2 hours of CSF collection. Hence, rapid examination is recommended
- Haemorrhage
- Increased bilirubin as in patients with jaundice
- Traumatic taps
- Carotenoids (dietary intake)
- Metastatic melanoma
- Rifampicin therapy.

Pyogenic meningitis: The following are the features:
- CSF pressure increases to more than 180 mm of water
- Proteins increase with fibrinous coagulum to 100–500 mg/dl
- Sugar reduced to less than 40 mg/dl
- In centrifuged deposit bacteria are present in 60–80% of the cases
- Cell count is very high, polymorphs range between 1000 and 10000 cells/cmm
- Chlorides are reduced and may fall below 110 mmol/L.

Tuberculous meningitis: The following are the features:
- Pleocytosis with lymphocytes—100 to 600 cells/cmm
- Proteins elevated to 100–500 mg/dl, may exceed 2 g/L as the disease progresses
- Glucose lowered to 30–45 mg/dl
- Bacteria are present, but extremely difficult to demonstrate
- ZN staining and auramine staining can be applied
- Pressure is increased
- Opaque and on standing forms cobweb
- Chlorides fall progressively, may be below 100 mmol/L.

Viral meningitis: The following are the features:
- Normal to moderate increase in CSF pressure
- Cell count 5–300 cells/cmm and sometimes more than 1000 cells and lymphocytes predominate
- Proteins—30–100 mg/dl
- Glucose—normal/reduced.

Abnormal Cells in CSF

Relative pleocytosis
- Atypical forms consistent with immunoblasts may be confused with leukaemia
- Nuclei have smooth outlines.

Acute leukaemia may show blast cells in CSF.

Chronic leukaemia—mature or immature cells may be present.

Lymphoma: Cell types vary with degree of differentiation.

Carcinoma cells: Cells are larger with atypical features.

Primitive neuroectodermal cells: Cells are in clusters with rosettes.

Exercise 77

Synovial Fluid

Synovial fluid microscopy is of great value in distinguishing inflammatory from non-inflammatory arthropathies.

Synovial fluid is a transudate of plasma from synovial blood vessels along with high molecular weight saccharide rich molecules (hyaluronic acid) produced by type B synoviocytes; type A synoviocytes are phagocytes.

Synovium is a tissue lining the synovial tendon sheaths, bursae, and diarthodial joints except for the articular surfaces. It is composed of one to three cell layers that form a discontinuous surface overlying fatty, fibrous or periosteal joint tissue.

Synovial fluid acts as a lubricant, adhesive and provides nutrients for the avascular articular cartilage.

Synovial fluid differs from the other body fluids because of the following reasons:
i. Synovial joints are rarely affected by the neoplastic processes.
ii. Crystals and matrix fragments are to be studied to understand the disease process.
iii. Diagnostic information can be obtained from recognition and quantification of cell types.

The normal quantity of synovial fluid is about 4 ml. It is pale yellow, clear and has thick mucoid consistency. It is acellular except for a few synovial lining cells and has debris, possibly representing fragments from cartilage.

In a patient with bacteremia or with local sepsis sterile joint is not aspirated.

Examination of synovial fluid should be done under following headings:
- Gross examination
- Nucleated cell count
- Wet preparation
- Cytocentrifuge preparation.

Gross Examination

Collect synovial fluid with sterile disposable needles and plastic syringes. Syringe is heparinised with 25 U of sodium heparin/ml of synovial fluid. Oxalate, ethylenediamine tetra-acetic acid (EDTA) and lithium heparin anticoagulants should be avoided as they form crystal artifacts and may mislead during examination.

Separate the specimen into three parts
1. 5 to 10 ml into sterile tube for microbiological study.
2. 2 to 5 ml for microscopic examination.
3. 5 ml is allowed to clot.

Examination of fresh synovial fluid is preferred. It can be refrigerated for 24–48 hours. No fixatives are added and noted for the following:

Colour

- Normal synovial fluid is pale yellow
- Red or orange coloured in haemarthrosis

- Cream to white coloured in inflammatory arthropathies
- Coloured by bacterial chromogen in septic arthritis.

Clarity

- Normal synovial fluid is clear
- As the number of cells/particles increase, the synovial fluid becomes opalescent to frankly opaque. Examination for clarity gives a clue to cellularity and/or crystals content of the synovial fluid.

Viscosity

Normal synovial fluid has thick mucoid consistency due to complex saccharides. The length of mucoid strands of the fresh synovial fluid may stretch up to 2 cm before they break. In inflammatory diseases, the viscosity falls due to enzymatic digestion and altered synthesis of saccharides.

Mucin Clot Test

- Mix synovial fluid and dilute solution of acetic acid (5% acetic acid). A white precipitate is formed in about one minute. A good clot is formed in normal synovial fluid.
- In inflammatory joint disease, there will be poor clot formation (due to digestive enzymes).
- Non-inflammatory joint diseases exhibit a good mucin clot.
- Haemorrhage dilutes the synovial fluid and prevents clot formation.

Nucleated Cell Count

- The synovial fluid is well-agitated to achieve uniform distribution of cells.
- It is diluted to a known concentration with normal saline containing methyl violet.
- Diluted fluid is placed in a Neubauer counting chamber and cells are counted.
- Manual counting is preferred over to automated counting due to high viscosity and danger of producing mucin clot.
- In inflammatory joint diseases more than 1000 cells/cmm are present. In non-inflammatory joint diseases the cell counts will be less than 1000 cells/cmm.
- Cells count more than 20000 cells/cmm are found in clinical conditions like rheumatoid arthritis, septic arthritis and reactive arthritis.

Wet Preparation

- Synovial fluid often contains small particles. For wet preparation, the specimen is agitated. Aspirate the particles with a glass pipette and place a large drop on a clean slide. The drop is gently squeezed flat beneath a coverslip and viewed unstained under the microscope. For optimal results, the microscope condenser diaphragm should be nearly closed to produce diffuse light, such that the unstained particles including crystals are clearly visible. Fragments of tissue can be from joint associated structures including cartilage, meniscus and ligament.
- Monosodium urate crystals are needle-shaped, highly birefringent and 5–30 µ in length. These are found in gout along with high cell counts.
- Calcium pyrophosphate dihydrate crystals (pseudogout) accumulate with increasing age in joints containing fibrocartilage such as knee joint. The crystals are associated with high cell counts. Patient usually has monoarthritis. The crystals may be also found in osteoarthritis.
- *Hydroxy apatite:* Crystals of hydroxy apatite indicate damage to the calcified zone of cartilage or underlying sub-articular bone. These crystals are seen in non-inflammatory osteoarthritis and rheumatoid arthritis. Sometimes, the crystals are too small to be seen with microscope. Staining with Alizarin red will produce birefringent bright red colour which can be easily visualised.
- *Lipids:* In inflammatory joint diseases and haemarthrosis various lipids enter the

synovial fluid. The different lipids have different shapes; cholesterol are notched plates and cholesterol esters are spherical.
- Steroids with intra-articular injection may remain for 10 weeks and may mislead the diagnosis.
- Non-crystalline, cellular and non-cellular particulate material may be encountered: These may be:
  - Clustered chondrocytes from cartilage as in osteoarthritis
  - Fragments of meniscal fibrocartilage—collagen fibrils and chondrocytes
  - In prosthetic surgery and prosthetic failure—foreign body from prosthetic origin will be seen.

Cytocentrifuge Preparation

- Synovial fluid is cytocentrifuged by diluting the fluid down to 400 cells/cmm with isotonic saline. In case of septic arthritis, the synovial fluid is diluted to a concentration of 1200 cells/cmm to identify the bacteria. Organisms are usually gram-positive bacteria. Gram-negative organisms are difficult to identify.
- In inflammatory arthropathies (gout, septic arthritis, and rheumatoid disease) polymorphs predominate.
- In non-inflammatory arthropathies (trauma/osteoarthritis), macrophages lymphocytes and synoviocytes predominate.

The following cellular elements can be observed in synovial fluid:
  i. Neutrophils.
  ii. Lymphocytes.
  iii. Plasma cells.
  iv. *Reider cells:* These cells are observed in rheumatoid arthritis, 15 µ in size, N : C ratio is 6 : 1, nucleus is lobed and have symmetrical lobes seen around a pale attenuated central region.
  v. *Mott cells:* These cells resemble plasma cells and they contain intracytoplasmic Russel bodies; seen in rheumatoid arthritis.
  vi. *Macrophages:* These are often observed in non-inflammatory arthropathies and implanted prosthesis.
  vii. *Cytophagocytic macrophages/mononuclear cells:* These have phagocytic apoptotic neutrophils seen in seronegative spondyl arthropathies (psoriasis, inflammatory bowel diseases, Behçet's disease, ankylosing spondylitis).
  viii. *Synoviocytes:* These are large mononuclear cells seen in non-inflammatory arthropathies.
  ix. *Eosinophils:* These are observed in intra-articular haemorrhage, arthrography and parasitic infection.
  x. *Mast cells:* These are found in non-inflammatory and seronegative spondyl arthropathies.
  xi. *Neoplastic cells:* These are rare to find.
  xii. LE cells
  xiii. *Tart cells:* These are observed in rheumatoid disease.
  xiv. *Dohle body cells:* These are macrophages or neutrophils with intracytoplasmic inclusions with aggregates of cytoskeletal microfibrils.
  xv. *Ragocytes:* These are seen in rheumatoid arthritis and inflammatory arthropathies. In rheumatoid arthritis, these cells may account per 70–95% of the nucleated cell counts. The cell is a macrophage or neutrophil, cytoplasm has refractile granules with partially closed condenser diaphragm. The granules are larger than conventional neutrophil granule and are identified on size and refractility. These cells were first recognised in rheumatoid arthritis and hence called ragocytes.

Exercise 78: Sampling, Cytopreparatory Techniques and Cytology of Oral Cavity and Alimentary Tract (Oesophagus, Stomach and Duodenum)

Collection of Material from Oral Cavity

- Imprint smears from biopsy, exfoliative cytology and abrasive cytology are used.
- Immediate biopsy is of help in early diagnosis; imprint smears before putting the biopsy in formalin are indicated.
- The exfoliated cells are smeared on a slide with the help of a cotton tipped applicator while scraped material obtained from wooden spatula are much superior.
- Fix the wet smears for Pap stain and air dry for MGG stain.

Specimen Collection from Alimentary Tract

Following are the different procedures:

- With the flexible fibreoptic endoscope, brushings and salvage cytology materials are obtained.
- After endoscopic biopsy of the lesions suspected of being malignant, the material present on the external surface of biopsy forceps that was dislodged during withdrawal of the forceps through the biopsy channel is retrieved and processed. The channel is flushed with saline and cellular material is collected and processed.
- Material obtained by brushings is directly smeared on the slides. From lavage, washings and salvage material, sediment/cytocentrifuge/filter preparations are prepared and studied.
- Touch/imprint smears from the biopsy are done before the biopsy is dropped into a fixative.
- Transmural FNA is valuable when lavage and brushings are not useful.
- Endoscopic retrograde cholangiopancreatography (ERCP) is a combined radiological and endoscopic procedure that is performed under fluoroscopic control. Endoscope can be passed into the second part of duodenum and the papilla of Vater is cannulated. Brush which is protected by a sheath can be advanced into the obstructed area, vigorously brushed and smears are prepared with the material obtained on the brush.

Blind Procedure to Retrieve the Material from Oesophagus by Abrasive Technique

The use of brushes passed through nasogastric tubes is not in use. For abrasive cytology, a balloon-like device is used for obtaining the material from oesophagus. The device is swallowed in deflated state and passed into the stomach. The tube is inflated and pulled through gastroesophageal junction and rubbed along the entire length of the oesophageal mucosal surface. At the level of cricoid, the balloon is deflated and removed. Direct smears are made from the tissue on the external surface or rinse the tissue on the external surface in saline, prepare sediment/cytocentrifuge preparations. Wet fixed smears are stained with Pap stain and air dried ones with MGG stain.

Histology, normal cytology and abnormal cytology of oral cavity, oesophagus and other parts of alimentary tract.

The oral cavity is lined by stratified squamous epithelium. The hard palate, gingiva, dorsal aspect of tongue are lined by keratinised stratified squamous epithelium; oesophagus, floor of mouth, lateral and ventral surface of tongue are lined by non-keratinised stratified squamous epithelium.

The cells normally seen in the oral cavity are keratinised surface epithelial cells, non-keratinised stratified squamous epithelial cells, parabasal cells and immature prickle cells.

Lip, tongue, floor of the mouth, palate, gingiva, buccal mucosa and oropharynx are the sites of cancer. About 90% of these cancers are squamous cell carcinomas. Early diagnosis and treatment is the most effective way of combating the oral cancers. Immediate biopsy/exfoliative cytology/abrasive cytology with toluidine blue stain, Pap stain or MGG stain can identify the dysplastic/malignant cells.

Malignant Oral Lesions

Squamous cell carcinoma is the most common malignant tumour with following features:
- Polygonal cells with hyperchromatic central nuclei
- Orangeophilic or cyanophilic cytoplasm
- Enlarged nuclei, variation in nuclear size and shape (pleomorphism)
- Prominent irregular nuclear borders
- Increased N/C ratio
- With nucleoli
- Abnormal chromatin pattern and distribution.

The oesophagus is lined by a non-keratinised stratified squamous epithelium. Distal 1 to 2 cm of oesophagus has simple columnar epithelium with or without mucous cells. The entire length of the oesophageal lamina propria has glandular cells which produce neutral mucins. The submucosa has glandular structures with acidic mucin.

Cytology of Oesophagus

In the cytological specimens of oesophagus, the superficial and intermediate types of squamous cells predominate. The glandular cells in brushings/washings are from the distal part of the oesophagus or from the stomach.

Malignant Neoplasms of Oesophagus, Stomach and other Parts of GI Tract

In oesophagus, squamous cell carcinoma or adenocarcinoma are the commonly occurring malignancies. In stomach and other parts of GI tract, adenocarcinoma is the commonest malignancy. Other rare malignancies also can be encountered.

Squamous cell carcinoma: The histological features are similar to squamous cell carcinomas in other sites.

Adenocarcinoma: The cytological features include:
  i. Small cell aggregates.
  ii. Large hyperchromatic nuclei with small nucleoli/prominent nucleoli.
  iii. Cytoplasm is vacuolated and filled with mucin.
  iv. Increased N/C ratio.
  v. Signet ring cell carcinomas—round cells with clear to foamy cytoplasm which has mucin and hyperchromatic eccentric nuclei with contours angulated or pointed.

Exercise 79

Sampling, Cytopreparatory Techniques and Cytology of Respiratory Tract

Sputum Sample

Sputum is a specialised product of respiratory tract. For sputum study, fresh early morning sample is produced by deep cough. Sputum is collected and brought immediately to the laboratory without adding any fixative. It is examined for tissue fragments and blood tinged areas. Smears from these blood tinged areas and randomly selected areas are fixed in 95% ethyl alcohol.

Pre-fixed Sputum Sample

If it is not possible to transport unfixed sample to the laboratory immediately, the patient is instructed to expectorate into a wide mouthed small jar, half-filled with 70% ethyl alcohol.

Disadvantages
a. Preservation is only fair as alcohol cannot penetrate the mucous.
b. Mucous may become rubbery producing greater difficulties in preparing the smears.

Sputum Pre-fixed with Alcohol and Carbowax (Saccomanno)

It involves collection of sputum in a mixture of 50% ethyl alcohol and 2% polyethylene glycol (carbowax). The specimen is broken in a food blender and smears are prepared from the centrifuged cell button.

Disadvantages
a. Tissue fragments and fungal fragments are disrupted.
b. Secretory vacuoles in the cells are exploded.
c. Cell clusters may be dispersed, e.g. small cell carcinoma.

Induced Sputum

Sputum may be induced in those patients who cannot produce sputum spontaneously by deep coughing. The inhalation of vapours stimulates mucous production, one such method is heated solution of 15% sodium chloride and 20% propylene glycol is inhaled for 20 minutes. Sputum is collected fresh and sent to the laboratory immediately.

Bronchoscopy

Bronchi are directly visualised and sampled for tissue and cells.

Bronchial Aspirates and Washings

Bronchial aspirates can be collected from the bronchoscope which enables the examiner to obtain specimens by means of a suction apparatus that aspirates secretion.

Washings from the visualised areas may also be collected by instilling 3 to 5 ml of normal saline/balanced salt solution through the bronchoscope and re-aspirating the resulting material. From the washings, sediment/cytocentrifused smears and cell blocks are prepared. Smears are immediately fixed in 95% ethyl alcohol.

Bronchial Brushings

With the flexible bronchoscope, the examiner may visualise smaller bronchi; brush a suspected lesion and send the material for laboratory examination. Smear preparation and staining are similar to bronchial aspirates and washings.

Bronchoalveolar Lavage (BAL)

This involves infusion and aspiration of sterile saline/balanced salt solution in the distal segments of the lung via a fiberoptic bronchoscope. A bronchoscope is advanced until it is wedged into a subsegmental bronchus. Sterile normal saline/balanced salt solution is introduced and re-aspirated. Usually around 50 to 100 ml of fluid in aliquots of 20 to 30 ml is instilled separately up to three subsegmental areas of the lung, the fluid will be retained for 5 to 10 seconds and recovered by aspiration. The smears are prepared similar to the washings. BAL specimens are submitted fresh because microbiological/immunological studies or chemical analysis may be requested.

BAL is of value in detecting lung diseases and opportunistic infections in immunocompromised hosts.

Fine Needle Aspiration Cytology (FNAC)

The cytology of respiratory tract has been revolutionised by:

 i. Radiological imaging techniques, making possible the precise visualisation and localisation of masses in the lungs.
 ii. Sampling of such lesions by inserting a needle is possible.

The needle attached to a syringe is passed through the chest wall or bronchial wall into the pulmonary mass visualised by fluoroscopy, computed tomography or bronchoscopy. The aspirated material is examined by conventional techniques.

Indications of FNAC

Suspected in-operable lung cancers.
- Patient who refuses exploratory thoracotomy for suspected lung cancer.
- Multiple pulmonary masses.
- Patient who fails to respond to appropriate antituberculous therapy.
- Suspected infectious disease.

Contraindications

- Uncontrollable cough
- Non-cooperative patient
- Patients with haemorrhagic disease and those on anticoagulant therapy
- Pulmonary hypertension
- Pulmonary hydatid cyst.

Transbronchial Fine Needle Aspiration (TBFNA)

It is a modification of needle aspirates, for the cases in which the neoplasm has not invaded through the mucosa into the bronchial lumen; thus, the neoplasm is not accessible through sputum or bronchial brushings.

This procedure involves inserting a flexible needle through the fibreoptic bronchoscope penetrating the wall and aspirating cytological material lying beyond.

The Wang disposable needle is deviced for this purpose and is most commonly employed for TBFNA. It consists of a 120 cm long double lumen retractable needle system. A central stylet is surrounded by two polythene sheaths, the inner of which is tipped with a 22 guage 13 mm long needle. The needle is protected by an outer sheath while traversing the bronchial tree and the stylet provides rigidity necessary for guidance. When the aspiration site is reached, the stylet is retracted and the proximal end of the catheter is attached to a 20 ml syringe. A vacuum is created by drawing the plunger and while this is maintained, a series of rapid passes into the lesion are made with the needle. The suction is then released; the catheter and the needle with cellular material *in situ* are withdrawn through the channel of bronchoscope.

Preparation of smears: After the procedure, the needle and syringe are separated. The syringe is refilled with air and attached to the needle and the contents of the needle are expelled on a slide; smears are prepared by gently laying one more slide over the material permitting weight of upper slide to spread the material, pulling the slides apart and quickly dropping into 95% ethyl alcohol. The remaining aspirate is put into 10 ml of normal saline and processed for direct smears, cytocentrifuge smears and cell blocks.

Complications: There are a few reported complications such as pneumothorax or haemorrhage; the patient needs observation after the procedure.

Percutaneous FNA

Under fluoroscopic/CT/US control, the needle is inserted with great accuracy to a predetermined depth and in predetermined direction. Obtain the material from the periphery as the centre may be necrotic. Local anaesthetic is injected down to pleura and the needle is inserted with breath held and advanced under fluoroscopic or other imaging control. 20 to 25 gauge needles can be used. Larger needles are available. Larger the bore, greater is the risk. A fresh sterile needle is required for each separate percutaneous pass. Needle with syringe is withdrawn and smears are prepared. Patient needs to be observed for any complications.

Complications: Pneumothorax, haemorrhage, air embolism, bacteremia and anaphylactic shock are immediate complications. Late complications are lung abscess and tumour seeding of needle tract.

Normal Histology and Cytology of Respiratory Tract

Normal Histology

- The major portion of upper and lower respiratory tract is lined by pseudo-stratified ciliated columnar epithelium which covers portion of nasal cavities, sinuses, portion of larynx and tracheo-

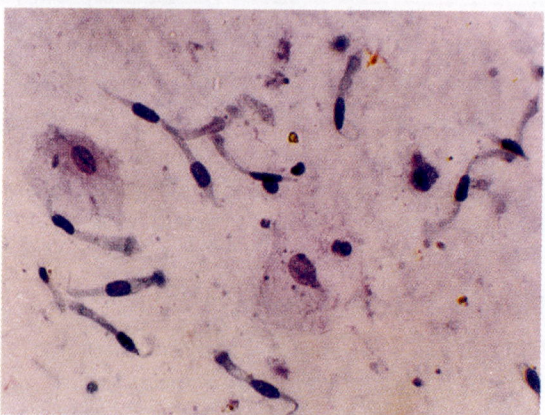

Fig. 5.3: Photomicrograph of ciliated columnar epithelial cells

bronchial tree. Between the epithelial cells, basal cells/reserve cells and goblet cells are present (Fig. 5.3).
- Alveoli are lined by type I pneumonocytes; these are flattened cells and line about 90% of the alveolar surface. Type II cells are cuboidal and have prominent nucleoli; these cells are the source of chemical substance that coats the alveoli and prevents their collapse during expiration. They are also involved in the repair of alveolar epithelium.

Normal Cytology

- Expected normal cellular elements include bronchial epithelial cells (columnar cells, goblet cells, basal/reserve cells) and alveolar macrophages.
- Ciliated bronchial columnar cells are long and slender columnar-shaped with one blunt end bearing a prominent terminal plate fringed with cilia. The basal portion is tapered and rests on a basement membrane. Oval nucleus is present in the lower portion. Nuclear chromatin is finely stipled and nucleoli are indistinct. Such cells are seen in groups and sheets.
- *Goblet cells:* These are mucous producing cells of bronchial epithelium, cytoplasm is vacuolated. These are numerous in chronic bronchitis and bronchiectasis.

- *Basal cells:* These are rarely found and are small cells with little cytoplasm and dark nuclei.
- *Bronchiolar and alveolar cells:* These are small cells with central to eccentric nuclei and vacuolated cytoplasm.
- *Alveolar macrophages:* These have plentiful pale vacuolated cytoplasm and eccentric oval/reniform nuclei with prominent nucleoli. Cytoplasm has black to brown dust or carbon particles. Sometimes, haemosiderin pigment may be present which stains yellow brown with Pap stain and blue black with MGG stain is indicative of chronic extravasation of erythrocytes (as in haemorrhage and CVC lung).
- In sputum, bronchial secretions and lavage specimens, the cellular components are epithelial cells and alveolar macrophages. Non-cellular components may be observed are: Curschmann's spirals, calcospherites, corpora amylacea and Charcot-Leyden crystals.
- Sputum examination has high diagnostic value in centrally located tumours such as squamous cell carcinoma and small cell carcinoma. Bronchial brushings and washings are of higher diagnostic value.
- Sputum examination should be performed over a period of three to five consecutive days which enhances the detection rate of malignant cells.

BAL is useful in
- Detection of microorganisms
- Interstitial lung diseases
- Airway diseases—chronic bronchitis, cystic fibrosis
- Pulmonary haemorrhage
- Acute inflammatory disease
- Malignancy
- Opportunistic infections in immunocompromised patients.

Percutaneous FNA is diagnostic in
- Peripherally placed tumours
- To confirm metastatic lesions
- To differentiate from infectious cavitatory lesions
- In unresectable tumours prior to radiation/chemotherapy.

Transbronchial FNA is useful in
- Submucosal or peribronchial lesions
- Mediastinal or hilar lymph nodes
- Friable endobronchial lesions with inadequate biopsy.

Cytology in Inflammations

- Aspirations of lung in infections are not usually done; however, in unresolved localised pneumonia aspirations can be undertaken to rule out malignancy. In pneumonia and lung abscess cases FNA shows purulent material; microscopy shows abundant cellular debris, numerous polymorphs and alveolar macrophages. In such cases especially in older patients, malignancy has to be ruled out. Thick necrotic material may be aspirated in squamous cell carcinoma.
- In FNA material, granulomas can be found. The differential diagnosis of granulomas include tuberculosis, sarcoidosis, Wegener's granulomatosis and fungal infection.
- Acid-fast bacilli in FNA material may be uncommonly found.
- Actinomycosis presents with solitary or multiple abscesses and sulphur granules (colony of organisms) are seen with naked eye in the aspirates; microscopy shows gram-negative bacteria.
- *Pneumocystis carinii* is usually diagnosed by BAL although organisms may be found in sputum, bronchoscopic specimen and FNA material. Morphological identification of organisms is necessary; honeycomb aggregates are highly typical and GMS stain demonstrates the yeasts.

Cytology in Neoplasms

Squamous Cell Carcinoma

i. FNA material is usually obtained at the periphery of the mass, as centre may be necrotic.

ii. Microscopy shows malignant pleomorphic cells singly or in irregular sheets.
iii. The malignant cells may be caudate/tadpole/spindle forms.
iv. The keratinised cells have orangeophilic cytoplasm in Pap-stained smears and blue cytoplasm in MGG-stained smears. Non-keratinised cells have hyperchromatic pleomorphic nuclei with opaque cytoplasm and needs to be differentiated from adenocarcinoma.

Small Cell Carcinoma

i. Frequently seen in males, occurs in the central location and has short survival.
ii. They are often symptomatic with clinical evidence of ectopic hormone production.
iii. At the time of diagnosis, about two-thirds of the cases have detectable metastasis.
iv. These can be grouped into oat cell carcinoma, intermediate cell and combined small/large cell type. In oat cell carcinomas, in FNA the cells are in clusters or in dispersed pattern. Cells have scant cytoplasm, nucleus is angulated, pleomorphic with finely granular, diffusely dispersed chromatin (salt and pepper) and has inconspicuous nucleoli. Nuclei are fragile and show nuclear moulding. In intermediate group the cells are larger, cytoplasm is more, nuclei are large and nucleoli are present. Squamous cell carcinoma or adenocarcinoma in combination with small cell tumours are called combined tumours. These should be treated as small cell tumours as they have aggressive course.
v. Small cell tumours have to be differentiated from carcinoid tumours.

Adenocarcinoma: Different histological patterns such as acinar, papillary, bronchiolo-alveolar and solid patterns can be encountered.

The cells are arranged in papillae, three-dimensional cell balls/clusters/acini. Nuclei are eccentrically placed, pleomorphic, hyperchromatic and appear to bulge from the periphery of the cluster. Cytoplasm is vacuolated, basophilic and many have fine lacy pattern. In Pap stain the vacuoles appear pale pink and with MGG stain magenta pink or purple coloured.

Large anaplastic cells, multinucleated malignant cells can be encountered in different histological patterns.

With poorly differentiated adenocarcinomas, the distinction from poorly differentiated squamous cell carcinoma is difficult and special stains are of help in such instances.

For metastatic lung lesions, primary malignancies from GIT, breast, female genital system, prostate, kidney, thyroid, etc. have to be considered.

Exercise 80

Sampling, Cytopreparatory Techniques and Cytology of Urinary Tract

The following sampling techniques may be used for urinary tract diseases.

- *Urine:* Voided urine is the specimen of choice in male patients because of simple collection procedure and satisfactory results. Catheterised sample is preferred for female patients. Hydration of patients, collection of the second voided urine sample in the morning and collection of three successive morning specimens have been recommended. Most of the times, single specimen is sufficient, but needs prompt fixation by collecting 50 to 100 ml of urine in equal amounts of 50% ethyl alcohol. Isopropyl alcohol also may be used.
- *Bladder washing:* Bladder washing with normal saline or Ringer's solution is performed at cystoscopy along with a biopsy procedure. This yields highly cellular specimen and contains more cell clusters than voided urine. This procedure is recommended whenever cystoscopy is performed and the sample is also used for flow cytometry studies. Fixation procedure is similar to urine samples.
- Washing and brushing samples of ureters and renal pelvis may be obtained by retrograde catheterisation.

Sample Preparation

- Direct smears are prepared after centrifugation of urine for 10 minutes at 1200 RPM and stained with Pap stain.
- Sample may be cytocentrifuged for monolayered, uncrowded and well-preserved cellular smears concentrated onto centre of the slide.
- Saccomanno blending technique can be used. For details refer to sampling techniques of respiratory tract. The sediment smears are prepared; smears are put in 95% ethanol for 10 minutes to dissolve carbowax and stained by Pap stain.
- Cell blocks from visible sediment or tissue fragments are prepared.
- Filter preparations provide greater cellularity and good cellular details than sediment smears.

Normal Histology, Normal and Abnormal Cytology of Urinary Tract

The diagnosis and accuracy of the urothelial neoplasms depend upon several factors such as grade of carcinoma, type of specimen, collection method and cytopreparatory technique.

Consideration must be given to the following facts of urinary cytology:
  i. It is effective in low grade tumours.
  ii. It can detect cancer cells in high-risk groups.
  iii. It helps in monitoring of patients with urothelial neoplasms.
  iv. It is an inexpensive and noninvasive procedure.

Indications

Urinary cytology helps in diagnosis of urinary tract lesions in:
  i. Symptomatic patients with gross/microscopic haematuria.

ii. Asymptomatic patients exposed to known carcinogens.
iii. To identify recurrences.
iv. For monitoring urothelial tumours under treatment.
v. For follow-up of conservatively treated patients.

Normal Histology and Cytology of Urinary Tract

Normal Histology

Transitional epithelium lines the urinary bladder and other excretory passages, namely, renal pelvis, ureter and portions of urethra.

Transitional epithelium is multilayered up to seven layers thick; composed of large often binucleated superficial cells (umbrella cells) measuring 20–50 μ. Intermediate pyramidal cells are smaller and elongated. Even smaller cuboidal cells with scant cytoplasm are located on the basement membrane.

The prostatic segment of male urethra is lined by transitional epithelium but short membranous and long cavernous portions of the urethra are lined by stratified or pseudo-stratified columnar epithelium. The epithelium near the meatus is stratified squamous epithelium.

The epithelium of the female urethra near the bladder is transitional; remaining part is usually stratified squamous epithelium with interposed areas of pseudostratified columnar epithelium.

Normal Cytology

Transitional epithelial cells are present in all the specimens (urine/washings/catheterised). They occur singly or in the form of loosely cohesive clusters or sheets. They can be large, often multinucleated superficial cells, the intermediate pyramidal cells and the cuboidal basal cells. Cytoplasm of these cells is opaque, granular or vacuolated.

Squamous cells may be seen in the urine from metaplastic squamous cells and especially in females, these cells may be originating from the trigone of bladder or as a contaminant from vagina.

Renal tubular cells may be rarely found.

Abnormal Cytology of Urinary Tract

Non-neoplastic abnormalities include:
- Nonspecific and bacterial infection
- Diverticulosis
- Endometriosis
- Viral infection
- Malakoplakia
- Cytological changes associated with calculi.

Neoplastic conditions include

Kidney tumours: Most commonly renal cell carcinoma is encountered.

Tumours of pelvis of the kidney, ureter, bladder and urethral tumours. These include:
- Transitional cell papilloma
- Transitional cell carcinoma
- Squamous cell carcinoma
- Adenocarcinoma.

Cytology in transitional cell papilloma: The features include:
- Cluster of small elongated epithelial cells.
- The nuclei are slightly hyperchromatic.

Cytology in transitional cell carcinoma: The features include:
- Abnormal cells with enlarged hyperchromatic irregular nuclei and the chromatin is coarsely granular.
- N/C ratio is high, nucleus has prominent multiple nucleoli.
- Cells are seen singly/small clusters or papillae. Similar cells may be seen in urothelial dysplasia and transitional cell carcinoma *in situ*.

Cytology in squamous cell carcinoma

This neoplasm in urinary tract is associated with *Schistosoma haematobium*. Urine or other preparations show keratinising or non-keratinising malignant squamous cells.

Cytology in adenocarcinoma: The features are similar to adenocarcinoma in other sites.

Exercise 81

FNAC of Thyroid, Salivary Gland and Breast Lesions

Fine needle aspiration (FNA) is done as an adjunct to biopsy in neoplastic and non-neoplastic lesions of salivary gland, thyroid, breast and other masses.

Direct smears and sediment smears are prepared from any fluid or discharge obtained from these areas; Pap and MGG-stained slides are studied.

Cytology of Thyroid Gland

Follicular cells are present in flat sheets. Nuclei of these cells are uniform; cytoplasm is poorly outlined, fragile and often lost. Single cells appear as bare nuclei and these have to be distinguished from lymphocytes (Fig. 5.4a).

Background has colloid which stains light blue to purple on MGG stain and pale pink to dark orange in Pap stain. Depending on its thickness, colloid forms a membrane-like coat on the slide often with folds and cracks. Thin colloid mimics protein rich fluid including serum. Colloid may be easily washed during processing particularly in alcohol fixed smears.

In fine needle aspirations of different lesions of thyroid, following cytological features may be encountered:

In colloid goitre a few follicular cells arranged in sheets and singly and thin layer of colloid are present. With cystic change haemosiderin laden macrophages, follicular cells and viscous globular colloid are seen.

Thyroglossal cyst shows macrophages; it may contain cholesterol crystals and inflammatory cells.

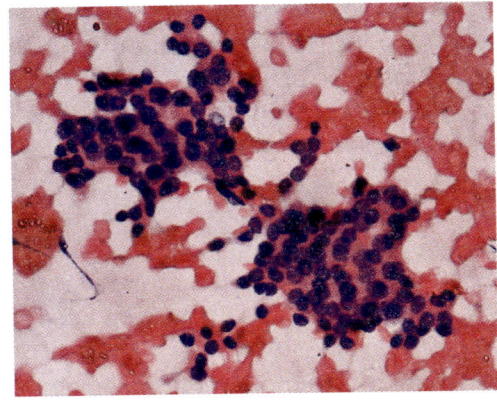

Fig. 5.4a: Microphotograph of cytology in multinodular goitre with hyperplastic nodule (Pap stain)

de Quervain's thyroiditis is accompanied by pain. FNA is rarely done in these cases and shows a few follicular cells, giant cells and epithelioid cells.

Hashimoto's thyroiditis has cells having dense cytoplasm with central nucleus (Askanazy cells) and lymphocytes.

In follicular hyperplasia FNA is done in hot nodules to distinguish hyperplasia from adenoma. There is anisocytosis of follicular cells; they have abundant granular cytoplasm with numerous vacuoles. The vacuoles stain pink with MGG stain and tend to gather peripherally. This suggests hyperfunction with pinocytosis of thyroglobulin (fire flares).

Follicular neoplasms show high cellularity. There is lack of colloid; follicular cells are in monolayered sheets, show microfollicles or macrofollicles. The nuclei are uniform, round or oval.

In follicular carcinoma, the cells have poorly outlined cytoplasm, nuclei may show moderate anisocytosis. Adenoma or carcinoma can be distinguished on histology. However, following features suggest follicular carcinoma:
i. High cellularity.
ii. Crowding of cells.
iii. Nucleoli in more than 75% of the cells.
iv. Irregular nuclear chromatin and nuclear membrane.

Aspiration material in papillary carcinoma shows papillae (Fig. 5.4b). Nuclei of these cells have peripheral clumping of chromatin with intranuclear inclusions. Longitudinal grooves and inclusions are appreciated in alcohol fixed Pap smears and not in MGG-stained smears. Psammoma bodies may be present.

Hürthle cell adenomas have cellular smears with single cell population. The cells have anisocytosis and prominent nucleoli without being malignant. Capsular and vascular invasion distinguishes Hürthle cell adenoma from Hürthle cell carcinoma.

Medullary carcinoma has plasmacytoid cells in loose aggregation or single cells with eccentric nuclei. These can present as frankly malignant neoplasms with prominent nuclei. Background may show amyloid.

"The Bethesda system for reporting thyroid cytology (TBSRTC) 2017" is followed for uniform reporting.[29]

Cytology of Salivary Gland

Normally, the acinar cells are in three dimensional clusters with eccentric nuclei having abundant foamy cytoplasm; ductal cells are rarely observed.

In acute/chronic sialadenitis, FNA is usually not performed.

Aspiration material of pleomorphic adenoma shows epithelial cells and chondromyxoid stroma. The epithelial cells are in clusters and in the form of ducts. Myoepithelial cells in the background have plasmacytoid appearance. Squamous metaplasia may be seen. The chondromyxoid stroma has fibrillary appearance which stains deep pink on MGG stain and grey pink with Pap stain (Fig. 5.5a).

In adenolymphoma (Warthin's tumour), the FNA smears have epithelial cells and lymphoid cells including follicular centre cells. Epithelial cells are in flat sheets, often have cystic component with macrophages and background has debris.

In adenoid cystic carcinoma, there are three dimensional clusters of cells which are small with scant cytoplasm; they have hyperchromatic nuclei and prominent nucleoli. There are holes with globules containing basement membrane material which stains magenta pink with MGG stain and pale pink with Pap stain.

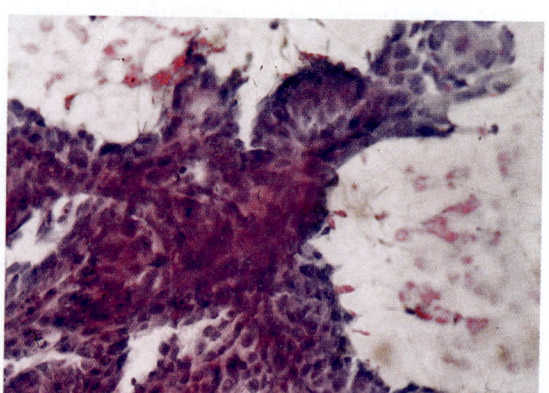

Fig. 5.4b: Microphotograph of cytology in papillary carcinoma, thyroid (Pap stain)

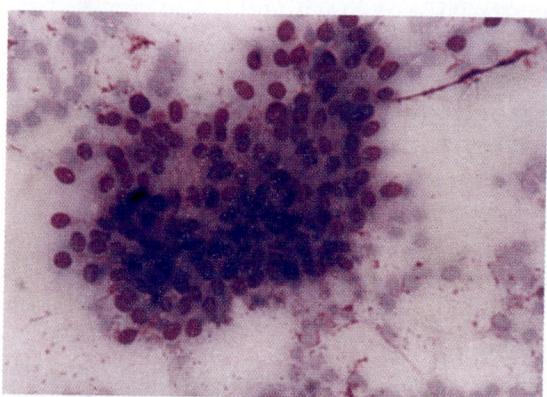

Fig. 5.5a: Microphotograph of cluster of epithelial cells in pleomorphic adenoma, background is myxoid (MGG stain)

In mucoepidermoid carcinoma there are three types of cells.
  i. Mucus secreting cells
  ii. Squamous cells
  iii. Intermediate cells

The background has debris and mucoid material.

Acinic cell tumour has serous cells which have granular/non-granular or clear cytoplasm. It is delicate, vacuolated and fragile. The nuclei are medium-sized and show little pleomorphism. The background is clean.

Carcinoma in pleomorphic adenoma is commonly adenocarcinoma or anaplastic carcinoma. Other varieties have been described including mucoepidermoid, adenoid cystic carcinoma and squamous cell carcinoma. "The Milan system for reporting salivary gland cytopathology 2018" is followed for uniform reporting.[30]

Cytology of Breast

In case of postpubertal breast, the functioning component is composed of branching network of ducts with enclosed fibro-fatty stroma and a peripheral component of terminal duct lobular unit (TDLU). The TDLU is composed of small ducts lined by two layers of cells that include the inner ductal epithelial cells and the outer myoepithelial cells. The TDLU is hormone dependent and usually carcinomas begin in this region.

Lactational breast has expanded acini with large secretory cells.

Large number of histiocytes with papillae favours papilloma.

Galactocoel has moderate cellularity, granular proteinaceous material, foamy histiocytes, and a few ductal cells with uniform nuclei.

Fibroadenoma has antler horn pattern with sheets of regular ductal cells, fragments of stroma and naked bipolar cells. Myxoid stroma may be present (Fig. 5.5b).

Fibrocystic disease has apocrine cells with granular cytoplasm and foamy macrophages.

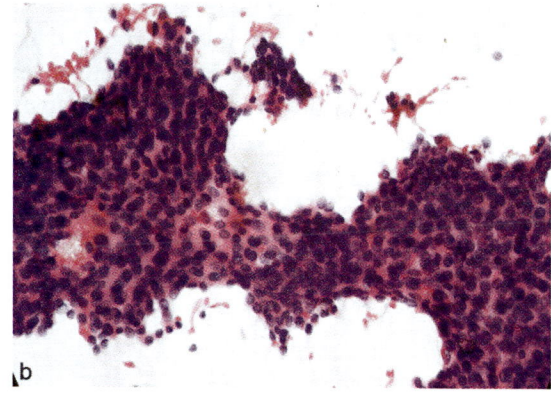
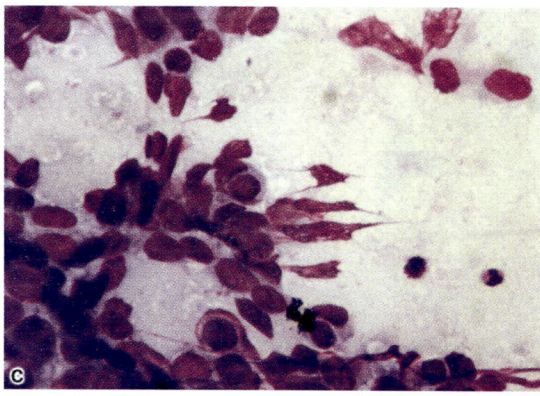

Figs 5.5b and c: (a) Microphotograph of fibroadenoma, (b) Pap stain, (c) to cluster of malignant cells in duct carcinoma, breast, MGG stain

Phyllodes tumour has increased cellularity with plenty of stromal cells.

Duct carcinoma *in situ* (high grade) has cellular aspirate. The cells are arranged in loose clusters and the background has necrotic debris. The cells show high N/C ratio and they are pleomorphic with vesicular nuclei having prominent nucleoli (Fig. 5.5c).

Aspirates from tubular carcinoma show small cells in tubules and cords. They have large nuclei with scant cytoplasm, nuclear chromatin is finely stippled.

In medullary carcinoma, aspirates show cells spread singly or in clusters with smooth bordered round nuclei having prominent nucleoli. Background has lymphoid infiltrate.

In mucinous carcinoma, cells are bland and uniform with eccentric nuclei. Background has mucin.

Papillary carcinoma has monotonous population of cells which are arranged in papillae and cells show minimal anisocytosis with clumped granular chromatin.

In infiltrating duct carcinoma, aspirates are cellular and the ductal epithelial cells show anisocytosis and pleomorphic hyperchromatic nuclei with smooth nuclear membrane (Grade I). As the grade increases, nuclear membrane becomes irregular with indentations, chromatin is clumped, shows nucleoli and increased mitosis. Areas of necrosis are present.

In lobular carcinoma, the cells are small, monomorphic, arranged singly or in files or in small groups and nuclei are regular.

"5 stage coding system (categories) proposed by Yokohama international congress of cytology" is followed for uniform reporting.[31]

Exercise 82

Cytology of Female Genital System

In the female genital system, the following cells can be observed:
- Vaginal and ectocervical cells
- Endocervical cells
- Cells from squamocolumnar junction
- Endometrial cells
- Tubal cells.

Vaginal and Ectocervical Cells

Vaginal and ectocervical epithelia have different types of epithelial cells.

The basal layer has one or two layers of cuboidal cells of 15 µm size. These cells have large nucleus of 8 to 10 µm, and scant cytoplasm. These are dividing cells. Abnormal increase of this layer is called basal cell hyperplasia.

Parabasal cells have several layers of polyhedral cells. These are 15–30 µm in diameter. The nucleus occupies a large part of the cell and is vesicular.

Intermediate cells are the inner ovoid and outer polyhedral cells. They are 15 to 40 µm in size; nucleus is 8 to 10 µm and has finely granular chromatin. Cytoplasm is basophilic and contains glycogen. Navicular cells are the intermediate cells; they have thick rolled edges and thinner centre. Glycogen accumulates in the centre around mid-secretory phase and early weeks of pregnancy.

Superficial cells are around 3 to 6 layers. They are flat polyhedral cells with pyknotic nucleus. The size of the cell is of 40 to 60 µm; nucleus is condensed and measures 5 to 6 µm. Cytoplasm is eosinophilic, occasionally it can be cyanophilic. These are oestrogen responsive cells.

Only basal cells divide. Rest of the cells undergo maturation, functionally and morphologically are differentiated into parabasal, intermediate and superficial cells which are continuously exfoliated.

Endocervical Cells

Endocervical epithelium consists of single layer of tall columnar epithelium; they are 30 µm in height and more than 8 µm in diameter. Size of these cells varies with hormones. During oestrogenic phase, they are smaller and cytoplasm is opaque. With progesterone effect, they become larger, have clear cytoplasm and are distended with mucous.

During proliferative phase, the mucous produced by endocervical cells is capable of crystallising into fan-like structure. As ovulation approaches, mucous becomes liquefied and facilitates easy penetration of sperms. Endocervical cells also line endocervical glands which are simple tubular glands penetrating into the stroma of cervix. These cells occur singly or in parallel arrays or in clusters with honeycomb appearance.

Squamocolumnar Junction

This is the area where endocervical epithelium meets the stratified squamous epithelium of ectocervix. This is also known as transformation zone (T zone). This zone is important in understanding the neoplastic events.

Transformation zone position varies with age. At puberty, it is on the surface of ectocervix. In young females and childbearing age, it is at the level of external os. During menopause, it recedes up and is present in the endocervical canal.

Metaplastic Cells

The columnar epithelial cells of endocervix are replaced by squamous epithelium and these cells originate from the reserve cells.

Stroma of the Cervix

It consists of fibroblasts and smooth muscle cells which are elongated and vary in size.

Endometrial Cells

These cells can be in the vaginal smears or obtained by aspiration or direct scraping of the endometrium. The glandular and surface epithelial cells are columnar or cuboidal and the smaller cells are from the stroma. Normally, up to 12 days of the menstrual cycle, the stromal and glandular cells may be seen in the vaginal smears. After 12 days of menstrual cycle and in postmenopausal women, presence of these cells is abnormal. During menstruation, the cells are isolated or in clusters; the epithelial cells are seen surrounding the smaller stromal cells.

Exodus

This is seen on 5th to 7th days of menstruation and is comprised of cluster of endometrial cells surrounded by numerous macrophages. It is assumed that the macrophages are modified endometrial stromal cells that acquire a phagocytic property.

Proliferative Phase

In this phase, the cuboidal endometrial epithelial cells are arranged in palisading or honeycombing pattern or singly. Nuclei have fine granular chromatin and small nucleoli are evident.

Secretory Phase

The glandular cells increase in size; they have large nuclei and cytoplasm is vacuolated because of the presence of glycogen. The stromal cells are seen as small epithelial like cells towards the end of the cycle; these cells become larger as the amount of glycogen increases and sometimes are recognised as decidual cells.

Postmenopausal Age Group

There is atrophy of glands and stroma which may take several years to be completed. The number and size of the glands are reduced and are lined by cuboidal or low columnar epithelial cells. The glands are surrounded by dense stroma. The glands may be cystic and the stroma has thick-walled arterioles.

Fallopian Tube

It has ciliated columnar epithelial cells and secretory cells. Cilia are more numerous during oestrogenic phase. The epithelium rests on loose connective tissue and smooth muscle. The cells may be found in vaginal and cervical smears and in peritoneal lavage.

Collection of Specimen for Cervical Smear

- Exfoliative cytology
- Abrasive cytology.

Exfoliative Cytology

In exfoliative cytology smear preparation is done by collection of cells desquamated from cervix and vagina which accumulate in the posterior and lateral fornices.

Abrasive Cytology

It is forceful removal of cells from the surface of ectocervix, endocervix and vagina by means of an instrument.

Vaginal Smear

Smears are prepared by taking material from the vaginal wall using spatula/glass pipette or tongue depressor. Besides, vaginal and ectocervical cells the smears may also contain mucous, leukocytes, macrophages and cellular debris. Less commonly, endocervical cells, cells of tubal, ovarian and peritoneal origin may be present.

Cervical Smear

The aim is to obtain cells from squamocolumnar junction. Majority of the times, cancer starts in this region. Abrasive cytology is superior to exfoliative cytology in detecting cancer of uterine cervix.

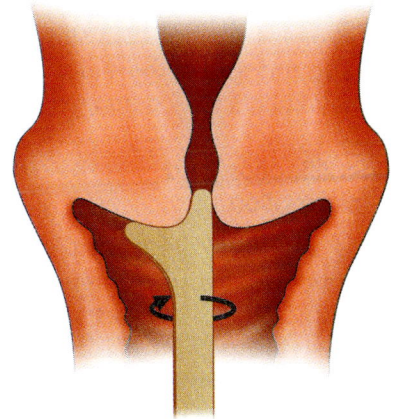

Fig. 5.7: Method of obtaining smears using Ayer's spatula

Different devices are available to obtain cervical smears (Fig. 5.6)
- Ayer's spatula.
- Cervical brush
- Others.

Ayer's Spatula

This is introduced into the cervical canal. The concave part must be in contact with the ectocervix; under pressure the spatula is completely rotated to sample the entire epithelial surface. The concave part collects material from ectocervix and the tip portion collects material from endocervix (Fig. 5.7).

Brushes

Several models are available. Complete rotation is done to obtain endocervical material. Smears obtained by brush must be accompanied by ectocervical smears obtained from a spatula which gives information about the ectocervix (Fig. 5.8).

Smear Preparation

Smear should be obtained during mid cycle because cell morphology can be easily interpreted. Smear should not be obtained during menstruation. After visualising the cervix, collect the material from the cervix and place the instrument on the surface of glass

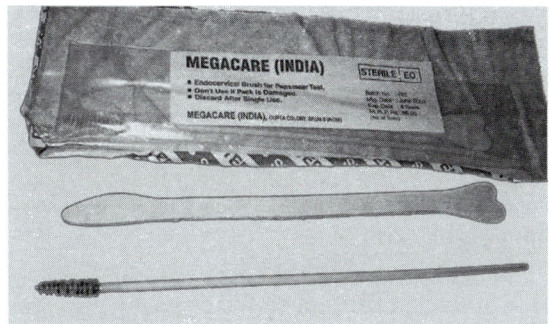

Fig. 5.6: Devices for cervical smear

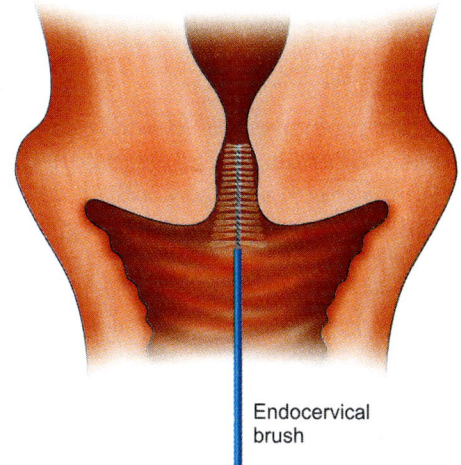

Endocervical brush

Fig. 5.8: Method of obtaining endocervical material using cytobrush

slide. Prepare a smear by passing the instrument along the length of the slide. All the surfaces of spatula or brush should touch the glass slide and spread the material evenly. Circular movements may damage the cells.

Smear Identification and Clinical Information

Before the smear is prepared write the patient's name with pencil or diamond pencil. Pertinent clinical data is entered; age, date of last menstrual period (LMP), onset of menopause, past and present history or any treatment given is noted in the request form.

Fixation of Smears

Fix the smears in alcohol or ether-alcohol for 15 minutes. Spray fixative also can be used. These smears are stained with Pap stain.

Screening of Smears

- Screen under X10.
- Any abnormalities re-examine under X40.
- Abnormal or unusual cells are marked with ink dots or circled.

Bethesda System of Reporting of Pap Smears (Bethesda 2014)[32]

Specimen Type

Indicate conventional smear (Pap smear) or liquid-based preparation or other.

Specimen Adequacy

Satisfactory for evaluation (describe presence or absence of endocervical/transformation zone component and any other quality indicators, e.g. partially obscuring blood, inflammation, etc.).

Unsatisfactory for Evaluation (Specify Reason)

Specimen rejected/not processed (specify reason)/specimen processed and examined, but unsatisfactory for evaluation of epithelial abnormality because of (specify reason).

General Categorisation (Optional)

- Negative for intraepithelial lesion or malignancy
- *Other:* See interpretation/result (e.g. endometrial cells in a woman 45 years of age)
- *Epithelial cell abnormality:* See interpretation/result (specify 'squamous' or 'glandular' as appropriate).

Interpretation/Result

Negative for Intraepithelial Lesion or Malignancy

Non-neoplastic cellular variations
- Squamous metaplasia.
- Keratotic changes
- Tubal metaplasia
- Atrophy
- Pregnancy-associated changes.

Reactive cellular changes associated with:
- Inflammation (includes typical repair)
- Lymphocytic (follicular) cervicitis
- Radiation
- Intrauterine contraceptive device (IUD)
- Glandular cells status posthysterectomy.

Organisms
- Trichomonas vaginalis
- Fungal organisms morphologically consistent with Candida spp.
- Shift in flora suggestive of bacterial vaginosis
- Bacteria morphologically consistent with Actinomyces spp.
- Cellular changes consistent with herpes simplex virus
- Cellular changes consistent with cytomegalovirus.

Other Findings

Endometrial cells (in a woman 45 years of age).

Epithelial Cell Abnormalities

Squamous cell
- Atypical squamous cells
  – of undetermined significance (ASC-US)
  – cannot exclude HSIL (ASC-H)

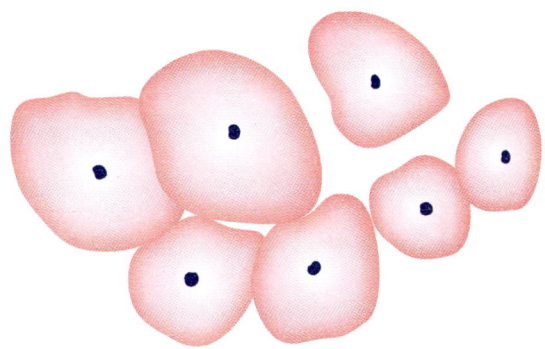

Fig. 5.9a: Schematic diagram of normal squamous epithelial cells

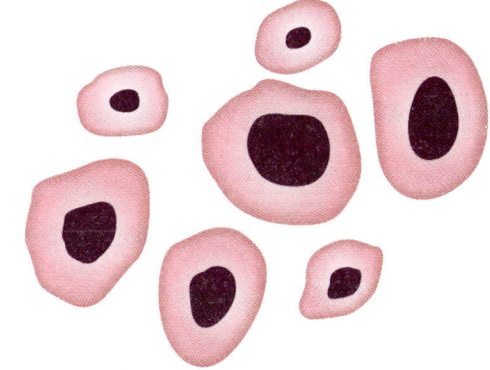

Fig. 5.10a: Schematic diagram of malignant squamous epithelial cells

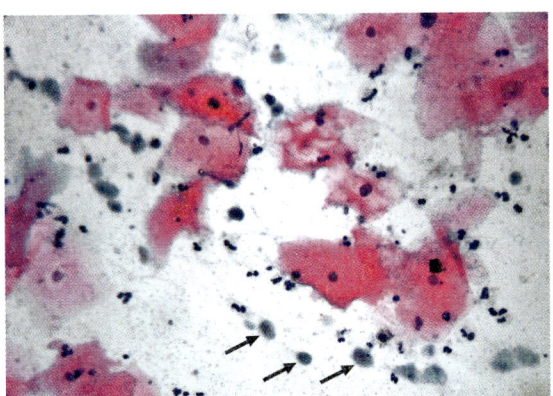

Fig. 5.9b: Photomicrograph of *Trichomonas vaginalis* organisms (arrows). Photograph by Dr Karle

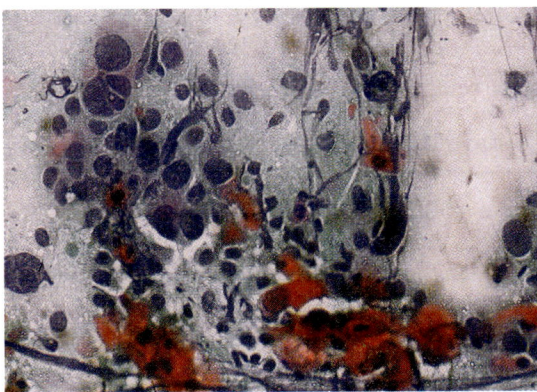

Fig. 5.10b: Photomicrograph of malignant squamous epithelial cells

- Low-grade squamous intraepithelial lesion (LSIL) (encompassing: HPV/mild dysplasia/CIN 1)
- High-grade squamous intraepithelial lesion (HSIL) (encompassing: moderate and severe dysplasia, CIS; CIN 2 and CIN 3)
- Squamous cell carcinoma.

Glandular cell
- Atypical
- Endocervical adenocarcinoma *in situ*
- Adenocarcinoma.

Other Malignant Lesions

Adjunctive testing

Computer—assisted interpretation of cervical cytology

Educational notes.

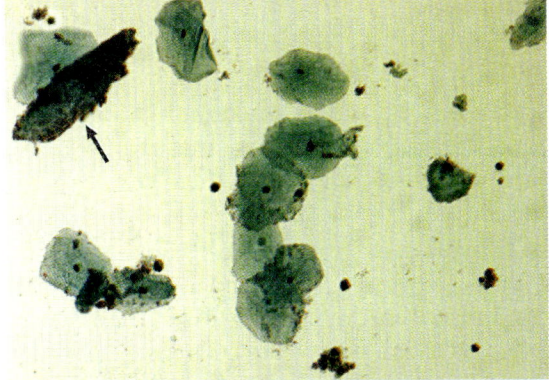

Fig. 5.9c: Photomicrograph of *Gardnerella vaginalis* (arrow-clue cell)

Exercise 83

Hormone Cytology

The evaluation of endocrinological condition of a female patient by means of study of vaginal cells is actually one of the earliest diagnostic applications of cytology. Although newer techniques and correlative studies are now available, it is still the consensus that with certain limitations, the technique is an efficient, inexpensive and rapid method for establishing hormonal condition of a patient as well as for assessing ovarian function from puberty to menopause and in old age. Hormonal cytology is also used to estimate time of ovulation, to determine ovarian dysfunction, to assess placental function or dysfunction in obstetrics, to assist in hormonal therapy and follow hormonal treatment.

Specimen Collection

The optimal site for obtaining a smear for hormonal evaluation is lateral vaginal wall. The specimen should consist of recently shed cells and should not have been forcefully scraped. The material is collected by lightly dipping the applicator into the secretion without forceful scraping or by aspiration.

Fixation

Smears are fixed immediately while still wet in 95% ethanol for at least 15 minutes or by spray fixative. Papanicolaou or Shorr stains are applied.

Shorr Stain

The staining solution consists of:
Ethyl alcohol 50%   100 ml
Biebrich scarlet (water soluble) 0.5 g
Orange G   0.25 g
Fast green FCF   0.075 g
Phosphotungstic acid   0.5 g
Phosphomolybdic acid   0.5 g
Glacial acetic acid   1.0 ml

Procedure of staining: Keep the smears for 1 minute in Shorr staining solution, carried through 70, 80, 95% alcohol, absolute alcohol, xylene and then mounted.

Results
Most mature cells   Orange red
Less mature cells   Deep green to pale green

Squamous Cell Types for Hormonal Evaluation

Superficial cells: These are polygonal with cynophilic or eosinophilic cytoplasm, nucleus is pyknotic.

They are flat cells and exhibit more or less prominent lines within the cytoplasm apparently caused by prekeratin. Most of the cells lie singly. The least mature cells are folded, sometimes crowded and exhibit translucent cytoplasm.

The nuclei of superficial cells have pyknotic nuclei (compressed small nuclei with condensed chromatin) of lesser than 6 μm, whereas the intermediate cells have vesicular nuclei (larger oval or round nucleus).

Intermediate cells: Mature cells contain non-pyknotic vesicular nuclei. The cell is as large as superficial cell but the nucleus is not pyknotic. Intermediate cells exhibit cytoplasmic infoldings and crowding. However, the most mature intermediate cells are flat and lie singly. In the presence of bacillus vaginalis, these cells exhibit cytolytic changes.

Basal and parabasal cells: These cells are small, oval or round immature squamous epithelial cells. They have large nucleus and cytoplasm is usually cyanophilic. These cells do not exhibit cytolysis as observed in intermediate cells.

Other Cells Unrelated to Hormonal Condition

i. *Anucleated squames:* These are not normally found. If they are found, the reason could be either the smear is taken from the distal third of vagina or from ectocervix with area of leukoplakia.

ii. *Metaplastic cells:* These are the cells with prominent cellular borders; they have intracytoplasmic vacuoles and the nucleus is usually situated in the centre of the cell. These are similar in size to parabasal cells. Presence of metaplastic cells indicates that the smears are taken from cervix. They are rarely found in vaginal smears in case of vaginal adenosis with exposure to diethylstilbestrol.

iii. Histiocytes.

iv. *Epithelial cells exhibiting inflammatory changes:* The cells have prominent nucleoli, perinuclear halo and disturbed staining reaction.

v. Glandular cells.

vi. Precursor or malignant cells.

Cellular Indices for Hormonal Assessment and Reporting Procedure

Karyopyknotic index (KPI): This is the ratio of superficial cells to intermediate cells regardless of staining characters. It is generally carried out by counting a minimum of 300 cells.

Disadvantages
a. 300 cells form a relatively small sample.
b. Bright field microscopy does not permit a critical differentiation between pyknotic and vesicular nuclei.

Maturation index (MI): This is the percentage of parabasal, intermediate and superficial (P/I/S) cells. It gives more information than KPI.

With rare exceptions, only one or two cell types occur in hormonal pattern:
1. Parabasal cells alone
2. Parabasal cells and intermediate cells
3. Intermediate cells alone
4. Intermediate and superficial cells
5. Superficial cells alone. Usually superficial cells occur with admixture of intermediate cells.

MI like any other index is meaningless, when the assessment is made on only one smear.

Eosinophilic index (EI): This is the ratio of mature eosinophilic cells to mature cyanophilic cells regardless of the nuclear appearance. EI is not difficult to assess, it is also the index, which is most often altered by artifacts such as pseudoeosinophilia due to poor fixation, poor staining or changes due to the influence of vaginal pH. The EI, if determined without assessing the KPI or MI, is of limited value.

Folded cell index (FCI): This is the ratio of folded mature cells to flat mature cells regardless of staining and nuclear appearance. A high FCI is usually found when the KPI is low and *vice versa*. Folded squamous cells are usually less mature than are flat cells that have lost the tendency to fold.

Crowded cell index (CCI): This is the ratio of mature cells in clusters of four or more to cells lying in clusters of three or less. This is relatively difficult index to assess, because cell clusters often contain so many cells that they do not tend themselves to accurate counting. Moreover, this index is usually parallel to FCI.

Cytological Patterns

Infancy and Childhood

The cytological patterns during the first day of infancy are similar to the patterns of mother at the time of delivery. Mostly, intermediate cells and certain percentage of superficial cells are seen. The cell patterns in infant are characterised by absence of leukocytes, erythrocytes and bacterial flora. The pattern changes with increasing age of the infant.

MI at birth	0/85/15
MI during first two weeks	20/80/0
MI during 3 to 4 weeks	90/10/0

In young girls: The main aim of studying vaginal cytology in young girls is in infections such as Trichomonas and less commonly in cases of precocious puberty or ovarian tumours.

Menstrual Cycle

Menstrual period: The smears are characterised by the presence of blood, desquamated endometrial cells (singly or in clusters) and polymorphs. The squamous cells of intermediate type dominate; these cells are in clumps with folded cytoplasm.

Proliferative (follicular) phase: It consists of occasional erythrocytes with a few leukocytes, good number of superficial cells and a few intermediate cells. Exodus may be present.

At the time of ovulation: This period represents height of cellular maturity for a given patient. At the time of ovulation, superficial cells dominate. RBCs and leukocytes disappear. Background is clean.

Secretory phase (luteal phase): There is reduction of superficial cells which are replaced by intermediate cells with folded cytoplasm. Rarely navicular cells are observed. Polymorphs are numerous. KPI is reduced. Shortly before the onset of menstruation, the pattern consists predominantly of folded and crowded intermediate cells with cytolytic features.

Menopause and Postmenopause

During this period there is decrease in steroid hormones. Menopause occurs in progressive manner and events are reflected in the cervicovaginal smears.

Early menopause: Resembles postovulatory phase with low levels of oestrogen. Intermediate cells dominate. Superficial cells are still present.

With passage of time (a few months to years): Intermediate cells increase and a few navicular cells and parabasal cells in variable proportion are present. Because of increase in intermediate cells, Papanicolaou called this as crowded menopause.

With major decrease in oestrogen activity (atrophy): Good number of parabasal cells, scanty intermediate and superficial cells and inflammatory cells are present.

With decrease in endocervical mucous: There will be dryness of epithelia. Because of dryness, parabasal cells appear flattened and appear larger with large nucleus. Variation in size and shape, pyknosis, karyorrhexis and increased eosinophilia may also be observed. All these features cause diagnostic problems.

In advanced menopause: Blue bodies may be seen which denote condensed mucous or degenerated parabasal cells and these can be mistaken for cancer cells.

Pregnancy

During pregnancy no cyclic effects of hormones are seen. As pregnancy progresses, progesterone levels are increased. During first six weeks, the smears are of pre-menstrual type with slight oestrogen effect. The classical smears of pregnancy show numerous intermediate cells with navicular cells. It may take 3 to 5 months to achieve complete replacement by the intermediate cells (MI of 0/100/0). Decidual cells may be observed. These are large cells with abundant faintly vacuolated cytoplasm, seen singly or in sheets with large nucleus and small nucleoli.

Sometimes, decidual cell nucleus may be hyperchromatic and mimic carcinoma cells. Endometrial and endocervical cells may be observed with hyperchromatic multilobate nucleus which mimic carcinoma cells. These cells most likely represent Arias-Stella phenomenon.

Postpartum Period

After delivery navicular cells and cytolysis disappear. The smears are predominantly atrophic with inflammatory cells and coccoid cells after delivery. Varying degree of atrophy persists for several months. Later, oestrogenic pattern or mixed patterns are observed.

Exercise 84

Barr Body

In 1949, Barr and Bertram noted tiny dark granule adjacent to the nuclear membrane in the neuronal nuclei of the female but not the male cats. This represents X chromosome that is condensed and is inactive in females.

In 1961, Lyon proposed X inactivation in somatic cells of females, the inactivated X is observed in interphase of cells. Thus, Barr body is an inactivated X, heterochromatin, planoconvex body beneath the nuclear membrane observed in interphase (Fig. 5.11).

Number of Barr bodies will be determined by the number of X chromosomes and to get the number of Barr bodies 'n-1' formula is used where 'n' represents number of X chromosomes. Barr bodies can be observed in female individuals with two X chromosomes; in these females, one Barr body will be observed, whereas in a 3X individuals, two Barr bodies will be observed.

Shorr/Orcein/Pap-staining is used for staining the Barr bodies. Buccal smears or vaginal smears after scraping are used for Barr body study.

Orcein Staining for Barr Bodies

Orcein stain

Orcein	1 g
Glacial acetic acid	45 ml
Distilled water	55 ml

Fast green solution

Fast green	0.03 g
Ethyl alcohol	100 ml

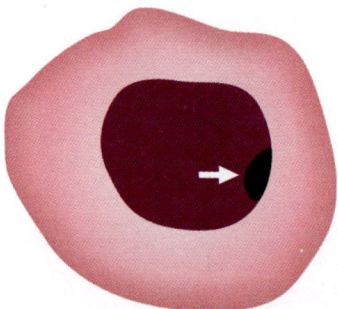

Fig. 5.11: Schematic diagram of Barr body (arrow)

Procedure of Staining

Smears are fixed in 95% alcohol for 20 to 30 minutes, hydrated (80%, 70%, 50% alcohol), stained for 5 minutes in Orcein stain followed by distilled water wash for 10 to 15 seconds; dehydrated and stained with fast green solution for 1 minute; dip in 95% alcohol, clear and mount.

SIMILES IN PATHOLOGY

1. **Ant hill:** Actinomycosis or fungal infections
2. **Anchovy sauce:** Appearance of exudate/pus in amoebic liver abscess
3. **Antler horn pattern:** Cytology in fibroadenoma
4. **Butterfly pattern of rash:** Malar rash in SLE (Lupus erythematosus)
5. **Bread and butter appearance:** Fibrinous pericarditis in rheumatic heart disease
6. **Bite cells:** RBCs in G6PD haemolytic anaemia
7. **Banana-shaped/boot-shaped heart:** Shape of heart in hypertrophic cardiomyopathy
8. **Banana-shaped gametocytes:** *P. falciparum* gamatocytes in RBCs
9. **Button hole appearance:** Valves in rheumatic heart disease.
10. **Chicken wire collagen:** Perivenular collagen in alcoholic cirrhosis
11. **Chicken wire appearance:** Anastomosing capillaries in oligodendroma and chondrosarcoma and liposarcoma.
12. **Crab:** For cancer
13. **Cigar-shaped bundles:** Arrangement of *M. leprae* organisms in lepromatous leprosy
14. **Cartwheel-shaped nuclei:** Nuclei of plasma cells (chromatin arrangement)
15. **Cobble stone appearance:** Mucosa in Crohn's disease
16. **Cheese like material:** Necrotic material in tuberculosis
17. **Caterpillar appearance:** Wavy nuclei of Anitschkow cells in RHD
18. **Coraline thrombus:** Propagating thrombus
19. **Current jelly:** Postmortem clot due to stagnant blood, no time for separation of cells and plasma, red coloured giving jelly like appearance
20. **Chicken fat:** Postmortem clot due to stagnant blood slowly formed (blood separates into layers, lower red coloured due to RBCs, upper plasma layer) which is yellow or pale coloured
21. **Coffee bean:** Nuclei with grooves, seen in cells of granulosa cell tumour and Brenner's tumour.
22. **Cartwheel appearance:** Cell arrangement in MFH, nucleus of plasma cell
23. **Comedo appearance:** Necrotic material in DCIS (comedo carcinoma)
24. **Cambium layer:** Embryonal carcinoma
25. **Carrot-shaped nuclei:** Medulloblastoma
26. **Crumple tissue paper appearance:** Cytoplasm of Gaucher cells
27. **Cribriform pattern:** Adenoid cystic carcinoma, cribriform DCIS, prostatic carcinoma
28. **Cob web:** Appearance of CSF due to increased proteins in tuberculous meningitis
29. **Chinese letter:** Curvilinear bony trabaculae (woven bone) in fibrous dysplasia of bone
30. **Club-shaped deformity:** Gross appearance of osteoclastoma
31. **Cannon ball appearance:** X-Ray appearance of metastatic lesions in lung
32. **Dumbell-shaped:** Asbestos bodies
33. **Dilapidated brick wall appearance:** Acantholytic cells in Hailey Hailey disease (familial benign chronic pemphigus)
34. **Envelope-shaped crystals:** Oxalate crystals
35. **Egg shell-crackling:** Thinned cortex of osteoclastoma, with pressure gives egg shell, crackling
36. **Exodus ball:** Endometrial cells, 6 to 10 days of menstrual cycle.
37. **Elephantiasis:** Filariasis obstructing lymphatics
38. **Fern like pattern:** Cervical mucin due to oestrogen activity
39. **Fish mouth appearance:** Valves in rheumatic heart disease.
40. **Fishnet pattern:** Immunofluorescence in pemphigus vulgaris
41. **Fried egg appearance:** Cells of oligodendroglioma
42. **Flea bitten kidney:** Kidney in RPGN and Malignant HT
43. **Grape-like structures:** Vesicular mole, gross appearance.
44. **Gritty sensation:** Dystrophic calcification on necrosis in carcinoma breast
45. **Hair with flag sign:** Hair of PEM patients.
46. **Horseshoe kidney:** Both kidneys joined at the lower pole
47. **Hosepipe or lead pipe appearance:** Intestine in Crohn's disease due to transmural inflammation and fibrosis
48. *Hair on end appearance:* Bones in thalassaemia due to widening of medullary cavity
49. **Herring bone pattern:** Cell arrangement in fibrosarcoma, similar to skeleton of herring fish.
50. **Honeycomb:** Gross appearance in bronchiectasis, lung in Hamman-Rich syndrome
51. **Hobnail:** Macronodules in postnecrotic cirrhosis

52. **Holly leaf:** RBCs in sickle cell anaemia
53. **Helmet cells:** Broken RBCs in hemolytic anaemia
54. **Hair-like structures:** Pilocytic astrocyoma
55. **Indian file:** Arrangement of cells, one behind the other in lobular carcinoma breast
56. **Jigsaw puzzle appearance:** Paget's disease of bone, cylindroma
57. **Leonine facies:** Nodular skin lesions on face in lepromatous leprosy
58. **Laennec's cirrhosis:** Alcoholic cirrhosis (micronodules)
59. **Lines of Zahn:** Gross appearance of surface of thrombus (elevated areas of platelets and depressed areas of red cells, WBCs and fibrin)
60. **Leaf like:** Stromal overgrowth, ductal epithelium stretched over it giving leaf appearance in phyllodes tumour of breast.
61. **Lardaceous spleen:** Amyloidosis involving sinusoids of spleen
62. **Schiller dual body:** In yolk sac tumour
63. **Needle-shaped crystals:** Gout (monosodium urate crystals)
64. **Rhomboid-shaped crystals:** Triple phosphate crystals
65. **Millet seeds:** Lesions in Miliary tuberculosis
66. **Sago:** Lesions of spleen in amyloidosis involving lymphoid follicles and terminal arteriole
67. **Tapioca appearance:** Lesions of spleen in amyloidosis involving lymphoid follicles and terminal arteriole
68. **Nutmeg:** CVC liver, gross appearance
69. **Maple syrup:** Smell of urine in enzyme deficiency involving metabolism of branched chain amino acids.
70. **Ochronosis:** Ocher like (yellowish) discolouration due to accumulation of homogentisic acid in connective tissues
71. **Psammoma body:** Dystrophic calcification in whorled appearance observed in papillary carcinoma thyroid, serous papillary carcinoma ovary, psammomatous meningioma
72. **Onion peal/skin appearance:** X-ray appearance of periosteal reaction with new bone in Ewings sarcoma
73. **Sirenomalia (mermaid appearance):** Anomalies of lower spine and lower limbs, partial or complete fusion of lower limbs
74. **Rice water:** Stools in cholera
75. **Sickle:** Shape of RBCs in sickle cell HA
76. **Potato tumour:** Gross appearance of carotid body tumour
77. **Signet ring:** Malignant cells in mucinous carcinoma
78. **Portwine colour:** Urine in porphyria
79. **Orphan Annie eye:** Appearance of nuclei with peripheral clumping of chromatin in cells of papillary carcinoma thyroid.
80. **Rubbery feel:** Hodgkin's disease, feel of the lymph nodes
81. **Owl eye:** RS cells in Hodgkin disease, mirror image (similar looking) nuclei
82. **Punched out osteolytic lesions:** Bone in multiple myeloma due to osteoclastic activity
83. **Swiss cheese appearance:** Gross appearance in cystoglandular hyperplasia, adenomyosis
84. **Tadpole cells:** Cells in syringoma and individual cells with tapered cytoplasm in squamous cell carcinoma
85. **Staghorn calculi:** Renal stones in pelvis, composed of struvite (magnesium ammonium phosphate) or calcium carbonate apatite
86. **Moth eaten appearance:** Vacuolated cytoplasm in necrosis
87. **Starry sky pattern:** Tingible body macrophages in Burkitt lymphoma
88. **Navicular cells:** Progesterone effect on cervical cells especially in pregnancy
89. **Onion skin appearance:** Touch receptor also called Pacinian corpuscle, blood vessels in malignant HT, X-ray of periosteal reaction in Ewing's sarcoma
90. **Pallisading:** Peripheral cells in BCC
91. **Safety pin appearance:** *Donovanosis C. granulomatis* organisms
92. **Storiform pattern:** Arrangement of cells in Fibrosarcoma and fibroma
93. **Spider like cells:** Lipoblasts in liposarcoma
94. **Zebra bodies:** Lamellated inclusions in neuronal lysozymes mucopolysaccharidosis/gangliosidosis
95. **Rosettes and florets:** Homer Wright rosettes (cell arrangement around neuropil) in medulloblastoma/neuroblastoma/PNET, flexner Wintersteiner rosettes in retinoblastoma, ependymal rosettes with cell arrangement around a tubular lumen.
96. **Mutton or chicken leg appearance:** Gross appearance of osteosarcoma
97. **Soap bubble appearance:** Osteoclastoma, adamantinoma
98. **Saddle embolus:** Thromboembolus obstructing the main pulmonary trunk
99. **Turkish towel appearance:** Adenomyosis, gross appearance.

100. **Tree bark:** Syphilitic aortitis classically seen in ascending aorta, intima showing scars and furrows due to end-arteritis of vasavasorum, inflammation with predominantly plasma cells and other chronic inflammatory cells and destruction of media which is replaced by fibrosis.
101. **Tigered heart:** Fatty heart in chronic ischaemia showing alternate dark coloured normal muscle with pale coloured muscle with fat accumulation.
102. **Thrush breast heart:** Fatty heart with normal dark coloured muscle alternating with light coloured muscle with fatty change appearing like patches on chest of bird called Thrush.
103. **Portwine-stained skin areas:** This is due to hemangiomas or anomalies of blood vessels. It may be component of Sturge Weber syndrome.
104. **Peau d' Orange:** Over lying skin in carcinoma breast, appears like skin of orange due to obstructed lymphatics.
105. **Targetoid appearance:** Arrangement of tumour cells in concentric manner around normal ducts in lobular carcinoma breast
106. **Turbon tumour:** Numerous dome-shaped nodules on scalp in cylindromas
107. **Tombstone appearance:** Coagulative necrosis
108. **Spider naevi/angioma:** Due to excess oestrogen or cirrhosis and portal hypertension, there is failure of sphincteric muscle surrounding the cutaneous arteriole, central portion has dilated arteriole
109. **Splinter haemorrhage:** Haemorrhages below nail in bacterial endocarditis
110. **Salt and pepper appearance:** Nuclei in carcinoid tumour
111. **Strawberry like uterine cervix:** Erythematous punctate and papillaeform appearance in trichomonas vaginalis infection.
112. **Zell ballen:** Cell arrangement in paraganglioma or pheochromocytoma

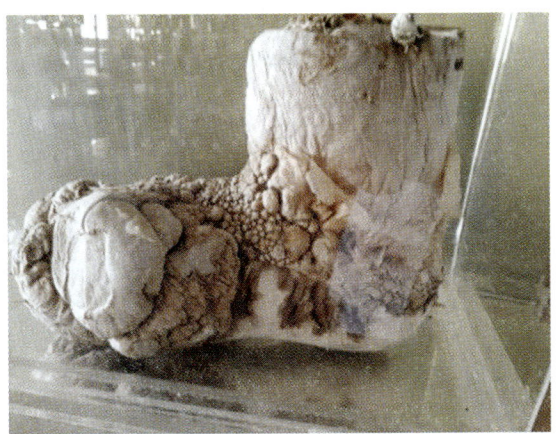

Elephantiasis foot (Filariasis)

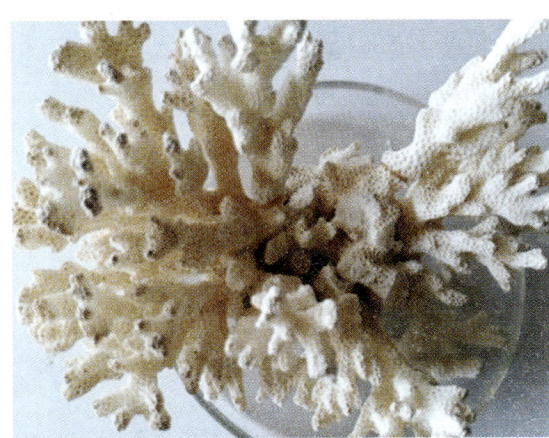

Corals (Coraline thrombus)

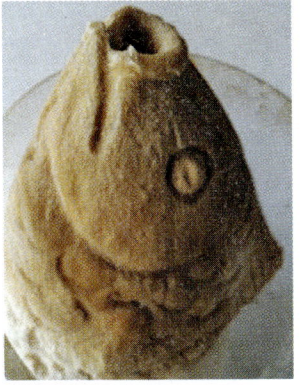

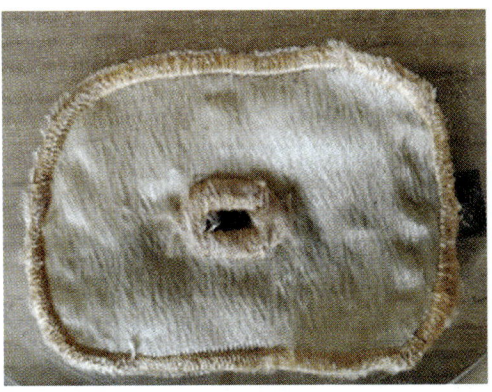

Fish mouth /button hole: Valves in rheumatic heart disease

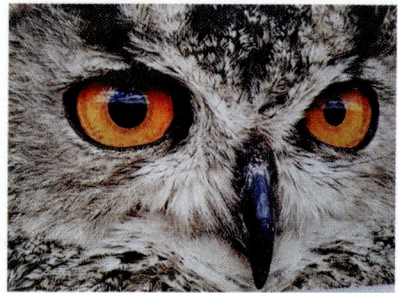

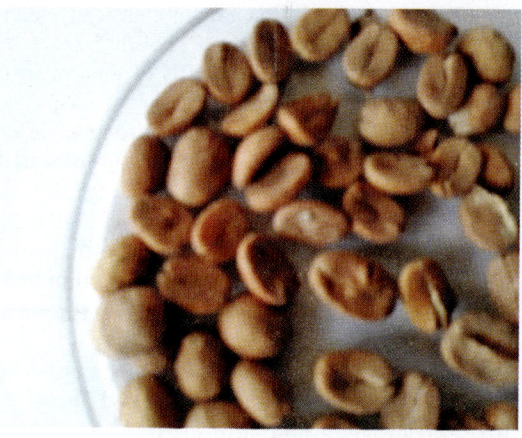

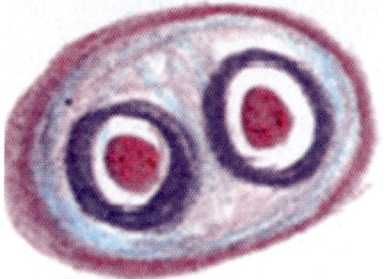

Coffee bean: Nuclei with grooves, cells of Granulosa cell tumour and Brenner's tumour.

Owl eye: Mirror image nuclei of RS cells

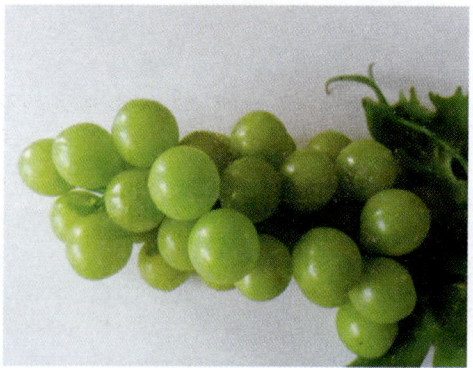

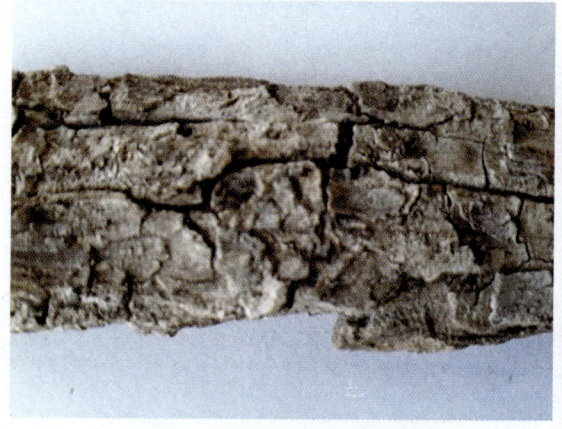

Grape-like structures: Vesicular mole, gross appearance

Tree bark: Syphilitic aortitis

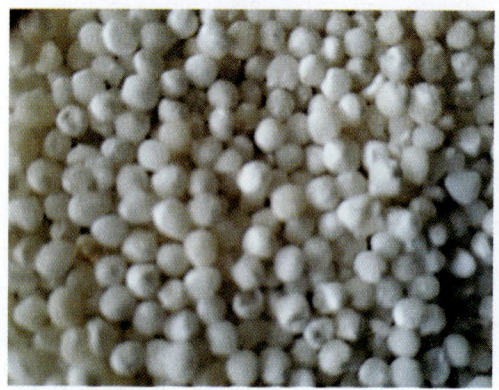

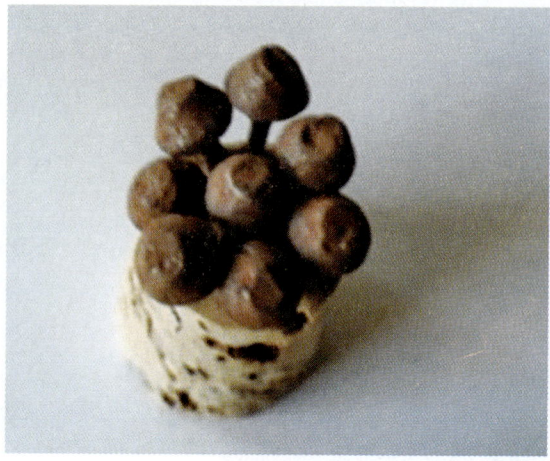

Sago: Spleen in amyloidosis

Hobnail: Macronodules in postnecrotic cirrhosis

Similes in Pathology

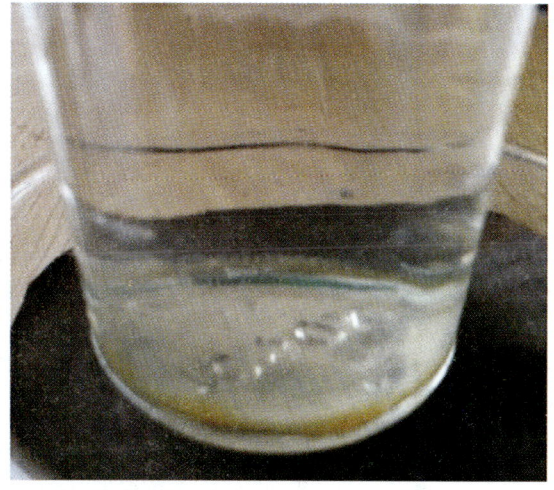

Rice water: Stools in cholera

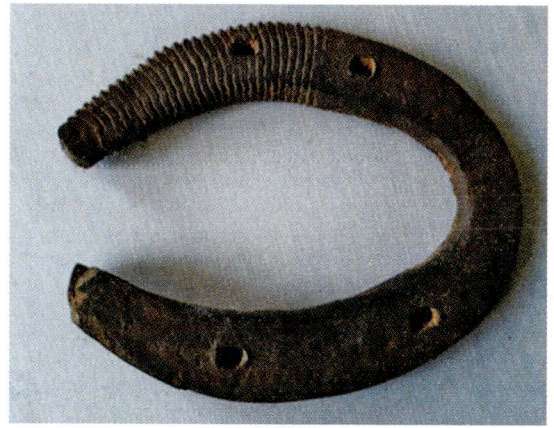

Sickle: Shape of RBCs in sickle cell HA

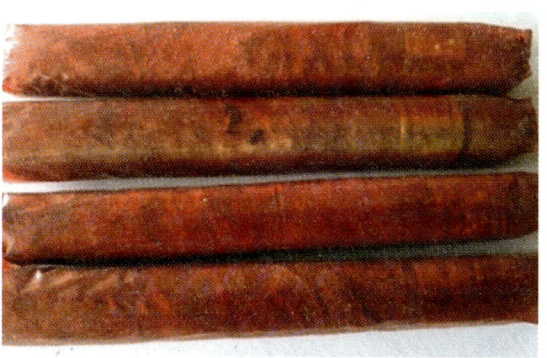

Cigar bundle: Arrangement of Lepra bacilli

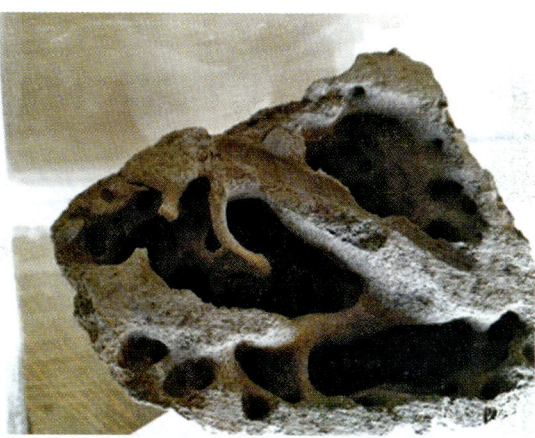

Ant hill: Actinomycosis or fungal infections

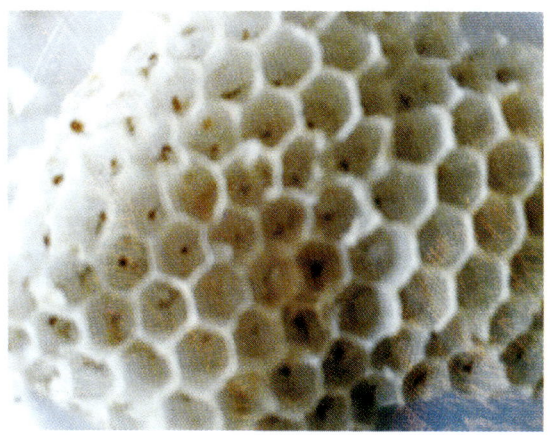

Honeycomb: Gross appearance in bronchiectasis

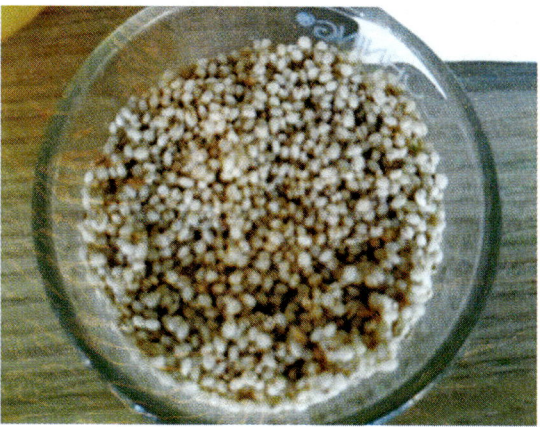

Millet seeds: Tiny lesions in Miliary tuberculosis

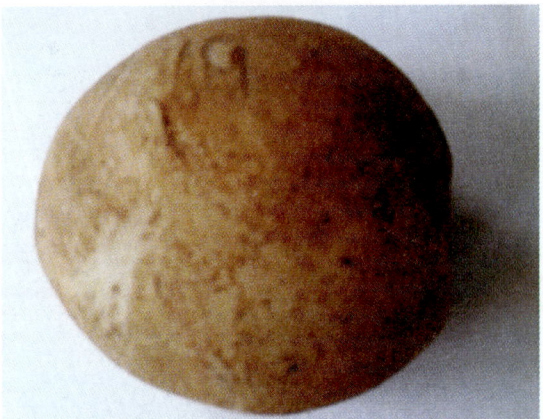

Potato tumour: Gross appearance of carotid body tumour

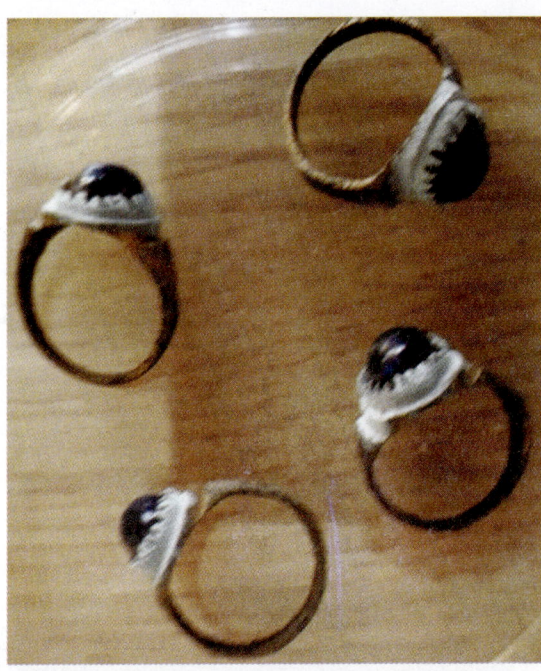

Signet ring: Malignant cells in mucinous carcinoma

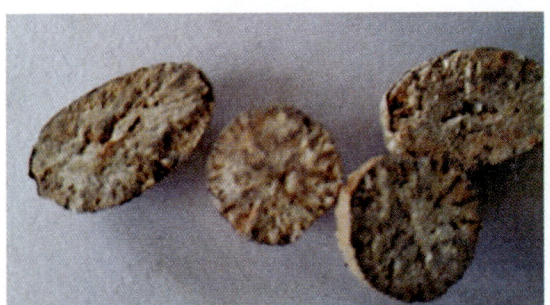

Nutmeg: CVC liver, gross appearance

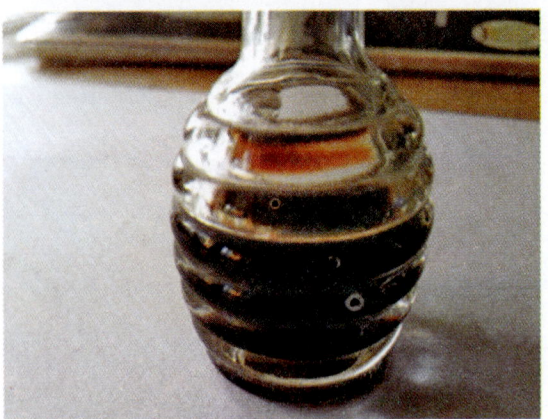

Portwine colour: Urine in porphyria

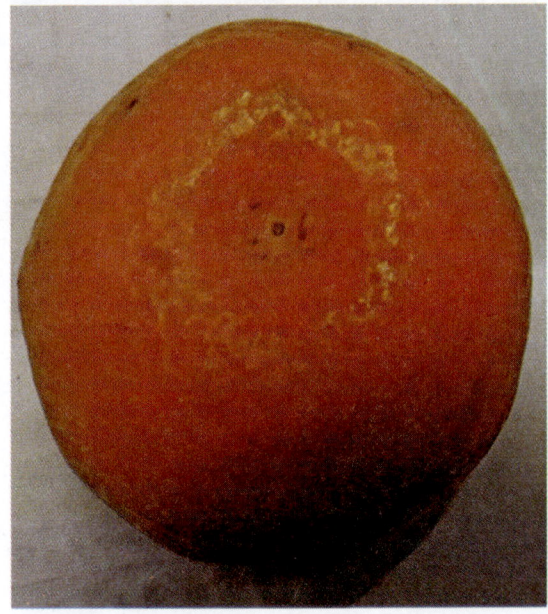

Peau d' Orange: Skin in breast carcinoma

KNOW YOUR SCIENTISTS

1. **Hippocrates (460–377 BC):** He was a Greek physician. He is called the father of medicine. He established the basic principles of medicine.
2. **Aulus cornelius celsus (25 BC–50 AD):** He was a Roman physician, first described the four cardinal signs of inflammation (rubor, calor, tumour and dolor).
3. **William Harvey (1578–1657):** Established circulation of blood.
4. **Giovanni B. Morgagni (1682–1771):** He conducted 700 postmortems with clinicopathological correlations and described morbid anatomy.
5. **John Hunter and William Hunter:** Described inflammation, defense mechanism and repair mechanism. Also wrote a book on Venereal diseases.
6. **Mathew Baillie:** Described morbid anatomy.
7. **Thomas Hodgkin (1798–1866):** Described the reasons for enlargement of Lymph nodes, spleen and liver.
8. **Carl Von rokitansky (1804–1878):** Conducted 30,000 autopsies, described endocarditis, lobar pneumonia, bronchopneumonia, anomalies like Rokitansky Ascoff sinuses and septal defects of heart.
9. **Rudolf virchow (1821–1902):** Virchow is father of cellular pathology or modern pathology. On his name are Virchow's method of autopsy, Virchow cell and Virchow triad which are described by him.
10. **Paul Ehrlich (1854–1915):** He is a German scientist, first identified mast cells and his prodigious laboratory talent led to the use of aniline dyes as metachromatic stains.
11. **Friedrich von Recklinghausen (1833–1910):** He is remembered for 'multiple neurofibromatosis'. Neurofibromatosis type I which is due to mutation of NF1 gene located on chromosome 17q11.2 is named after him.
12. **Sternberg and Reed:** These two scientists described the RS cells and histopathological changes in Hodgkin disease.
13. **Ludwig Aschoff (1866–1942):** Developed the concept of the reticuloendothelial system and described Aschoff cells, Aschoff sinus and Aschoff rule.
14. **Nikolai Anitschkov (1885–1964):** Described the histopathology of the heart in rheumatic fever.
15. **Paul Klemperer (1884–V1964):** Introduced the concept of collagen disease and described the LE cell phenomenon.
16. **Albert Coons (1912–1978):** He is known for revolutionary discoveries of fluoresceinlabelled antibodies.
17. **George Kohler (1946–1995):** George Kohler was awarded nobel prize in physiology in 1984 along with other two scientists for the work on immune system and production of monoclonal antibodies.
18. **Dr. James Holmer Wright:** He demonstrated that multiple myeloma is a tumour of plasma cells, that platelets arise from megakaryocytes, spirochetes can be identified in syphilis and neuroblastoma is of nerve cell lineage and contains 'Homer Wright' rosettes.
19. **George Papanicolaou (1883–1962):** He was a pioneer in cytopathology and early cancer detection, and inventor of the "Pap smear".
20. **Watson and Crick:** Described the structure of DNA and revolutionised genetic study.
21. **Karl Landsteiner (1868–1943):** In 1900 Karl Landsteiner (Austrian physician), discovered A, B and O blood groups. AB blood group was discovered in the year 1902 by A. Decastello and A. Sturli.
22. **James Paget (1814–1899):** He was a surgical pathologist, prepared catalogue of pathology museum of the Royal College of Surgeons in 1882.
23. **Julius Cohnheim (1839–1884):** He was a pathologist from Germany, described migration of leukocytes in inflammation.
24. **Richard Bright (1789–1858):** He was a physician from England, described Bright disease.
25. **Gregor Johann Mendel (1822–1884):** Experiments on green peas and discovered the fundamental laws of inheritance.
26. **DL Romanowsky (1861–1921):** Developed stain to stain blood cells. He used two basic stains methylene blue and eosin.
27. **Barry Marshall and Robin Warren:** In 2005, Barry Marshall and Robin Warren were awarded the Nobel Prize in Physiology for their pioneering work on *Helicobacter pylori*.
28. **JB Chatterjee:** Macrocytic anaemia.
29. **James Paget:** Described Paget's disease of breast and bone.
30. **VB Khanolkar:** Worked on leprosy, demonstrated bacilli in nerves and worked on cancer research

31. **Thomas Addison:** Described Addisonian anaemia (Pernicious Anaemia) and Addison's disease (Adrenal insufficiency)
32. **Richard Bright:** Bright disease (Nephritis)
33. **Rene Laennec:** Alcoholic cirrhosis and stethoscope
34. **Jean Baptiste Bouillaud:** Worked on rheumatic fever
35. **Percivol Pott:** Pott's puffy tumour, Pott's fracture, Pott's spine and scrotal cancer in chimney sweepers.
36. **BK Aikat:** Worked on tropical splenomegaly.
37. **Antonie van Leeuwenhoek:** Used microscope to observe bacteria.
38. **Robert Koch:** Physician and founder of modern microbiology. Discovered tuberculous bacilli in the year 1882 and described Koch's postulates. Causative agent for Anthrax was discovered.
39. **Dr Bhende and colleagues:** Invented Bombay blood group in Bombay.
40. **Dr Dharmendra:** Worked on Leprosy. Published book on leprosy.

PEARLS TO REMEMBER

Anaemias
1. Red cells normally survive for 120 days.
2. Anticoagulant of choice in haematology laboratory are: EDTA, double oxalate, 3.2% or 3.8% trisodium citrate and heparin.
3. Warm antibodies in HA are: IgG antibodies.
4. A person with haemoglobin of 15 gm/dl % will have PCV of 45%.
5. Low MCV and High RDW: Iron deficiency anaemia.
6. A unit of packed red cells will increase Hb by 1 gm/dl.
7. Fanconi Anaemia: AR disease with bone marrow failure. 90% of these cases have aplastic anaemia.
8. PNH: Absence of GPI-linked proteins with reduced anchorage of decay accelerating factors are unusually sensitive to complement mediated lysis.
9. G6PD is required to generate NADPH.
10. NADPH protects RBCs from oxidative stress.
11. In sickle cell anaemia, there is substitution of valine for glutamic acid in 6th position of beta chains.
12. At less pH and low oxygen tension, Hb-S cells begin to sickle.
13. Cryohemolysis more than 20% is seen in HS.
14. In HS, there is spectrin deficiency.
15. DDs for Normocytic Normochromic Anaemia
    i. Acute blood loss
    ii. Haemolytic anaemia
    iii. Chronic renal failure (erythropoietin deficiency)
    iv. Anaemia of chronic disorders: Infections
    v. Microangiopathic HA
    vi. Autoimmune HA
    vii. Transfusion reactions
    viii. Burns
16. DDs for Microcytic Anaemia (Pnemonics TICS)
    i. Iron deficiency anaemia
    ii. Thalassemia
    iii. Anaemia of chronic diseases
    iv. Sideroblastic anaemia
17. DDs for Macrocytic Anaemia
    i. B_{12} deficiency
    ii. Folic acid deficiency
    iii. MDS
    iv. Alcohol
    v. Chronic liver disease (cirrhosis)
    vi. Congenital BM failure (Schwamann-Diamond syndrome—BM dysregulation, sketetal abnormalities and exocrine pancreatic insufficiency)
    vii. Hypothyroidism
    viii. Reticulocytosis

Leukaemias
1. B lymphoid markers: CD10, CD19, CD79
2. T cell markers: CD2, CD3, CD7
3. M6 leukaemia has myelofibrosis
4. T cell ALL can manifest as mediastinal mass of thymic origin.
5. CML: Massive spleen, increased basophils and eosinophils, immature WBCs specifically myelocytes, t(9:22) Philadelphia chromosome.
6. CML phases: Chronic phase, accelerated phase and blast crisis.
7. Chronic phase: Less than 10% myeloblasts in bone marrow.
8. Accelerated phase: Myeloblasts in bone marrow are between 11 and 19%.
9. Blast crisis: Blasts in bone marrow more than 20%.

Multiple Myeloma and Plasma Cell Disorders
1. Plasma cell neoplasms: There is clonal proliferation of plasma cells.
2. Plasmacytoma is multiple myeloma (MM) occurring in soft tissue
3. Punched out lesions of MM are due to: IL-6.
4. POEMS syndrome: Polyneuropathy, organomegaly, endocrinopathy, monoclonal gammopathy and skin changes.
5. CRAB features for MM: Calcium elevated, renal insufficiency, anaemia and bony osteolytic lesions.
6. BJ proteins in urine: These are light chain gamma globulins excreted in plasma cell dyscrasiasis.
7. Increased ESR more than 100 mm at the end of first hour is characteristic in MM and other plasma cell dyscrasiasis.
8. Waldenstrom macroglobulinaemia (WM): IgM producing malignant plasma cell disease presents with anaemia and hyperviscocity features.
9. M band on serum electrophoresis is diagnostic in MM and WM.
10. MUGS : Clonal plasma cells <10% .

Myeloproliferative Disorders

1. Primary myelofibrosis: Prefibrotic and fibrotic phases. Prefibrotic phase can have Leuko-erythroblastic blood picture, tear drop cells and splenomegaly.
2. BCR-ABL negative and JAK2 mutations positive disorders are: PV. ET, PMF, CML.
3. PV: Hb more than 16.5 gm% for men and 16 gm% for females, panmyelosis, JAK2 positive.
4. ET: Platelet counts more than 4.5 L cells/cmm, increased megakaryocytes in BM, JAK2 positive.

Myelodysplastic Syndrome (MDS)

1. MDS is a stem cell malignancy.
2. The cells in MDS are dysplastic.
3. MDS presents with ineffective blood cell production.
4. MDS can occur in old age with 5q deletion.
5. Monosomy 7, 5q deletion and other chromosomal abnormalities are known in MDS.
6. ALIP is observed in MDS.
7. Neutrophils with hypogranularity, hypolobulation or hypersegmentation can be present in MDS.
8. Micromegakaryocytes are observed in MDS.

Haemorrhagic Disorders

1. Idiopathic thrombocytopenic purpura (ITP) is an acquired disorder with thrombocytopenia due to antibody formation.
2. Megakaryocytes increased which are often in clusters. Often hypogranular and hypolobulation present. Cytoplasm is basophilic.
3. The monoclonal antibody specific immobilisation of platelet antigen (MAIPA): Positive (50–65%) in ITP.
4. Hermansky Pudlak syndrome: Albinism and platelet dysfunction.
5. PGI_2 and NO produced by endothelial cells have antiplatelet effect.
6. Glanzmann thrombasthenia: AR, GP IIb/IIIa receptor deficient or dysfunctional. These genes present on chromosome 17. With dysfunction or deficiency, there is defective aggregation of platelets.
7. Factor II, VII, IX , X and protein C and S are vitamin K dependent factors.
8. von Willebrand disease: AD with spontaneous bleeding from mucous membranes, platelet count is normal.
9. A newborn with bleeding from umbilical cord is: Factor X and XII deficiency.
10. A female with haemathrosis is probably due to Factor VIII inhibitors.
11. DIC has: FDPs, prolonged PT, APTT and reduced platelet count.
12. vWF produced from endothelium.
13. Factor VIII is always in combination with vWF.
14. Protein C, thrombomodulin, and thrombin produce activated protein C. This along with protein S inactivates FVa and FVIIIa.
15. Protein C cannot cleave Factor Leiden Va.
16. Heparin like molecules from endothelium activate Antithrombin III. This binds thrombin and inactivates vitamin K dependent activated factors.
17. Antiphospholipid antibody syndrome: Presence of antibodies against phospholipid binding plasma proteins. The syndrome presents with recurrent abortions.
18. PT: Assesses coagulation mechanism by extrinsic pathway and deficiency of common pathway (Factor VII, X, V , II and I).
19. APTT: Assesses coagulation mechanism by intrinsic pathway and deficiency of common pathway. (FXII, XI, IX, VIII, X, V, II and I).
20. PT normal and APTT prolonged in FVIII, IX, pre-kallikrein, HMWK deficiency and with presence of inhibitors.
21. PT increased in defects of FV, VII, X and fibrinogen deficiency.

Blood Grouping and Transfusion Medicine

I. Important points regarding blood groups

1. Antigens are present on the wall of RBCs.
2. ABO and Rh are important blood groups.
3. IgM antibodies are present in ABO system. These IgM antibodies can be also be present in other rare blood groups (MNSs, P).
4. IgG antibodies may be produced in O blood group patients.
5. IgG antibodies can be produced in Rh system with immunological sensitisation.
6. IgG antibodies can be also produced with immunological sensitisation in other blood group systems such as Kell, Duffy, Kidd, MNSs and Lutheran.
7. IgG antibodies produce HDN and haemolytic transfusion reactions.
8. Compatible blood needs to be given to save the life.

II. Donation of blood and blood components

1. 8 ml per kg body weight blood can be donated.
2. The plasma volume and platelets are replaced within 48 hours, granulocytes and other elements of plasma (proteins, etc.) within

7 days, red blood cells in 56 days and iron lost is replaced in 8 weeks.
3. Plasmapheresis can be done at an interval of 48 hours.
4. Platelet apheresis at an interval 48 hours
5. Red blood cells/whole blood used within 35 days with CPDA1.
6. Platelets are used within 5 days.
7. FFP and cryoprecipitate can be used up to one year.

III. Blood and blood components
1. One unit of whole blood will increase Hb by 1gm/dl and PCV by 3%.
2. 1 unit of packed red cells has 250 mg of iron.
3. Iron that can be removed by the body is 1 mg/day.
4. One unit of single donor platelets (SDP) will increase platelet count by 30,000–60000 platelets/cmm.
5. One unit of random donor platelets (RDP) will increase the platelet count by 4,000–6000 platelets/cmm.
6. Preserve the platelets at 22–24°C in agitator.
7. Transfuse platelets if platelet count is less than 10,000 cells/cmm with antibodies to platelets, platelet transfusion may not be of use.
8. Platelet increase is observed after 1 hour and again at 20–24 hours of platelet transfusion.
9. Preserve the whole blood/PRBCs at 1–6°C.
10. FFP once collected from the Blood Bank can be preserved at 1–6°C and has to be used within 12 hours.
11. Do not transfuse unless clear indication is present. Some of the indications are given below:
    - Chronic Anaemias with Hb less than 6 gm/dl.
    - Less than 7 gm/dl when patient is symptomatic and undergoing surgery.
    - Less than 8 g with CVS problems.
    - With 6–10 g/dl only when severe bleeding or complications of inadequate hypoxia are expected.
    - Blood loss of 30–40% of circulating blood volume.
    - In anaemia/severe heart or pulmonary disease/when bleeding continues with 15–30% blood loss.
    - In Obstetrics patients Hb less than 7 g/dl, not amenable to timely therapies antenataly.
    - In concealed haemorrhage with abruptio placenta, to replenish the concealed blood loss irrespective of symptoms.

IV. Important points to keep in mind regarding neonatal transfusion
- In neonates 10–20 ml/kg body weight blood can be given.
- Blood less than 7 days is preferred for neonatal transfusion.
- In neonates only antigen grouping is done.
- Blood to be given to neonate should be compatible with mother's serum.
- If mother's and baby's group are the same, use Rh negative blood of baby/mother's ABO group. If not the same use 'O' Rh negative blood.
- In neonates, rate of transfusion should be less than 10 ml/kg/hour.

V. The common causes of transfusion of ABO incompatible blood are:
- Errors in blood request form
- Taking wrong sample into prelabelled sample tube
- Incorrect labelling of the sample tube sent to the blood bank
- Inadequate checks of the blood against the identity of the patient while starting a transfusion

VI. Prevention of errors:
1. Correctly label the blood samples and request forms.
2. Place the patient's blood sample in the sample tube.
3. Always check the blood against the identity of the patient at the bedside before transfusion.
4. Proper identification of the patient from sample collection through to blood administration, proper labelling of samples and products is essential. Prevention of nonimmune haemolysis requires adherence to proper handling, storage and administration of blood products.

VII. Different types of donors:
- Voluntary donors
- Replacement donors
- Autologous donors

Voluntary donor is one who donates blood for storage at a blood blank for transfusion to an unknown recipient.
- A greater percentage of better quality of blood comes from voluntary donors.
- These donors are very important because the incidence of blood transmitted infections is much less in blood drawn from these volunteers.

Replacement donor is a person, often a family member, donates blood for transfusion to a specific individual.
- The donor is selected by the recipient.
- Since there is pressure to donate, they may give blood even if there is risk behaviour.

Autologous donor is a person who donates blood to be stored and is transfused back to the donor at a later stage, usually during and/or after surgery.

VIII. Criteria for donor selection:

Age: 18–65 years

Minimum body weight: 45 kg

A person can donate 8 ml/kg body weight (up to 450 ml every three months)

Haemoglobin (Hb): 12. 5 gm% or above or Hct equal to more than 38%.

Donor screening: Involves registration, consent of the donor, demographic information, medical history, limited physical examination and simple laboratory tests.

Demographic information: It should be complete and correct so that the donor can be informed of any laboratory testing abnormality.

1. Donor's full name
2. Father's/Husband's name
3. Age
4. Gender
5. Phone number
6. Residential address

Medical History

1. History of any long-term illness.
2. Any medication if patient is taking.
3. Allergy to any substance/medication, etc.

Physical Examination

A qualified practitioner of medicine or blood bank Officer will examine for the following:
- *General appearance:* A donor should be healthy.
- *Pulse:* 60–100 beats/minute.
- *Temperature:* 37°C.
- *Blood Pressure:* Systolic pressure: 100–140 mm Hg
  Diastolic pressure: 60–90 mm Hg.
- Respiratory, cardiovascular, gastrointestinal, etc. systems should be normal and no problems should be detected by a rapid physical examination.

Informed Consent: If the donor has successfully passed the history, physical examination, prior to donation, informed consent is required.

IX. Laboratory tests: Following are the tests done on a unit of blood donated.

1. Haemoglobin estimation
2. Blood grouping and crossmatching
3. Screening for unwanted antibodies
4. Screening for transfusion transmissible infections: Indian Govt. regulatory authorities for Blood Bank recommends following 5 tests to be mandatory. These are mentioned below:
   - HIV 1 and 2
   - Hepatitis B
   - Hepatitis C
   - Syphilis
   - Malaria

Tests must be performed at each donation regardless of number of earlier donations.

There are temporary deferrals or permanent deferrals for blood transfusion.

Introduction and History of Pathology

1. Hippocrates: Father of medicine. He established the basic principles of medicine.
2. Aulus Cornelius celsus described the four cardinal signs of inflammation (rubor, calor, tumour and dolor).
3. William Harvey established circulation of blood.
4. Giovanni B. Morgagni conducted 700 post-mortems with clinico-pathological correlations and described morbid anatomy.
5. Huntarian museum at the Royal College of Physicians and surgeons is named after John Hunter and William Hunter.
6. Thomas Hodgkin described the reasons for enlargement of lymph nodes, spleen and liver.
7. Carl Von Rokitansky conducted 30,000 autopsies.
8. Migration of Leukocytes in Inflammation is described by Julium Cohnheim.
9. Karl Landsteiner discovered A, B and O blood groups. AB blood group was discovered by A. Decastello and A. Sturli.
10. Pap smear is named after George Papanicolaou.
11. Monoclonal antibodies production credit goes to George Kohler.
12. Albert Coons is known for discovery of fluorescein-labelled antibodies.
13. Combination of methylene blue and eosin are named after Romanowsky.
14. Gregor Johann Mendel discovered the fundamental laws of inheritance
15. Barry Marshall and Robin Warren discovered *Helicobacter pylori.*

Cell Injury

1. Moth eaten appearance is due to: Enzymatic digestion of cell organelles.
2. In Fenton reaction, ROS develop when ferrous iron is converted to ferric ion.
3. Superoxide dismutase takes off superoxide which in combination with hydrogen molecule gets converted to H_2O_2 and oxygen.
4. Anti-oxidants are endogenous and exogenous anti-oxidants (vitamins A, E, C and Beta-carotenes) block the formation of free radicals.
5. Superoxide dismutase protects brain from injury by ROS.
6. Ionising radiation produces cell injury by release of free radicals especially OH ions.
7. During lactation breast hyperplasia is seen.
8. Breast enlargement during puberty and pregnancy are examples of hyperplasia.
9. Skeletal muscle of limbs in athletes is an example of hypertrophy due to increased muscle activity.
10. Myocardial fibres undergo only hypertrophy. No hyperplasia is seen as they are permanent cells.
11. Wear and tear pigment is lipofuscin which is yellow brown coloured.
12. Brown colour in brown atrophy of heart is due to deposition of wear and tear pigment, i.e. lipofuscin.
13. Undigested material from lipid peroxidation is lipofuscin.
14. Metaplasia can be epithelial or mesenchymal, reversible, occurs at stem cell level.
15. Commonest metaplasia in respiratory tract is ciliated pseudostratified columnar epithelium changes to stratified squamous epithelium.
16. Ducts of salivary glands with glandular epithelium may undergo metaplasia to stratified squamous epithelium due to chronic irritation by stones.
17. In Barrett's oesophagus, squamous epithelium changes to columnar epithelium.
18. Osseous and mesenchymal metaplasia can be seen in leiomyomas and fibromas.
19. In cloudy degeneration, the parenchymal cells affected are rich in mitochondria.
20. Chaperones are responsible for proper protein folding.
21. Dutcher bodies are cytoplasmic inclusions found in the nucleus (intranuclear inclusions) of plasma cells
22. Mott cells plasma cell with multiple Russell bodies.
23. Plasma cell with eosinoplilic cytoplasmic inclusion is: Russell body.
24. Neurofibrillary tangles are seen in: Amyloidosis brain.
25. Amyloid gives green birefringence with polarising microscope.
26. Fatty heart is encountered in diphtheria and chronic ischaemia.
27. Mallory hyaline refers to damaged intermediate filaments.
28. Programmed cell death refers to apoptosis, observed in embryogenesis, deletion of autoreactive T cells and virus infected cells.
29. Characteristic of apoptosis is chromatin condensation.
30. Anti-apoptotic molecules are: Bcl2 and Bcl-XL. These are present on the outer mitochondrial and ER membranes. These prevent leakage of cytochrome C into cytosol.
31. BAX and BAK are pro-apoptotic.
32. Cytochrome C binds to APAF1 and activates caspase 9.
33. With failure of calcium pump, influx of calcium activates many enzymes.
34. In cell injury, there is ATP depletion, ribosomes detach from rough endoplasmic reticulum with reduction in protein synthesis.
35. Death receptors are TNFR and FAS-l.
36. Initiator caspase in intrinsic pathway: Caspase 9.
37. Initiator caspase in extrinsic pathway: Caspase 8.
38. Fat saponification is seen in: Chronic pancreatitis and traumatic injury to fat.
39. Wet gangrene is combination of coagulative and liquefactive nacrosis.
40. Coagulative necrosis: Organ is mummified, blackish coloured and microscopy shows tomb stone appearance.
41. Fragmentation of nucleus: Karryorrhexis
42. Fading with basophila of nucleus is referred to as: Karryolysis.
43. Pyknosis: Shrinkage of nucleus.
44. Autophagy: Self destruction. Cell eats its own contents.
45. Hyperplasia is increase in number of cells in organ or tissue. This type of adaptation occurs in tissues which can undergo division.
46. Physiological causes of hyperplasia

1. Hormonal stimulus can cause proliferation of the glands and stromal tissue:
   a. Breast during puberty and pregnancy
   b. Uterus in pregnancy
   c. Prostate enlargement called benign prostatic hyperplasia (BPH) or nodular prostatic hyperplasia (NPH)
2. Compensatory hyperplasia which occurs after portion of tissue is resected or diseased as in liver, lung and kidney.
47. The pathological causes of hyperplasia
    i. Endometrial hyperplasia due to excess estrogen hormone
    ii. Skin epithelium with HPV infection which causes hyperplasia of stratified squamous epithelial cells causing papilloma (Viral Wart).
    iii. Skin epithelium in Psoriasis.
    iv. Pancreatic islet cell hyperplasia in infants of diabetic mothers.
48. Hypertrophy is an increase in the size of the cells resulting in increased size of the organs. In hypertrophy, there are no new cells.
49. Physiological causes of hypertrophy
    i. Uterus during pregnancy: Estrogen stimulates smooth muscle cells to undergo hypertrophy and hyperplasia.
    ii. Skeletal muscle of limbs in athletes: Skeletal muscles undergo hypertrophy due to increased muscle activity.
50. Pathological causes of hypertrophy
    i. Hypertrophy of heart due to increase in demand as in hypertension or aortic valve incompetence/stenosis.
51. Atrophy is shrinkage in size of the cell, due to loss of cell substances.
52. Physiological causes of atrophy
    i. Involution of branchial cleft, thyroglossal duct, and notochord.
    ii. Involution of Wolffian duct and Mullerian duct in females and males respectively
    iii. Atrophy of ovary, endometrium after menopause and atrophy of other tissues in old age.
    iv. Old age (senile atrophy).
53. Pathological causes of atrophy
    i. Disuse atrophy of limb: Decreased workload (immobilisation of limb in plaster cast in fracture of limb bones)
    ii. Loss of innervation
    iii. Loss of blood supply
    iv. Pressure atrophy
    v. Lack of nutrients
    vi. Reduced hormones
    vii. Loss of endocrine stimulation.
54. Metaplasia is a reversible change in which one adult cell type (epithelial or mesenchymal) is replaced by another adult cell type.
55. Epithelial metaplasia
    i. Respiratory epithelium (ciliated pseudo-stratified columnar epithelium) changes to stratified squamous epithelium in habitual cigarette smokers and vitamin A deficiency.
    ii. Endocervical epithelium may be change to stratified squamous epithelium.
    iii. Ducts of salivary glands with glandular epithelium may undergo metaplasia to stratified squamous epithelium due to chronic irritation by stones.
    iv. Ducts of pancreatic glands may change to stratified squamous epithelium due to stones.
    v. Transitional epithelium of bladder and pelvis of kidney may change to stratified squamous epithelium due to irritation by renal stones.
    vi. Endometrial metaplasia may show different type of epithelia.
    vii. The lower end of oesophagus which is usually lined by stratified squamous epithelium may change to columnar epithelium due to reflux oesophagitis (Barrett's oesophagus).
56. Mesenchymal metaplasia: The undifferentiated cells transform into other adult mesenchymal cells. Cartilagenous metaplasia or osseous metaplasia are more common.
    i. In old scars, necrotic areas, myositis ossificans foci of bone may develop.
    ii. Foci of bone may develop in the walls of diseased arteries destroyed by injury or inflammation.
    iii. In laryngeal and bronchial cartilage of old people, cartilage may undergo ossification.
    iv. Fibromas may show osseous metaplasia.
    v. Uterine leiomyoma may undergo osseous and mesenchymal metaplasia.
57. Though the metaplastic epithelium has survival advantages, the important protective mechanisms are lost, such as:
    i. Mucous secretion
    ii. Ciliary clearance of particulate matter as in respiratory tract.

58. The metaplastic epithelium may predispose to malignant transformation, if it is not reversed back or the causative agent is not removed.
59. Degenerations are retrogressive changes in the cells due to direct action of the injurious agents.
60. Hyaline degeneration is glassy, amorphous and homogenous material which stains pink/eosinophilic with H & E stain.
61. Physiological conditions with hyaline degeneration are:
    i. Arteries of atrophic uterus
    ii. Colloid in multinodular goitre
    iii. *Corpora amylacea* in prostate
    iv. *Corpora albicans* in ovary
62. Extracellular hyaline:
    i. Collagen in:
        a. Old scar tissue
        b. Keloid
        c. Thickened capillaries and vessels
    ii. Fibroma
    iii. Vessel wall in
        a. Diabetes mellitus
        b. Hypertension
    iv. KW lesions of kidney in diabetes mellitus
    v. Hyalinsation of islets of Langerhans in diabetes mellitus.
63. Intracellular Hyaline
    i. Mallory hyaline: damaged prekeratin intermediate filaments. Commonly seen in fatty change, hepatitis or cirrhosis due to alcohol, Wilson's disease, Indian childhood cirrhosis, primary biliary cirrhosis, non-alcoholic steatohepatitis (NASH), hepatocellular carcinoma, etc.
    ii. Councilman bodies: Seen in yellow fever
    iii. Russel bodies: These represent immunoglobulins in plasma cells.
    iv. Epithelial hyaline: These are commonly seen in epithelium of the proximal tubules due to excess absorption of plasma proteins.
    v. Zenker's degeneration: Striated muscles of diaphragm, abdomen and thigh muscles show hyaline change in typhoid fever.
64. Abnormal accumulation of triglycerides within the parenchymal cells is refered to as fatty change.
65. Stains for demonstration of fat
    i. Oil red 'O'—fat stains red
    ii. Sudan III/IV—fat stains orange to red
    iii. Osmium tetroxide— with alpha naphthylamine reaction phospholipids are stained orange red; cholesterol and triglycerides are stained black.
    iv. Neutral fat is stained black with 1% osmic acid in saturated bichlorides or mercury.
66. Fatty change heart: Prolonged moderate hypoxia as seen in severe anaemia results in focal intracellular fat deposits, grossly, this gives yellowish appearance to the affected myocardial fibres and the normal fibres remain darker and red brown ('tigered' or 'Thrush breast' effect). The myocardial fibres are uniformly and diffusely affected due to some toxins, e.g. diphtheria. The anaemia is more severe and profound.
67. Amyloid is an abnormal proteinaceous substance deposited extracellularly in various organs.
68. Special stains for amyloid
    i. H & E stain—amyloid stains homogenous and pale pink
    ii. PAS stain—amyloid stains magenta pink
    iii. Van Gieson—amyloid stains yellow to yellow brown
    iv. Iodine (Gram's or Lugol's)—amyloid stains Mahagony brown turning to blue or violet with application of dilute sulphuric acid
    v. Metachromatic stains (e.g. 1% methyl violet, 1% toluidine blue)—amyloid stains pink, other tissues stain violet
    vi. Congo red—amyloid stains orange
    vii. Congo red with polarisation: Apple green birefringence
    viii. X-ray diffraction: Cross beta pleated structure
    ix. Fluorescence with thioflavin T and S
69. Apoptosis is a process that helps to eliminate unwanted cells, by an internally programmed series of events, the process is tightly regulated and the cells are destined to die.
70. Necrosis has a spectrum of morphological changes that follow cell death in a living tissue, largely resulting from progressive degradative action of enzymes on lethally injured cells. The damage caused is irreversible.

Inflammation

1. Acute inflammation has vasodilatation, oedema, and inflammatory response.
2. Chronic inflammation has inflammation and repair occurring at the same time.

3. ICAM1 and VCAM1 are responsible for adhesion of neutrophils.
4. Pro-inflammatory cytokines are IL-1, TNF and chemokines.
5. Pain is caused by : PGE_2, bradykinin, histamine, serotonin and neuropeptide.
6. Fever: IL-1, IL-8, TNF and PGE_2.
7. Cytokines: Signaling molecules produced by many cells.
8. Chemotaxis: C5a, LTB4, IL-8, PAF, 5-HETE
9. Chemokines are chemo-attractants for leukocytes.
10. CXC, CC, XC and CX3C are important chemokines. These mediate G protein-coupled receptors.
11. IL-8 is a CXC chemokine.
12. CC chemokine is monocyte attractant protein (MCP1), eotaxin, macrophage inflammatory protein 1 alpha
13. Platelet aggregation is by TXA2 and PAF.
14. Vasoconstriction is by TXA2, LTB4, LTC4, LTD4 and C5a.
15. Vasodilatation: Histamine, serotonin, bradykinin and C3a.
16. Increased vascular permeability: Histamine, serotonin, C3a, C5a, LTC4, D4 and E4
17. C3a, C5a and C4a act as: Anaphylatoxins.
18. Inflammation is reaction of a living tissue to an injurious agent. Inflammation tries to eliminate, dilute or neutralize the harmful agents.
19. Vascular Changes of inflammation are:
    i. The changes in vascular flow and caliber
    ii. Increased vascular permeability
20. The cellular events in inflammation
    i. Margination, rolling, pavementation, adhesion and transmigration
    ii. Chemotaxis
    iii. Recognition and attachment
    iv. Phagocytosis/Engulfment
    v. Killing and degradation
21. The chemical mediators of inflammation are:

    Cell derived
    i. Vasoactive amines—histamine, serotonin
    ii. Lysosomal component
    iii. Platelet activating factor
    iv. Cytokines
    v. NO and O2 metabolites
    vi. Arachidonic acid metabolites.

    Plasma Derived
    i. The kinin system
    ii. The clotting system
    iii. The fibrinolytic system
    iv. The complement system
22. Leukocytes express many types of toll like receptors which identify toll proteins present on the microbes.
23. TLRs are present on neutrophils, macrophages, natural killer cells, epithelial cells and endothelial cells. Most important amongst these TLRs is TLR-4 which can bind LPS binding proteins on microbes and activate potent cytokines like IL-1 and TNF.
24. Granulomatous inflammation is a chronic inflammation characterised by focal collection of epithelioid cells (modified macrophages), giant cells and mantle of lymphocytes.
25. Morphological patterns of inflammation
    i. Serous inflammation
    ii. Fibrinous inflammation
    iii. Suppurative or purulent inflammation
    iv. Abscess
    v. Gangrene
    vi. Ulcer.

Cell Cycle and Wound Healing

1. Labile cells: Epithelial cells lining different tracts, endometrium, bone marrow cells.
2. Continuously dividing cells are labile cells.
3. Liver, kidney and pancreatic cells are stable cells.
4. Neuronal and cardiac muscle cells are permanent cells.
5. If regeneration cannot occur, the injured cells are replaced by connective tissue.
6. Regeneration of liver is triggered by cytokines and growth factors. Surviving cells or progenitor cells proliferate.
7. VEGF drives angiogenesis.
8. Important growth factors for connective tissue are: PDGF, TGF beta, FGF2
9. TGF beta is important growth factor for formation of connective tissue.
10. Myofibroblasts are fibroblasts which have features of smooth muscle cells, including presence of actin filaments.
11. Myofibroblasts are involved in wound contraction.
12. Scar is remodeled by matrix metalloproteases which are dependent on zinc.
13. The granulation tissue is oedematous, reddish, velvety and formed in 3 days of wound healing.
14. In wound healing initial collagen formed is type III, which is later replaced by type I.

15. An excessive amount of granulation tissue is called 'Proud flesh'.
16. Excess production of ECM is encountered in hypertrophic scar and keloid which are abnormalities tissue repair.
17. The cell cycle phases
    i. Gap1 (G1) phase: This is pre-DNA synthetic phase.
    ii. DNA synthesis phase (S phase): DNA synthetic phase lasts for 6–8 hours.
    iii. Gap2 (G2) phase: This is pre-mitosis phase, lasts for 2–4 hours.
    iv. Mitosis (M) phase: This is mitosis phase, and lasts for a short-time (usually 1 hour).
18. Steps of wound healing by first intention
    i. Haematoma formation and above this scab forms.
    ii. Within 24 hours, neutrophils appear at the incision margin. The neutrophils migrate towards the fibrin clot. There is hyperaemia. The inflammatory cells remove clot and debris if any.
    iii. The epithelial cells (basal cells) at the cut edge, show increased mitotic activity within 24–48 hours.
    iv. By 3rd day, neutrophils are replaced by macrophages and granulation tissue is formed.
    v. By day 5, epidermis recovers normal thickness.
    vi. By the 2nd week, there is continued collagen accumulation, deposition and regression of vascular channels. The leukocyte infiltration, oedema, vascularity are reduced.
    vii. By the end of first month, the tensile strength of the wound increases. The connective tissue is devoid of inflammatory cells and surface is covered by normal epidermis.
19. Wound healing by second intention
    i. The tissue destruction is more and edges are ragged.
    ii. The edges cannot be approximated due to extensive loss of tissue.
    iii. As bleeding is heavy, large clot or hematoma formation is present.
    iv. Inflammation is more intense, necrotic debris and exudate formed is more.
    v. Epithelial cells migrate to replace the dead cells within a few days.
    vi. Larger amount of granulation tissue is formed to fill the large defect.
    vii. A large amount of collagen is laid down.
    viii. In 4–6 weeks, there is wound contraction, large skin defects are reduced to 5–10% of their original size by wound contraction.
20. Factors influencing wound healing
    Local factors:
    i. Location of wound on joints and bones
    ii. Intervening tissue or foreign body have necrotic debri
    iii. Type of tissue
    iv. Mechanical: variables local pressure, movement.
    v. Wound dehiscence
    vi. Infection
    vii. Growth factors

    General factors (Systemic factors):
    i. Age: Older the age delay in healing
    ii. Nutrition status: Vitamin C deficiency, lack of zinc and protein energy malnutrition cases have delayed wound healing.
    iii. Blood supply: Atherosclerosed blood vessels and tissues with less blood supply have delayed wound healing.
    iv. Exogenous cortico-steroids/increased glucocorticosteroids retards wound healing
    v. Diabetes and some haematological disorders: Diabetes has decreased phagocytic and chemotactic activity of inflammatory cells. Agranulocytosis leads to susceptibility of infection.
    vi. Radiation energy: Ultraviolet rays, X-rays in small doses stimulate wound healing whereas large doses delay healing.
    vii. Smoking delays healing.
    viii. Environmental temperature: Wound healing is slow in cold weather.
21. Steps of healing of fracture bone (simple fracture)
    i. Hematoma formation
    ii. Inflammatory reaction
    iii. Granulation tissue formation
    iv. Provisional callus formation (Procallus/soft tissue callus/callus composed of cartilage and woven bone)
    v. Callus formation
    vi. Remodelling.

Haemodynamic Disorders

1. Transudate is protein poor while exudate is protein rich.
2. Platelet GPIb binds to subendothelial collagen via vWF.
3. Platelet IIb/IIIa binds fibrinogen.
4. Normal endothelium releases factors which inhibit platelet aggregation. These are: Prostacyclin (PGI_2), NO and ADPase.
5. Normal endothelium has anticoagulant properties.
6. Thrombomodulin binds thrombin and activates protein C which is a inhibitor of Va and VIIIa.
7. Heparin like molecules activate antithrombin III which binds thrombin inactivate activated coagulation factors.
8. Protein C is a tissue factor pathway inhibitor.
9. Protein C requires protein S as cofactor.
10. Activated endothelial cells down regulate thrombomodulin, thus increased thrombin activity.
11. Stasis and turbulence are produced in aneurysms and atherosclerotic plaques.
12. DVT is associated with hypercoagulable state with bedrest and immobilisation.
13. Most pulmonary emboli are silent as they are small.
14. Factor V Leiden is resistant to cleavage and inactivation by protein C. These have increased risk of thrombosis.

Infectious Diseases

1. Defects in complements are prone for infections: Early complement deficiencies: organisms like S. pneumococci, late complement deficiencies: Neisseria infections.
2. Defects of Toll like receptors are prone for: pyogenic infections.
3. Mutations of receptors: IL-12, TNF Gamma and transcription factor STAT-1 impair generation of TH1 cells and are associated with atypical mycobacterial infections.
4. Gp of HIV 120 binds CD4 and CCR4 on T cells and CCR5 chemoreceptor on macrophages.
5. Koplic spots are pathognomonic of measles.
6. West Nile Virus is an arthropod borne virus, proliferates in skin dendritic cells and lymph nodes, can cross blood brain barrier and can infect neurons too.
7. CMV show cytoplasmic and nuclear basophilic inclusions.
8. Shingles occurs in varicella zoster virus (VZV) infection, virus has latent infection in dorsal root ganglia and spreads to sensory nerves.
9. Dengue fever is arbovirus infection spread by aedes aegypti mosquitoes. Dengue haemorrhagic fever has increased vascular permeability with plasma leakage and shock.
10. Ghon focus: 1 to 1.5 cm, subpleurally present in lower portion of the upper lobe or upper portion of the lower or middle lobe.
11. Apical tuberculosis on X-ray is called Simon's focus.
12. Rhinoscleroma: Chronic inflammatory cells, vacuolated histiocytes containg organisms (Mikulicz cells), plasma cells with Russel bodies and lymphocytes.
13. Fernandez and Mitsuda reactions are examples of delayed HS reaction in tuberculoid leprosy.
14. Destruction of vomer bone causes collapse of nasal bridge.
15. Syphilitic osteochondritis and periostitis affects all bones.
16. Eighth nerve deafness in syphilis is due to meningovascular syphilis.
17. Cryptococcus is yeast and has gelatinous capsule.
18. Aspergillus: Acute angle branching, septate, 5 to 10 micron in thickness.
19. Mucormycosis: Non-septate hyphae, right angle branching, variable width (6 to 50 microns).
20. Leishmania donovani: pro-mastigote forms in sandfly, amastigote in macrophages of host cells.

Calcification

1. Metastatic calcification occurs in normal tissues with increased calcium levels.
2. Dystrophic calcification occurs in dead and dying tissues.
3. Increased bone catabolism occurring in multiple myeloma is an example of metastatic calcification.
4. Metastatic pulmonary calcification is a common complication of MM.
5. Intracellular deposits of calcium initially start in damaged mitochondria.
6. Intracerebral calcification (dystrophic calcification) occurs in toxoplasmosis.
7. Fibro-siderotic nodules with calcification are Gandy Gamna bodies.

8. Phlebolith in pelvis can be confused with stones in the ureters.
9. Psammoma bodies can be seen in papillary carcinoma thyroid, serous carcinoma ovary, psammomatous meningioma, etc.

Pigment Dsorders

1. Lipofuscin is a wear and tear pigment. It is brownish granular and intracellular pigment. It is seen in brown atrophy.
2. Ochronosis is AR disease with absence of homogentisic acid oxidase, homogentisic acid is deposited in tissues as brown or black pigment.
3. Hemosiderin is stained by Perl's or Prussian blue stain.
4. Haemozoin is a haemoglobin derived pigment-stained with Romonwosky stains (Giemsa, wright, etc.) and methylene blue stain.

Hypersensitivity Reactions

1. Type I HS: Anaphylaxis, allergies and asthma,
2. Type II HS: AIHA, Goodpasture syndrome, HDN, drug reactions and graft rejection.
3. Antibody mediated destruction and phago-cytosis (Type II HS) occurs in: Transfusion reactions, HDN, AIHA, drug reactions.
4. Type III HS: Kidney in SLE, AGN, serum sickness, Arthus reaction.
5. Arthus reaction: Localised tissue reaction with vasculitis due to exposure of an antigen in a case with previously formed antibodies.
6. T cell-mediated (Type IV) HS reaction: Tuberulosis, sarcoidosis, etc.
7. Asthma is type I HS reaction
8. Type I is IgE antibody-mediated.
9. Type II HS is antibody dependent cell-mediated cytotoxicity (ADCC).

Autoimmune Disorders

1. MHC molecule (HLA): Class I expressed on all nucleated cells and platelets. Peptides derived from virus or tumour antigens are displayed on the surface and recognised by CD8 T lymphocytes.
2. Class II HLA display peptides derived from microbes or soluble proteins recognised by CD4 T cells.
3. Anergy: T cells have CD28 and APC B7. APC without B7 is rendered anergic. No immune reaction occurs.
4. Regulatory T cells: Prevent immune reactions against self reactive T cells.
5. Self-tolerance: Central and peripheral, breakdown leads to AI.
6. T cells recognising self-antigens undergo apoptosis.
7. Polymorphisms of NOD2 are associated with Crohn's disease.
8. Diagnostic of SLE: Anti-DNA (Double stranded) antibodies and Anti-Smith Antibodies.
9. SLE: Low levels of complement, DNA-Anti-DNA complexes, antibodies to RBCs, white cells, platelets, APLA positive.
10. Libman Sack's endocarditis is seen in SLE.
11. Sjögren's syndrome: Inflammation of lacrimal gland and salivary gland.
12. Salivary gland in Sjögren's disease has lymphocytic and plasma cell infiltrate and ductal cell hyperplasia.
13. Sjögren's syndrome has high incidence of B cell lymphoma.

Genetic Disorders

1. Fragile X syndrome patient is inactive, mental retardation, macro-orchidism, FMR1 gene mutations, CGG repeats are hypermethylated.
2. Gaucher's disease: Splenomegaly, hepato-megaly, failure to thrive, may have CNS manifestations.
3. DiGeorge syndrome: T cell markers are absent.
4. Child with failure to thrive, splenomegaly and diarrhoea suggests galactosaemia.
5. Niemann-Pick (NP) disease is due to: Deficiency of enzyme sphinomyelinase.
6. NP is a lipid storage disorder.
7. In NP disease bone marrow, liver, spleen have foamy RE cells or macrophages.
8. NP is a AR disease.
9. Type Ia (von Gierke's disease) is most type of glycogen storage disease.
10. Maple syrup urine disease, there is defect in metabolism of branched chain amino acids (valine, leucine and isoleucine). Urine smells of maple syrup, sweetish odour.
11. Cystic fibrosis: There is CFTR gene mutation with disruption of chloride channels, glands have thick and sticky mucus and allows growth of organisms.
12. If both the parents have CFTR gene, there will be 25% chance to get the disease, 25% normal and 50% chance to be carriers.

Neoplasia

1. Common malignant tumours in Indian males: Oral cancer and lung cancer.
2. Common malignant tumour in Indian females: Breast and cervical cancer.
3. Common malignancies in whites: Carcinoma colon and malignant melanoma.
4. Common malignancy in USA: Lung cancer, Ca colon and malignant melanoma.
5. Common malignancy in Japan: Gastric cancer.
6. Schistosomiasis is common in: Africa and middle east countries.
7. C-kit mutations are seen in: GIST.
8. Microsatellite instability seen in: HNPCC.
9. Choristoma is normal cells in abnormal location.
10. Hamartoma is normal cells in excessive number in normal location
11. VHL tumour suppressor gene is mutated in: Angiomatosis and haemangioblastoma. VHL gene is on chromosome 3 and AD.
12. RET proto-oncogene is associated with: MEN type 2.
13. Mutation of PAX7 seen in Rhabdomyosarcoma.
14. CA 15.3 is a breast cancer marker.
15. CA19.9 is a marker for pancreatic cancer.
16. CEA is a tumour marker for colonic cancer.
17. AFP is tumour marker for yolk sac tumour.
18. HTLV causes T cell lymphoma and leukaemia.
19. DNA viruses causing cancer are HPV, HBV, EBV, human herpesvirus 8
20. Oncogenic RNA viruses: HCV and HTLV-1.
21. Only action of promoter carcinogens cannot initiate malignancy.
22. Action of initiator carcinogens cause mutations.
23. Aflatoxin1 from Aspergillus flavus causes HCC.
24. Asbestosis produces mesothelioma and lung cancer.
25. RB and p53 are tumour suppressor genes.
26. Telomerase is responsible for limitless replicative activity in cancers.
27. The most common oncogenic DNA viruses causing cancer are:
    i. Human Papillomavirus (HPV): HPV commonly produces warts, and squamous cell carcinoma of cervix and skin.
    ii. Epstein-Barr virus (EBV): EBV is implicated in Burkitt's lymphoma, patients of organ transplantation, Hodgkin's lymphoma, nasopharyngeal carcinoma.
    iii. Hepatitis B virus (HBV): Hepatocellular carcinoma
    iv. Kaposi's sarcoma herpesvirus (KSHV, human herpesvirus 8)
28. The oncogenic RNA viruses are:
    i. Human T cell leukaemia virus (HTLV-1): It causes T cell leukaemia and lymphoma in Japan and the Caribbean region.
    ii. HCV: Hepatocellular carcinoma.
29. Application of initiator in chemical carcinogenesis may cause mutational activation of genes such as RAS. Subsequent application of promoter leads to clonal expansion of initiated cell. These are pharbol esters, hormones, phenols and benzopyrines, azo dyes and aflatoxins.
30. Application of promoters alone does not cause mutations. However, act on a mutated cell.
31. Asbestos produces malignant mesothelioma and lung carcinoma. Crocidolite fibres have greater risk than shorter and thicker Amosite and flexible chrysolite fibres for mesothelioma and lung cancer.
32. Aflatoxin B1, a natural product of fungus *Aspergillus flavus* is known to produce hepatocellular carcinoma.
33. Preneoplastic conditions include disorders that are associated with a significantly increased risk of cancer and these are:
    i. Chronic atrophic gastritis of pernicious anaemia
    ii. Solar keratosis
    iii. Oral lichen planus
    iv. Oral submucous fibrosis
    v. Endometrial hyperplasia
    vi. Chronic gastritis
    vii. Ulcerative colitis
    viii. Adenomatous polyps of colon
    ix. Xeroderma pigmentosum
    x. Epidermolysis bullosa hereditaria
34. Mucin secreting adenocarcinomas of pancreas, lung and GIT can have:
    a. Nonbacterial thrombotic endocarditis (marantic endocarditis).
    b. Hypercoagulability leading to venous thrombosis.
    c. Trousseau's syndrome (migratory thrombosis in superficial veins and uncommon site).
35. Syndromes which can occur in lung carcinoma are:
    a. Hypercalcaemia (non-small cell carcinoma/squamous cell carcinoma).
    b. SIADH (non-small cell carcinoma/squamous cell carcinoma).

c. Carcinoid (small cell carcinoma).
d. Venous thrombosis (Trousseau phenomenon).
e. Hypertrophic osteoarthropathy and clubbing of the fingers.
f. Dermatomyositis.
g. Myesthenia gravis.
h. Acanthosis nigricans.
i. Hypoglycemia.
36. Paraneoplastic syndromes which can occur in breast carcinoma are:
a. Hypercalcaemia
b. CNS and nerve disorders.
37. Paraneoplastic syndromes which can occur in renal cell carcinoma are:
a. Polycythemia.
b. Hypercalcaemia.

Lymph Nodes

1. Nodular lymphocyte predominant HD: Express Pan B markers: CD19, CD20, PAX5, LCA, MUM1, CD15 and 30 negative
2. RS cells are CD15 and CD30 positive.
3. Lacunar RS cells are present in nodular sclerosis HD
4. Prognosis in nodular sclerosis HD: Good
5. Prognosis in mixed cellularity HD: Intermediate
6. EBV causes HD and nasopharyngeal carcinoma.
7. Favourable prognosis is seen in NLPHD and NSHD.
8. Worst prognosis is seen in LDHD.
9. SLL may present as lymphocytosis, monoclonal gammapathy, or hypogammaglobulinaemia.
10. Richter syndrome: Transformation of SLL to large cell lymphoma which is aggressive type of lymphoma.
11. PAX5 positive in RS cells and B cell lymphomas.
12. In follicular lymphoma, t(14:18)(q32:q21) places Bcl-2 close to IgH, thus over expression of Bcl-2.
13. t(2:5)(p23:q35), involves ALK (thyrosine kinase gene) close to nucleophosmin (NPM) with increased activity of thyrosine kinase.
14. t(8:14) in Burkitt's lymphoma, c-myc proto-onogene of chromosome 8 moves to chromosome 14 close IgH region.
15. t(11;14) Cyclin D1 overexpressed. And Cyclin D1 on chromosome 11 is placed near IgH on chromosome 14.
16. Mantle zone lymphoma is CD5 positive and CD23 negative.
17. SLL cells are: CD20 +, CD5+ and CD23+.
18. Follicular NHL cells are: Pan B cell markers +, CD10 + (CALLA+), Bcl-2+, Bcl-6 + in high grade follicular lymphoma.
19. DLBCL CD20+, CD30+, Ki-67+, Bcl-2 overexpressed, Bcl-6 +.
20. Myc overexpressed in Burkitt Lymphoma. Express B cell markers, CD10 and Bcl-6.
21. Germinal centre cell markers are: CD10 and Bcl-6.
22. Lymphoblastic lymphoma: Common in children and adults, aggressive, T cell markers present in 85% of the cases. They are TDT +, CD1+, CD2+ and CD7+.
23. T cell rich DLBCL: B cells are less than 10%.
24. Peripheral T cell and NK cell lymphoma are highly aggressive with poor prognosis. Cells express CD2+, CD3+, CD45 RO+, CD5+ and CD7+.
25. Anaplastic large cell lymphoma: CD30+, Ki-1+.
26. Mantle zone lymphoma: CD5+, Cyclin D1+ due to t(11:14).

Respiratory Diseases

1. Nasopharyngeal carcinoma is associated with EBV.
2. Type II pneumocytes synthesise surfactant.
3. Type I pneumocytes are flat and occupy 95% of the alveolar surface.
4. Type II cells are involved in repair mechanisms and can produce Type I cells.
5. Histoplasma capsulatum produce granulomas can undergo necrosis and cavitation. Disseminated histoplasmosis occurs in immunocompromised hosts.
6. *Pneumocystis carinii* pneumonia usually occurs when CD4 T cell count is below 200 cells/cmm.
7. Simon's focus: Apical tuberculosis
8. Infraclavicular lesion in tuberculosis is known as Assman focus.
9. Schaumann bodies and asteroid bodies are seen in sarcoidosis.
10. Non-caseating granulomas are seen in sarcoidosis.
11. Most common cause of nosocomial pneumonia is *Staphylococcus aureus*.
12. Commonest cause of lung abscess is aspiration.
13. Bronchial artery is the source of haemoptysis in TB.
14. Hyaline membrane is made of fibrin and necrotic cells.
15. Deep vein thrombosis (DVT) is the commonest cause of pulmonary thromboembolism.
16. Creola bodies are seen in bronchial asthma.

17. Crushmann spirals are mucus plugs. Also present are eosinophils and Charcot Leyden Crystals.
18. Asthma has increased sensitivity to variety of stimuli with episodic bronchoconstriction.
19. Atopic asthma is IgE-mediated.
20. For nonatopic asthma is respiratory infection (viral) and inhaled pollutants are common triggers. Family history in nonatopic asthma is not available. TH2 cells are activated to normal harmless antigens of the environment which produce cytokines which promote B cells and inflammation.
21. LTC4, D4 and E4 and acetylcholine cause bronchoconstriction. Histamine, prostaglandin D2 and PAF also induce brochoconstriction.
22. Eosinophils are the cells found in asthma.
23. Reid index is increased in chronic bronchitis. Normal Reid index is 0.4, whereas its value increases in chronic bronchitis. Reid index is ratio of the thickness of the submucous glands to the thickness between the epithelium and the cartilage.
24. Bronchiectasis affects vertical air passages of lower lobes bilaterally with involvement of left side more frequent than right.
25. Chronic bronchitis: Persistent cough for 3 consecutive months for at least two years.
26. Chronic bronchitis has hyperplasia of mucous glands, goblet cell hyperplasia, chronic inflammation and bronchiolar wall fibrosis.
27. Smoking, pollutants and genetic predisposition plays role in emphysema.
28. Patients with anti-protease alpha1-anti-trypsin deficiency have tendency for emphysema. Severe alpha-1-anti-trypsin deficiency (PiZZ) is autosomal co-dominantly inherited disorder. Normal individuals are PiMM and PiMZ state is associated with moderate deficiency of Alpha-1-anti-trypsin deficiency.
29. Alpha-1-anti-trypsin is produced by liver and by neutrophils during inflammation.
30. Smoking and pollutants are cause of inflammation and release of elastases.
31. With loss of elastic recoil of the lung parenchyma, there is functional obstruction during expiration (functional outflow obstruction).
32. Panacinar emphysema is common with alpha-1-antitrypsin deficiency.
33. Both emphysematous and normal acini are present in centri-acinar emphysema. Heavy smokers and chronic bronchitis patients have centriacinar emphysema.
34. Bronchiectasis: Causes include bronchial obstruction, infection and ciliary dyskinesia (Kartageners syndrome). The airways are dialated.
35. Restrictive lung diseases are characterised by inflammation and fibrosis.
36. Goodpasture's syndrome is antibodies to non-collagenous domain of alpha-3 chain of collagen IV. There is necrotising haemorrhagic interstitial pneumonitis.
37. Nuclear molding, necrosis and high mitotic count is present in small cell carcinoma lung.
38. Azzopardi effect is present in small cell carcinoma. Dark blue DNA material from necrotic tumour cells encrusts the inner surface of the vessel.
39. Cancerous suppressor gene deletions are: 3p, 9p and 17p.
40. TTF1 is positive in thyroid neoplasms and lung carcinomas.
41. Adenocarcinoma lung express TTF1 and CK7 and SCC express P63 and CK5/6.
42. EGFR mutations are associated with adeno-carcinomas in non-smokers.
43. Lung carcinomas with paraneoplastic syndromes: ADH-inducing hyponatremia, ACTH producing Cushing syndrome, parathormone related peptide inducing hypercalcaemia, calcitonin producing hypocalcaemia, gonado-tropins inducing gynaecomastia and serotonin and bradykinin causing carcinoid syndrome.
44. Simple coal worker pneumoconiosis has macules and nodules. Progressive lesions have scars.
45. Amphiboles (chrysotile, amosite, crocidolite) are dangerous and act as initiators and promoters of cancer.
46. Asbestos bodies: Golden brown fusiform rods are asbestos fibres surrounded by iron containing proteinaceous material.
47. The most dangerous particle size for causation of pneumoconiosis is 1–5 microns.
48. Most common lesion in asbestosis is benign pleural plaques.
49. Bronchogenic carcinoma is the commonest asbestos related cancer.
50. Heart-failure cells are the hemosiderin laden macrophages.
51. Malignant mesothelioma is not associated with smoking.
52. Byssinosis: Occupational lung diseases due to textile fibres like: Cotton, hemp or linen fibres, etc.

53. Bagassosis: Occupational lung disease causing hypersensitivity pneumonitis due to inhalation of sugarcane dust.
54. Caplan syndrome is co-existence of pneumoconiosis with cavitating rheumatoid nodules.

Vascular Diseases

1. Hyaline arteriosclerosis is characteristic of benign nephrosclerosis.
2. Hyperplastic arteriosclerosis: Seen in malignant hypertension, onion skin, concentric and laminated thickening of vessel wall are common features, can also have necrotising arteriolitis.
3. Mycotic aneurysms are due to infective aetiology (bacterial, fungal, etc.)
4. Ischaemia because of endarteritis to media and loss of elastic fibres with scarring is characteristic of syphilitic aneurysm.
5. Marfan syndrome is due to mutation of fibrillin which is required for elastic tissue synthesis.
6. Older individuals with large vessel involvement is characteristic of giant cell arteritis
7. Vasculitis of small vessels of lung tissue is seen in Wegeners.
8. Pulseless disease occurring below 50 years is Takayasu arteritis.
9. Immune complex deposits in vessel wall with inflammation are seen in: PAN.
10. Young male smokers commonly have TAO or Buerger's disease.

Gastrointestinal Disease: Oesophagus

1. Aetiology of GERD: Smoking, decreased physical activity, increased abdominal pressure, delayed gastric emptying, oestrogen therapy.
2. GERD has basal cell hyperplasia, elongated papillae, intra-epithelial eosinophils and venular dilatation, bile crystals may be present.
3. CMV can affect oesophagus and rest of GIT. Multiple, superficial serpeginous or oval ulcers are present.
4. CMV has intranuclear eosinophilic and sometimes basophilic intracytoplasmic inclusions.
5. Barrett oesophagus: There is metaplasia of squamous epithelium of lower esophagus which is replaced by columnar epithelium.
6. Bile acids act as tumour promoter in Barrett oesophagus.
7. Barrett oesophagus is associated with adenocarcinoma.
8. Plummer-Vinson syndrome is associated with carcinoma oesophagus.
9. Carcinoma oesophagus is more common in upper and middle portion of oesophagus.
10. Risk factors for oesophageal carcinoma: Alcohol, tobacco, HPV infection, Barrett oesophagus, nitrate and nitroso compounds, radiation exposure, etc.

Gastrointestinal Disease: Stomach and Intestinal Lesions

1. Peptic ulcer is most commonly located in first part of duodenum (anterior wall more often affected) and stomach (more commonly on lesser curvature) usually at antral and corpus junction. Majority are solitary. These are usually less than 2 cm. They may penetrate the muscle tissue. Round to oval, sharply punched out, with straight walls, margins are usually levelled. Base is smooth and clean, converging mucosal folds are present. The blood vessels at the margins may be thrombosed.
2. Cushing's ulcer: Seen in burns and acute erosive gastritis. Ischaemia and breakdown of protective mucosal barrier play role.
3. B_{12} is absorbed from distal ileum.
4. Syndromes associated with polyposis of intestine: Turcot's syndrome, Gardener syndrome, PJ syndrome, adenomatous polyposis, HNPCC, Lynch syndrome, Cowden syndrome.
5. Increased levels of 5-hydroxy-indole-acetic acid its excretion in urine is seen in carcinoid syndrome. Presents with flushing, diarrhoea and intermittent abdominal cramps.
6. Leukoplakia and erythroplakia can undergo malignant transformation.
7. CEA is tumour marker for adenocarcinoma colon, lung, ovary, pancreas and breast.
8. Carcinoid is most commonly arises from Midgut.
9. Intestinal biopsy is diagnostic in celiac disease and fatty diarrhoea.
10. Sites of gastric ulcer: Lesser curvature and antrum (common), anterior and posterior wall and greater curvature (less common).
11. Ulcerative colitis predisposes to colonic carcinoma.

Lesions of liver

1. Hepatitis C: Spreads by blood and blood products
2. Hepatitis B: Spreads by blood and blood products

3. Fibrolamellar variant of HCC has good prognosis.
4. Adenomas of liver enlarge and cause symptoms and have malignant potential.
5. Right lobe of liver is prone for abscess due to the streaming effect of superior mesenteric artery.
6. E. multilocularis is endemic in US and likely to be fatal.
7. E. granulosus is common in certain parts of Europe and resectable without peritoneal soilage.

Lesions of Breast

1. Ductal epithelium has two layers.
2. Milk line runs from axilla to inguinal region. Ectopic breast tissue can be present in this line.
3. Fat necrosis of breast can mimic carcinoma and presents as painless mass.
4. Fibrocystic disease is associated with: Epithelial hyperplasia, cystic change, fibrosis, adenosis, chronic inflammation, apocrine metaplasia and fibroadenomatoid change.
5. Phyllodes tumour has proliferating stroma more than the epithelial component having leaf-like appearance.
6. Mondor disease is thrombophlebitis of breast and contiguous tissue.
7. Fibroadenoma is oestrogen responsive benign capsulated tumour which occurs in reproductive life.
8. Low grade phyllodes is similar to FA, but more cellular and mitotically active.
9. High grade phyllodes has high cellularity, high mitotic rate, nuclear pleomorphism stromal overgrowth and infiltrative borders.
10. Bilatality and multicentricity is more common with lobular carcinoma.
11. A breast carcinoma patient, has five times more risk of developing carcinoma in contralateral breast.
12. DCIS is limited to ducts and LCIS to lobules.
13. DCIS can be detected by mammography.
14. Atypical ductal and lobular hyperplasia has increased risk of malignancy.
15. Oestrogen hormone therapy: Increases risk of carcinoma breast.
16. Radiation exposure increases risk of breast malignancy.
17. With longer duration of breastfeeding, there is reduced risk of carcinoma breast.
18. Mutation of BRCA1 and BRCA2 are seen in familial breast cancers.
19. BRCA1 is located on chromosome 17q21 and BRCA2 on 13q12.3.
20. Mucinous, medullary, colloid, tubular, apocrine, secretary carcinomas have good prognosis.
21. Medullary carcinoma breast has pushing borders, tumour cells grow in syncytial pattern and surrounding stroma is infiltrated with lymphocytes.
22. Metaplastic carcinoma: Pain present.
23. Sentinel lymph node (LN): First LN to receive tumour cells.
24. ER positive and HER2 negative cancers are most common and occur in elderly age.
25. HER2 positive and ER, PR negative breast carcinoma is common in younger females.
26. Triple negative breast carcinoma (basal like) occur in young females, as well as in African females.
27. Luminal A: ER and PR positive and has good prognosis.
28. Luminal B: ER and PR positive HER2 variable, higher histological grade than luminal A tumours.
29. Basal like: Poor prognosis, triple negative.
30. Medullary BRCA1 positive, ER and PR negative, HER2 negative. However has good prognosis.

Female Genital System: Cervix

1. Carcinoma cervix is one of the leading causes of cancer death in women in the world.
2. According to latest data the estimated new cases of cervical cancer are: 5,00,000 in the year 2018.
3. With oestrogen spinnbarkeit test is positive. Mucous can withstand stretching up to 10 cm.
4. Presence of fern test positive after 21 days of menstrual cycle suggests: Anovulatory cycle.
5. Abnormal Pap smears followed by biopsy after abnormal colposcopic biopsy can detect cervical cancer in early stages.
6. Persistent infection with high-risk HPV is the important causative factor in carcinoma cervix.
7. HPV-16 is the most common type of HPV causing carcinoma cervix, LSIL and HSIL.
8. HPV infect immature basal cells of the stratified squamous epithelium or immature metaplastic epithelial cells. Viral replication occurs in mature cells.
9. Damage to the epithelium is necessary for HPV to gain entry into the cells.

10. Viral oncoproteins E6 and E7 interfere with the activity of the tumour suppressor genes.
11. E7 binds to active RB gene and degrades it.
12. E7 also inhibits p21 and p27 cyclin dependent kinase inhibitors. This enhances cell cycle progression and impairs DNA repair ability.
13. E6 protein binds to p53 and degrades it.
14. E6 upregulates telomerase, with immortalisation.
15. E6 and E7 prevent cell cycle arrest.
16. Ki 67 activity normally limited to the basal layer. In high-risk HPV infection, Ki-67 expression extends to upper portion of stratified squamous epithelium.
17. P16 and Ki-67 suggest-high risk HPV infection.
18. Koilocytes: Squamous epithelial cells with perinuclear halo, peripheral condensation of cytoplasm, and hyperchromatic moderately enlarged nucleus. These are superficial or intermediate squamous cells.
19. LSIL and HSIL are caused by high-risk HPV.
20. Features of dyskeratosis are increased cell size, clumping of chromatin, irregular nuclear borders, hyperchromatic nucleus.
21. Recombinant HPV vaccine prepared from highly purified virus like particles is available for HPV types 6, 11, 16, 18, 31, 33, 45, 52 and 58.
22. Patients of CIN I are followed up for 6 and 12 months and if negative both times, thereafter every three years Pap smear is repeated.
23. In carcinoma *in situ*, atypia is limited to the epithelium and basement membrane is intact.
24. Squamous cell carcinoma is the most common histological type followed by adenocarcinoma.
25. Microinvasion of squamous cell carcinoma cervix (Stage I a1): Invasion is not deeper than 3 mm and not wider than 7 mm.
26. Stage Ia2 squamous cell carcinoma cervix: Depth more than 3 mm and not deeper than 5 mm and horizontal not more than 7 mm.
27. Women with normal cervical cytology and high-risk HPV-DNA positive, cervical Pap smears repeated after 6 to 12 months.
28. For abnormal Pap smears colposcopy done, biopsied from aceto-white area.
29. LSIL is followed up and for HSIL conisation is done.
30. Cytoplasmic glycogen is absent in cancerous squamous cells of ectocervix (Lugol or Schiller test positive).
31. Lymph node metastasis seen in carcinoma cervix.
32. Pap smears in squamous cell carcinoma show: necrosis, tadpole cells, atypical tumour cells.
33. Sarcoma botryoides (embryonal Rhabdomyosarcoma) of cervix/vagina is a highly malignant tumour occurring in children. Microscopy has undifferentiated cells seen below the epithelium (similar to cambium layer of plants) and has poor outcome.

Female Genital System: Uterus and Placenta

1. Metaplasia in endometrium: Papillary, squamous, tubal (ciliated tall columnar epithelium), mucinous, granular cell, etc.
2. Endometriosis: Endometrial tissue in abnormal location. Encountered in ovaries, tubes and outer surface of uterus and intestine, uterine ligaments, urinary bladder and ureters, scar tissue after uterine surgery.
3. Infertility can be because of fallopian tube tuberculosis.
4. Leiomyoma: Common benign smooth muscle tumour. Can undergo mucoid/myxoid degeneration, red degeneration, etc. Other histological variants: Cellular leiomyoma, bizarre leiomyoma, epithelioid leiomyoma, angioleiomyoma, leiomyolipoma, intravascular leiomyoma.
5. Leiomyoma is oestrogen sensitive tumour. Can cause infertility, bleeding, rarely polycythemia, pain, etc.
6. Pecoma: Uncommon mesenchymal tumour, perivascular epithelioid cell neoplasm (PEComa).
7. Simple hyperplasia has 1% chance while complex hyperplasia with atypia has about 28% chance of going for endometrial carcinoma.
8. Endometrial cancer is common in nulliparous, elderly age, common in Jews, predisposing factors: HT, obesity, DM.
9. Patient of endometrial carcinoma is an elderly lady with H/O abnormal bleeding.
10. Risk factors for endometrial carcinoma are oestrogen excess as with anovulatory cycles, polycystic ovaries, use of oestrogen agonists, HRT treatment, obesity, DM, etc.
11. Type I endometrial (Endometrioid) carcinoma has microsatellite instability and PTEN and beta catenin gene mutations.
12. Type I endometrial carcinoma are estrogen dependent and endometrioid type.
13. Type II endometrial carcinoma are non-estrogen dependent, non-endometrioid, aggressive and

have poor prognosis. Alterations of p53, human epidermal growth factor –2/neu, p16 and E-cadherin. Serous and clear cell histological types are most common.

Female Genital System: Ovary

1. Turner's syndrome: 45XO, short statured female, web neck, cubitus valgus, shield-like chest, renal abnormalities, streak gonads, etc.
2. Stein Leventhal syndrome: It is polycystic ovarian syndrome with anovulatory cycles, high levels of LH, oestrogen, androgens, insulin resistance and hyperinsulinaemia. They can have increased BMI, facial hair and acne.
3. Risk factors for ovarian carcinoma: Age 40–60 years, family history, BRCA1 and 2 mutations, nulliparity, streak ovaries, obesity, etc.
4. Screening test for detection of Epithelial Ovarian tumours: Serum CA-125.
5. CA-125 also helps in detection of recurrence and monitoring with treatment.
6. Lynch syndrome: AD, with HNPCC, carcinoma endometrium and carcinoma ovary.
7. Yolk sac tumour has Schiller-Duval bodies.
8. Call-Exner bodies are present in granulosa cell tumour.
9. Patients of sex-cord tumours can have: Precocious puberty, AUB, postmenopausal bleeding. They also can have hyper-oestrogenic effects and sometimes with androgen effects.
10. Arrhenoblastoma is sex cord stromal tumour.
11. Granulosa cell tumours can have: Precocious puberty, endometrial hyperplasia and endometrial carcinoma.
12. Granulosa cell tumour produces oestrogen and can produce endometrial hyperplasia, endometrial carcinoma and breast carcinomas.
13. Inhibin is a marker for stromal tumours.
14. Feminisation and sex cord masculinisation are encountered in sex cord stromal tumours.
15. Germ cell tumours occur in young females. Teratoma is common germ cell tumour followed by Dysgerminoma.
16. AFP is raised in yolk sac tumour.
17. Krukenburg tumour is secondaries in ovaries from malignant tumour of breast, GIT, pancreas, spread occurs through transcoelomic spread or retrograde lymphatics. Microscopy has signet ring cells which are PAS positive.

Male Genital System

1. Anaplastic seminoma has worse prognosis.
2. Spermatocytic seminoma has good prognosis.
3. Verrucous carcinoma: Broad fonts, well-differentiated squamous cell carcinoma and rare metastasis.
4. Schiller-Duval bodies are seen in endodermal sinus tumour.
5. AFP is raised in endodermal sinus tumour.
6. LDH and gamma glutamyl transpeptidase (GGT) in testicular tumours are markers for bulk disease.
7. Raised LDH in testicular tumours has poor prognosis.
8. AFP is elevated in yolk sac tumour, HCC and hepatoblastoma.

Endocrinology

1. MEN I: AD, parathyroid tumours, pancreatic islet cell tumours and anterior pituitary hyperplasia or adenoma.
2. MEN 2A: AD, medullary carcinoma thyroid, thyroid hyperplasia, pheochromocytoma, Hirschsprung disease, lichen amyloidosis.
3. MEN 2B: Medullary carcinoma thyroid, pheochromocytoma, mucosal or GI neuromas, Marfanoid body features.

Renal System

1. Kidneys remove waste and excess water, maintain electrolyte balance, hormone produced by the kidneys helps to regulate blood pressure, help in RBC production, and keep our bones strong.
2. Microalbuminuria is excretion of 30–300 mg/day of albumin in urine.
3. Polycythemia and hypercalcaemia are the paraneoplastic features in renal cell carcinoma.
4. Major cause of papillary necrosis is analgesic nephropathy.
5. Michaelis-Gutmann bodies are seen in malacoplakia.
6. Tamm-Horsfall protein secreted by the thick ascending loop of Henle forms the matrix of all casts.
7. Subepithelial deposits are seen in: PSGN (Humps), MGN, RPGN, Heymann nephritis.
8. Subendothelial deposits are seen in lupus nephritis, MPGN I.
9. Membranous deposits are seen in: MPGN II.
10. Mesangial deposits are seen in: IgA nephropathy.
11. Kidney in RPGN is enlarged, pale, often have petechial haemorrhages (Flea bitten Kidney).
12. Causes of nephrotic syndrome: Primary: MGN, MCD, FSGS, MPGN, IgA nephropathy.

13. Causes of nephrotic syndrome: Secondary causes: DM, amyloidosis, drugs, infections, malignant diseases, hereditary nephritis
14. The normal urine albumin creatinine ratio (ACR) in young adults is <10 mg/g (<1 mg/mmol).
15. Urine albumin creatinine ratio of 10–30 mg/g (1–3 mg/mmol) is considered high.
16. Alport syndrome has deafness, corneal dystrophy and hematuria.
17. Most common cause of nephrotic syndrome in children is MCD.
18. Most common cause of nephritic syndrome in adults is FSGS.
19. Serum antibodies to alpha 3NC1 domain of collagen IV are seen in Goodpasture syndrome.
20. LM features of MPGN are glomeruli large, hypercellular, GBM is double contoured, tram track appearance or shows duplication.
21. Adult polycystic disease PKD1 is on chromosome 16 and ADPKD2 on chromosome 4.

Lesions of Bone

1. Multiple enchondroma: Ollier's disease
2. Ollier's disease: Nonhereditary, childhood disease with enchondromatosis, risk of visceral and bone cancers
3. Muffucci's disease: Multiple enchondromas, skeletal deformities, abnormal vascular lesions and has IDH1 mutation.
4. Gardener syndrome is GI polyps (FAP), multiple osteomas, epidermoid cysts, desmoid tumours, and other benign tumours.
5. Aneurysmal bone cyst (ABC): 10 to 20 years of age, accentric expansion, metaphysis involved, blood-filled spaces with thin shell of reactive bone. Plump fibroblasts, reactive woven bone and multinucleated osteoclastic giant cells are present. Pain and swelling are common symptoms. Rearrangements of 17p13 with NFkB increased activity
6. Metaphysial fibrous defect: Painful, fibrous tissue with irregularly scattered osteclasts.
7. Fibrous dysplasia: Bone is thinned out, expanded, curved fish hook bony trabaculae or resembling C and Y Chinese characters (Woven bone).
8. Rice bodies: Causes include tuberculous bursitis or arthritis, rheumatoid arthritis, tenosynovitis, inflammatory athritis.
9. Gout: Preserve in alcohol to appreciate needle-shaped urate monohydrate sodium crystals. These are refrictile crystals.
10. Pseudogout: Deposition of calcium pyrophosphate dihydrate crystals in joint cavities.
11. Paget disease: Also called osteitis deformans, three phases: Initial lytic phase, osteoclastic and osteoblastic phase and osteosclerotic phase. Mutations of RANK and inactivating mutations of OPG are known.
12. Osteoid osteoma: Cortex, less than 2 cm, nocturnal pain, relieved by aspirin, reactive bone present around nidus.
13. Osteoblastoma: Osteoblastoma similar to osteoid osteoma, however, larger than 2 cm. Pain is not relieved by aspirin.
14. Osteosarcoma (OS): Bimodal age peak, below 20 years of age and above 60 years of age.
15. Variants of osteosarcoma: Depending on location: Periosteal OS, parosteal OS, intramedullary OS, intracortical OS or surface OS.
16. Histological variants OS: Conventional OS (about 90%), telangiectatic OS, small cell OS, fibroblastic OS, chondroblastic OS, giant cell rich OS
17. Osteosarcoma risk factors: Familial Paget's disease, NF type1, p53/RB gene mutations, INK4a inactivation.
18. Osteosarcoma: X-ray characteristic with sunburst appearance and Codman's triangle.
19. Chondrosarcoma has osteolytic lesion with splotchy calcification or arcs and ring form of calcification or spotty calcification.
20. Variants of chondrosarcoma (CS): Clear cell CS, myxoid CS, dedifferentiated CS, mesenchymal CS.
21. Giant cell tumour: Epiphysis involved, 20–40 years age group.
22. Giant cell tumour (GCT): RANKL (receptor activator of nuclear factor) overexpressed, epiphysial tumour, RANKL inhibitor denosumab is the adjuvant therapy used in recent years. Rarely metastasise and a locally malignant tumour.
23. Ewings sarcoma: Childhood bone tumour, aggressive tumour.
24. Ewings sarcoma: t(11;22)(q24:q12) with this translocation EWS-FLI1 fusion gene formed.
25. Metastasis to bone: Most common primaries are from breast, lung, thyroid and kidney.
26. Giant cell lesions of bone
    i. Gaint cell tumour of bone
    ii. Chondroblastoma
    iii. Osteosarcoma
    iv. Simple bone cyst
    v. Aneurysmal bone cyst

    vi. Osteoid osteoma
    vii. Osteoblastoma
    viii. Non-ossifying fibroma
    ix. Giant cell reparative granuloma
    x. Brown tumour of hyperparathyroidism.
27. Cystic bone lesions
    i. Solitary (simple, unicameral) bone cyst (SBC)
    ii. Aneurysmal bone cysts (ABC)
    iii. Giant cell tumour of bone
    iv. Adamantinoma
    v. Intraosseous ganglion cyst
    vi. Epidermal cyst in bone
    vii. Hydatid cyst of bone
28. Painful tumours
    i. Osteoid osteoma
    ii. Osteoblastoma
    iii. Chondroblastoma
    iv. Reparative granuloma
    v. Glomus tumour
    vi. Aneurysmal bone cysts (ABC)
    vii. Metaphysial fibrous defect

Lesions of Central Nervous System

1. Co-deletion of chromosome 1p and 19q is seen in oligodendroglioma.
2. Isocitrate dehydrogenase 1 and 2 (IDH1 and IDH2) are found in infiltrating astrocytomas and oligodendrogliomas.
3. Isocitrate dehydrogenase (IDH) mutation in diffuse gliomas have favorable prognosis, compared with IDH wild-type tumours.
4. Medulloblastoma with alterations in the WNT pathways is associated with a significantly indolent prognosis.
5. RELA fusion-positive are seen in ependymoma.
6. The NF1 gene is located on chromosome 17q11.2, which encodes for a protein known as neurofibromin.
7. Microglia are derived from monocyte lineage, also called gitter cells or Hortega cells.

Skin Lesions

1. Precancerous conditions of skin: Xeroderma pigmentosa, Bowen's disease, bowenoid papulosis
2. Pautrier abscess are seen in: Mycosis fungoides.
3. 'Row of tombstone' seen in: Pemphigus vulgaris.
4. Fishnet with IF is seen in: Pemphigus vulgaris.
5. Acantholytic cells in pemphigus are derived from: Stratum spinosum.
6. Café au lait spots are seen in: NF1 or von Recklinghausen disease.
7. Lepra cells are macrophages seen in lepromatous leprosy.
8. Turbon tumour: Dermal cylindroma of scalp.
9. Langerhans' cell histiocytosis expresses CD1a and langerin.

Normal Values

Haematology		*Normal range*
Hb	Men	13.5 to 15.5 gm%
	Women	12.5 to 13.5 gm%
	Newborn	16 to 18 gm%
	10 to 12 years of age	12 to 13 gm%
MCV		80–98 fl
MCH		26–34 pg
MCHC		31–37 gm/dl
RDW		11.5–14.5%
Platelet count		1.5 to 4 lakh cells/cmm
RBC count	Males	4.5 to 5.5 million cells/cmm
	Females	3.8 to 4.8 million cells/cmm
Reticulocyte count		0.5 to 2.0%
Total leukocyte count		4000–11000 cells/cmm
Adults		4000–11000 cells/cmm
At birth		10000–25000 cells/cmm
1–3 years		6000–18000 cells/cmm
4–7 years		6000–18000 cells/cmm
8–12 years		4500–13500 cells/cmm
Absolute eosinophil count		40–440 cells/cmm

Differential count	*Adults*	*Children*
Neutrophils	60–70%	20–30%
Lymphocytes	20–40%	60–70%
Monocytes	02–08%	02–08%
Eosinophils	01–08%	01–08%
Basophils	00–01%	00–01
PCV	Males	47 ± 7 (40–54%)
	Females	42 ± 5 (37–47%)
ESR (Westergren's method)	Males	5 to 15 mm/1st hour
	Females	5 to 20 mm/1st hour
Bleeding time		2–7 minutes
Clotting time		4–9 minutes
Hess/tourniquet test	Less than 10 petechiae	Negative/normal

Biochemistry

Urea		16–45 mg/dl
Serum creatinine		0.6–1.2 mg/dl
RBS		60–160 mg/dl
FBS		90–110 mg/dl
PPBS		90–140 mg/dl
Uric acid		2–7 mg/dl
SGOT (AST)		5–45 IU/L
SGPT (ALT)		5–40 IU/L
GGT		9–48 U/L
Alkaline phosphatase		20–80 IU/L (adults)
Total bilirubin		0.1–1.3 mg/d
Direct bilirubin		0.1–0.4 mg/dl
Indirect bilirubin		0.2–0.8 mg/dl
Calcium, serum		9–11 mg/dl
Cholesterol		150–250 mg/dl
HDL cholesterol		30–60 mg/dl
LDL cholesterol		80–150 mg/dl
Triglycerides		75–160 mg/dl
Creatine kinase	Male	25–90 U/L
	Female	10–70 U/L
Total proteins		6–8 gm/dl
Albumin		3.5–5.0 gm/dl
Globulin		1.8–3.6 gm/dl
Thyroxine (T_4), serum		5.1–14.1 µg/dl
Triiodothyronine (T_3), serum		85–202 µg/dl
TSH		0.3 and 4 mIU/L
Haemoglobin A_{1c}	>6.5 %	4–6.5%
Serum iron	Male	27–138 µg/dl
	Female	33–102 µg/dl
Serum ferritin	Male	29–248 µg/L
	Female	10–150 µg/L
TIBC	Male	174–351 µg/dl
	Female	194–372 µg/dl
Plasma transferrin	Male	194–348 µg/dl
	Female	181–416 µg/dl
Free erythrocyte protoporphyrin		17–27 µg/dl

References

1. Gale E, Torrance J, Bothwell T. Quantitative Estimation of Total Iron Stores in Human Bone Marrow. J Clin Invest 1963 Jul;42:1076–82.
2. Manglani M, Lokeshwar MR, Vani VG, et al. NESTROFT. An effective screening test for beta thalassemia trait. Indian pediatrics 1997; 34: 702–7.
3. Arber DA, et al. The 2016 revision of the WHO classification of myeloid neoplasms and acute leukemia. Blood 2016;127:2391–405.
4. Rajkumar SV, Dimopoulos MA, Palumbo A, et al. International Myeloma Working Group updated criteria for the diagnosis of multiple myeloma Lancet Oncol 2014;15(12):e538–48.
5. Zumla A. Geraint James D. Granulomatous Infections: Etiology and Classification. In: Clinical infectious Diseases 1996;23:146–58
6. Dey NC, Grueber HLE & Dey TK. Medical Mycology, Ist Central edition, 2006, New Central Book Agency(P) Ltd. Kolkata, India.
7. Modified from Stary HC, Chandler AB, Dinsmore RE, et al. A definition of advanced types of atherosclerotic lesions and a histological classification of atherosclerosis: a report from the Committee on Vascular Lesions of the Council on Arteriosclerosis, American Heart Association. Circulation 1995; 92:1355–74.
8. Travis WD et al. The WHO classification of tumours of Lung, Pleura, Thymus and heart. 5th ed. Lyon, France, IARC press, 2015.
9. Classification of salivary gland neoplasms, 4th Ed. Of the WHO classification of Head and Neck tumours. 2017.
10. Lauren's classification, Acta Pathol Microbiol Scand 1965; 64; 31–49.
11. Lauwers GY, et al. Classification of tumours of the digestive system 4th Ed, Lyon: IARC;2010.
12. Odze RD, Goldblum JR. Surgical pathology of the GI tract, liver, biliary tract and Pancreas 2nd Ed. 2009, Saunders Elsevier, Philadelphia.
13. Dasgupta A, Singh N and Bhatia A. Abdominal Tuberculosis: A Histopathological Study with Special Reference to Intestinal Perforation and Mesenteric Vasculopathy, 2009.
14. Lakhani S, et al. WHO classification of histological typing of tumours of the Breast, 4th ed, Lyon: IARC; 2012.
15. Fleming ID, Cooper JS, Henson DE, Hutter RVP, Kennedy BJ, Murphy GP, et al., editors. American Joint Committee on Cancer staging manual. 5th edition. Philadelphia: JB Lippincott, 1997.
16. Friedman RJ, et al. Volume of malignant melanoma is superior to thickness as a prognostic indicator. Preliminary observation. Dermatologic clinics.1991;9:643–8.
17. New classification system of endometrial hyperplasia WHO 2014. Geburtsh Frauenheilk. 2015; 75:135–6.
18. Endometrial hyperplasia, Lacey JV Jr. et al. *J Clin Oncol*.2010;28:788–92 .
19. Kurman RJ, et al. The WHO classification of tumours of female reproductive organs. Lyon: IARC;2014.
20. Classification of Testicular tumours: From The 2016 WHO Classification of tumours of the urinary system and male genital organs, 4th edition, IARC.
21. Moore RA. Benign Hypertrophy of prostate: A morphological study. J Urol 1943;50: 680–710.
22. Desai SS and Nirmala A Jambhekar Pathology of Ewing's sarcoma/PNET: Current opinion and emerging concepts Indian J Orthop. 2010 Oct-Dec; 44(4): 363–8.
23. 2016 WHO Classification of mature lymphoid, histiocytic and dendritc neoplasms, From WHO classification of tumours of haemopoietic and Lymphoid tissues, Lyon, IARC, 2016.
24. Louis DN et al. The 2016 WHO classification of tumours of the CNS: A summary. Acta Neuropathol Springer Verlag Berlin Heidelberg 2016.
25. Cohen A, Holmen S and Colman H. Curr Neurol Neurosci Rep 2013; 13: 345–54, Chen JR, Yao Y, Xu HZ et al. Medicine (Baltimore) 2016:95; e2583.
26. Tateishi K et al. Neurosurgery 2017:64;134–8.
27. Faulker C. et al. J Neuropath Exp. Neurol. 2015;74:867–72.

28. Moore WG, Berman JJ. Performance Analysis of Manual and Automated Systemized Nomenclature of Medicine (SNOMED) Coding. Am J Clin Pathol 1994;101:253–6.
29. Ali SZ, Cibas ES, eds. The Bethesda System for Reporting Thyroid Cytopathology, 2nd ed. Cham, Switzerland: Springer; 2017.
30. Faquin WC, Rossi ED, eds. The Milan System for Reporting Salivary Gland Cytopathology. Cham, Switzerland: Springer; 2018.
31. Field AS, Schmitt F, and Vielh P. 5 stage coding system (categories) proposed by Yokohama International Congress of cytology. Acta Cytologica 2017;61:3–6.
32. Nayar R, Wilber DC. The Pap Test and Bethesda. Acta Cytologica 2015;59:121–32.

Book References

Haematology

1. Brown BA, Hematology Principles and Procedures. Lea & Febriger, 1993.
2. Dacie JV, Lewis SM, Practical Haematology. 8 ed.. Edinburg: Churchill Livingstone, 1994.
3. Firkin F, Chesterman C, Penington D, Rush B, de Gruchy's climical Hematology in Medical practice. 6th adapted ed. 2013, Wiley. India Pvt. Ltd.
4. Hillyer CD, Silberstein LE, Ness PM, Anderson KC, eds. Blood Banking and Tranfusion medicine - Basic principles & practice, Philadelphia: Churchill Livingstone, 2003.
5. Mollison PL, Engelfriet CP, Contreras M, Blood transfusion in clinical Medicine. 10th ed. Blackwell Science, 1997.
6. Rodak BF, Diagnostic Hematology. Philadelphia: WB Saunders Company, 1995.
7. Rudmann SV, Textbook of blood banking and transfusion medicine. Philadelphia: W.B. Saunders Company, 1995.
8. Wintrobe's Clinical Hematology 12th Ed. 2009 Wolter Kluwer Health/Lippincott Williams and Wilkins.

Clinical Pathology

1. Frankel S, Reitman S, Sonnenwirth AC, eds. Gradwohl's Clinical Laboratory Methods and diagnosis. 7th ed. St.Louis: The CV Mosby Company, 1970.
2. Godkar PB and Godkar DP, Textbook of Medical Laboratory Technology. 2nd ed. India: Bhalani Publishing House, 2003.
3. Henry JB, Clinical diagnosis and management by laboratory methods. 20th ed. Philadelphia: W.B. Saunders, 2001.
4. Fine LG and Salehmoghaddam S. Chapter Proteinuria In: Clinical Methods Walker KH, Hall DW, and Hurst WJ (Editors), 3rd ed., Emory University School of Medicine, Atlanta, Georgia, Boston:Butterworths; 1990.
5. Satyanarayana U, Biochemistry. 2nd ed. India: Books and Allied (P) Ltd, 2004.

General Pathology and Systemic Pathology

1. Damjanov J, Linder J, Anderson's Pathology. 10th ed. St. Louis: Mosby, 1996.
2. Cotran RS, Kumar V, Collins T, Robins and Cotran Pathologic Basis of Disease. 8th ed. Saunders Elsevier. 2010.
3. Fuster V., Alexander WR, O Rourke RA, Hurst's The Heart, 10th ed. (International ed.), The McGraw-Hill Companies Inc. 2001.
4. Rubin R, Stayer DS (Editors). Rubin's Pathology. (Clinico-pathologyic Foundation of Medicine) 5th ed. Wolter Kluwer Health/Lippincott Williams and Wilkins, 2008.
5. Rosai J, Rosai and Ackerman's Surgical Pathology. 10th ed. St. Louis: Mosby, 2011.
6. Underwood JCE, Cross SS (Editors) General and Systemic Pathology, 5th ed. Churchill Livingstone Elsevier, 2009.

Histopathology Techniques

1. Bancroft JD, Gamble M, Theory and Practice of Histopathological Techniques. 5th ed. London: Churchill Livingstone, 2002.
2. Culling CFA, Handbook of Histopathological techniques. 2nd ed. London: Buttherworths and co. Ltd, 1963.
3. Drury RAB, Wallington EA, Carleton's histological technique. 5th ed. Oxford: Oxford University Press, 1980.

Cytology

1. Bibbo M, Comprehensive Cytopathology. 2nd ed. Philadelphia: WB Saunders company, 1997.
2. Gray Winifred, McKee GT, Diagnostic cytopathology. 2nd ed. Churchill Livingstone, 2003.
3. Kini SR, Colour atlas of differential diagnosis in Exfoliative and Aspiration cytopathology. Baltimore: William and Wilkins, 1999.
4. Koss LG, Diagnostic cytology and its histopathological basis. 4th ed. Philadelphia: JB Lippincott, 1992.
5. Naib Z, Cytopatholgy. 4th ed. Boston: Little, Brown and Company, 1996.
6. Orell SR, Sterrett GF, Whitaker D, Fine Needle Aspiration Cytology. 4th ed. Australia: Churchill Livingstone, 2005.
7. Young JA, Fine Needle Aspiration Cytopathology. 1st ed. London: Blackwell Scientific Publication, 1993.

Index

A
Absolute eosinophil count 22
Accessing procedures in surgical pathology 311–313
   coding 313
   gross room 311
   principles of grossing 312
   receiving of specimens 311
   record keeping 312
   storage and filing of slides 313
Actinomycosis 156
Acute
   lymphoblasic leukemia 56–59
   myeloblastic leukemia 56–59
Ameloblastoma 293
Amyloidosis 141–143
Anticoagulants 10–11
   double oxalates 10
   EDTA 10–11
   heparin 11
   tri-sodium citrate 11
Appendicitis 149–151
Atherosclerosis 187
Automation in haematology 74–78

B
Barr body 384
Basal cell carcinoma 267
Bleeding time 67–68
   Duke's method 67
   Ivy's method 67
   modified Ivy's method 67
Blood collection 8–9
   capillary 8
   venous 9
Blood groups 31–35
   ABO blood grouping 31–33
   ABO subgroups 32–33
   Bombay blood group 33
   cross matching 35
   Rh typing 33–34
   weak D phenotype (Du phenotype) 34
Breast carcinoma 247
Buffer for peripheral smear 73

C
Capillary
   haemangioma 183
   resistance test (Hess/tourniquet test) 68
Cavernous haemangioma 183
Cell counts 17–20
Cell injury 133–138
   adaptations 134
   apoptosis 135
   degenerations 134
   differences between dry gangrene and wet gangrene 138
   gangrene 137–138
   necrosis 136
Cerebrospinal fluid 356–358
Chronic
   appendicitis 150
   lymphocytic leukemia 59–63
   myeloid leukemia 59–63
   venous congestion (lung, liver and spleen) 161–163
Cleaning of glasswares
Clot
   lysis time 68
   retraction 68
Clotting time 67
Capillary tube method 67
   Lee and White's method 67
Collection of urine 82
Colloid goiter 296
Composition of urine 82
Congenital heart diseases 191–194
Coomb's test 35
   direct 35
   indirect 35
Criteria to evaluate screening tests 343
Cytological fixatives 316, 341
Cytology of
   female genital system 375–379
   oral cavity and alimentary tract 362–363
   respiratory tract 364–368
   thyroid, salivary gland and breast lesions 371–374
   urinary tract 369–370
Cytopreparatory techniques 347–348

D

Decalcification 330
Differential leukocyte count 23–25
  basophilia 25
  eosinophilia 24
  lymphocytosis 24
  lymphopenia 25
  monocytosis 24–25
  neutropenia 25
  neutrophilia 23
Duct carcinoma *in situ* 246

E

Erythrocyte sedimentation rate (ESR) 28–30
  factors influencing ESR 29
  Westergren's method 28
  Wintrobe's method 29

F

Factors involved in fixation 316
Fatty change liver 139–140
Fibroadenoma 244
Fibrocystic disease 245
Filariasis 117–118
Fixation 129–132, 314
  aims 129
  classification of fixatives
  cytological 316
  microanatomical 315
FNAC 349
Foetal haemoglobin 51–52
  acid elution method 51–52
  alkali haematin method 51
Formaldehyde 315
Formalin based fixatives 315
  bouins fluid 315
  picric acid containing fixative 315
  postchroming and secondary fixation 314
  vapour fixation 315
Fractional test meal (FTM) 102
Frozen section 329

G

Gastric ulcer/duodenal ulcer/peptic ulcer 222
Glucose tolerance test 101
Granulation tissue 159–160
Gynaecomastia 246

H

Haematocrit 26–27
Haematoxylin and eosin (H&E) staining 320–321
  acid alcohol 320–321
  blueing 321

  differentiation 321
  Ehrlich's haematoxylin 320
  eosin for H&E staining 321
  Harri's haematoxylin 320
  Mayer's haematoxylin 320
  mordant 321
  ripening 321
  steps of H&E staining 320
Haemoglobin electrophoresis 54
Haemoglobin estimation 14–16
  cynmethaemoglobin method 15
  Sahli's method 14
  specific gravity method 16
Haemolytic anaemia 44
Haemopoiesis 3–7
Heart
  cardiomayopathy 199
  congenital anomalies 191–194
  infective endocarditis 194–196
  pericarditis 201
  pleural effusion 201
  rheumatic fever and RHD 196–198
Hodgkin disease 299
Hormone cytology 380–383
  infarction 166–170
  iron deficiency anaemia 37–39
  lung/pulmonary 169
  myocardial 167–169

I

Inflammation 144
  cardinal signs 144
  causative agents 144
  cellular phenomenon 146
  chemical mediators 147
  definition 144
  different types of giant cells 149
  granulomatous inflammation 148
  morphological patterns 148
  vascular phenomenon 145
Instruments 109–114
  bone marrow needle 109–110
  Esbach's albuminometer 113
  liver biopsy needle (vim Silverman's needle) 111–112
  lumbar puncture needle 110–111
  Ryle's tube 112–113

L

LE cell phenomenon 70–71
Leprosy 158–159
Leukemias 56–63
  acute 56–59
  chronic 59–63

Lipoma 184
Liver function tests 105–106
Lysing fixatives 342

M

Malaria 115–117
Malignant melanoma 269
Mature cystic teratoma 285
Megaloblastic anaemia 39–43
Meningitis 154
Microscopy 92
    casts 93–95
    cells 93
    crystals 95
    parasites 96
    urine sediment 92–93
Microtomes and microtomy 322–328
    adhesives 325
    embedding media 325
Microtome knife 326
    honing 327–328
    section cutting 323
    stropping 328
Microtomes 322
Mucinous cystadenoma ovary 285
Multiple myeloma 64–65
Myocardial infarction 167–169

N

Neoplasia 176–182
    AD and AR diseases with cancer 180
    chemical 178
    diagnosis of malignancy 180
    etiology 176
    paraneoplastic syndrome 181–182
    pre-neoplastic lesions 179
    virus and cancer 176
    X-linked diseases 180
Neubauer counting chamber 17
Neurofibroma 186
Nodular hyperplasia of prostate 290
Non-Hodgkin lymphoma 302
Non-invasive breast carcinoma 246
Normal blood picture 36

O

Oedema 170–172
    cardiac 170
    pathophysiology 171–172
    renal 171
Oliguria 81
Osmotic fragility (OF) 52–54
    Dacie method 52
    NESTROF test 53–54
    Sanford method 52
Osteoclastoma 294
Osteomyelitis 292
Osteosarcoma 293

P

Packed cell volume (haematocrit) 26–27
Papilloma 266
Peripheral smear (blood film) preparation and
        staining 12–13
Phyllodes tumour 244
Physical examination 83–85
    appearance 83
    colour 83–84
    odour 84
    reaction 84
    specific gravity 84–85
Platelet count 18
Pleomorphic adenoma 219
Pleural, pericardial and peritoneal fluids 352–455
Pneumonia 151–154
Polyuria 81
Pregnancy test 98
Preparation 12–13
    Romanowsky stains 12, 72–73
    staining procedure 13
Preservation of urine 82–83
Processing 318
    automatic processing 130
    block making 319
    clearing 318
    dehydration 318
    embedding 319
    impregnation 319
    manual processing 131
    steps of processing 129
Prostatic
    carcinoma 291
    intraepithelial neoplasia 290
Pulmonary infarction 169
Pyogenic meningitis 154

R

RBC count 18–19
Reagent strips 96–97
    asbestosis 216–217
    bilirubin 97
    Caplan's 215
    coal workers pneumoconiosis 214
    glucose 96
    haemoglobin and myoglobin 97
    ketone bodies 97

pleural diseases 218
pneumoconiosis 213–218
proteins 96
silicosis 215
tumours 218
urobilinogen 97
Red cell indices 21
Renal function tests 103–104
Respiratory tract
Pulmonary tuberculosis 202
 asthma 207–209
 bronchiectasis 209–210
 chronic bronchitis 204
 emphysema 205
 obstructive pulmonary diseases 204
Restrictive lung diseases 210–211
 lung carcinoma 211–213
Reticulocyte count 49
Rhinoscleroma 157–158
Rhinosporidiosis 156–157
Romanowsky stains 72

S

Schwannoma 184–186
Semen analysis 99–100
Seminoma 288
Serous cystadenoma ovary 284
Shock 173–175
 cardiogenic 173
 hypovolemic 174
 organ changes 175
 septic 175
 stages 173
Sialadenitis 151
Sickling phenomenon 50
Special stains 333
 Masson trichrome stain 334
 PAS stain (periodic acid–Schiff stain) 334
 reticulin stain (Gordon and Sweet's method) 334
 theoretical aspects 336
 van Gieson stain 333
 Verhoeff stain 333

Spray fixation 341
Squamous cell carcinoma 266
Staining techniques in cytology 344–46
 diff-quick staining 346
 MGG staining 345
 Pap staining 344–345
Synovial fluid 359–361

T

Teratoma testis 288
Thrombosis 163–167
Thyroid function tests 107–108
Total leukocyte count 19–20
Tuberculous lymphadenitis 154–156
Types of urine samples 82

U

Urine examination 81–97
 anuria 81
 Benedict's test 86
 benzidine test 88
 causes for proteinuria 86
 causes of glycosuria 87
 causes of haematuria 89
 chemical examination 85–92
 Ehrlich's reagent 91
 Fouchet's reagent 90
 Fouchet's test 90
 Gerhardt's test 88
 Gmelin's test 90
 microalbuminuria 86
 reducing agents for Benedict's test 87
 Rothera's test 88
 tests for bile pigments 90
 tests for bile salts 90
 tests for glucose 86–88
 tests for ketone bodies 88
 tests for proteins 85–86
 tests for urobilinogen 91–92

V

Vascular pathology in HT 189–190